Growth Hormone Therapy in Pediatrics – 20 Years of KIGS

Growth Hormone Therapy in Pediatrics

20 Years of KIGS

Editors

Michael B. Ranke   Tübingen
David A. Price   Manchester
Edward O. Reiter   Springfield, Mass.

128 figures and 133 tables, 2007

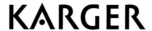

Basel · Freiburg · Paris · London · New York ·
Bangalore · Bangkok · Singapore · Tokyo · Sydney

Prof. Michael B. Ranke
Paediatric Endocrinology Section
University Children's Hospital
University of Tübingen
Tübingen, Germany

Dr. David A. Price
Royal Manchester Children's Hospital
Pendlebury, Swinton
Manchester, UK

Prof. Edward O. Reiter
Baystate Children's Hospital
Tufts University School of Medicine
Springfield, Mass., USA

'Growth Hormone Therapy in Pediatrics – 20 Years of KIGS' was supported by an unrestricted educational grant from Pfizer Endocrine Care.

Library of Congress Cataloging-in-Publication Data

Growth hormone therapy in pediatrics – 20 years of KIGS / editors, Michael B. Ranke, David A. Price, Edward O. Reiter.
 p. ; cm.
 Includes bibliographical references and index.
 ISBN 978-3-8055-8256-8 (hard cover : alk. paper)
 1. Dwarfism, Pituitary – Hormone therapy. 2. Growth hormone releasing factor – Physiological effect. I. Ranke, Michael B. II. Price, David A. (David Anthony), 1943– III. Reiter, Edward O.
 [DNLM: 1. Pfizer International Growth Database. 2. Growth Disorders–drug therapy. 3. Adolescent. 4. Child. 5. Databases, Factual. 6. Growth Hormone – therapeutic use. 7. Infant. 8. Longitudinal Studies.
WS 104 G8836 2007]
RC658.7.G78 2007
618.92'47–dc22   2007005269

Bibliographic Indices. This publication is listed in bibliographic services.

Disclaimer. The statements, options and data contained in this publication are solely those of the individual authors and contributors and not of the publisher and the editor(s). The appearance of advertisements in the book is not a warranty, endorsement, or approval of the products or services advertised or of their effectiveness, quality or safety. The publisher and the editor(s) disclaim responsibility for any injury to persons or property resulting from any ideas, methods, instructions or products referred to in the content or advertisements.

Drug Dosage. The authors and the publisher have exerted every effort to ensure that drug selection and dosage set forth in this text are in accord with current recommendations and practice at the time of publication. However, in view of ongoing research, changes in government regulations, and the constant flow of information relating to drug therapy and drug reactions, the reader is urged to check the package insert for each drug for any change in indications and dosage and for added warnings and precautions. This is particularly important when the recommended agent is a new and/or infrequently employed drug.

All rights reserved. No part of this publication may be translated into other languages, reproduced or utilized in any form or by any means electronic or mechanical, including photocopying, recording, microcopying, or by any information storage and retrieval system, without permission in writing from the publisher.

© Copyright 2007 by S. Karger AG, P.O. Box, CH–4009 Basel (Switzerland)
www.karger.com
Printed in Switzerland on acid-free paper by Reinhardt Druck, Basel
ISBN 978-3-8055-8256-8

Contents

	Contributors	IX
	Preface	XV
1 KIGS	**KIGS: Structure and Organization** Patrick Wilton	1
2 Review	**Assessment of Growth and Puberty** Gary E. Butler	6
3 KIGS	**Diagnosis of Children with Short Stature: Insights from KIGS** Kenji Fujieda, Toshiaki Tanaka	16
4 KIGS	**Data Analyses within KIGS** Anders Lindberg, Michael B. Ranke	23
5 KIGS	**The KIGS Aetiology Classification System** Michael B. Ranke	29
6 Review	**Growth Hormone Deficiency: Growth Hormone Tests and Growth Hormone Measurements** Susan R. Rose	38
6 KIGS	**Growth Hormone Testing in KIGS** Maïthé Tauber	47
7 Review	**Growth Hormone Deficiency and Modalities of Birth** Angel Ferrández-Longás, Esteban Mayayo, José Ignacio Labarta, Agustin Romo	56
7 KIGS	**Modalities and Characteristics at Birth: Commentaries Based on KIGS Data** Michael B. Ranke	60
8 Review	**The Role of Insulin-Like Growth Factors in Growth Hormone Deficiency** Anders Juul	70
8 KIGS	**Insulin-Like Growth Factor 1 Levels in Patients within the KIGS Database** Michael B. Ranke	83

9 Review   **Neuroimaging in Growth Hormone Deficiency**
Mohamad Maghnie, Natascia di Iorgi, Andrea Rossi, Roberto Gastaldi,
Paolo Tortori-Donati, Renata Lorini 93

10 Review   **Characteristics of Idiopathic Growth Hormone Deficiency at the Start of Growth Hormone Therapy and the Response to Growth Hormone**
Herwig Frisch 108

10 KIGS   **Idiopathic Growth Hormone Deficiency in KIGS: Selected Aspects**
Michael B. Ranke, Edward O. Reiter, David A. Price 116

11 Review   **Growth Hormone Deficiency: Puberty and Final Height**
Edward O. Reiter, Wayne S. Cutfield 136

11 KIGS   **Growth Hormone Treatment to Final Height in Idiopathic Growth Hormone Deficiency: The KIGS Experience**
Wayne S. Cutfield, Georgios Karagiannis, Edward O. Reiter 145

12 Review   **The Transition from Childhood to Adulthood: Managing Those with Growth Hormone Deficiency**
Helena Gleeson, Peter E. Clayton 163

12 KIGS   **Effect of Prior Pediatric Growth Hormone Replacement on Serum Lipids and Quality of Life in Young Adults with Reconfirmed Severe Growth Hormone Deficiency: The Combined KIGS and KIMS Experiences**
Mitchell E. Geffner, Peter Jönsson, John P. Monson, Roger Abs, Václav Hána,
Charlotte Höybye, Maria Koltowska-Häggström 176

13 KIGS   **Who Stops Growth Hormone in KIGS – and Why?**
Michael B. Ranke 183

14 Review   **Congenital Growth Hormone Deficiency**
Primus E. Mullis 189

14 KIGS   **Growth Hormone Deficiency of Known Origin within KIGS (Code No. 2.1.1–2.1.6)**
Michael B. Ranke, Hanna Karlsson 202

15 Review/KIGS   **Growth Hormone Treatment of Children with Previous Craniopharyngioma: The KIGS Experience**
David A. Price 207

16 Review/KIGS   **Growth Hormone Treatment in Rare Disorders: The KIGS Experience**
Feyza Darendeliler 213

17 Review   **Childhood Brain Tumours and Growth Hormone Treatment**
Andreas Jostel, Stephen M. Shalet 240

17 KIGS   **KIGS Patients with Acquired Growth Hormone Deficiency (Code No. 2.2 ff.)**
Michael B. Ranke 250

18 KIGS   **Growth Hormone Treatment of Children with Previous Leukaemia and Lymphoma: The KIGS Experience**
David A. Price, Hanna Karlsson 261

19 Review — **Growth Hormone, Langerhans Cell Histiocytosis and Neurofibromatosis**
Michel Polak 269

19 KIGS — **Growth Hormone Treatment in Neurofibrosis Type 1 Involving Central Nervous System Tumours and Pituitary Langerhans Cell Histiocytosis within KIGS**
Michael B. Ranke, Wayne S. Cutfield 277

20 Review — **Growth and GH Treatment in Patients with Juvenile Idiopathic Arthritis**
Paul Czernichow 286

20 KIGS — **The KIGS Experience with Growth Hormone Treatment of Juvenile Rheumatoid Arthritis**
Edward O. Reiter 292

21 Review — **Cystic Fibrosis – Growth Hormone Treatment**
Dirk Schnabel 296

21 KIGS — **The KIGS Experience with Growth Hormone Treatment of Cystic Fibrosis**
Edward O. Reiter 304

22 Review — **Idiopathic Short Stature: Definition, Spontaneous Growth and Response to Treatment**
Jan M. Wit 309

22 KIGS — **Short- and Long-Term Response to Growth Hormone in Idiopathic Short Stature: KIGS Analysis of Factors Predicting Growth**
Michael B. Ranke, Anders Lindberg, David A. Price, Feyza Darendeliler, Kerstin Albertsson-Wikland, Patrick Wilton, Edward O. Reiter 319

23 Review — **Turner Syndrome – Growth Hormone Treatment**
Ron G. Rosenfeld 326

23 KIGS — **Turner Syndrome within KIGS Including an Analysis of 1146 Patients Grown to Near Adult Height**
Michael B. Ranke, Anders Lindberg 332

24 Review — **Noonan Syndrome**
Christopher J.H. Kelnar 340

24 KIGS — **Short Stature in Noonan Syndrome: Results of Growth Hormone Treatment in KIGS**
Barto J. Otten, Kees Noordam 347

25 Review/KIGS — **Growth Hormone Treatment in Skeletal Dysplasias: The KIGS Experience**
Thomas Hertel 356

26 Review — **Prader-Willi Syndrome and Growth Hormone Treatment**
Ann Christin Lindgren 369

26 KIGS — **Effects of Growth Hormone Treatment in Children Presenting with Prader-Willi Syndrome: The KIGS Experience**
Maïthé Tauber 377

27 Review | **Growth and Growth Hormone Treatment in Children Born Small for Gestational Age and with Silver-Russell Syndrome**
Wayne S. Cutfield, Edward O. Reiter on behalf of the KIGS International Board 389

27 KIGS | **KIGS 20 Years: Children Born Small for Gestational Age**
David B. Dunger 400

28 Review/KIGS | **Growth Hormone Treatment in Short Children with Chronic Kidney Disease**
Otto Mehls, Anders Lindberg, Richard Nissel, Elke Wühl, Franz Schaefer, Burkhard Tönshoff, Dieter Haffner 407

29 Review/KIGS | **Predicting Growth in Response to Growth Hormone Treatment – The KIGS Approach**
Michael B. Ranke, Anders Lindberg 422

30 Review/KIGS | **Adverse Events Reported in KIGS**
Patrick Wilton 432

31 Review | **Progress and Challenges in Understanding the Psychology of Growth Delay**
Brian Stabler, Louis E. Underwood 442

32 Review | **Growth Hormone and Brain Function**
Fred Nyberg 450

33 Review | **Review of Methods for Body Composition Assessment in Children**
Jonathan C.K. Wells 461

34 Review | **Metabolic Effects of Growth Hormone**
Ulla Feldt-Rasmussen 477

35 Review | **The Growth Plate**
Ola Nilsson 485

36 Review | **Pharmacogenetics of Growth Hormone Therapy**
Linda B. Johnston, Adrian J.L. Clark 500

Author Index 509
Subject Index 511

Contributors

Dr. Roger Abs
Department of Endocrinology
University Hospital Antwerp
Wilrijkstraat 10
BE–2650 Edegem (Belgium)
Tel. +32 3 821 3885
Fax +32 3 821 4185
E-Mail roger.abs@uza.be

Prof. Kerstin Albertsson-Wikland
Paediatric Growth Research Centre
Department of Paediatrics
Queen Silvia Children's Hospital
Sahlgrenska
Academy of Gothenburg University
SE–416 85 Gothenburg (Sweden)
Tel. +46 31 343 5165
Fax +46 31 848 952
E-Mail kerstin.albertsson-wikland@pediat.gu.se

Prof. Gary E. Butler
Department of Paediatrics and Growth
Institute of Health Sciences
University of Reading
London Road
Reading RG1 5AQ (United Kingdom)
Tel. +44 118 378 6863
Fax +44 118 378 6862
E-Mail g.e.butler@reading.ac.uk

Prof. Adrian J.L. Clark
Department of Endocrinology
William Harvey Research Unit
John Vane Science Centre
Charterhouse Square
Barts and the London Queen Mary
School of Medicine
London EC1M 6BQ (United Kingdom)
Tel. +44 207 601 7078
Fax +44 207 601 8505
E-Mail a.j.clark@qmul.ac.uk

Prof. Peter E. Clayton
Department of Child Health and
Paediatric Endocrinology
University of Manchester
Oxford Road
Manchester M13 9PT
(United Kingdom)
Tel. +44 161 922 2585
Fax +44 161 922 2583
E-Mail peter.clayton@manchester.ac.uk

Prof. Wayne S. Cutfield
Liggins Institute
University of Auckland
2-6 Park Avenue
Grafton, Auckland (New Zealand)
Tel. +64 9 373 7599 (ext. 84476)
Fax +64 9 373 7497
E-Mail w.cutfield@auckland.ac.nz

Prof. Paul Czernichow
Department of Endocrinology and
Growth Diseases
Hôpital Necker
149 rue de Sèvres
FR–75015 Paris (France)
Tel. +33 1 44 49 48 01
Fax +33 1 44 49 48 00
E-Mail paul.czernichow@nck.aphp.fr

Prof. Feyza Darendeliler
Department of Pediatrics
Istanbul Faculty of Medicine
Istanbul University
TR–34390 Capa – Istanbul (Turkey)
Tel. +90 212 635 11 89
Fax +90 212 533 13 83
E-Mail feyzad@istanbul.edu.tr

Prof. David B. Dunger
Department of Paediatrics
Addenbrooke's Hospital
University of Cambridge
Hills Road, Level 8, Box 116
Cambridge CB2 2QQ
(United Kingdom)
Tel. +44 1223 762 944
Fax +44 1223 336 996
E-Mail dbd25@cam.ac.uk

Prof. Ulla Feldt-Rasmussen
Department of Medical
Endocrinology PE-2132
Rigshospitalet
Copenhagen University Hospital
Blegdamsvej 9
DK–2100 Copenhagen (Denmark)
Tel. +45 35 45 23 37
Fax +45 35 45 22 40
E-Mail ufeldt@rh.dk

Prof. Angel Ferrández-Longás
Hospital Infantil Universitario Miguel Servet
Av. Isabel la Católica 3
ES–50009 Zaragoza (Spain)
Tel. +34 976 765 649
Fax +34 976 765 633
E-Mail aferrandezl@salud.aragon.es

Prof. Herwig Frisch
St. Anna Children's Hospital
Kinderspitalgasse 6
AT–1090 Vienna (Austria)
Tel. +43 1 401 700
Fax +43 1 401 70 710
E-Mail herwig.frisch@meduniwien.ac.at

Prof. Kenji Fujieda
Department of Pediatrics
Asahikawa Medical College
2-1-1-1 Midorigaoka, Higashi
Asahikawa 078-8510, Hokkaidou
(Japan)
Tel. +81 166 682 481
Fax +81 166 682 489
E-Mail ken-fuji@asahikawa-med.ac.jp

Dr. Roberto Gastaldi
Department of Pediatrics
IRCCS Giannina Gaslini
University of Genova
Largo Gerolamo Gaslini 5
IT–16147 Genova (Italy)
Tel. +39 010 563 6691
Fax +39 010 377 6778
E-Mail gastaldiro@hotmail.com

Dr. Mitchell E. Geffner
The Saban Research Institute
Children's Hospital Los Angeles
4650 Sunset Blvd.
Los Angeles, CA 90027 (USA)
Tel. +1 323 669 7032
Fax +1 323 953 1349
E-Mail mgeffner@chla.usc.edu

Dr. Helena Gleeson
Department of Endocrinology
Christie Hospital NHS Trust
Wilmslow Road
Withington
Manchester M20 4BX
(United Kingdom)
Tel. +44 161 860 0696
Fax +44 161 446 3772
E-Mail helena.gleeson@btinternet.com

Prof. Dieter Haffner
University Hospital of Pediatric and
Adolescent Medicine
Rembrandtstrasse 17–18
DE–18075 Rostock (Germany)
Tel. +49 381 494 7001
Fax +49 381 494 7002
E-Mail dieter.haffner@med.uni-rostock.de

Dr. Václav Hána
3rd Department of Internal Medicine
Faculty of Medicine 1
Charles University
U nemocnice 1
CZ–128 08 Prague 2 (Czech Republic)
Tel. +420 22496 2919
Fax +420 22491 9780
E-Mail vhana@lf1.cuni.cz

Dr. Thomas Hertel
Department of Paediatrics
Odense University Hospital
Sdr. Boulevard 29
DK–5000 Odense C (Denmark)
Tel. +45 65 41 45 60
Fax +45 65 911 862
E-Mail thomas.hertel@ouh.fyns-amt.dk

Dr. Charlotte Höybye
Department of Endocrinology,
Metabolism and Diabetes
Karolinska University Hospital
SE–171 76 Stockholm (Sweden)
Tel. +46 8 517 75379
Fax +46 8 517 73096
E-Mail charlotte.hoybye@karolinska.se

Dr. Natascia di Iorgi
Department of Pediatrics
IRCCS Giannina Gaslini
University of Genova
Largo Gerolamo Gaslini 5
IT–16147 Genova (Italy)
Tel. +39 010 563 6002
Fax +39 010 377 6778
E-Mail natasciadiiorgi@ospedale-gaslini.ge.it

Mr. Peter Jönsson
Pfizer Endocrine Care
KIGS/KIMS/ACROSTUDY
Medical Outcomes
Vetenskapsvägen 10
SE–191 90 Sollentuna (Sweden)
Tel. +46 8 550 529 34
Fax +46 8 550 526 80
E-Mail peter.j.jonsson@pfizer.com

Dr. Linda B. Johnston
Department of Endocrinology
William Harvey Research Unit
John Vane Science Centre
Charterhouse Square
Barts and the London Queen Mary
School of Medicine
London EC1M 6BQ (United Kingdom)
Tel. +44 20 7882 6242
Fax +44 20 7882 6197
E-Mail l.b.johnston@qmul.ac.uk

Dr. Andreas Jostel
Department of Endocrinology
Christie Hospital
Wilmslow Road
Manchester M20 4BX
(United Kingdom)
Tel. +44 161 446 3668
Fax +44 161 446 3772
E-Mail andreas.jostel@man.ac.uk

Dr. Anders Juul
University Department of Growth
and Reproduction
Rigshospitalet, Section 5064
Blegdamsvej 9
DK–2100 Copenhagen (Denmark)
Tel. +45 35 45 5085
Fax +45 35 45 6054
E-Mail ajuul@rh.dk

Mr. Georgios Karagiannis
Pfizer Endocrine Care
KIGS/KIMS/ACROSTUDY
Medical Outcomes
Vetenskapsvägen 10
SE–191 90 Sollentuna (Sweden)
Tel. +46 8 550 529 38
Fax +46 8 550 526 80
E-Mail georgios.karagiannis@pfizer.com

Ms. Hanna Karlsson
Pfizer Endocrine Care
KIGS/KIMS/ACROSTUDY
Medical Outcomes
Vetenskapsvägen 10
SE–191 90 Sollentuna (Sweden)
Tel. +46 8 550 529 39
Fax +46 8 550 526 80
E-Mail hanna.karlsson@pfizer.com

Prof. Christopher J.H. Kelnar
Department of Paediatric
Endocrinology
Section of Child Life and Health
University of Edinburgh
20 Sylvan Place
Edinburgh EH9 1UW (United Kingdom)
Tel. +44 131 536 0611
Fax +44 131 536 0821
E-Mail chris@kelnar.com

Dr. Maria Koltowska-Häggström
Pfizer Endocrine Care
KIGS/KIMS/ACROSTUDY
Medical Outcomes
Vetenskapsvägen 10
SE–191 90 Sollentuna (Sweden)
Tel. +46 8 550 529 16
Fax +46 8 550 526 80
E-Mail maria.koltowska-haggstrom@pfizer.com

Prof. José Ignacio Labarta
Hospital Infantil Universitario Miguel Servet
Av. Isabel la Católica 3
ES–50009 Zaragoza (Spain)
Tel. +34 976 765 500 (ext. 3475)
Fax +34 976 566 234
E-Mail jilabarta@solunet.es

Mr. Anders Lindberg
Pfizer Endocrine Care
KIGS/KIMS/ACROSTUDY
Medical Outcomes
Vetenskapsvägen 10
SE–191 90 Sollentuna (Sweden)
Tel. +46 8 550 529 37
Fax +46 8 550 526 80
E-Mail anders.lindberg@pfizer.com

Dr. Ann Christin Lindgren
Pediatric Endocrinology Unit
Department of Woman and
Child Health
Astrid Lindgren Children's Hospital
Karolinska Hospital
SE–171 76 Stockholm (Sweden)
Tel. +46 733 380816
Fax +46 8 517 777 39
E-Mail ann.christin.lindgren@ki.se

Dr. Renata Lorini
Department of Pediatrics
IRCCS Giannina Gaslini
University of Genova
Largo Gerolamo Gaslini 5
IT–16147 Genova (Italy)
Tel. +39 010 563 6654
Fax +39 010 377 3210
E-Mail renatalorini@ospedale-gaslini.ge.it

Prof. Mohamad Maghnie
Department of Pediatrics
IRCCS Giannina Gaslini
University of Genova
Largo Gerolamo Gaslini 5
IT–16147 Genova (Italy)
Tel. +39 010 563 6574
Fax +39 010 353 8265
E-Mail mohamadmaghnie@
ospedale-gaslini.ge.it

Dr. Esteban Mayayo
Hospital Infantil Universitario Miguel
Servet
Av. Isabel la Católica 3
ES–50009 Zaragoza (Spain)
Tel. +34 976 765 636 (ext. 3378 or 3376)
Fax +34 976 566 234
E-Mail emayayo@salud.aragon.es

Prof. Otto Mehls
University Hospital of Pediatric and
Adolescent Medicine
Im Neuenheimer Feld 151
DE–69120 Heidelberg (Germany)
Tel. +49 6221 564 503
Fax +49 6621 564 501
E-Mail otto.mehls@med.uni-
heidelberg.de

Prof. John P. Monson
The London Clinic Centre for
Endocrinology and Diabetes
145 Harley Street
London W1G 6BJ (United Kingdom)
Tel. +44 793 972 0284
Fax +44 207 616 7791
E-Mail j.p.monson@qmul.ac.uk

Prof. Primus E. Mullis
Department of Paediatric
Endocrinology, Diabetology and
Metabolism
University Children's Hospital
Inselspital
CH–3010 Bern (Switzerland)
Tel. +41 31 632 9552
Fax +41 31 632 9550
E-Mail primus.mullis@insel.ch

Dr. Ola Nilsson
Pediatric Endocrinology Unit, Q2:08
Department of Woman and
Child Health
Karolinska Institutet
Karolinska University Hospital
SE–171 76 Stockholm (Sweden)
Tel. +46 8 517 762 26
Fax +46 8 517 751 28
E-Mail ola.nilsson@ki.se

Dr. Richard Nissel
University Hospital of Pediatric and
Adolescent Medicine
Rembrandtstrasse 17–18
DE–18075 Rostock (Germany)
Tel. +49 381 494 7025
Fax +49 381 494 7002
E-Mail richard.nissel@med.uni-
rostock.de

Dr. Kees Noordam
Department of Metabolic and
Endocrine Disorders
Radboud University Medical Centre
PO Box 91-01
NL–6500 HB Nijmegen
(The Netherlands)
Tel. +31 24 361 4429
Fax +31 24 366 8532
E-Mail c.noordam@cukz.umcn.nl

Prof. Fred Nyberg
Department of Pharmaceutical
Biosciences
Uppsala University Biomedical Center
PO Box 591
Husargatan 6
SE–751 24 Uppsala (Sweden)
Tel. +46 18 471 4166
Fax +46 18 501 920
E-Mail fred.nyberg@farmbio.uu.se

Dr. Barto J. Otten
Department of Metabolic and
Endocrine Disorders
Radboud University Medical Centre
PO Box 91-01
NL–6500 HB Nijmegen
(The Netherlands)
Tel. +31 24 361 4429
Fax +31 24 366 8532
E-Mail b.otten@cukz.umcn.nl

Prof. Michel Polak
Service d'Endocrinologie Pédiatrique
INSERM EMI 363
Hôpital Necker-Enfants Malades
149 rue de Sèvres
FR–75015 Paris (France)
Tel. +33 1 44 49 48 02
Fax +33 1 44 38 16 48
E-Mail michel.polak@nck.aphp.fr

Dr. David Anthony Price
Royal Manchester Children's Hospital
Hospital Road
Pendlebury, Swinton
Manchester M27 4HA
(United Kingdom)
Tel. +44 161 727 2584
Fax +44 161 727 8387
E-Mail rmpdap@btinternet.com

Prof. Michael B. Ranke
Paediatric Endocrinology Section
University Children's Hospital
University of Tübingen
Hoppe-Seyler-Strasse 1
DE–72076 Tübingen (Germany)
Tel. +49 7071 298 3417
Fax +49 7071 294 157
E-Mail mlranke@med.uni-tuebingen.de

Prof. Edward O. Reiter
Baystate Children's Hospital
Tufts University School of Medicine
759 Chestnut Street
Springfield, MA 01199 (USA)
Tel. +1 413 794 5060
Fax +1 413 794 3623
E-Mail edward.reiter@bhs.org

Dr. Agustin Romo
Hospital Infantil Universitario Miguel Servet
Av. Isabel la Católica 3
ES–50009 Zaragoza (Spain)
Tel. +34 976 765 500 (ext. 3240)
Fax +34 976 566 234
E-Mail aromo@salud.aragon.es

Prof. Susan R. Rose
Division of Endocrinology
Cincinnati Children's Hospital Medical Center
University of Cincinnati, MLC 7012
3333 Burnet Avenue
Cincinnati, OH 45229 (USA)
Tel. +1 513 636 4744
Fax +1 513 636 7486
E-Mail susan.rose@cchmc.org

Prof. Ron G. Rosenfeld
Lucile Packard Foundation for Children's Health
(Stanford University)
400 Hamilton Avenue
Suite 340
Palo Alto, CA 94301 (USA)
Tel. +1 650 724 6930
Fax +1 650 498 2619
E-Mail ron.rosenfeld@lpfch.org

Dr. Andrea Rossi
Department of Neuroradiology
IRCCS Giannina Gaslini
University of Genova
Largo Gerolamo Gaslini 5
IT–16147 Genova (Italy)
Tel. +39 010 563 6002
Fax +39 010 376 1017
E-Mail andrearossi@ospedale-gaslini.ge.it

Prof. Franz Schaefer
University Hospital of Pediatric and Adolescent Medicine
Im Neuenheimer Feld 151
DE–69120 Heidelberg (Germany)
Tel. +49 6221 563 2396
Fax +49 6221 564 203
E-Mail franz.schaefer@med.uni-heidelberg.de

Dr. Dirk Schnabel
Department of Pediatric Endocrinology and Diabetology
University Children's Hospital, Charité
Humboldt University Berlin
Augustenburger Platz 1
DE–13353 Berlin (Germany)
Tel. +49 30 450 566 343
Fax +49 30 450 566 947
E-Mail dirk.schnabel@charite.de

Prof. Stephen M. Shalet
Department of Endocrinology
Christie Hospital
Wilmslow Road
Manchester M20 4BX
(United Kingdom)
Tel. +44 161 446 3667
Fax +44 161 446 3772
E-Mail stephen.m.shalet@man.ac.uk

Prof. Brian Stabler
Department of Psychiatry
CB 7160
School of Medicine
The University of North Carolina at Chapel Hill
Chapel Hill, NC 27599 (USA)
Tel. +1 919 933 3689
E-Mail brian_stabler@med.unc.edu

Dr. Toshiaki Tanaka
Department of Clinical Laboratory Medicine
National Center for Child Health and Development
2-10-1 Ohkura, Setagaya-ku,
Tokyo 157-8535 (Japan)
Tel. +81 3 5494 7120
Fax +81 3 5494 7136
E-Mail tanaka-t@ncchd.go.jp

Prof. Maïthé Tauber
Department of Endocrinology
Hôpital des Enfants
330 avenue de Grande-Bretagne
TSA 70034
FR–31059 Toulouse Cedex 9 (France)
Tel. +33 5 34 55 85 51
Fax +33 5 34 55 85 58
E-Mail tauber.mt@chu-toulouse.fr

Prof. Burkhard Tönshoff
University Hospital of Pediatric and
Adolescent Medicine
Im Neuenheimer Feld 151
DE–69120 Heidelberg (Germany)
Tel. +49 6221 563 9310
Fax +49 6221 564 203
E-Mail burkhard.toenshoff@
med.uni-heidelberg.de

Dr. Paolo Tortori-Donati
Department of Neuroradiology
IRCCS Giannina Gaslini
University of Genova
Largo Gerolamo Gaslini 5
IT–16147 Genova (Italy)
Tel. +39 010 563 6002
Fax +39 010 376 1017
E-Mail paolotortori@ospedale-
gaslini.ge.it

Prof. Louis E. Underwood
Department of Pediatrics
CB 7039
3341 Med Biomolecular Building
The University of North Carolina at
Chapel Hill
Chapel Hill, NC 27599 (USA)
Tel. +1 919 323 0354
Fax +1 919 966 2423
E-Mail louis_underwood@med.unc.edu

Dr. Jonathan C.K. Wells
Childhood Nutrition Research Center
Institute of Child Health
30 Guilford Street
London WC1N 1EH (United Kingdom)
Tel. +44 207 905 2389
Fax +44 207 831 9903
E-Mail J.Wells@ich.ucl.ac.uk

Dr. Patrick Wilton
Pfizer Inc.
235 East 42nd Street
New York, NY 10017-15755 (USA)
Tel. +1 212 733 1007
Fax +1 212 309 4693
E-Mail patrick.wilton@pfizer.com

Prof. Jan Maarten Wit
Department of Paediatrics, J6S
Leiden University Medical Center
Albinusdreef 2
PO Box 9600
NL–2300 RC Leiden (The Netherlands)
Tel. +31 71 526 2824
Fax +31 71 524 8198
E-Mail j.m.wit@lumc.nl

Dr. Elke Wühl
University Hospital of Pediatric and
Adolescent Medicine
Im Neuenheimer Feld 151
DE–69120 Heidelberg (Germany)
Tel. +49 6221 563 9318
Fax +49 6221 564 568
E-Mail elke.wuehl@med.uni-
heidelberg.de

Preface

Since its inception in 1987, KIGS (Pfizer International Growth Database) has established itself as a major pharmacoepidemiological survey investigating growth hormone (GH) treatment in children with short stature. Today, more than 62,000 patients from more than 50 countries are enrolled in KIGS, and a considerable number of them have been followed to final height. Over the years, KIGS has become a major source of documentation of growth disorders and their treatment with recombinant GH.

During the past 20 years, the worldwide social, economical and medical structures have changed considerably. The idea of evidence-based medicine, which was part of the founding idea of KIGS, has become a globally accepted principle. The increasingly available information as a result of the new and ubiquitously available media has created a higher level of information and openness in the world of medicine and the public domain. With regard to GH, our understanding of its role in child development beyond growth and our concepts of treatment have expanded. Several new indications for GH treatment, such as chronic renal insufficiency, Prader-Willi syndrome and small for gestational age, were added to its traditional role of replacement in various forms of GH deficiency. The effects of GH on body composition, metabolism and child development have been recognised as additional important elements of GH treatment. The concept of responsiveness has emerged, and today, as a consequence of the development of new treatment algorithms, GH therapy can be individualised and optimised. The KIGS system has, by various means, accompanied, promoted and documented all of these developments over the past 20 years.

The present volume attempts to expand on the accounts given in the books published after 5 and 10 years. We are grateful for the contributions of many experts who have summarised the global experience in a multiplicity of areas of growth and GH treatment. Part of the extensive information accumulated in the KIGS database was analysed and gives an additional reflection of the various aspects from within KIGS. We hope that all of this information will stimulate the participants within KIGS to further support this unique and evolving quest to improve the long-term efficacy and safety of GH treatment in children and adolescents.

The editors are grateful for the continuing support and encouragement by Pfizer and the KIGS team, in particular Margaretha Lindell, Anders Lindberg, Georgios Karagiannis and Hanna Karlsson who have made the realisation of this book possible. We would also like to express our gratitude for the encouragement and endorsement the KIGS project received from Annika Wallström, Rolf Gunnarsson, Olivier Guilbaud and Patrick Wilton. We greatly appreciate the scientific support of the members of the Strategic Advisory Board: Kerstin Albertsson-Wikland, Magda Vanderschueren-Lodeweyckx, Pierre Chatelain, Marc Maes, Wayne Cutfield, Chris Cowell, Feyza Darendeliler, Angel Ferrandez-Longas, Maïthé Tauber, David Dunger and Mitchell Geffner. In particular, we would like to acknowledge the efforts taken by all participating physicians in contributing data for the analyses within KIGS. We are also grateful to Karger for their committed editorial support.

Michael B. Ranke, Tübingen, Germany
David A. Price, Manchester, UK
Edward O. Reiter, Springfield, Mass., USA

KIGS: Structure and Organization

Patrick Wilton

The KIGS database was initiated in December 1987 at the request of pediatric endocrinologists and health authorities [1]. The main objective of KIGS at this initial stage was to document the long-term efficacy and safety of recombinant growth hormone (GH) therapy. Since 1987, KIGS has registered more than 60,000 children from 50 different countries, who have been treated with GH for various growth disorders. The heterogeneity within the database, which includes patients of different ethnic origins and cultures who have been exposed to different treatment modalities, has made it possible to gain a better understanding of the use of GH in actual clinical practice around the world and has provided new insights beyond the scope of traditional, randomized clinical trials.

Background

The rationale behind the initiation of KIGS was to build a database consisting of a large cohort of children who had been prescribed GH and who could be followed over a period sufficiently long to allow general conclusions to be drawn regarding the long-term efficacy and safety of GH treatment in the population of children with growth-related disorders.

KIGS was originally intended to be a postmarketing surveillance (PMS) trial. However, at this time, PMS trials did not enjoy wide acceptance. Moreover, discrepancies in local regulations surrounding these trials in different countries precluded a homogeneous framework for the study. Therefore, it was decided to obtain permission to run KIGS as a registry according to Swedish law, with local adaptation to specific regulations in each country. Thus, depending on the local situation, KIGS is defined as a database drawing on a large cohort of patients with short stature originating in different set-ups in different countries, a noninterventional survey, a phase IV clinical trial or a PMS trial.

The low incidence of growth-related disorders, long treatment periods and low frequency of adverse drug reactions reported in clinical trials, the difficulties of establishing a parallel control group of untreated GH-deficient children because of ethical considerations and the desire for a prospective follow-up study made the database definition a logical choice. In addition to being a base for pharmacoepidemiological evaluations,

Pfizer Inc., 235 East 42nd Street, New York, NY 10017-15755 (USA)

the KIGS database is also intended to function as a signaling system for new adverse drug reactions. The terminology and accepted structures for this type of activity did not exist at the time KIGS was initiated, but this monitoring function has become common practice in the years since the inception of KIGS [2–6]. In order to lower the known risk of selection bias, it was decided to leave the reporting of patients to the discretion of the treating physician, while at the same time encouraging participants to include all patients receiving GH (Genotropin, Pfizer) as a prescribed drug.

The set goal of following 500 children for a period of 5 years was revised several times during the initial stages of KIGS because of the great interest in the project. The number of reported children more than tripled during the early phase as more countries joined (table 1). It was then decided to abandon the idea of limiting enrollment to a fixed number of children because a large cohort would provide a better basis from which to generalize to the total population of GH-deficient children.

Table 1. Enrollment in KIGS from 1987 to 2006

Year	Countries	Patients
1987	3	500
1989	14	5,000
1994	35	15,000
1999	44	30,000
2006	>50	62,000

Scientific Organization

The overall structure of KIGS includes the International Board which meets once a year and consists of local coordinators who are the KIGS physicians elected or nominated from participating countries. Each country is entitled to have 1 local coordinator per 1,000 patients registered. The local coordinator may be nominated for a certain period or may alternate with colleagues according to a predefined scheme. In order to be able to have a regular member on the International Board, a participating country must have more than 25 patients included in the database. Countries with fewer than 25 patients may send an observer, who, however, cannot take part in votes.

The International Board elects members of the Strategic Advisory Board who serve as scientific advisors to the Pfizer Endocrine Care, KIGS Medical Outcomes group.

Reporting of Data in KIGS

KIGS is open to all children with growth failure associated with GH deficiency or other causes who have been prescribed GH (Genotropin). All children are subclassified according to the diagnosis. Appropriate use of the KIGS Aetiology Classification List provides KIGS physicians with a tool to classify the diagnosis in a standardized way. This facilitates the difficult task of processing data from a large sample of heterogeneous patients.

Clinics with complete reporting of all children treated with GH (Genotropin) are routinely compared with clinics with less complete reporting in order to detect the influence of a possible selection bias. Much effort is also put into convincing participating clinics to report all their children receiving GH (Genotropin). This places high demands on the data-collecting process, which must be accommodated to fit into everyday clinical practice. This means balancing the number of variables collected against the desire for detailed information required to produce scientifically interesting analyses. The core data registered in the KIGS database are reported case report forms (CRFs) which, in the majority of cases, nowadays are electronic and include patients' medical history, diagnostic procedures, auxology, concomitant medication, laboratory measurements and adverse events reports.

In the case of a more specific and advanced investigation, the KIGS physician may wish to report more detailed information on specific forms in order to contribute to more extensive analysis. Additional data have been collected for certain subgroups of patients within KIGS, including Turner syndrome, brain tumors, Langerhans cell histiocytosis, neurofibromatosis, septooptic dysplasia and Fanconi anemia.

The KIGS Database

The KIGS database was developed to handle an indefinite number of patients. The main objectives in designing the architecture of the database were:
1. to build flexibility and easy access to the system
2. to develop efficient procedures for monitoring and verification of data
3. to provide for subsequent statistical analyses
4. to support all KIGS physicians with feedback relating to individual patients.

The considerations behind the original structure of the database have been described previously [1]. The original rationale and logic still hold today, even though more sophisticated software and technical solutions are now available. Since 2005, a web-based system, endoKIGS, is in use for KIGS.

Data Management

Guidelines or protocols represent the key to a successful research project. However, equally important is the transformation from guidelines to operating procedures. One of the more critical aspects of this process involves data capture, which includes data collection, quality control and data processing. In addition to clinical and statistical expertise, this also requires a wide range of organizational, data management and computing skills.

Data Collection
Data collection is the process in which patient information is transferred from hospital files onto CRFs. In long-term surveys, it is of great importance for the data collected to be identical to the data collected in routine clinical practice. A major achievement in data collection occurred with the introduction of electronic processes. The traditional CRF as a paper form requesting information has now been replaced by computerized programs and electronic transmission. In any case, whether paper forms or electronic spreadsheets are used, the design of the data collection sheet is one of the key success factors in obtaining high-quality data.

Quality Control
Quality control begins the moment a new country or a new clinic is introduced to the KIGS system. Thorough education and explanation are needed in order for all personnel to fully understand the importance of gathering complete and accurate data. Ensuring that the personnel understand this aspect of data collection is the responsibility of the reporting physicians. Whenever a large form requests a lot of information, it is easy to skip over items that are not immediately available, on the ground that most of the information is being provided and a few missing values will not matter. However, failure to provide complete information has significant implications for carrying out scientific analyses of data. If we assume, for example, that there is a 99% likelihood of having a variable completed on the CRF and that 100 observations for each patient are used to perform a particular analysis, some types of statistical analysis require complete patient data in order to be completed. Thus, patients whose CRFs have even one missing item

must be excluded from analysis. The proportion of patients with complete data can then be calculated and the somewhat surprising result is that the data for fewer than 40% of patients can be used. Thus, the importance of reporting complete data needs to be emphasized repeatedly.

The data collection phase, in which outcome parameters are clearly defined and variables are standardized, is another important part of quality control. All variables are described in a data dictionary that defines the parameters included in the CRFs, the data entry screens and the database. The dictionary includes the name of the variable in the database, its description, type (e.g., multiple choice, numerical data or free text) and outcomes of the variable. Ranges and interrelations of variables are also described, as well as coding systems for free text [7].

KIGS physicians and staff involved in the process of transmitting information to the KIGS database are continuously trained by personnel from the local KIGS conduct team in connection with their regular visits in order to reduce variability. A preliminary assessment of the data is performed at this stage when the CRFs are screened for completeness and translation/coding of all text fields.

Data verification is also part of quality control and needs to be initiated from the very beginning. The use of specifically designed computer programs makes it possible not only to enter data at the clinic, but also to apply range controls and simple consistency checks when data are entered. This process includes tracing incomplete variables, out-of-range data and inconsistencies. The process is further complicated by the fact that corrections need to be done on different levels in order to maintain conformity.

Data Processing
Automatic data processing has traditionally been the last step in the overall conduct of a survey or a clinical trial where the variables were introduced in software packages for statistical analysis. However, modern technology has revolutionized not only the statistical analyses utilized, but also the entire chain of data capture. Personal computers are now available in almost every hospital, and electronic transmission via the Internet is common. This introduces new concepts not only in terms of the speed of data collection, but above all, with regard to quality control. The objectives of data processing are to guarantee accuracy, prevent the introduction of errors and ensure the completeness of the data collected, which is the responsibility of the reporting physician.

A web-based system, endoKIGS, has replaced KGS (Pfizer Growth System), a software program for advanced patient management introduced in 1990. endoKIGS facilitates data entry on site with electronic CRFs that mimic the paper-based forms. Range controls are performed on numerical data, and pull-down menus display available codes for text variables. Electronic signatures have replaced the time-consuming process of printing out paper CRFs which needed to be signed to validate the accuracy of the data.

The KIGS team in each country is responsible for monitoring the data before they are transmitted to the main database. In the past, this was usually an inefficient and time-consuming manual process, which is now considerably improved by the new web-based endoKIGS.

The Future

Another important function of KIGS is the development of response prediction models. Such models also represent a new strategic direction for observational studies. The development of such models requires large patient numbers and long experience in analyzing this type of information. The introduction of these prediction models will most probably introduce a paradigm shift in the use of GH. Prediction models will enable the physician to set a clear goal for the outcome of treatment, as well as to make it possible, through close monitoring and frequent treatment adjustments, to optimize outcome in the most cost-effective way. Deviations from the predicted response may also serve as an early warning of concomitant disease or noncompliance or the necessity of re-evaluating the initial diagnosis. The large number of patients with different diagnoses in KIGS has made it possible to develop prediction models for all major subgroups of growth failure. However, the acceptance and use of these models is dependent on the accessibility of modeling in clinical practice when decisions are made regarding treatment regimens. Therefore, the prediction models will be included in endoKIGS, easily accessible for each investigator.

Since the initiation of the KIGS survey, the general attitude towards prospective, observational cohort studies has progressed significantly. Many health authorities now have firm regulations in place and request long-term follow-up studies of a large cohort of patients in order to grant market authorization.

When cohort observations are provided with an appropriate design, they represent excellent tools with which to study current medical practice in varying clinical settings and to generate new hypotheses that can then be evaluated in controlled clinical trials. In addition, cohort observations are essential for signaling adverse drug reactions in rare disorders.

The fact that almost all health authorities request long-term follow-up in connection with market authorization will increase demands on the pharmaceutical industry in terms of competence, structure and resources. However, this will also mean a unique opportunity for different societies to perform meta-analyses and complete audits. This will require increased collaboration among pharmaceutical companies in order to agree on a common data structure permitting meta-analyses.

In summary, 20 years of experience with the KIGS database have led to a genuine understanding of the difficulties in establishing a structure that will provide unbiased patient inclusion, complete reporting of patient information and immediate signaling of adverse drug reactions.

This knowledge was used when the database for follow-up of adults with GH deficiency treated with GH, KIMS, was developed, and recently, when a database, ACROSTUDY, for follow-up of patients treated for acromegaly with a GH receptor blocking analog, pegvisomant, was initiated.

References

1 Wallström A, Trulsson L: The Kabi International Growth Study: rationale, organisation and development; in Ranke MB, Gunnarsson R (eds): Progress in Growth Hormone Therapy – 5 Years of KIGS. Mannheim, J&J Verlag, 1994, pp 1–9.
2 Wertheimer AL, Andrews KB: An overview of pharmacoepidemiology. Pharm World Sci 1995;17:61–66.
3 Winterer G, Herrmann WM: Effect and efficacy: on the function of models in controlled phase III trials and the need for prospective pharmacoepidemiological studies. Pharmacopsychiatry 1996; 29:135–143.
4 Edwards JR: Who cares about pharmacovigilance? Eur Clin Pharmacol 1997; 53:83–88.
5 Figueiras F, Tata B, Takkouche J, Gestal-Otero J: An algorithm for the design of epidemiologic studies applied to drug surveillance. Eur J Clin Pharmacol 1997;53:445–448.
6 Schäfer H: Post-approval drug research: objectives and methods. Pharmacopsychiatry 1997;30(suppl):4–8.
7 Van Es GA: Research practice and data management. Neth J Med 1996;48:38–44.

Assessment of Growth and Puberty

Gary E. Butler

Our understanding of the process of human growth has accelerated rapidly over the last 20 years, especially with the opportunity to intervene in many situations where growth is abnormal. Whenever we attempt to alter growth by way of a treatment, such as with growth hormone, the major challenge is to prove that a real effect has taken place and that we have actually changed a child's endogenous trajectory, be it pathological or not. This depends on repeated accurate measurement of growth, comparison with the appropriate reference standards and the correct use of input parameters in the calculation of predicted growth. There are still many gaps in our understanding, as well as challenges to perform these assessments correctly, and this chapter examines some of the recent advances and highlights where difficulties still arise and further research is needed.

Department of Paediatrics and Growth
Institute of Health Sciences
University of Reading
London Road
Reading RG1 5AQ (UK)

Growth References

A plethora of different growth charts is available in the parts of the world where growth hormone treatment is given to children. Charts not only vary from country to country in format, but in some cases, competing standards are available within individual countries, often of quite different construction and quality. It is also recognised that within any one nation state, there can be significant variations in stature and weight between different regions, and even nowadays, between rural and urban populations, although the marked differences previously noted have mostly disappeared. Today, with increased migration to the 'old' world and movement of people across national boundaries, so that immigrants now form a significant proportion of any population, the notion of a single nation state of homogeneous background is no longer tenable.

Given all these considerations, which growth charts should be used? To answer this question, we need to understand which standards are currently in use throughout the world. In a recent survey of 178 countries [1], weight for age alone was the only growth parameter assessed in over half of the respondents. Two thirds of the charts in use covered the pre-school period only. The most common references used in 68% of countries were the National Centre for Health Statistics/World Health Organisation (WHO) 2000 charts [2]. This contrasted with European countries which tended to use local standards. Of the growth charts in use, 63% classified growth using percentiles, whereas 20% used Z (standard deviation, SD) score parameters. Therefore, which is the most appropriate set of growth standards and which factors should determine this decision?

The WHO expert committee recognised that there was a problem with growth standards produced from retrospective measurements taken from local communities, as these merely reflected how children actually grow rather than how they should grow in ideal circumstances. The lack of representation of an ideal growth pattern and a misunderstanding of normal growth has led to misinterpretation of 'normal' growth. An example of this is the growth of breast-fed infants, which is regarded as pathological when compared with 'normal' standards comprised of mainly bottle-fed infants. Therefore, a multi-centre growth reference study was established in 6 countries worldwide (India, Norway, United States, Ghana, Oman and Brazil), and longitudinal data from birth to 5 years of age were collected prospectively in 8,440 children, breast-fed and reared in optimal circumstances. The resulting standards are made available for weight, length/height, weight for height and body mass index [2]. These charts are currently recommended for international use, having been designed in a way to facilitate the recognition of the normal growth pattern. Currently, they only cover up to 5 years of age. Thereafter, the current National Centre for Health Statistics/WHO standards are recommended. Should we therefore all change to these new charts? Do they convey any advantage for western European countries? Are we seeing the end of local and national growth standards? This new type of growth standard is the first of its kind and is the beginning of a new era. However, we need to know how they perform in both community and specialist practice. Furthermore, although constructed from data from a diverse mix of countries worldwide, are they actually suited to the task in every location? Pilot studies are needed to provide evidence before major changes in established practice should occur.

Use of Growth Charts

Paediatricians and paediatric endocrinologists are actually the minority users of growth charts. In the main, charts are used for screening of individuals within populations, and hence, non-specialists should be able to determine easily whether a child's growth is normal or not. This was attempted when producing the UK 1990 growth standards [3] by the addition of a 0.4th centile (–2.7 SD) with the intention of providing a clear cut-off point to aid identification of abnormal growth. This had the additional benefit of reducing referrals of short normal children to medical services who were normal by definition but simply lying in the lowest 2% of the population. Similarly, at the top end, the 99.6th centile (+2.7 SD) for height and weight may aid detection of abnormality of oversized children and reduce referrals of those who are constitutionally tall, or come from large families.

Two thirds of growth charts currently available display centile lines of different intervals, the lowest variably being the 5th, 3rd, 2nd and/or 0.4th centile. The new WHO standards are available in SD and centile format. So what is the advantage of one over the other? SD scores (Z scores) are valuable for comparisons across groups and for longitudinal evaluation of individual or group data to detect trends. However, the principle of SD scores is less well understood by the majority of users of growth charts, so percentiles should be the preferred format for general and community use. Where centile bands are spaced in equal portions of SDs (0.7 SD as in the UK 1990 charts), rapid estimation of individual SD scores can be achieved by visual inspection. Routine calculations of SD scores for individuals of groups require access to the reference data, which are not widely available, and indeed, those derived from the newer mathematical smoothing models used to construct centile lines, e.g., the LMS method [3], are complex and require computerised calculations. Paediatric endocrinologists may have ready access to the required programs, but the decision by the WHO to offer the new charts in both centile and SD formats should widen the access and use of these standards and promote further understanding of the differences.

Inherent and Unresolved Problems of Growth Charts

Growth during mid-childhood is relatively steady and in the main predictable, and deviations outwith one centile (or SD) band on the distance chart can often suggest abnormal growth. The greatest difficulties come in the first year of life on account of inequalities in perinatal health, diverse feeding patterns and tracking of growth, all of which can cause significant crossing of centile bands before the infant's growth pattern establishes itself along any one particular channel. An appreciation of this is important, and an attempt to portray normal growth in optimal circumstances has been made with the new WHO charts (see above).

Another unresolved problem found with all existing growth charts is the representation of the normal variations of growth that can occur during puberty. Charts constructed from cross-sectional data result in the paradox that no child exhibiting a normal pubertal growth spurt will continue growing along a single centile line or band on this type of chart, and if they do so, it demonstrates abnormal growth. Even longitudinal style charts are hampered in the display of normal adolescent growth on account of the wide variations in total pubertal growth which are known to be unpredictable. Attempts to represent variations of growth not only in terms of amplitude but also tempo result in a growth chart covered with many crossing centile lines. That can cause considerable confusion even to the experienced user. This difficulty has yet to be satisfactorily resolved.

One further unmet challenge in handling growth data at adolescence is the calculation of SD scores. Population SD data are produced by fitting average (50th centile) curves to the data, and SDs of height or weight are available for males or females having an adolescent growth spurt exactly at the 50th centile tempo only. This causes significant difficulty in the comparison of individuals and groups whose tempo of puberty is faster or slower than the mean. Most clinical interest in SD scores centres around patients or groups of patients with delayed puberty. At present, SDs taking into account different stature centiles and pubertal stages are not available. An attempt to tackle this has been made by extending the childhood growth curve into the pubertal period using the Karlberg infancy-childhood-puberty model [4] to try to describe growth in the absence of puberty, but this is only an estimate. Therefore, at present, determination of individual or group changes in growth as the result of disease or an intervention during adolescence can only be represented by mean height velocity changes, categorised by sex, stature and pubertal stage.

Disease-Specific Growth Charts

Once a child has been diagnosed with a condition which is recognised to cause a different growth trajectory from the norm, reference to disease-specific growth charts can be helpful. Quite a wide range of these growth charts is available, and the most well known are for Turner and Down syndrome. They have been produced from mixed cross-sectional and longitudinal growth data from sufficient numbers of affected, untreated children for accurate centile distributions calculated. In rarer conditions, the centile distributions may be less reliable, having been calculated from smaller numbers of patients from differing sources, and therefore, may have methodological limitations. As with standard charts, they generally represent growth in a cross-sectional format, but their most valuable function is to reassure the patients or their families that although their growth is different from the norm, it could be within the acceptable range for any defined condition.

There is also evidence to suggest that the target height centile of the parents on the standard charts can be similar to the target height centile of the affected child on the disease-specific charts and may therefore help to ascertain whether any affected child is growing acceptably, given what is known about its primary condition. These charts play no part in screening for abnormal growth.

Height Velocity Assessment and Calculation

Perhaps the one single area in the field of growth that has caused the most controversy is calculation and interpretation of height velocity. This is partly due to measurement error which is magnified when two height values are used to calculate the velocity. Traditionally, the interval over which height velocity is calculated has been no less than 1 year to minimise the impact of measurement error and to control for seasonal variation of growth. Although properly calibrated equipment and trained measurers can help reduce this error, it is the inherent variability of the child which is at the root of the problem and the appreciation that there is no such thing as absolute stature – height is a composite measurement which varies from hour to hour throughout the day. However, if serial growth estimations are taken, and sequential height velocity values calculated, then measurement error, generally estimated to be no more than 0.3 cm in experienced hands, is not magnified, but actually, its influence diminishes, and much greater diagnostic certainty can be placed on the series of height velocity values and the pattern of height velocity [5].

When serial estimates of height velocity are presented graphically, rhythmic variations can be seen, the pattern of which depends on the frequency of measurement and the frequency of calculation of height velocity. This phenomenon is called 'aliasing'. In clinical practice, if height measurements are taken 2–3 times a year and annualised height velocity is calculated, it is possible to see a cyclical pattern in normal childhood growth [5] with spurts in the prepubertal period that are significantly greater than can be accounted for by measurement error or any pathology (fig. 1). The previously identified single mid-childhood spurt, temporarily associated with adrenarche, has been shown to be artefactual, as it was demonstrated in longitudinal growth studies with an infrequent (annual) measurement schedule only. The finding of multiple prepubertal spurts has led to reconsideration of the description of individual growth and the determination of normal and abnormal upper and lower acceptable values, as individual variability can be large [6]. Ideally, the demonstration of abnormal growth would consist of calculating a height velocity that is above or below the specific range determined for a child of that stature range at that particular point in time, as shorter children generally grow more slowly than taller ones and vice versa. We would then be able to demonstrate that interventions such as growth hormone treatment would produce a greater increment than what would have happened spontaneously if it were successful. On an individual basis, this has proven to be an unmet challenge.

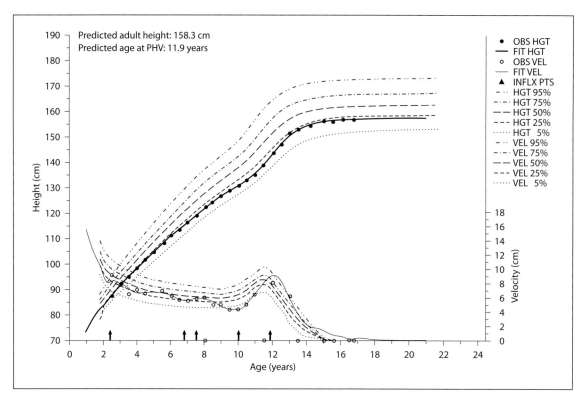

Fig. 1. Height velocity curve for 1 girl [5] showing raw height velocity values (circles) and a fitted non-parametric curve (AUXAL) [6] demonstrating prepubertal growth spurts, the wide variability in prepubertal height velocity values and take-off for the adolescent spurt. The background is the Tanner-Davies US standards. PHV = Peak height velocity; OBS HGT = observed height; FIT HGT = fitted height; INFLX PTS = points of inflexion – peaks and troughs in velocity; VEL = velocity.

However, in groups of children of a similar age distribution, it is still acceptable to continue calculating either mean annual height velocity or mean annual height velocity SD scores. Yet again, there is no satisfactory way of effecting appropriate height velocity comparisons during the adolescent growth spurt unless they are controlled for sex and puberty stage (and ideally stature as well), but attempts to calculate height velocity SD scores, especially individual ones, are inappropriate.

Further Discussion of Analyses of Growth during Puberty

The Age of the Onset of Puberty

In clinical practice, paediatric endocrinologists are often involved with manipulation of the timing and progress of puberty to achieve optimal growth results. However, it is important to appreciate trends in populations and how these vary in different parts of the world when referring to the norm. Ten years ago, it was suggested from a research survey of office-based paediatricians in the United States of America [7] that the onset of puberty in girls was getting earlier, especially in those of African-American background. However, recent evidence suggests that the picture is far from clear [8]. Studies from the United States [9, 10] have confirmed that there is a decrease in the age of onset of puberty of between 0.5 and 1 year with the onset of breast development in African-Americans between 8.9 and 9.6 years and in white girls between 10 and 10.2 years. Age at menarche shows a less marked fall from 12.2 to 12.0 years in black and from 12.9 to 12.6 years in white girls, but the age of attainment of adult height has not advanced, with girls still continuing to grow up to the ages of 16.5 and 17 years, respectively. This suggests a very different change in the tempo and pattern of growth in contemporary US children compared with existing standards.

The situation in boys is even more complicated, with less clear-cut trends. Evidence of earlier sexual maturation is seen in Hispanic-American boys [11, 12] but not in white or African-American boys. However, timing of achievement of Tanner stage 5 has not been recorded as different across the racial groups nor does it differ from current standards.

The situation in Europe appears mixed. Despite the great prevalence of obesity, a trend towards early sexual maturation has not been demonstrated in recent studies from Denmark [13] and Greece [14], whereas there is a suggestion that the onset of puberty in both sexes has decreased by 1 year in Northern Italy [15] but less in Sweden [16]. No clear patterns are emerging. In some countries, the timing of the onset of puberty may be subject to a downward secular trend, but the overall effect on the subsequent milestones of puberty seems to be less marked. This has important social and cultural corollaries in that although the age at which children start puberty may be declining, the age of attainment of fertility is not. This phenomenon also prompts a re-examination of our understanding of the tempo of growth during adolescence.

Determination of the Clinical Onset of Puberty
A major difficulty of obtaining reliable estimates of population secular trends is the accurate determination of the clinical onset of puberty. This may be more confusing in girls on account of confusion between true breast development and pseudo-breast development seen in the current trend towards greater levels of obesity. To determine pubertal stages in large populations of children, self-rating has been advocated as accurate in comparison with hormonal estimates [17], whereas others have not found this reliable [18].

In boys, parallel estimations of clinical assessment of the initial testicular volume increase with the rise in testosterone have confirmed that the onset of male puberty is determined by an increase in the testicular volume to 3 and not 4 ml as currently considered [19, 20]. What difference does this make in the analysis of the adolescent growth spurt? When analysing longitudinal data for calculation of total pubertal growth, the dip in height velocity prior to puberty is frequently used as the starting point. This is usually referred to as a take-off. However, this time point may not necessarily be associated with the clinical onset of puberty, and difficulties with underestimating the age at take-off, hence over-estimating the size of the pubertal growth spurt, are seen when parametric (fitted) growth models are used for this purpose [16, 21]. It may be possible to overcome this problem by using some of the newer non-parametric (flexible) growth modelling programs which can describe individual growth variation more accurately [6], but accurate parallel pubertal staging and an appreciation of the direct link between the phases of puberty and growth is also required.

Pubertal Growth in Late Maturers and Short Individuals
There is considerable variation of growth in height and weight between individuals at adolescence, and the difference between spontaneous

growth and induced pubertal growth needs to be appreciated when calculations of success of growth-promoting treatment interventions are considered. Issues which confound these assessments are discussed above. Although some phenomena about adolescent growth are well described and appreciated, some of the subtle variants in growth at puberty are sometimes forgotten.

Longitudinal studies of normal children have demonstrated that later maturing individuals will have a pubertal growth spurt of lower intensity and lower peak velocity than earlier maturers. That is not the case for weight, where the intensity of adolescent weight gain is independent of the timing of puberty. In children who are short but do not demonstrate a delay in the onset of puberty, a normal intensity pubertal growth spurt will be seen, despite their short stature, and this needs to be appreciated when attempts are being made to predict the size of the pubertal growth spurt and adult height [22].

Prediction of Adult Height

One of the greatest challenges facing paediatric endocrinologists is the prediction of adult height. Objectively, the simplest way to attempt predicting a child's adult height is by taking into account their parental heights; but what are the main obstacles that we encounter doing this? The first is the accuracy of measurement (discussed above), and secondly, even if accurate measures are recorded, they may not always be from the child's biological parents. Parents' heights should be measured at the earliest available opportunity, ideally at the time of antenatal assessment. The taking of the measurements personally is important, as recent studies confirm the long-held belief that reported parental heights are inaccurate, especially those for males, on account of exaggeration of self-reported or partner-reported stature [23].

Target Height

The debate continues as to the best method of calculation of target height and whether this should be a simple calculation based on parental heights or a computational analysis using parental height SD scores. Discussion has continued as to whether this should include a correction for parents of disparate stature, or simply make an allowance for the phenomenon of assortative mating which describes the fact that individuals will link up with partners of similar physique and stature and thus make prediction of target height easier. The issue of the secular trend towards increased stature must also be taken into consideration. The importance of accurate prediction of adult height is highlighted when height predictions are made in comparison with actual final height in studies of short children with growth hormone. Failure to account for the regression to the mean, assortative mating and secular trend may lead to a serious under-estimate of predicted adult height, and therefore, an over-estimate of the effects of growth-promoting therapies. Whereas a number of formulae have been derived to control for these factors, the simplest and most practical approach taking into account secular trends may be the one using parental height SD scores alone, which has the advantage of being independent of sex differences, and thus, no correction is needed [24]. These SD scores are calculated from current growth standards (which are representative of the population heights in their own generation), and a correction factor of 0.7 is used to allow for current secular trends. The confidence intervals of this method and indeed all other methods of prediction are approximately ±10 cm.

The Use of Bone Age to Predict Adult Height

Many attempts have been made to use the assessment of bone age to assist with calculating predicted adult height. Although the initial reference standards were derived from normal population, in recent years, the methodology has been expanded to include extremes of stature; however, the unpredictability of the adolescent growth spurt still confounds the situation, particularly when it is of abnormal shape or duration. The commonly used methods of prediction of adult height in clinical practice are the Tanner-Whitehouse 2 (TW2) [25], recently superceded by the TW3 method [26], and the Bayley-Pinneau method [27] based on estimating the bone age using the Greulich and Pyle standards of skeletal maturation [28]. Published studies have suggested that the Bayley-Pinneau method may be preferable in children with short stature [29] and constitutional growth delay of growth and puberty using suitable corrections [30], although advocates for the TW2 method using single observers of bone age estimation claim equal efficacy [31]. The Bayley-Pinneau method may also be the most accurate for children with growth hormone deficiency [32]. National preferences often decide which method is employed.

Similar discussions have taken place in final height prediction in constitutionally tall children in the decision process as to whether growth-limiting therapy should be considered. Generally, height prediction is less accurate for tall compared with short children, and even more inaccurate in boys. The Bayley-Pinneau method seems to give a reasonably accurate prediction in girls, although the actual final height is over-estimated [33]. The errors found in the prediction of adult height for children with short and tall stature suggest that presently, there is no single ideal method.

Bone age predictions have also been applied to Turner syndrome in girls who have received growth hormone treatment. Again, reports of outcomes using the different methods vary [34, 35], but prediction of the long-term response to growth hormone treatment seems best achieved when treatment parameters, especially the first year growth response and the natural log of the weekly growth hormone dose, are taken into consideration [36].

Predicting Adult Height in Children with Disability

Growth predictions have also been attempted in children with mobility impairment who are either unable to be measured using standard auxological techniques or have other disabilities or deformities. Of these, the most promising approach to height prediction comes from measuring ulna length [37], which appears to be superior to calculating predicted adult height using arm span.

Conclusions

The science of auxology has considerably contributed to our understanding of human growth over the last century, with increased focus over the last 20 years following the wide-spread availability of biosynthetic growth hormone. The principal objective of growth-promoting therapy is to normalise a child's growth, and the onus is on ourselves to ensure that this therapy is used effectively, efficiently and wisely. Accurate assessment of a child's growth and calculation of growth potential still requires the development of new and more refined methods. Although our understanding of growth has advanced enormously, the biggest challenge is to devise new tools suitable for use in routine clinical practice.

References

1 De Onis M, Wijnhoven TMA, Onyango AW: Worldwide practices in child growth monitoring. J Pediatr 2004;144: 461–465.
2 www.who.int/childgrowth.
3 Cole TJ, Freeman JV, Preece MA: British 1990 growth reference centiles for weight, height, body mass index and head circumference fitted by maximum penalized likelihood. Stat Med 1998;17:407–429.
4 Karlberg J, Fryer JG, Engstrom I, Karlberg P: Analysis of linear growth using a mathematical model. 2. From 3 to 21 years of age. Acta Paediatr Scand Suppl 1987;337:12–29.
5 Butler GE, McKie M, Ratcliffe SG: The cyclical nature of prepubertal growth. Ann Hum Biol 1990;17:177–198.
6 Bock RD: Multiple prepubertal growth spurts in children of the Fels Longitudinal Study: comparison with results from the Edinburgh Growth Study. Ann Hum Biol 2004;31:59–74.
7 Herman-Giddens ME, Slora EJ, Wasserman RC, Bourdony CJ, Bhapkar MV, Koch GG, Hasemeier CM: Secondary sexual characteristics and menses in young girls seen in office practice: a study from the Pediatric Research in Office Settings network. Pediatrics 1997;99:505–512.
8 Herman-Giddens ME: Recent data on pubertal milestones in United States children; the secular toward earlier development. Int J Androl 2006;29: 241–246.
9 Kaplowitz P: Pubertal development in girls: secular trends. Curr Opin Obstet Gynaecol 2006;18:487–491.
10 Biro FM, Huang B, Crawford PB, Lucky AW, Striegel-Moore R, Barton BA, Daniels S: Pubertal correlates in black and white girls. J Pediatr 2006;148:234–240.
11 Sun SS, Schubert CM, Liang R, Roche AF, Kulin HE, Lee PA, Himes JH, Chumlea WC: Is sexual maturity occurring earlier among US children? Adolesc Health 2005;37:345–355.
12 Himes JH: Examining the evidence for recent secular changes in the timing of puberty in US children in light of increases in the prevalence of obesity. Mol Cell Endocrinol 2006;254–255:13–21.
13 Juul A, Teilmann G, Scheike T, Hertel NT, Holm K, Laursen EM, Main KM, Skakkebaek NE: Pubertal development in Danish Children: comparison of recent European and US data. Int J Androl 2006;29:247–255.
14 Papadimitriou A, Stephanou N, Papantzimas K, Glynos H, Philippidis P: Sexual maturation of Greek boys. Ann Hum Biol 2002;29:105–108.
15 Castellino N, Bellone S, Rapa A, Vercellotti A, Bonotti M, Petri A, Bona G: Puberty onset in Northern Italy: a random sample of 3597 Italian children. J Endocrinol Invest 2005;28:589–594.
16 Liu YX, Wikland KA, Karlberg J: New reference for the age at childhood onset of growth and secular trend in the timing of puberty in Swedish children. Acta Paediatr 2000;89:637–643.
17 Rapkin AJ, Tsao JC, Turk N, Anderson M, Zeltzer LK: Relationships among self-rated Tanner staging, hormones and psychosocial factors in healthy female adolescents. J Pediatr Adolesc Gynecol 2006;19:181–187.
18 Desmangles JC, Lappe JM, Lipaczewski G, Haynatzki G: Accuracy of pubertal Tanner staging self-reporting. J Pediatr Endocrinol Metab 2006;19:213–221.
19 Ankarberg-Lindgren C, Norjavaara E: Changes of diurnal rhythm and levels of total and free testosterone secretion from pre to late puberty in boys: testis size of 3 ml is a transition stage to puberty. Eur J Endocrinol 2004;151:747–757.
20 Butler GE, Walker RF, Walker RV, Teague P, Riad-Fahmy D, Ratcliffe SG: Salivary testosterone levels and the progress of puberty in the normal boy. Clin Endocrinol 1989;30:587–596.
21 Martin DD, Hauspie RC, Ranke MB: Total pubertal growth and markers of puberty onset in adolescents with GHD: comparison between mathematical growth analysis and pubertal staging methods. Horm Res 2005;63:95–101.
22 Mulligan J, Bailey BJ, Voss LD, Betts PR: Pubertal growth of the short normal girl. Horm Res 1999;52:261–268.
23 Cizmecioglu F, Doherty A, Paterson WF, Young D, Donaldson MDC: Measured versus reported parental height. Arch Dis Child 2005;90:941–942.
24 Hermanussen M, Cole J: The calculation of target height reconsidered. Horm Res 2003;59:180–183.
25 Tanner JM, Landt KW, Cameron N, Carter BS, Patel J: Prediction of adult height from height and bone age in childhood. A new system of equations (TW Mark II) based on a sample including very tall and very short children. Arch Dis Child 1983;58:767–776.
26 Tanner JM, Healy MJR, Goldstein H, Cameron N: Assessment of Skeletal Maturity and Prediction of Adult Height (TW3) Method, ed 3. Singapore, Saunders, 2001.
27 Bayley N, Pinneau SR: Tables for predicting adult height from skeletal age revised for Greulich and Pyle standards. J Pediatr 1952;40:423–441.
28 Greulich WW, Pyle SI: Radiographic Atlas of Skeletal Development of the Hand and Wrist. Stanford, Stanford University Press, 1959.
29 Maes M, Vandeweghe M, De Caju M, Ernould C, Bourguignon JP, Massa G: A valuable improvement of adult height prediction methods in short normal children. Horm Res 1997;48:184–190.
30 Sperlich M, Butenandt O, Schwarz HP: Final height and predicted height in boys with untreated constitutional growth delay. Eur J Pediatr 1995;154: 627–632.
31 Kelly BP, Paterson WF, Donaldson MD: Final height outcome and value of height prediction in boys with constitutional delay in growth and adolescence treated with intramuscular testosterone 125 mg per month for 3 months. Clin Endocrinol (Oxf) 2003; 58:267–272.
32 Cacciari E, Cicognani A, Pirazzoli P, Zucchini S, Salardi S, Balsamo A, Cassio A, Pasini A, Carla G, Tassinari D, Gualandi S: Final height of patients treated for isolated GH deficiency: examination of 83 patients. Eur J Endocrinol 1997;137:53–60.

33 De Waal WJ, Greyn-Fokker MH, Stijnen T, van Gurp EA, Toolens AM, de Munick Keizer-Schrama SM, Aarsens RS, Drop SL: Accuracy of final height prediction and effect of growth-reductive therapy on 362 constitutionally tall children. J Clin Endocrinol Metab 1996;81:1206–1216.

34 Van den Broeck J, Massa GG, Attanasio A, Matranga A, Chaussain JL, Price DA, Aarskog D, Wit JM: Final height after long term growth hormone treatment in Turner syndrome. European study case. J Pediatr 1995;127:729–735.

35 Sas TC, de Muinck Keizer-Schrama SM, Stijen T, van Teunenbroek A, Hokken-Koelega AC, Waelkens JJ, Massa GG, Vulsma T, Gerver WJ, Reeser HM, Delemarre-van de Waal HE, Jansen M, Drop SL: Final height in girls with Turner's syndrome treated with once or twice daily growth hormone injections. Dutch Advisory Group on Growth Hormone. Arch Dis Child 1999;80:36–41.

36 Ranke MB, Lindberg A, Chatelain P, Wilton P, Cutfield W, Albertsson-Wikland K, Price DA, KIGS International Board, Kabi International Growth Study: Prediction of long-term responses to recombinant human growth hormone treatment in Turner syndrome: development and validation of mathematical models. KIGS International Board. Kabi International Growth Study. J Clin Endocrinol Metab 2000;85:L4212–L4218.

37 Gauld LM, Kappers J, Carlin JB, Robertson CF: Height prediction from ulna length. Dev Med Child Neurol 2004;46:475–480.

Diagnosis of Children with Short Stature: Insights from KIGS

Kenji Fujieda[a]   Toshiaki Tanaka[b]

The 20 years of KIGS (Pfizer International Growth Database) data now available offer the opportunity to evaluate long-term trends in the approaches to the diagnosis and categorization of the different aetiologies of short stature. In this chapter, we aim to describe the characteristics of patients whose data are documented in KIGS and to survey both the diagnoses recorded in KIGS and the development of KIGS data in terms of diagnostic categories over time.

Methods

In chapter 5 of this book [pp. 29–37], Ranke presents the most up to date Aetiology Classification List used in KIGS, building on the system he presented in earlier studies [1, 2]. There are three main diagnostic groups: (1) idiopathic growth hormone deficiency (GHD), (2) organic GHD, and (3) other causes of short stature, and these three main groups can be subdivided into specific diagnoses that document over 50 causes of GHD and more than 60 other causes of short stature. Many patients in the 'other causes of short stature' category receive this diagnosis rather than a more general diagnosis of idiopathic or organic GHD. A patient with Turner syndrome, for example, would be classified in the Turner syndrome category, but may also have GHD.

Results

In January 2006, there were 55,028 patients registered in the KIGS database. The proportion of patients in each of the main diagnostic categories (idiopathic GHD, organic GHD, and other causes of short stature) has remained reasonably constant despite the great increase in the number of registered patients (fig. 1). However, there has been a steady change in the proportion of patients in the idiopathic GHD category from 45% in 1993 to 51% in 2006, at the expense of both of the other main categories. A key variation that occurs across the diagnostic categories is in the ratio of males to females: idiopathic GHD 2.1, organic GHD 1.5, and other causes of short stature (including girls with Turner syndrome) 0.8.

Idiopathic GHD

In 2006, the idiopathic GHD category contained 28,088 patients, with a history of perinatal trau-

[a]Department of Pediatrics, Asahikawa Medical College
2-1-1-1 Midorigaoka, Higashi
Asahikawa 078-8510, Hokkaidou (Japan)
[b]Department of Clinical Laboratory Medicine
National Center for Child Health and Development
2-10-1 Ohkura, Setagaya-ku, Tokyo 157-8535 (Japan)

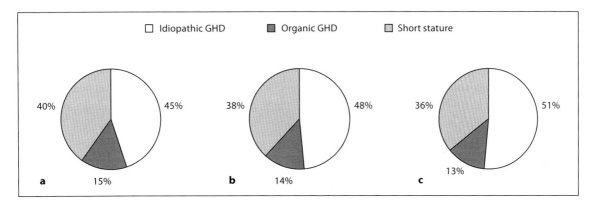

Fig. 1. Distribution of the three main diagnostic categories of patients treated with GH registered in KIGS: idiopathic GHD, organic GHD and other causes of short stature in January 1993 (**a**), March 1998 (**b**) and January 2006 (**c**).

Table 1. Congenital forms of GHD (KIGS Aetiology Classification List No. 2.1)

Code	Description	1993, cases	1998, cases	2006, cases
2.1.1	Genetic causes of GHD	18 (6.9)	75 (9.1)	279 (11.8)
2.1.2	Central malformation	215 (82.7)	639 (77.9)	1,679 (71.3)
2.1.3	Complex syndrome with congenital GHD	8 (3.1)	31 (3.8)	88 (3.7)
2.1.4	Prenatal infection	5 (1.9)	10 (1.2)	20 (0.8)
2.1.5	Bioinactive GH syndromes	12 (4.6)	55 (6.7)	173 (7.3)
2.1.6	Functional GHD	2 (0.8)	10 (1.2)	116 (4.9)
	Total	260	820	2,355

Figures in parentheses are percentages.

ma confirmed in only 758 (2.7%). However, for 7,086 patients (25.2%) in this category, no such history was reported, while in 66.7% of patients, a perinatal history was not recorded. The disturbed GH secretory pattern (neurosecretory dysfunction), i.e. diagnostic category 1.2, was used to classify the remaining 1,499 patients (5.3%) in the main idiopathic GHD category.

Organic GHD
When assessed in 2006, the organic GHD category contained 7,137 patients, with 4,782 patients (67.0%) having acquired GHD and 2,355 (33.0%) patients classified with congenital aetiologies. Congenital GHD mainly resulted from central malformation (71.3%) (table 1), primarily empty sella syndrome and septo-optic dysplasia (34.4 and 27.7%, respectively) (table 2). However, there have been small but steady increases in the proportions of patients in the groups with genetic causes of GHD and functional GHD since the 1993 analysis.

Table 3 shows the sub-categories for patients with acquired GHD. The two main sub-categories each contain a similar proportion of patients: specific pituitary-hypothalamic tumours (37.4%) and other cranial tumours (32.2%). As with organic GHD, comparisons of proportions of pa-

Table 2. Central malformation as the cause of GHD (KIGS Aetiology Classification List No. 2.1.2)

Code	Description	1993, cases	1998, cases	2006, cases
2.1.2.1	Septo-optic dysplasia	70 (32.6)	151 (23.6)	466 (27.7)
2.1.2.2	Empty sella syndrome	64 (29.8)	240 (37.6)	578 (34.4)
2.1.2.3	Solitary central maxillary incisor syndrome	4 (1.9)	11 (1.7)	18 (1.1)
2.1.2.4	Midline palatal cleft	31 (14.4)	49 (7.7)	91 (5.4)
2.1.2.5	Arachnoid cyst	9 (4.2)	21 (3.3)	55 (3.3)
2.1.2.6	Congenital hydrocephalus	16 (7.4)	37 (5.8)	76 (4.5)
2.1.2.9	Others	21 (9.8)	130 (20.3)	395 (23.5)
	Total	215	639	1,679

Figures in parentheses are percentages.

Table 3. Acquired GHD (KIGS Aetiology Classification List No. 2.2)

Code	Description	1993, cases	1998, cases	2006, cases
2.2.1	Tumours of the pituitary-hypothalamic area			
	Craniopharyngioma	253 (24.2)	610 (23.8)	1,140 (23.8)
	Germinoma	84 (8.0)	185 (7.2)	336 (7.0)
	Hamartoma	5 (0.5)	16 (0.6)	26 (0.5)
	Others	58 (5.5)	149 (5.8)	287 (6.0)
2.2.2	Cranial tumours distant from the pituitary-hypothalamic area			
	Astrocytoma	47 (4.5)	130 (5.1)	227 (4.7)
	Ependymoma	36 (3.4)	80 (3.1)	141 (2.9)
	Glioma	31 (3.0)	115 (4.5)	145 (3.0)
	Medulloblastoma	142 (13.6)	350 (13.7)	754 (15.8)
	Nasopharyngeal tumour	11 (1.1)	27 (1.1)	68 (1.4)
	Others	56 (5.3)	118 (4.6)	206 (4.3)
2.2.3	Treatment for malignancy outside the cranium			
	Leukaemia	174 (16.6)	402 (15.7)	694 (14.5)
	Lymphoma	13 (1.2)	34 (1.3)	60 (1.3)
	Solid tumour	11 (1.1)	40 (1.6)	101 (2.1)
2.2.4	Other causes of acquired GHD			
	Head trauma	41 (3.9)	78 (3.0)	121 (2.5)
	Central nervous system infection	14 (1.3)	26 (1.0)	45 (0.9)
	Hydrocephalus (not congenital)	15 (1.4)	27 (1.1)	61 (1.3)
	Granulomatous disease	1 (0.1)	7 (0.3)	7 (0.1)
	Histiocytosis	35 (3.3)	91 (3.6)	158 (3.3)
	Vascular anomaly	3 (0.3)	7 (0.3)	16 (0.3)
	Others	17 (1.6)	71 (2.8)	189 (4.0)
	Total	1,047	2,563	4,782

Figures in parentheses are percentages.

Table 4. Causes of short stature other than GHD (KIGS Aetiology Classification List No. 3)

Code	Description	2006, cases
3.1	Idiopathic short stature	5,035 (25.4)
3.2	Clinically defined syndromes with chromosomal aberrations	7,283 (36.8)
3.3	Clinically defined syndromes without chromosomal aberrations	1,649 (8.3)
3.4	Intrauterine growth retardation without stigmata	2,187 (11.0)
3.5	Intrauterine growth retardation with minor dysmorphic stigmata	230 (1.2)
3.6	Skeletal dysplasia	522 (2.6)
3.7	Disorders of bone metabolism	38 (0.2)
3.8	Disorders in specific systems	2,226 (11.2)
3.9	Endocrine disorders (not GHD) Precocious puberty (n = 92) Thyroid disorder (n = 55) Adrenal disorder (n = 54) Others (n = 162)	363 (1.8)
3.10	Metabolic disorders	80 (0.4)
3.11	Iatrogenic short stature	128 (0.6)
3.12	Psychogenic short stature	55 (0.3)
	Total	19,796

Figures in parentheses are percentages.

tients in 1993, 1998 and 2006 demonstrated stability. This stability was also shown across the same time period in the proportions of patients with non-cranial tumours and other causes of acquired GHD.

Other Causes of Short Stature
In total, 19,796 patients were found to be classified in the 'other causes of short stature' category in the 2006 analysis of KIGS. Clinically defined syndromes with chromosomal aberrations (including Turner syndrome), idiopathic short stature and disorders in specific systems were the three sub-categories containing the most patients (36.8, 25.4 and 11.2%, respectively) (table 4). Turner syndrome accounted for the majority of the patients with clinically defined syndromes with chromosomal aberrations (82.0%), while Silver-Russell syndrome and Noonan syndrome were the largest sub-groups of patients with clinically defined syndromes without chromosomal aberrations (28.1 and 25.3%, respectively) (table 5).

The idiopathic short stature category contained 5,035 patients. Of these, 1,210 (24.0%) had a family history of short stature, while constitutional delay of growth and adolescence (CDGA), with or without a family history of this condition, was seen in 167 patients (3.3%); a combination of the two aetiologies was seen in 108 patients (2.1%).

Intrauterine growth retardation without stigmata was the classification for 2,187 (11.0%) patients with causes of short stature other than GHD. In total, 522 patients were classified within the skeletal dysplasia category (table 6), and the largest number of patients was included under hypochondroplasia (n = 169; 32.4%).

The renal disorders group contained the largest number of patients in the disorders of specific systems category (n = 1,649; 74.1%); chronic inflammatory disorders (n = 164; 7.4%), pulmonary disorders excluding cystic fibrosis (n= 98; 4.4%) and chronic anaemias (n = 94; 4.2%) were the next largest groups (table 7).

Among the other categories within the 'other causes of short stature' group, 363 patients (1.8%) were classified under endocrine disorders other than GHD (table 4). Within this classification, the main subgroups were precocious puberty (25.3%), thyroid disorders (15.2%) and adrenal disorders (14.9%).

Discussion

The number of patients registered in KIGS has continued to increase over the 8 years since the analysis in 1998, further contributing to its power as an analytical tool evaluating GH treatment of children. The proportions of patients within the three main categories, idiopathic GHD, organic GHD and other causes of short stature, have remained reasonably constant since the 1993 analysis of KIGS, although there has been a trend for an increasing proportion of patients to be placed within the idiopathic GHD category. This may reflect changes in patient selection, diagnostic criteria, or the availability of treatment during this time. In addition, the geographical scope of KIGS has expanded, as more countries have started registering patients in the database, and this may have affected the proportions of patients being categorized in the main diagnostic groups.

The gender bias in the ratio of males to females observed in the 1998 analysis remains, with the 'other causes of short stature' category, containing girls with Turner syndrome, still the only one in which boys were not found to predominate (males to females ratio 0.8). However, in the idiopathic short stature group, within this category, the imbalance is present (males to females ratio 2.1). In the other main categories (id-

Table 5. Clinically defined syndromes without chromosomal aberrations (KIGS Aetiology Classification List No. 3.3)

Code	Description	2006, cases
3.3.1	Silver-Russell syndrome	464 (28.1)
3.3.2	Noonan syndrome	417 (25.3)
3.3.3	Von Recklinghausen syndrome (neurofibromatosis)	212 (12.9)
3.3.4	Cornelia de Lange syndrome	18 (1.1)
3.3.5	Prader-Willi syndrome[1]	229 (13.9)
3.3.6	Williams syndrome	14 (0.8)
3.3.8	Rubenstein syndrome	11 (0.7)
3.3.9	Others	284 (17.2)
	Total	1,649

Figures in parentheses are percentages.
[1] Patients with Prader-Willi syndrome who had identifiable chromosomal aberrations (n = 906) were included in group 3.2 (table 4). No patients were included in group 3.3.7.

Table 6. Skeletal dysplasia (KIGS Aetiology Classification List No. 3.6)

Code	Description	2006, cases
3.6.1	Achondroplasia	88 (16.9)
3.6.2	Hypochondroplasia	169 (32.4)
3.6.3	Osteogenesis imperfecta	31 (5.9)
3.6.9	Others	234 (44.8)
	Leri-Weill dyschondrosteosis (n = 50)	
	Metaphyseal chondrodysplasia (n = 28)	
	Spondyloepiphyseal dysplasia (n = 25)	
	Pseudoachondroplastic dysplasia (n = 16)	
	Langer-Giedion syndrome (trichorhinophalangeal syndrome) (n = 15)	
	Others (n = 100)	
	Total	522

Figures in parentheses are percentages.

Table 7. Disorders in specific systems (KIGS Aetiology Classification List No. 3.8)

Code	Description	2006, cases
3.8.1	Cardiac disease	36 (1.6)
3.8.2	Pulmonary (except cystic fibrosis)	98 (4.4)
3.8.3	Liver disorders	35 (1.6)
3.8.4	Intestinal disorders	84 (3.8)
3.8.5	Renal disorders	1,649 (74.1)
	Renal hypoplasia/dysplasia/aplasia (n = 387)	
	Primary nephritic syndrome (n = 110)	
	Others (n = 1,152)	
3.8.6	Chronic anaemias	94 (4.2)
3.8.7	Chronic inflammatory disorders	164 (7.4)
3.8.8	Muscular disorders	9 (0.4)
3.8.9	Neurological disorders	57 (2.6)
	Spina bifida (n = 13)	
	Myelomeningocele (n = 6)	
	Others (n = 38)	
	Total	2,226

Figures in parentheses are percentages.

iopathic and organic GHD), the over-representation of boys was consistent with the previous analysis (2.1 and 1.5, respectively). The over-representation of boys within the organic GHD category may occur because girls are more likely to exhibit precocious puberty, affecting a category that should otherwise have an equal number of boys and girls.

Two possible explanations for the gender bias were discussed previously when the imbalance was highlighted following the 1998 analysis. The first explanation was genetic, and the second suggested that the bias may result from more boys than girls being presented for treatment because of the difference in the social acceptability of girls and boys being short. The genetic explanation would involve (1) genes on the Y chromosome, (2) recessive alleles of genes on the X chromosome, or (3) the 'dose' of an X chromosome gene. Although genes have been identified that may be implicated in growth failure in Turner syndrome [3, 4], and may also be involved in idiopathic short stature, there is no general awareness of an over-representation of boys among children with short stature. In addition, there is a gender bias of 1.5 (males to females ratio) among children treated with GH for GHD caused by treatment for leukaemia. There is no gender bias among the patients who develop leukaemia, thus genetic variation would not appear to explain the difference in this case.

With the explanation of 'social acceptability', although more likely than the genetic explanation, the idiopathic and organic GHD categories should exhibit similar degrees of bias, but this is not the case (2.1 and 1.5, respectively). If the imbalance among patients with idiopathic GHD is genuine, it may occur if, for example, boys are being initiated on treatment at a higher mean age than girls, indicating that some boys with CDGA may be receiving an incorrect diagnosis of GHD. CDGA occurs more commonly in boys than in girls and can result in poor peak GH responses which then spontaneously normalize during puberty.

It is encouraging to note a decrease in the occurrence of idiopathic GHD associated with perinatal trauma as documented in KIGS. While the frequency of occurrence of this association between perinatal trauma and idiopathic GHD did not change significantly between 1993 (5.5%) and 1998 (6.0%), by 2006, the prevalence had reduced to 2.7%. As perinatal trauma is preventable, this is an important reduction.

In the 1998 analysis of KIGS, a relative stability was observed in the proportions of patients with organic GHD registered in KIGS after treatment for leukaemia, lymphoma and solid tumours. The 2006 analysis demonstrates that this stability has been maintained over time, indicating an important continuity in approach in this patient group. Reiter [5] provided a detailed review of the demography of patients with central nervous system neoplasms treated with GH in KIGS in an analysis of the database in 2004.

Conclusions

The key feature revealed by the 2006 analysis of KIGS and its comparison with previous analyses is the change from relative stability of the proportions of patients in each of the three main categories between 1993 and 1998 to a trend towards categorization of patients in the largest group, i.e. idiopathic GHD. However, the gender biases seen previously have been maintained, indicating that the factors that lead to the biases, whether resulting from genetics, social acceptability or other influences, still affect the proportions of males and females being presented for GH treatment.

The wealth of data collected within KIGS continues to provide an important opportunity to monitor and evaluate the use of GH in children. The volume and quality of these data, the length of time that data have been collected and the steady growth rate of the database all contribute to the strength of the analyses that can be generated from KIGS and ensure their continued relevance to clinical practice.

References

1 Ranke M, Lindberg A, Guilbaud O: Prediction of growth in response to treatment with growth hormone; in Ranke MB, Gunnarsson R (eds): Progress in Growth Hormone Therapy: 5 Years of KIGS. Mannheim, JJ Verlag, 1994, pp 97–111.
2 Ranke M: The KIGS aetiology classification system; in Ranke MB, Wilton P (eds): Growth Hormone Therapy in KIGS: 10 Years' Experience. Heidelberg, Johann Ambrosius Barth Verlag, 1999, pp 389–401.
3 Ellison JW, Wardak Z, Young MF, Gehron Robey P, Laig-Webster M, Chiong W: PHOG, a candidate gene for involvement in the short stature of Turner syndrome. Hum Mol Genet 1997;6:1341–1347.
4 Rao E, Weiss B, Fukami M, Rump A, Niesler B, Mertz A, Muroya K, Binder G, Kirsch S, Winkelmann M, Nordsiek G, Heinrich U, Breuning MH, Ranke MB, Rosenthal A, Ogata T, Rappold GA: Pseudoautosomal deletions encompassing a novel homeobox gene cause growth failure in idiopathic short stature and Turner syndrome. Nat Genet 1997;16:54–63.
5 Reiter EO: The demography of central nervous system neoplasms in growth hormone-treated patients found in the KIGS database. Pfizer International Growth Database Report No 22, Annual Report, 2004, pp 1–7.

Data Analyses within KIGS

Anders Lindberg[a]   Michael B. Ranke[b]

Anthropometry and its analysis are the basis for establishing a correct diagnosis in abnormally growing children. The principles of assessing growth have been outlined by Preece [1] in the account after 5 years of KIGS and by Butler [this vol., pp. 6–15]. Since contributions to the KIGS database come from more than 50 countries, it is evident that diagnoses of growth disorders are primarily based on analyses which take into consideration appropriate national references. However, data analyses from KIGS for this account of 20 years could not be based upon the existing variability of references and could not take into consideration the diversity in the field. The members of the International Board of KIGS together with the KIGS statisticians had to decide on the tools to be used and the path of data analysis in order to make a uniform analysis possible. In addition, certain modifications of analyses were made compared with those published previously from KIGS in order to account for methodological progress. We hope that the analytical strategy chosen and outlined here will be accepted by the reader as a reasonable compromise between potentially other possible strategies.

Anthropometrical Standards in Healthy Children

The establishment of references for anthropometrical parameters in healthy children – such as height and weight – is methodologically complex and demands a process which has to take into consideration a multitude of aspects [2]. (1) The population investigated must be ethnically homogenous and balanced according to social variability. Potential selection biases need to be avoided. (2) The survey must cover the entire age range and must include a sufficient number of individuals. (3) The relevant anthropometrical parameters need to be measured with high precision in the same cohort. (4) Data collected should be limited to a narrow time frame in order to avoid possible secular influences. (5) Sex and stages of pubertal development need to be considered. (6) The highest standards have to be applied to the statistical processing of data. (7) Some anthropometrical parameters, such as height velocity, require the collection of longitudinal data. (8) The results must be published – numerically and graphically – in a useful format. There are only a few national studies which take into consideration all (or most) of these considerations. Unfortunately, the large and multidimensional growth studies inaugurated in several European countries (France, the Netherlands, Switzerland, Sweden, the UK) during the 1950s have not been

[a]Pfizer Endocrine Care
KIGS/KIMS/ACROSTUDY Medical Outcomes
Vetenskapsvägen 10, SE–191 90 Sollentuna (Sweden)
[b]Paediatric Endocrinology Section
University Children's Hospital, University of Tübingen
Hoppe-Seyler-Strasse 1, DE–72076 Tübingen (Germany)

continued into recent decades. Thus, if one wants to use normative references with a multitude of anthropometrical parameters documented beyond height and weight, the choice is limited. For this book, we have decided to no longer base the analysis of most of the postnatal anthropometrical data on the UK references [3, 4] but on the Swiss references [5]. Compared with age, children and adults in the Swiss population are taller than those of the formerly used UK population.

In children with growth disorders, pubertal onset is frequently delayed. Thus, if the height (or any other anthropometrical parameter) of such a child is compared with normal references on the basis of chronological age, the calculation shows a high deviation from normal. In accordance with previous analyses [6] and based on the infancy-childhood-puberty model by Karlberg et al. [7], we have extrapolated the Swiss prepubertal standards into the pubertal age range (fig. 1, table 1). These data were used for the growth analysis of children with delayed onset of puberty.

Size at Birth

Anthropometrical data at birth (weight, length, head circumference) are compared with Swedish references [8]. Since the Swedes are amongst the tallest of the Caucasian race, the references tend to be greater than those from other populations.

Body Mass Index

The body mass index [weight (kilograms)/height^2 (square metres)] allows to define weight in relation to height. It has become popular, since in children and adults, it has been shown to be a fairly good indicator of fat mass which allows to define the degree of obesity [9] and the resulting health risk in adult individuals. Body composition with regard to the relationship between fat mass and lean body mass is changing dramatically during childhood and is profoundly gender dependent. Within KIGS, the references published by Cole et al. [10] were used.

Height Velocity

Height velocity, either in terms of centimetres/year or change in height standard deviation score (SDS), was calculated based on Swiss references only if two measurements were done in intervals of 9–15 months.

Puberty Onset

Age at the onset of puberty was defined as the first visit at which Tanner breast stage 2 (B2) [11], unbiased by exogenous oestrogens, was documented in girls, or when marked by a max testicular volume of >3 ml in boys [12, 13]. For the evaluation of growth data, the time elapsed from a documented prepubertal to pubertal status had to be <6 months.

Near Adult Height

Near final (adult) height was assumed when height progressively slowed down and height velocity was <2 cm/year, or when bone age was ≥14 years in girls or ≥16 years in boys, respectively.

Bone Age

Bone age estimations using the standards of Greulich and Pyle [14] or Tanner et al. [15, 16] were provided by the referring physicians, and prediction of adult height was calculated using the tables of Bayley and Pinneau [17] or, when appropriate, the methods of Tanner et al. [15, 16].

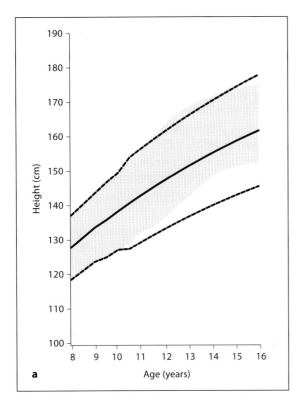
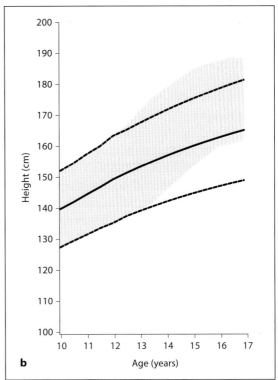

Fig. 1. Height extrapolation (50th, 3rd, 97th centiles) for female (**a**) and male (**b**) children with delayed puberty in comparison with normal Swiss references (shaded area) [5].

Table 1. Adjusted height references for boys and girls with delayed puberty

	Age, years	Height, cm	Adjusted height, cm		Age, years	Height, cm	Adjusted height, cm
Boys	10	140.2 ± 6.2	140.2 ± 6.2	Girls	9	133.6 ± 5	133.6 ± 5.0
	10.5	142.5 ± 6.3	142.5 ± 6.3		9.5	135.9 ± 5.5	135.9 ± 5.5
	11	145.0 ± 6.6	145.0 ± 6.6		10	138.4 ± 5.6	138.4 ± 5.6
	11.5	147.3 ± 6.7	147.3 ± 6.7		10.5	141.1 ± 6.0	140.8 ± 6.7
	12	149.9 ± 7.1	149.9 ± 7.1		11	144.3 ± 6.0	143.1 ± 6.8
	12.5	152.6 ± 7.4	151.9 ± 7.0		11.5	146.9 ± 6.6	145.3 ± 7.0
	13	155.9 ± 8.0	153.8 ± 7.2		12	150.2 ± 6.8	147.5 ± 7.1
	13.5	159.2 ± 8.6	155.7 ± 7.3		12.5	153.2 ± 6.7	149.5 ± 7.3
	14	162.9 ± 8.3	157.4 ± 7.4		13	155.7 ± 6.6	151.5 ± 7.4
	14.5	166.2 ± 8.1	159.0 ± 7.6		13.5	158.2 ± 6.3	153.4 ± 7.5
	15	169.7 ± 7.9	160.6 ± 7.7		14	160.1 ± 5.8	155.3 ± 7.7
	15.5	172.2 ± 7.5	162.1 ± 7.8		14.5	161.9 ± 5.8	157.1 ± 7.8
	16	174.4 ± 7.0	163.4 ± 8.0		15	162.7 ± 5.8	158.7 ± 7.9
	16.5	175.4 ± 7.0	164.7 ± 8.1		15.5	163.5 ± 5.6	160.4 ± 8.0
	17	176.2 ± 6.7	165.9 ± 8.2		16	164.0 ± 5.7	161.9 ± 8.1

Body Surface Area

The body surface area was calculated based on the formula of Dubois and Dubois [18].

Target Height

Target height (TH) is a child's predicted height based on the height of the parents, along with a (95%) confidence interval representing the likely range of final height [19]. There are several mathematical formulas which have been suggested for the calculation of TH.

Equation 1, suggested by Tanner et al. [20]: TH (centimetres) = [father's height (centimetres) + mother's height (centimetres)]/2 – 6.5 cm (girls)/+ 6.5 cm (boys); 95% confidence intervals: ±10 cm for boys and ±9 cm for girls.

Equation 2, suggested by Cole et al. [9]: TH SDS = (father's height SDS + mother's height SDS)/2.

Equation 3, suggested by Cole [21]: TH SDS = (father's height SDS + mother's height SDS)/1.61.

Equation 4, suggested by Hermanussen and Cole [19]: TH SDS = (father's height SDS + mother's height SDS) × 0.72; 95% confidence interval (sex independent): TH SDS ± 1.64 times population SD.

Equations 1 and 2 give similar but somewhat lower (0.5 SDS; 3.5 cm) results compared with equations 3 and 4. Within KIGS, for this book, equation 3 has been used.

Disease-Specific References

A variety of congenital growth disorders are characterised by a specific pattern of growth. The systematic study of typical, disease-specific growth relating to many disorders has been conducted during the past decades [for a review, see ref. 22, 23]. The need for such growth standards is evident for a variety of reasons: (1) patients, their parents and physicians need to be informed and counselled; (2) deviations from the disease-specific growth pattern are likely indications of additional diseases; (3) the growth pattern may help in understanding the pathogenesis of the underlying growth disorder; (4) the growth of an individual may be predicted and can be drawn into consideration before attempts to promote growth are made, and (5) effects of growth-promoting treatment can be evaluated.

In the light of the stringent criteria under which normal data for growth standards should be established (see above), it is reasonable to question whether a similar standard can be set with regard to syndromes associated with growth disorders. Mostly, the disorders are infrequent, which makes the data collection difficult. In many syndromes, the aetiology and the pathogenesis of the growth disorder are unclear. Recently, the genetic causes of many syndromes have been elucidated. However, in many instances, a specific genetic defect can only be found in part of the population with a syndrome, which is generally described by its specific pattern of symptoms, while in another phenotypically similar/identical fraction of individuals, this is not the case. Disease-specific references of the same disorder are also reported from various countries and ethnicities and do not consider possible secular trends in growth. Thus, the data collection in growth disorders is biased in many ways. Nevertheless, such references have been serving the medical community well. Within KIGS, it was decided to use certain references of specific growth disorders (table 2) for analytical purposes. The choice does not imply that the references used are 'better' than others. It is obvious that for example French height references for girls with Turner syndrome are more suitable for the analysis of French Turner girls within KIGS. However, for many syndromes, there are only a limited number of references (or even only one) available.

Table 2. List of default disease-specific references used for data analyses within KIGS

Disease	Anthropometrical parameter available	Reference
Turner syndrome	height, weight, sitting height	Ranke et al. [24], 1988 Ranke [25], 1998
Noonan syndrome	height	Ranke et al. [26], 1988
Prader-Willi syndrome	height	Hauffa et al. [27], 2000
Silver-Russell syndrome	height	Wollmann et al. [28], 1995

Lastly, the application of a specific reference in comparison with references from normal children appears to be a suitable way to illustrate growth within KIGS before and during growth hormone (GH) therapy.

Data Analysis

Means and SD versus Medians and Centiles
Group data can either be given as means and SD or medians and ranges. The former mode requires a Gaussian distribution. In addition, these parameters are sensitive to outliers, by which a single extreme value can distort the results. The default choice within KIGS is to calculate medians and centiles (e.g., 10th and 90th centiles), since this gives a robust estimate irrespective of the underlying distribution.

Standard Deviation Scores
An SDS (or Z score) expresses the distance of a data point to the mean of the reference as a multiple of the SD of the mean reference. The analysis is usually related to the chronological age and matched for gender [SDS = (subject parameter – mean of reference)/SD of reference]. For this book, the default settings of references used for SDS calculations are: (1) height [5], (2) height velocity [5], (3) weight [29], (4) body mass index [10], (5) sitting height [5], (6) birth weight and birth length [8], (7) specific diseases (table 2), and (8) insulin-like growth factor 1 [30].

Group Comparison
Non-parametric statistics (two-sided Wilcoxon rank sum test) were used to test for differences between groups when the distribution of data was unknown or skewed. In cases of a normal distribution of the data, Student's t test was applied. In order to compare proportions, Fisher's exact test was used. Significance was considered at the 5% level ($p < 0.05$), unless otherwise specified. The principles of regression analysis are outlined in the chapter by Ranke and Lindberg [this vol., pp. 422–431].

Missing Data
Missing data points can be of two types: (1) not available and (2) not applicable (e.g., testis size in girls). Missing values of type 1 are considered in, for example, frequency analyses, while missing values of type 2 are excluded from all analyses. No missing value was replaced by extrapolation or any other statistical method to deal with missing values. However, if a Tanner stage B3 was reported, e.g., 6 months after stage B1, without the time at appearance of B2, then the onset of B2 was calculated as in between B1 and B3. Such interpolations were only done for pubertal stages, GH doses and the number of GH injections.

In the absence or incorrectness of essential data, <5% of all cases could not be considered for analysis. However, information on adverse events was always completely reported.

GH Dose

Long-term GH doses were calculated as mean doses over the selected time frame applied. Thus, every change in dose and weight was considered. Periods without GH were not included in the denominator.

Computer Programmes

The SAS® version 8 for Sun Solaris was used for all analyses.

References

1 Preece MA: The assessment of growth; in Ranke MB, Gunnarsson R (eds): Progress in Growth Hormone Therapy – 5 Years of KIGS. Mannheim, J&J Verlag, 1994, pp 10–36.
2 Tanner JM: A History of the Study of Human Growth. Cambridge, Cambridge University Press, 1981.
3 Tanner JM, Whitehouse RH, Takaishi M: Standards from birth to maturity for height, weight, height velocity, and weight velocity: British children, 1965 II. Arch Dis Child 1966;41:613–635.
4 Tanner J, Whitehouse R: Clinical longitudinal standards for height, weight and height velocity, weight velocity and the stages of puberty. Arch Dis Child 1976;51:170–179.
5 Prader A, Largo RH, Molinari L, Issler C: Physical growth of Swiss children from birth to 20 years of age. First Zurich longitudinal study of growth and development. Helv Paediatr Acta Suppl 1989;52:1–125.
6 Price DA, Ranke MB: Final height following growth hormone treatment; in Ranke MB, Gunnarsson R (eds): Progress in Growth Hormone Therapy – 5 Years of KIGS. Mannheim, J&J Verlag, 1994, pp 129–144.
7 Karlberg J, Fryer JG, Engström I, Karlberg P: Analysis of linear growth using a mathematical model. From 3 to 21 years of age. Acta Paediatr Scand Suppl 1987;337:12–29.
8 Niklasson A, Ericson A, Fryer JG, Karlberg J, Lawrence C, Karlberg P: An update of the Swedish reference standards for weight, length and head circumference at birth for given gestational age (1977–1981). Acta Paediatr Scand 1991;80:756–762.
9 Cole TJ, Bellizzi MC, Flegal KM, Dietz WH: Establishing a standard definition for child overweight and obesity worldwide: international survey. BMJ 2000;320:1240–1243.
10 Cole TJ, Freeman JV, Preece MA: Body mass index reference curves for the UK, 1990. Arch Dis Child 1995;73:25–29.
11 Tanner JM: Growth at Adolescence. Oxford, Blackwell, 1962.
12 Zachmann M, Prader A, Kind HP, Haflinger H, Budlinger H: Testicular volume during adolescence. Helv Paediatr Acta 1974;29:61–72.
13 Ankarberg-Lindgren C, Norjavaara E: Changes of diurnal rhythm and levels of total and free testosterone secretion from pre to late puberty in boys: testis size of 3 ml is a transition stage to puberty. Eur J Endocrinol 2004;151:747–757.
14 Greulich WW, Pyle SI: Radiographic Atlas of Skeletal Development of Hand and Wrist, ed 2. Stanford, Stanford University Press, 1959.
15 Tanner JM, Landt KW, Cameron N, Carter BS, Patel J: Prediction of adult height from height and bone age in children. A new system of equations (TW Mark II) based on a sample including very tall and very short children. Arch Dis Child 1983;58:767–776.
16 Tanner JM, Healy MJR, Goldstein H, Cameron N: Assessment of Skeletal Maturity and Prediction of Adult Height (TW3) Method, ed 3. Singapore, WB Saunders, 2001.
17 Bayley N, Pinneau S: Tables for predicting adult height from skeletal age. J Pediatr 1952;40:423–441.
18 Dubois D, Dubois EF: A formula to estimate the approximate surface area if height and weight be known. Arch Int Med 1916;17:863–871.
19 Hermanussen M, Cole J: The calculation of target height reconsidered. Horm Res 2003;59:180–183.
20 Tanner JM: Fetus into Man. London, Open Books, 1978.
21 Cole TJ: Some questions about how growth standards are used. Horm Res 1996;45(suppl):18–23.
22 Hall JG, Froster-Iskenius UG, Alanson JJE: Handbook of Normal Physical Measurement. Oxford, Oxford University Press, 1989.
23 Ranke MB: Disease-specific standards; in Johnston FE, Zemel B, Eveleth PB (eds): Human Growth in Context. London, Smith-Gordon, 1999, pp 159–168.
24 Ranke MB, Stubbe P, Majewski F, Bierich JR: Spontaneous growth in Turner's syndrome. Acta Paediatr Scand Suppl 1988;343:22–30.
25 Ranke MB: Turner and Noonan syndrome: disease-specific growth and growth promoting therapies; in Kelnar CJH, Savage MO, Stirling HF, Saenger P (eds): Growth Disorders. London, Chapman & Hall Medical, 1998, pp 623–640.
26 Ranke MB, Heidemann P, Knupfer C, Enders H, Schmaltz AA, Bierich JR: Noonan syndrome: growth and clinical manifestations in 144 cases. Eur J Pediatr 1988;148:220–227.
27 Hauffa BP, Schlippe G, Roos M, Gillessen-Kaesbach G, Gasser T: Spontaneous growth in German children and adolescents with genetically confirmed Prader-Willi syndrome. Acta Paediatr 2000;89:1302–1311.
28 Wollmann HA, Kirchner T, Enders H, Preece MA, Ranke MB: Growth and symptoms in Silver-Russell syndrome: review on the basis of 386 patients. Eur J Pediatr 1995;154:958–968.
29 Freeman JV, Cole TJ, Chinn S, Jones PR, White EM, Preece MA: Cross-sectional stature and weight reference curves for the UK, 1990. Arch Dis Child 1995;73:17–24.
30 Juul A, Dalgaard P, Blum WF, Bang P, Hall K, Michaelsen KF, Muller J, Skakkebaek NE: Serum levels of insulin-like growth factor (IGF)-binding protein-3 (IGFBP-3) in healthy infants, children, and adolescents: the relation to IGF-I, IGF-II, IGFBP-1, IGFBP-2, age, sex, body mass index, and pubertal maturation. J Clin Endocrinol Metab 1995;80:2534–2542.

The KIGS Aetiology Classification System

Michael B. Ranke

KIGS (Pfizer International Growth Database) is a worldwide pharmacoepidemiological survey. Its main objectives are both to study the efficacy of Genotropin®, a recombinant human growth hormone (GH), in treating various growth disorders and to monitor adverse events that may occur during GH treatment. In order to optimally fulfill these tasks, it is of great importance to obtain information on the patients enrolled in the survey that is as detailed and complete as possible. One of the most important pieces of information required is the exact diagnosis of the patients treated, since both the effects of treatment and any concomitant adverse events may vary accordingly.

To fulfill this goal, the KIGS Strategic Advisory Board has developed the KIGS Aetiology Classification List to allow the participating physicians to classify diagnoses in a standardized way. The appropriate use of this diagnostic code facilitates the difficult task of processing data from a large, heterogeneous group of patients.

Underlying Philosophy of the KIGS Aetiology Classification List

A formal coding system of diagnoses must fulfill a number of prerequisites.
1 It should allow classification of all patients in question.
2 There should be latitude for accommodating further developments in aetiologies and pathogenetic aspects.
3 The diagnoses listed should be well defined in order to preclude misclassifications.
4 The classification should follow one general principle (e.g., nosology, aetiology, pathogenesis or symptomatology).
5 It should be easy to use.
6 It should serve the purpose for which it is designed in an optimal way.

In light of this (incomplete) list of demands, it is evident that no system for the classification of diseases can be ideal. The KIGS Aetiology Classification List (reproduced below) was designed to reflect the fact that GH is used for the promotion of growth in children with a variety of growth disorders [1]. The primary common link among the patients enrolled in KIGS is treatment with Genotropin.

The main problem of reviewing a classification system such as this is that one is required to

Paediatric Endocrinology Section
University Children's Hospital, University of Tübingen
Hoppe-Seyler-Strasse 1, DE–72076 Tübingen (Germany)

maintain continuity for the past and future use of the database and at the same time to integrate new developments in the understanding of causes of disorders. Therefore, the KIGS Aetiology Classification System will maintain its basic structure, which for historical reasons is based on the descriptive and clinical criteria. This approach is still valid in times when the molecular basis of many disorders is only partly disclosed and/or not always available to the investigators. The participants of the KIGS system are encouraged to give as much (clinical, anatomical, biochemical, genetic) information about their cases as possible. This will eventually allow an appropriate data analysis in groups/subgroups of patients.

We have added a few general and specific comments to make the KIGS Aetiology Classification List more useful to the investigator.

Hierarchy of Diagnoses

Treatment with GH to improve short stature is based on the presence of GH deficiency (GHD), various causes of short stature without proven abnormalities of the GH axis, or a combination of both. We assume that the responsiveness to GH is different in cases with genuine abnormalities of GH in comparison with other situations. In the case where GHD is present and the cause of short stature is commonly not associated with a disorder of the GH axis, the latter is considered to be ranking higher in the hierarchy of diagnoses. If, for example, GHD is also proven in Turner syndrome, the patient should primarily be classified under the diagnosis of Turner syndrome. In this instance, the patient should be secondarily classified as GHD. In general, if there is a combination of diagnoses encoded under both No. 3. ff. and No. 1. ff./2. ff. within the hierarchy of classifications, diagnoses defining primary diseases rank before states of GHD (e.g., disturbed GH secretory pattern).

Chromosomal, Molecular Genetic or Biochemical Definitions

The diagnosis of a disease may be based on one specific (pathognomonic) finding or a sum of phenotypical characteristics. The latter may be clinical, anthropometrical, biochemical or X-ray phenomenological. In the absence of a pathognomonic symptom/sign, diagnoses are often established based on scores which take empirical probability into consideration. One typical example for such an approach is the Noonan syndrome. Interestingly, mutations of the PTPN11 gene have been found to be associated in about 50% of the cases classified as Noonan syndrome on the basis of clinical criteria. Similarly, hypochondroplasia has been associated with FGFR3 mutations in about 70% of the cases. Thus, in cases in which these genetic defects have been documented, a specific diagnosis is proven. However, the absence of such genetic defects does not exclude the correctness of certain diagnoses, since genetic heterogeneity may result in very similar phenotypes. Thus, in any instance, the investigator should document on the case report forms (CRFs) how the diagnosis was established.

Growth Hormone Deficiency

Historically, GH was first and exclusively used to treat children with GHD [2]. An impaired secretion of GH in children is causally associated with impaired growth, changes of the anthropometrical characteristics (e.g., normal proportions, relatively large head) and the composition of the body (e.g., sarcopenia, excess of body fat), as well as functional abnormalities (e.g., hypoglycaemia). During the past decades, we have observed a multitude of methods which allow to distinguish various forms of GHD in terms of the underlying pathology and aetiology. However, this has led to a higher degree of complexity rather than uniformity in the ability to classify. Classi-

Table 1. Diagnostic tests and pattern of biochemical findings related to the level of disorder along the GH axis

Level of disorder	Diagnostic tests				
	standard GH stimulation tests	GHRH test	spontaneous GH secretion	IGF-1/ IGFBP-3	response of IGF to GH
Neurosecretory 'unit'	normal	normal	low	low	normal
Hypothalamus	low	normal	low	low	normal
Pituitary	low	low	low	low	normal
IGF-producing tissue	normal	normal	normal	low	low
Target tissue for IGF	normal	normal	normal	normal	normal

GHRH = GH-releasing hormone; IGFBP-3 = IGF binding protein 3.

fications based on functional investigations of GH secretion and action have allowed some degree of understanding of the level of pathogenesis of the GH axis (table 1).

Functional investigations include measurements of GH by means of various assays (immunoassays, bioassays), determination of GH levels after various exogenous stimuli, the analysis of spontaneously secreted/excreted GH, measurements of GH-dependent factors, such as insulin-like growth factor 1 (IGF-1), IGF binding protein 3 and acid-labile subunit, and the biochemical response to exogenous GH (e.g., IGF generation). In addition to the difficulty of conducting such functional tests, the limitations of standardization and normative data have hindered a concise interpretation of the obtained data and their interplay until today [see Tauber, this vol., pp. 47–55]. New imaging tools (computed tomography and magnetic resonance tomography) allow to describe qualitative and quantitative anatomical anomalies of the pituitary region [see Maghnie et al., this vol., pp. 93–107]. A higher resolution and functional imaging is likely to lead to a further dimension in describing more subtle abnormalities. Discoveries by means of molecular genetics allow to describe abnormalities in the development of the pituitary and its ability to produce and secrete GH and other trophic hormones [see Mullis, this vol., pp. 189–201]. Classification systems of GHD may also consider whether GHD is congenital and follows a certain pattern of inheritance, e.g., in isolated GHD [see Mullis, this vol., pp. 189–201], or whether it is acquired.

KIGS Aetiology Classification List No. 1.1 ff.: Idiopathic Growth Hormone Deficiency

Idiopathic GHD (i.e. no aetiology is established) is still the most common form of GHD. It appears trivial but nevertheless important to note that every reasonable effort should be made to exclude diagnoses other than GHD before treatment. The key diagnostic tools to establish the diagnosis are blood GH measurements collected under spontaneous condition or after physiological or pharmacological stimuli (e.g., arginine). In order to avoid falsely positive results, these tests should be conducted under strict standardization and under the least stressful condition for the child. Since it is assumed that test results are prone to be falsely low, at least two independent tests are required to confirm the diagnosis. A cut-off level of 10 µg/l GH in serum or plasma is accepted as a guideline. However, this cut-off level may vary according to the applied GH assay, the test procedures used and the normative references available. In my institution, for example, we have reduced the cut-off from 10 to 8 µg/l after introducing a more recent international reference preparation for GH (IRP 88/624, IRP 98/574) in the GH assay. It is obvious that today, all available methods should be applied to increase the likelihood of the diagnosis of GHD. Normal stature, normal height velocity and normal bone age are not completely excluding the diagnosis of idiopathic GHD, but make its presence unlikely. Likewise, normal/high-normal IGF-1 (IGF binding protein 3, acid-labile subunit) levels are not supportive of the diagnosis [3]. We are convinced that magnetic resonance imaging of the pituitary area is an essential part of the diagnostic process of GHD. A small anterior pituitary or a pituitary abnormality (code No. 2.1.2.7) is not an a priory proof of a disturbed GH secretion, but is likely to provide evidence that the established diagnosis of GHD is correct. With greater refinement in our diagnostic arsenal, less cases with GHD will be classified as idiopathic. However, at this point in time, it is too early to expand the spectrum of classifications, but it is of utmost importance that all parameters in support of a pathogenesis and/or aetiology are documented on the CRFs in order to allow for an appropriate analysis of the data.

KIGS Aetiology Classification List No. 1.2 ff.: Neurosecretory Dysfunction

The term 'neurosecretory dysfunction' describes a specific situation of GHD. In affected children, GH levels observed during stimulation tests are normal, but spontaneously secreted GH is low. This situation was first described in children who had been treated with X-ray therapy to the cranium as part of treatment for malignancy. In these cases, neurosecretory dysfunction appears to be intuitively understandable and can be seen as a special pathogenetic situation of organic GHD. However, this situation was also found in children without such a history ('idiopathic neurosecretory dysfunction'?). In the latter (code No. 1.2), the diagnosis should be established with the support of other indicators of GHD and with great care.

KIGS Aetiology Classification List No. 2.1.5: Bioinactive Growth Hormone Syndrome

In principle, the situation of bioinactive GH can be suspected in children clinically resembling the 'classical' GHD category, with low circulating IGF-1 levels but with normal GH secretion based on immunoassay measurements. Treatment with recombinant human GH leads to an increase in IGF levels and a growth response to GH. It can be assumed that one reason for bioinactive GH is a congenital structural abnormality of GH, which impairs/abolishes interaction with the GH receptor and subsequent signal transduction. Sophisticated methods (e.g., radioreceptor assay, bioassay and gene analyses) are required to prove such an entity [4]. Although this diagnosis has stimulated the scientific fantasy of a whole generation, little empirical evidence of its existence has emerged.

KIGS Aetiology Classification List No. 3.1: Idiopathic Short Stature

In a recent consensus meeting, the definition of idiopathic short stature (ISS) was re-evaluated and the following conclusions reached [5].

(1) Short stature is defined as a condition in which the height of an individual is 2 standard deviations below the corresponding mean height for a given age, sex and population group. Whether the height of a child is 'abnormal' from a purely statistical point of view or whether it is an indication of abnormal growth itself is a matter that needs to be clarified by applying additional criteria. At present, the term 'idiopathic short stature' is used to describe short stature for which no underlying pathogenesis of aetiology is known [see also Wit, this vol., pp. 309–318].

(2) The definition of ISS is based on the exclusion of other likely causes of short stature, as well as on the following minimal criteria: normal size (more than a standard deviation score of –2) for gestational age at birth; normal body proportions; no evidence of chronic organic disease; no psychiatric disease or severe emotional disturbance; normal food intake; no evidence of endocrine deficiency, and the tempo of growth throughout the growth process may be either slow or normal.

(3) The expert group came to the conclusion that only the subclassifications of ISS (before puberty) outlined below can be made with certainty.
– Familial short stature (FSS): the child is short in comparison with the relevant population, but remains within the expected range of height relating to his or her family.
– Non-FSS: the child is short in comparison with the relevant population and is below the range of height relating to his or her family.

It is obvious that in the future, many children in this category will no longer be classified 'idiopathic', since a specific defect explaining short stature will be found [6]. It has also been claimed that defects in the SHOX gene could cause ISS. However, it is my personal conviction that with careful clinical and X-ray analyses, such children will not classify as ISS. Today, short children with a defect in the SHOX gene will classify under bone dysplasias (code No. 3.6 ff.).

KIGS Aetiology Classification List No. 3.2.1–3.3.9

One of the problems with these disorders is the fact that in many of the diagnoses which are primarily made on the basis of clinical criteria, we are starting to discover small defects in chromosomes or genetic or epigenetic abnormalities. In addition, in subgroups with clinically well-established diagnoses, no such or different abnormalities of chromosomes or genes are found. A typical example for this is Prader-Willi syndrome, which can be documented under code No. 3.2.3 or 3.3.5. Irrespective of the result of genetic analyses, it is advisable to carefully document the basis of the established diagnosis on the CRFs.

KIGS Aetiology Classification List No. 3.4 ff. and 3.5 ff.: Intrauterine Growth Retardation

There is a subgroup of children with short stature and smallness for gestational age. Smallness at birth can either be the result of a retardation of intrauterine development starting from a normal size, or can be the result of smallness early on during prenatal development. The former situation is descriptively termed 'intrauterine growth retardation' (IUGR) and was used in the KIGS Aetiology Classification List to describe both situations (code No. 3.4 ff. and 3.5 ff.). More recently, for children, the term 'small for gestational age' (SGA) has become popular. It needs to be realized that both terms are purely descriptive. Primarily, nothing is said about the cause of short stature; thus, it is necessary to come to a consensus on the terminology for these children.

However, notably, any defined disorder with smallness at birth needs to be classified under the respective specific diagnosis. For example, children with Turner syndrome tend to be small at birth, but are classified under code No. 3.2.1. Likewise, Silver-Russell syndrome is an independent entity (code No. 3.3.1). In order to get more information on the possible cause of a short child born SGA, there is a specific CRF.

KIGS Aetiology Classification List No. 3.6 ff.: Skeletal Dysplasias

Skeletal dysplasias exist in a great variety. Often, the specific diagnosis can only be established by taking into account the clinical appearance during development and radiological findings [7]. Since with the advent of modern imaging techniques 'classic' paediatric radiologists have become rare, it seems advisable to seek a specialist's advice before making a diagnosis. Molecular genetic techniques provide a whole new array of tools for establishing specific diagnoses.

KIGS Aetiology Classification List No. 3.8 ff.: Disorders in Specific Systems

Growth disorder in these diseases may be caused by a multitude of factors. The extent of the disorder within an organ system, the possible cause of such a disorder (e.g., cardiac failure in a specific syndrome) and treatment modalities (e.g., steroids in inflammatory disorders) may all have an impact on growth. Therefore, it is of utmost importance to extensively document these components longitudinally during GH treatment. Similarly, this applies to KIGS Aetiology Classification List No. 3.9 ff. (endocrine disorders, not GHD), 3.10 ff. (metabolic disorders) and 3.11 ff. (iatrogenic short stature).

Specific lists for the classification of renal disorders have been developed [see Mehls, this vol., pp. 407–421].

KIGS Aetiology Classification List No. 3.12 ff.: Psychogenic Short Stature

Without doubt, these disorders represent situations of the utmost complexity. Documentation of the symptomatology – after exclusion of organic causes – and the application of standardized psychological inventories during follow-up are advised [8].

Concluding Remarks

A system for the classification of diseases of growth and other paediatric endocrine disorders is needed to meet the clinical and scientific demands of the international medical community. The KIGS Aetiology Classification List is an attempt to standardize the broad spectrum of growth disorders. It is hoped that it will serve both to classify patients followed in KIGS and as a nucleus for an extended system of classification of paediatric endocrine disorders.

A good notation has a subtlety and suggestiveness which at times make it seem almost like a live teacher.
Bertrand Russell

KIGS Aetiology Classification List

Idiopathic GHD (see comments)
1.1   Idiopathic GHD (classical form) (see comments)
1.2   Neurosecretory dysfunction (see comments)
1.3   Transient GHD

GHD of known origin ('organic' GHD)
Congenital form
Genetic cause of GHD (see comments)
2.1.1.1   GH gene defect (type IA, dominant or recessive) (specify)
2.1.1.2   GH gene defect (specify)
2.1.1.3   GH-releasing hormone gene defect (specify)
2.1.1.9   Others (specify)

Central malformation
2.1.2.1   Septo-optic dysplasia
2.1.2.2   Empty sella syndrome (including pituitary aplasia)
2.1.2.3   Solitary central maxillary incisor syndrome
2.1.2.4   Midline palatal cleft
2.1.2.5   Arachnoid cyst
2.1.2.6   Congenital hydrocephalus
2.1.2.7   Hypoplastic anterior pituitary, missing stalk and ectopic posterior pituitary (hemimegalencephaly)
2.1.2.9   Others (specify)

Complex syndrome with congenital GHD
2.1.3.1   Fanconi pancytopenia
2.1.3.2   Rieger syndrome
2.1.3.3   Ectrodactyly-ectodermal dysplasia-clefting syndrome
2.1.3.9   Others (specify)

Prenatal infection
2.1.4.1   Rubella
2.1.4.9   Others (specify)

Bioinactive GH syndrome (see comments)
2.1.5.1   Kowarski type
2.1.5.9   Others (specify)

Congenital form
Functional GHD
2.1.6.1   GH receptor defect (Laron type)
2.1.6.2   GH receptor/postreceptor defect (specify)
2.1.6.3   IGF resistance (specify)
2.1.6.9   Others (specify)

Acquired GHD
Tumour of the pituitary/hypothalamic area
2.2.1.1   Craniopharyngioma
2.2.1.2   Germinoma (dysgerminoma, pinealoma)
2.2.1.3   Hamartoma
2.2.1.9   Others (specify)

Cranial tumour distant from the pituitary/hypothalamic area
2.2.2.1   Astrocytoma
2.2.2.2   Ependymoma
2.2.2.3   Glioma
2.2.2.4   Medulloblastoma
2.2.2.5   Nasopharyngeal tumour
2.2.2.9   Others (specify)

Treatment for malignancy outside the cranium
Leukaemia
2.2.3.1.1 Lymphatic leukaemia
2.2.3.1.2 Myeloid leukaemia
2.2.3.1.3 Aplastic leukaemia
2.2.3.1.9 Others (specify)

Lymphoma
2.2.3.2.1 Hodgkin lymphoma
2.2.3.2.2 Non-Hodgkin lymphoma
2.2.3.2.9 Others (specify)
2.2.3.3   Solid tumour (specify)

Other causes of acquired GHD
2.2.4.1   Head trauma
2.2.4.2   Central nervous system infection
2.2.4.3   Hydrocephalus
2.2.4.4   Granulomatous diseases
2.2.4.5   Histiocytosis
2.2.4.6   Vascular anomaly
2.2.4.9   Others (specify)

Other causes of short stature (see comments)
ISS
FSS (see comments)
3.1.1.1   FSS occurring with normal timing of puberty
3.1.1.2   FSS occurring with delayed onset of puberty
3.1.1.3   FSS, onset of puberty unknown

Non-FSS (see comments)
3.1.5.1   Non-FSS occurring with normal timing of puberty
3.1.5.2   Non-FSS occurring with delayed onset of puberty
3.1.5.3   Non-FSS, onset of puberty unknown
3.1.9   Not possible to classify

Clinically defined syndrome with chromosomal aberration (see comments)
3.2.1   Turner syndrome (specify karyotype)
3.2.2   Down syndrome
3.2.3   Prader-Labhart-Willi syndrome (without chromosomal aberration 3.3.5)

Gonadal dysgenesis
3.2.4.1   Females (specify karyotype)
3.2.4.2   Males (specify karyotype)
3.2.9   Others (specify)

Clinically defined syndrome without chromosomal aberration
3.3.1   Silver-Russell syndrome
3.3.2   Noonan syndrome
3.3.3   von Recklinghausen syndrome (neurofibromatosis, type 1)
3.3.4   Cornelia de Lange syndrome
3.3.5   Prader-Labhart-Willi syndrome (with chromosomal aberration 3.2.3)
3.3.6   Williams syndrome
3.3.7   Bloom syndrome
3.3.8   Rubinstein syndrome
3.3.9   Others (specify)

SGA/IUGR with persisting short stature without stigma
3.4.1   Cause known (specify)
3.4.2   Cause unknown

SGA/IUGR with persisting short stature with minor dysmorphic stigma
3.5.1   IUGR due to prenatal infection (specify)
3.5.2   IUGR due to drugs (including smoking and alcohol) (specify)
3.5.9   Others (specify)

Skeletal dysplasia
3.6.1   Achondroplasia
3.6.2   Hypochondroplasia
3.6.3   Osteogenesis imperfecta (specify)
3.6.9   Others (specify)

Disorder of bone metabolism
3.7.1   Mucopolysaccharidosis (specify)
3.7.2   Mucolipidosis (specify)
3.7.9   Others (specify)

Disorder in specific systems
3.8.1   Cardiac disease (specify)
3.8.2   Pulmonary disorder, except cystic fibrosis (3.8.7.1) (specify)
3.8.3   Liver disorder (specify)

Intestinal disorder
3.8.4.1   Granulomatous disorder including Crohn's disease (specify)
3.8.4.2   Malabsorption (specify)
3.8.4.3   Exocrine pancreas, except cystic fibrosis (3.8.7.1) (specify)
3.8.4.4   Short bowel disorder (specify)
3.8.4.9   Others (specify)

		Corresponding EDTA numbers
Renal disorder		
Malformations (with or without pyelonephritis)		
3.8.5.1.1	Renal hypoplasia/dysplasia/aplasia including multicystic dysplasia	49, 60, 61, 63, 66
3.8.5.1.2	Obstructive uropathy, urethral valves, dysfunctional voiding, neurogenic bladder	21, 22, 29
3.8.5.1.3	Reflux nephropathy	24
3.8.5.1.4	Pyelonephritis without known underlying renal disease	20
3.8.5.1.9	Others (specify)	
Hereditary diseases		
3.8.5.2.1	Autosomal recessive polycystic kidney disease	42
3.8.5.2.2	Autosomal dominant polycystic kidney disease	41
3.8.5.2.3	Familial juvenile nephronophthisis	43
3.8.5.2.4	Cystinosis	52
3.8.5.2.5	Primary hyperoxaluria	53
3.8.5.2.6	Infantile nephrotic syndrome with onset before the age of 1 year (specify)	59
3.8.5.2.7	Hereditary glomerulonephritis (Alport syndrome)	51
3.8.5.2.9	Others (specify)	40, 49, 50, 54, 59
Glomerulopathies		
3.8.5.3.1	Primary glomerulonephritis including crescentic glomerulonephritis (specify)	10, 12, 13, 14, 15, 16, 19, 85
3.8.5.3.6	Primary nephrotic syndrome (specify)	11, 13, 14, 15
3.8.5.3.7	Lupus glomerulonephritis	84
3.8.5.3.9	Other secondary glomerulonephritis with or without nephrotic syndrome (specify)	76, 86, 89
Vascular disorders		
3.8.5.5.1	Vasculitis (specify)	73, 74
3.8.5.5.2	Hemolytic uremic syndrome	88
3.8.5.5.3	Post-ischaemic renal failure including post-septic, post-thrombotic (specify)	75, 90
3.8.5.5.9	Others (specify)	70, 79
Interstitial nephritis (if interstitial nephritis = pyelonephritis, see 3.8.5.1.4)		
3.8.5.6.1	Drug-induced nephropathy or nephropathy of unknown origin (specify)	30, 31, 32, 33, 39
3.8.5.6.2	Nephrocalcinosis and hypercalcaemic nephropathy	25, 93
3.8.5.6.9	Others (specify)	83, 92
Miscellaneous		
3.8.5.7.1	Kidney tumour (specify)	95
3.8.5.7.2	Traumatic or surgical loss of kidney	96
3.8.5.7.9	Others (specify)	99
3.8.6	Chronic anaemia (specify)	

Chronic inflammatory disorder
3.8.7.1   Cystic fibrosis
3.8.7.2   Other multiorgan disorder (specify)
3.8.7.3   Granulomatous disorder (specify)
3.8.7.9   Others (specify)

Muscular disorder
3.8.8.1   Duchenne muscular dystrophy
3.8.8.2   Congenital myotonia
3.8.8.9   Others (specify)
3.8.9   Neurological disorder (specify)

Endocrine disorder (not GHD)
3.9.1   Thyroid disorder
3.9.2   Adrenal disorder

3.9.3 Gonadal disorder
3.9.4 Diabetes mellitus
3.9.5 Precocious puberty (specify)
3.9.9 Others (specify)

Metabolic disorder
Disorder of carbohydrate metabolism
3.10.1.1 Glycogen storage disorder (specify)
3.10.1.9 Others (specify)

Disorder of lipid metabolism
3.10.2.1 Lipid storage disorder (specify)
3.10.2.9 Others (specify)

Disorder of amino acids
3.10.3.1 Phenylketonuria

3.10.3.9 Others (specify)
3.10.4 Disorder of calcium and phosphate metabolism, except renal disorder (3.8.5 ff.) (specify)
3.10.5 Bone metabolism disorder

Iatrogenic short stature
3.11.1 Medication (specify)
3.11.2 Total body irradiation, except irradiation treatment for tumours
3.11.9 Others (specify)

Psychogenic short stature
3.12.1 Psychosocial short stature
3.12.2 Anorexia nervosa
3.12.9 Others (specify)

References

1 Ranke MB: The KABI Pharmacia International Growth Study: Aetiology classification list with comments. Acta Paediatr Scand Suppl 1991;379:87–92.
2 Sizonenko PC, Clayton PE, Cohen P, Hintz RL, Tanaka T, Laron Z: Diagnosis and management of growth hormone deficiency in childhood and adolescence. 1. Diagnosis of growth hormone deficiency. Growth Horm IGF Res 2001;11:137–165.
3 Ranke MB (ed): Diagnostics of Endocrine Function in Children and Adolescents, ed 3. Basel, Karger, 2003.
4 Besson A, Salemi S, Deladoey J, Vuissoz JM, Eble A, Bidlingmaier M, Biurgi S, Honegger U, Fluck C, Mullis PE: Short stature caused by a biologically inactive mutant growth hormone (GH-C53S). J Clin Endocrinol Metab 2005;90:2493–2499.
5 Ranke MB: Towards a consensus on the definition of idiopathic short stature. Horm Res 1996;45(suppl 2):64–66.
6 Rosenfeld RG: The molecular basis of idiopathic short stature. Growth Horm IGF Res 2005;15(suppl A):S3–S5.
7 International nomenclature and classification of osteochondrodysplasias. International Working Group on Constitutional Diseases of Bone. Am J Med Genet 1997;79:376–382.
8 Blizzard RM, Bulatovic A: Psychosocial short stature: a syndrome with many variables. Baillieres Clin Endocrinol Metab 1992;6:687–721.

Growth Hormone Deficiency: Growth Hormone Tests and Growth Hormone Measurements

Susan R. Rose

Historical Context

In the mid 1900s, it became clear that a biologic factor critical for linear growth was missing in some short children. Pituitary-extracted growth hormone (GH) was administered to selected short children by the 1960s. Initially, GH deficiency (GHD) was inferred clinically or by bioassay (sulfation, urinary hydroxyproline). The first radioimmunoassay for GH was developed in the 1970s. It was only then found that circulating GH concentrations in serum were not measurable much of the time. In fact, serum GH concentrations were unmeasurable during most of the day and could only be detected after physiologic or pharmacologic stimuli. Physiologic stimuli that led to detectable GH levels included sleep, exercise and fasting. During sleep, GH levels were not constant but rather pulsatile. It was found that pharmacologic stimuli simulating fasting or stress could be used to test for the presence or absence of a significant rise in serum GH concentrations or stimulated peak GH. These stimuli included glucagon, arginine, insulin-induced hypoglycemia, clonidine-induced sleep and others.

Diagnosis of Growth Hormone Deficiency

The diagnosis of GHD relies heavily on auxologic and clinical criteria. Clinically, a child who has untreated GHD has short stature and slow growth velocity. He or she is well-nourished and has a facial phenotype resembling a younger child. Bone maturation (bone age, BA) is delayed, and insulin-like growth factor 1 (IGF-1) and IGF-binding protein 3 (IGFBP-3) values are low. The critical factor in evaluating a short child is determining the growth velocity (regardless of the absolute height). It is important to compare the child's height to the genetic potential conferred

Division of Endocrinology
Cincinnati Children's Hospital Medical Center
University of Cincinnati, MLC 7012
3333 Burnet Avenue
Cincinnati, OH 45229 (USA)

by the parents (midparental height or target height, the average of the parents' height percentiles). The ratio of weight for height can be helpful in identifying the cause of growth retardation in a short child. Endocrine disorders (including GHD, thyroid hormone deficiency or glucocorticoid excess) are usually associated with a relatively preserved weight gain in a short child. In contrast, most 'systemic' disorders resulting in poor linear growth are associated with greater impairment of weight gain than linear growth. Affected children tend to be thin for their height.

Laboratory evaluation of the short, slowly growing child should include serum-free thyroxine, thyrotropin (thyroid-stimulating hormone, TSH), karyotype in a short girl, IGF-1 (if the child is older than 4 years), IGFBP-3 and radiography for BA. However, even a profoundly delayed BA does not indicate a specific diagnosis, because most conditions that cause poor linear growth also cause a delay in BA. Normal thyroid function test results, delayed BA and low IGF-1 and IGFBP-3 values for age in a well-nourished child are consistent with a diagnosis of GHD. Determining IGF deficiency is more difficult if there is malnutrition, chronic renal and liver disease, or hypothyroidism [1–3]. After recognition of the diagnosis of GHD, the rest of the pituitary function must be evaluated to identify potential combined pituitary hormone deficiencies, such as TSH, adrenocorticotropic hormone (ACTH), prolactin or gonadotropin deficiencies, or diabetes insipidus. Depending on initial screening results, additional tests may be indicated, including GH stimulation tests, a low-dose ACTH test to assess for cortisol sufficiency, and measurement of the diurnal pattern of thyrotropin (the TSH surge test) that can confirm or exclude central hypothyroidism.

GHD can be congenital or acquired. Infants with congenital GHD often have a history of perinatal distress, breech delivery, cesarean section and/or low Apgar scores. GHD presenting in infancy may be associated with early prenatal embryologic malformations, including central nervous system malformations (e.g., septooptic dysplasia) or midface abnormalities (e.g., coloboma of the eye, midface hypoplasia, cleft palate and lip, or single central incisor). Congenital GHD can present with prolonged jaundice, hypoglycemia, micropenis (in males), or failure to thrive, with relatively normal growth velocity. Subsequent linear growth deceleration with normal weight gain typically develops after the first postnatal year. About 12% of children with congenital hypopituitarism have gene mutations that affect either the organization and development of the pituitary gland or one or more of the pituitary cell types.

Magnetic resonance imaging (MRI) in a child with GHD may be normal or may show interruption of the pituitary stalk and displacement of the posterior pituitary bright spot (ectopic posterior pituitary). The finding of an ectopic posterior pituitary on the MRI confirms a diagnosis of hypopituitarism [4]. Otherwise, MRI of the brain in GHD may show abnormal anatomy such as a small pituitary gland, pituitary stalk agenesis, empty sella, or sellar or suprasellar mass. Acquired GHD is most commonly idiopathic but may result from tumors (such as craniopharyngioma, glioma, germinoma), cranial radiation therapy, traumatic brain injury, hydrocephalus, central nervous system infection or surgical damage to the pituitary and hypothalamus. Acquired childhood GHD and postradiation GHD usually result from hypothalamic deficiency of GH-releasing hormone (GHRH), rather than pituitary deficiency of GH. In contrast, adult GHD most often results from pituitary adenoma or another primary pituitary insult. GHD is more difficult to recognize in adults who are no longer capable of linear growth. Metabolic effects of GHD include increases in body fat mass and cholesterol, as well as reductions in lean body mass, bone mineral density, cardiac function, stamina and quality of life.

Growth Hormone Measurements and Growth Hormone Stimulation Tests

GH stimulation tests remain the mainstay for the diagnosis of GHD [5]. A variety of stimulation tests are used in clinical practice. Each stimulus necessitates the use of a specific cutoff derived from normative data [6]. However, the biochemical definition of GHD has generally been considered to be a peak stimulated GH concentration <10 ng/ml (10 μg/l) in response to two GH stimulation tests such as arginine, insulin, clonidine or glucagon. Lower cutoff numbers (such as 5 or 7 ng/ml) were used prior to the availability of synthetic GH.

It is important to understand the regulation of GH secretion and IGF-1 production in order to interpret GH testing results. GH, a 191-amino-acid polypeptide, is secreted by the anterior pituitary in a pulsatile fashion. Conditions that increase GH concentrations include those that raise hypothalamic GHRH such as sleep, fasting, exercise, levodopa, apomorphine (dopamine agonist), clonidine (α2-adrenergic), tryptophan (serotonergic), elevated thyroid hormone, sex steroid, stress, dexamethasone, γ-aminobutyric acid, opioids, corticotrophin-releasing hormone, GH-releasing peptide (GH secretagogues), theophylline, phorbol esters, cholera toxin, forskolin, arachidonic acid, prostaglandins E_1 and E_2, prostaglandin I_2 (prostacyclin), interleukin 6 cytokines, vasoactive intestinal peptide, galanin, neurotensin, substance P, neuropeptide Y, motilin, pyrogen, vasopressin and Bovril (beef tea) [7, 8]. Most of these are not used as standard GH stimulation tests.

Lowering of hypothalamic somatotropin-release inhibiting hormone (SRIH) tone will also increase GH concentrations. Conditions that lower SRIH include pyridostigmine, cysteamine, clonidine, arginine, fasting, insulin-induced hypoglycemia, glucagon, atenolol, propranolol, GH-releasing peptide, γ-aminobutyric acid, galanin and β-endorphin [7, 8]. Of course, not all of these conditions are employed in the most commonly used GH stimulation tests. In children, standard GH stimulation tests include arginine, clonidine, glucagon, L-dopa and insulin. GH test combinations make use of these physiologic actions, such as arginine (inhibits SRIH) plus clonidine (stimulates GHRH), arginine plus GHRH, or fasting (stimulates GHRH) plus insulin (inhibits SRIH).

Clonidine does not seem to stimulate GH release in adults, while it is a potent secretagogue in children. L-Dopa is no longer available in the United States for GH stimulation testing. In addition, many pediatric endocrine practitioners have moved away from performing insulin tolerance tests (ITT) for safety reasons, patient discomfort or because of the labor intensity of appropriate medical monitoring when performing the ITT.

GH circulates protein bound in serum to all tissues, which produce IGF-1 in response. Many of the growth-promoting actions of GH are mediated by IGF-1. GH stimulates both IGF-1 and IGFBP-3 production by the liver. IGF-1 is carried through the circulation associated with IGFBPs. Growth effects of IGF-1 are mediated by both endocrine action of circulating free IGF-1 and by autocrine/paracrine action of IGF-1 synthesized within the growth plate. Circulating concentrations of IGF-1 are low during the first 5 years after birth. Serum IGF-1 levels rise during childhood and attain adult levels at the onset of sexual maturation [9, 10]. During puberty, IGF-1 levels rise to 2–3 times the adult range and correlate better with Tanner stage (or BA) than with chronological age. IGFBP-3 values (highly GH dependent) are not as low as those of IGF-1 in the young child, but also increase during childhood and adolescence. In adults, IGF-1 and IGFBP-3 levels cannot always distinguish between healthy and GH-deficient individuals [11]. Diagnosis of adult GHD depends on severe impairment of the peak GH response to stimulation tests.

Children with all degrees of GHD (peak GH responses to stimulation test <10 ng/ml) are treated with GH, whereas in adulthood, only patients with severe GHD (peak GH responses to stimulation test <3 ng/ml) are considered for GH replacement. Childhood GHD without organic cause may persist into adulthood in only 60–70% of individuals previously diagnosed with GHD [11, 12]. Thus, patients with childhood GHD require reevaluation at adulthood.

Standardization of Growth Hormone Assays

Variations in GH assay methodology influence the measured GH values. Serum GH assayed by different methods yield different results on the same samples [13, 14]. This variation among assay results can dramatically alter the assignment of the diagnostic category. Immunoradiometric assays (IRMA) yield results that are only 60–70% of values from the same sample assayed by radioimmunoassay. This may be because of the greater specificity of the monoclonal antibody used in IRMA. IRMA may only be measuring one form of the endogenous GH molecule, the 22-kDa form. Normally, about 75% of GH produced by the pituitary is of the 22-kDa form. The 20-kDa form typically adds 5–10% of pituitary GH [15]. The rest of the pituitary GH content includes inactivated forms of GH.

The greatest differences in measured GH values observed in Japan were due to the GH standard used [16]. As of April 2005, all GH kits in Japan began using the same recombinant human GH standard. This has permitted refinement of the stimulated peak GH diagnostic cutoff from 10 to 6 ng/ml. Thus, the choice of GH assay affects absolute resulting GH values. GH cutoff values used for diagnosing GHD should take into account the GH assay used as well as the potency of the stimulus, i.e. L-dopa is less potent than GHRH. Endocrine practitioners need to know what GH assay they are using at their institution, which GH standard is used, and how the GH assay is calibrated [17].

Spontaneous Growth Hormone Secretion

GH is typically secreted from the pituitary gland in a pulsatile fashion throughout 24 h, with the majority of pulses occurring at night [18, 19]. Most commonly, a random daytime serum GH concentration is low. The pulses represent the net interaction between two opposing hypothalamic peptides that regulate the synthesis and secretion of GH from the somatotrope: GHRH and somatostatin or SRIH. Pulses of GH result from decreases in tonic SRIH under continuous, steady GHRH secretion [19]. In addition, ghrelin secreted from the stomach during fasting modulates the GH pulses [20].

Spontaneous mean GH levels during puberty tend to be higher than in the childhood or adult years [21, 22]. Adolescents have larger pulses of GH than prepubertal children. The GH pulses in adolescents occur throughout the day and night, not just between 22.00 and 04.00 h as seen in childhood [18]. Twenty-four-hour integrated GH secretion is highest during adolescence, contributing to the high serum levels of IGF-1 characteristic of puberty. In addition, mean GH concentrations and GH pulse amplitude at night tend to be higher in girls than in boys at comparable stages of puberty [18].

Spontaneously occurring GH values can be evaluated for mean concentration, pulsatility, frequency, amplitude and total area under the curve [23]. The pulsatile GH pattern represents secretion plus metabolic clearance. The GH secretion rate can be determined using deconvolution to separate out clearance effects [24]. Factors affecting the rate of GH clearance include time of day, body size and estradiol concentration. Factors affecting mean GH values include pubertal maturation, gender and body mass index [18, 25]. Fasting causes amplitude modulation, perhaps mediated by a rise in ghrelin [26].

A discrepancy between 24-hour secretion and response to stimulation tests was described as common in children with short stature [27]. However, such a discrepancy is not so common when the physician employs developmentally appropriate control data (pubertal matched or bone age matched) [21, 28]. The wide range of spontaneous GH values in normal children and the overlap in values between those with GH abnormalities and controls make it difficult to identify short children with spontaneous GH values below the normal range. Some practitioners have used an arbitrary value for signifying a low mean 24-hour GH level (such as 3 ng/ml) instead of basing interpretations on values in controls (matched for pubertal stage). However, this practice can lead to calling children 'abnormal', whose mean night GH values actually fall into the lower half of normal prepubertal values [21, 28, 29]. Observed mean GH values in normal controls may be as low as 1.0 ng/ml. Thus, in most settings, evaluation of spontaneous GH secretion is neither practical nor sensitive in diagnosing GHD.

Growth Hormone-Releasing Hormone Tests and Combinations

Peak GH response to GHRH is much greater than that to the other GH stimulation agents. Children with indisputable GHD may mount quite 'normal' peak GH concentrations in response to GHRH [30]. This has been attributed to having a hypothalamic rather than pituitary deficiency. GHRH plus GH secretagogues or arginine may provide a more consistent response to stimulation than GHRH alone [30–32]. Thus, a diagnostic GH cutoff of 10 ng/ml does not apply to GHRH tests.

Biller et al. [33] correlated GH response in adults to ITT (0.07–0.1 unit/kg i.v.) and to GHRH (1 μg/kg i.v.) plus arginine (0.5 g/kg i.v.). If sensitive and specific, the GHRH plus arginine test would be an alternative to ITT for retesting of childhood GHD patients as they reach adulthood [11]. GHRH plus arginine is a good test for differentiating GHD from normal levels in adults with adult-onset GHD (who often have pituitary disease). However, as a clinical population, adult-onset GHD patients differ from adults with childhood-onset GHD (who often have hypothalamic disease). Thus, GHRH plus arginine may miss confirming the diagnosis of childhood-onset GHD in adulthood by being 'too potent a secretagogue'.

As a result, the GHRH plus arginine standard for persistent GHD in adulthood (after childhood GHD) should be the adult third percentile cutoff (16.5 ng/ml) [34]. Donaubauer et al. [35] suggested a 100% sensitivity and 97.5% specificity for this cutoff value after GHRH plus arginine in retesting childhood-onset GHD. This GH cutoff will not result in poor specificity, as long as it is only applied in patients who have a significant medical history that puts them at risk for adult GHD.

Limitations of Testing

Factors that can alter the response to GH stimulation tests include fasting, overweight, steroids, hyperglycemia, illness and lack of sleep. Stimulated GH has limitations in the process of making an accurate diagnosis of GHD. 'Normal' is arbitrary (over 7–10 mg/l) and does not take into account the nature of the pharmacologic test, the assay used, or the child's age, adiposity or pubertal stage. A high proportion of normal short children may be falsely considered to be GH deficient on the basis of low stimulated GH. Gonadal steroids, adrenal steroids, thyroid hormone and IGF-1 concentrations alter the amount of GH synthesized and stored in the somatotrope [36].

One issue is to insure appropriate diagnosis of GHD and to minimize false negatives. Another issue is how to avoid inappropriate diagnosis of GHD in a child with false-positive GH stimulation testing. Even if the GH peak is low after stimulation, a prepubertal child may not have 'true' GHD unless the IGF-1 is also below the range seen in normal children. Short children have relatively lower IGF-1 values than normally growing children, despite normal results on other standard tests of GH secretion. There remains an overlap between IGF-1 values in normal short children and values in GHD patients, particularly of organic cause [37].

In spite of these limitations, failure to respond to two GH stimulation tests remains the current world-wide gold standard for clinical decision making about GH therapy in GHD.

Testing Limitations in Special Situations

The GH cutoff should be adjusted for the patient's body mass index, with a higher numerical cutoff used if the patient is lean and a lower cutoff if the patient is obese or overweight [30, 38, 39]. In the obese patient, preceding GH stimulation testing by 24 h of hypocaloric diet may lead to more accurate GH testing [39–41].

Children who have had severe head injury may be at risk for hypothalamic pituitary deficits, similar to those observed in adults [42, 43]. However, standard GH stimulation tests administered in the first 6 months after injury may overestimate the frequency, as some deficiencies are no longer evident at 1 year after injury [44].

The evolving hypothalamic pituitary axis after irradiation represents a unique clinical challenge [45]. Children who are long-term survivors of cancer merit longitudinal monitoring of their growth and pubertal development because hormone abnormalities may progressively develop for up to 10 years after radiation therapy. After therapy for any cranial tumor, there should be careful monitoring of the growth rate at least every 6 months. If the growth rate is slow (including lack of pubertal growth spurt), there should be assessment for GHD, primary or central hypothyroidism, ACTH deficiency, precocious puberty or hypogonadism. Early diagnosis of GHD and central or mild hypothyroidism can permit rapid initiation of targeted therapy, coupled with a ready addition of gonadotropin-releasing hormone analogue therapy at the first sign of early puberty or a rapid tempo of puberty. Improvements in adult height during the past 25 years in childhood brain tumor survivors with GHD are attributed to earlier testing for GHD, earlier initiation of GH therapy, improved GH regimens, and use of gonadotropin-releasing hormone analogues [46].

GHD develops after sellar/suprasellar radiation doses, particularly in excess of 23 Gy [47]. TSH, gonadotropin or ACTH deficiencies develop particularly after 30+ Gy [48, 49]. After pituitary adenoma and surgery, it is not surprising that some patients have hormone deficiencies. Merchant et al. [50] have shown that after surgery for cranial tumors, hormone deficiencies may be present before irradiation. Children who initially have 'normal' hormone test results may progress to have lower GH secretion with time. After cranial irradiation, disordered GH secretion is evident with a decreased amplitude of GH pulses, although pulses continue [51].

The most appropriate way to manage GH replacement in the transition period to adulthood in adults previously treated for childhood GHD is controversial. The Growth Hormone Research Society [52] suggested that the retesting of GH status at adult height is unnecessary in the presence of severe organic GHD. Cranial irradiation falls into this etiological category. However, 35 (48%) of 73 patients with moderate childhood GHD after cranial irradiation and 12 (36%) of 33 patients with severe GHD in childhood did not fulfill the severe GHD biochemical criteria for GH replacement in adulthood [53]. Thus, the diagnosis of severe GHD in childhood secondary to irradiation should not be taken as irrefutable evidence of permanent severe organic GHD. Retesting of the GH status at adult height should be mandatory [53].

During the first 10 years after cranial irradiation, there was discordance between GH response to GHRH plus arginine compared with ITT [54]. In contrast, at more than 10 years after irradiation, there was greater concordance between patients' responses to the two tests, suggesting a progressive loss of GH reserve. Contrary to the findings of Darzy et al. [54], some patients with GHRH deficiency and GHD still have preserved somatotrope function 19 years after cranial irradiation. More patients with childhood-onset GHD after cranial irradiation need evaluation in order to validate the GH diagnostic cutoff of 16.5 ng/ml to GHRH plus arginine [34]. In 161 adults with evidence of radiation damage to the somatotropic axis, the GH response to arginine was more resistant to the effects of irradiation than the response to ITT [55]. Thus, arginine may be a less sensitive guide to the functional status of the GH axis [55].

A number of studies have shown that GH therapy does not add to the risk of tumor recurrence or second tumors or leukemia after brain tumors and has only a small excess risk of second malignancy after leukemia [56–59]. Thus, after completion of cancer therapy and evidence of a clear medical status in childhood cancer survivors, it is considered safe to use GH therapy for acquired GHD.

References

1 Juul A: Determination of insulin-like growth factor I in children: normal values and clinical use. Horm Res 2001; 55(suppl 2):94–99.
2 Juul A, Skakkebaek NE: Prediction of the outcome of growth hormone provocative testing in short children by measurement of serum levels of insulin-like growth factor I and insulin-like growth factor binding protein 3. J Pediatr 1997;130:197–204.
3 Nunez SB, Municchi G, Rose SR: Insulin-like growth factor-1 and insulin-like growth factor binding protein-3 compared with stimulated and overnight growth hormone in short children. J Clin Endocrinol Metab 1996;81: 1927–1932.
4 Maghnie M, Ghirardello S, Genovese E: Magnetic resonance imaging of the hypothalamus-pituitary unit in children suspected of hypopituitarism: who, how and when to investigate. J Endocrinol Invest 2004;27:496–509.
5 Wilson T, Rose SR, Cohen P, Rogol AD, the Drug and Therapeutics Committee of the Lawson Wilkins Pediatric Endocrine Society: Update of guidelines for the use of growth hormone in children. J Pediatr 2003;143:415–421.

6 Ghigo E, Bellone J, Aimaretti G, Bellone S, Loche S, Cappa M, Bartolotta E, Dammacco F, Camanni F: Reliability of provocative tests to assess growth hormone secretory status. Study in 472 normally growing children. J Clin Endocrinol Metab 1996;81:3323–3327.
7 Rose SR: Neuroendocrine basis for insufficient growth hormone and its assessment; in Savage MO, Bourguignon JP, Grossman AB (eds): Frontiers in Paediatric Neuroendocrinology. Oxford, Blackwell, 1994, pp 149–155.
8 de Gennaro Colonna V, Cella SG, Locatelli V, Loche S, Ghigo E, Cocchi D, Muller EE: Neuroendocrine control of growth hormone secretion. Acta Paediatr Scand Suppl 1989;349:87–92.
9 Cara JF, Rosenfeld RG, Furlanetto RW: A longitudinal study of the relationship of plasma somatomedin-C concentration to the pubertal growth spurt. Am J Dis Child 1987;141:562–564.
10 Veldhuis JD: Neuroendocrine control of pulsatile growth hormone release in the human: relationship with gender. Growth Horm IGF Res 1998;8(suppl B):49–59.
11 Aimaretti G, Baffoni C, Bellone S, Di Vito L, Corneli G, Arvat E, Benso L, Camanni F, Ghigo E: Retesting young adults with childhood-onset growth hormone (GH) deficiency with GH-releasing hormone-plus-arginine test. J Clin Endocrinol Metab 2000;85:3693–3699.

12 Loche S, Bizzarri C, Maghnie M, Faedda A, Tzialla C, Autelli M, Casini MR, Cappa M: Results of early reevaluation of growth hormone secretion in short children with apparent growth hormone deficiency. J Pediatr 2002;140: 445–449.
13 Chatelain P, Bouillat B, Cohen R, Sassolas G, Souberbielle JC, Ruitton A, Joly MO, Job JC: Assay of growth hormone levels in human plasma using commercial kits: analysis of some factors influencing the results. Acta Paediatr Scand Suppl 1990;370:56–61.
14 Celniker AC, Chen AB, Wert RM Jr, Sherman BM: Variability in the quantitation of circulating growth hormone using commercial immunoassays. J Clin Endocrinol Metab 1989;68:469–476.
15 Cooke NE, Ray J, Watson MA, Estes PA, Kuo BA, Liebhaber SA: Human growth hormone gene and the highly homologous growth hormone variant gene display different splicing patterns. J Clin Invest 1988;82:270–275.
16 Tanaka T, Tachibana K, Shimatsu A, Katsumata N, Tsushima T, Hizuka N, Fujieda K, Yokoya S, Irie M: A nationwide attempt to standardize growth hormone assays. Horm Res 2005; 64(suppl 2):6–11.

17 Juul A, Bernasconi S, Clayton PE, Kiess W, DeMuinck-Keizer Schrama S, Drugs and Therapeutics Committee of the European Society for Paediatric Endocrinology: European audit of current practices in diagnosis and treatment of childhood growth hormone deficiency. Horm Res 2002;58:233–241.

18 Rose SR, Municchi G, Barnes KM, Kamp GA, Uriarte MM, Ross JL, Cassorla F, Cutler GB Jr: Spontaneous growth hormone secretion increases during puberty in normal girls and boys. J Clin Endocrinol Metab 1991;73: 428–435.

19 Tannenbaum GS: Neuroendocrine control of growth hormone secretion. Acta Paediatr Scand Suppl 1991;372:5–16.

20 Koutkia P, Canavan B, Breu J, Johnson ML, Grinspoon SK: Nocturnal ghrelin pulsatility and response to growth hormone secretagogues in healthy men. Am J Physiol Endocrinol Metab 2004; 287:E506–E512.

21 Rose SR, Municchi G, Barnes K, Cutler GB: Overnight growth hormone concentrations are usually normal in pubertal children with idiopathic short stature – a clinical research center study. J Clin Endocrinol Metab 1996;81: 1063–1068.

22 Hartman ML, Veldhuis JD, Thorner MO: Normal control of growth hormone secretion. Horm Res 1993;40:37–47.

23 Sartorio A, De Nicolao G, Liberati D: An improved computational method to assess pituitary responsiveness to secretagogue stimuli. Eur J Endocrinol 2002;147:323–332.

24 Hartman ML, Faria AC, Vance ML, Johnson ML, Thorner MO, Veldhuis JD: Temporal structure of in vivo growth hormone secretory events in humans. Am J Physiol 1991;260:101–110.

25 Veldhuis JD, Anderson SM, Shah N, Bray M, Vick T, Gentili A, Mulligan T, Johnson ML, Weltman A, Evans WS, Iranmanesh A: Neurophysiological regulation and target-tissue impact of the pulsatile mode of growth hormone secretion in the human. Growth Horm IGF Res 2001;11(suppl A):25–37.

26 Hindmarsh PC, Brain CE, Robinson IC, Matthews DR, Brook CG: The interaction of growth hormone releasing hormone and somatostatin in the generation of a GH pulse in man. Clin Endocrinol (Oxf) 1991;35:353–360.

27 Shulman DI, Bercu BB: Evaluation of growth hormone secretion: provocative testing vs endogenous 24-hour growth hormone profile. Acta Paediatr Scand Suppl 1987;337:61–71.

28 Rose SR, Ross JL, Uriarte M, Barnes KM, Cassorla FG, Cutler GB Jr: The advantage of measuring stimulated as compared with spontaneous growth hormone levels in the diagnosis of growth hormone deficiency. N Engl J Med 1988;319:201–208.

29 Tanaka T: Growth hormone secretion and the therapeutic effects of human growth hormone: first Japanese results of the Kabi Pharmacia International Growth Study/International Cooperative Growth Study. Acta Paediatr Scand Suppl 1991;379:126–135.

30 Maghnie M, Cavigioli F, Tinelli C, Autelli M, Arico M, Aimaretti G, Ghigo E: GHRH plus arginine in the diagnosis of acquired GH deficiency of childhood-onset. J Clin Endocrinol Metab 2002;87:2740–2744.

31 Petersenn S, Jung R, Beil FU: Diagnosis of growth hormone deficiency in adults by testing with GHRP-6 alone or in combination with GHRH: comparison with the insulin tolerance test. Eur J Endocrinol 2002;146:667–672.

32 Vierhapper H, Nardi A, Bieglmayer C: The use of the pyridostigmine growth hormone-releasing hormone stimulation test to detect growth hormone deficiency in patients with pituitary adenomas. Metabolism 2002;51:34–37.

33 Biller BMK, Samuels MH, Zagar A, Cook DM, Arafah BM, Bonert V, Stavrou S, Kleinberg DL, Chipman JJ, Hartman MK: Sensitivity and specificity of six tests for the diagnosis of adult GH deficiency. J Clin Endocrinol Metab 2002;67:1186–1189.

34 Ham JN, Ginsberg JP, Hendell CD, Moshang T: Growth hormone releasing hormone plus arginine stimulation testing in young adults treated in childhood with cranio-spinal radiation therapy. Clin Endocrinol 2005;62:628–632.

35 Donaubauer J, Kiess W, Kratzsch J, Nowak T, Steinkamp H, Willgerodt H, Keller E: Re-assessment of growth hormone secretion in young adult patients with childhood-onset growth hormone deficiency. Clin Endocrinol (Oxf) 2003; 58:456–463.

36 Ho KY, Evans WS, Blizzard RM, Veldhuis JD, Merriam GR, Samojlik E, Furlanetto R, Rogol AD, Kaiser DL, Thorner MO: Effects of sex and age on the 24-hour profile of growth hormone secretion in man: importance of endogenous estradiol concentrations. J Clin Endocrinol Metab 1987;64:51–58.

37 Bussieres L, Souberbielle JC, Pinto G, Adan L, Noel M, Brauner R: The use of insulin-like growth factor 1 reference values for the diagnosis of growth hormone deficiency in prepubertal children. Clin Endocrinol 2000;52:735–739.

38 Corneli G, Di Somma C, Baldelli R, Rovere S, Gasco V, Croce CG, Grottoli S, Maccario M, Colao A, Lombardi G, Ghigo E, Camanni F, Aimaretti G: The cut-off limits of the GH response to GH-releasing hormone-arginine test related to body mass index. Eur J Endocrinol 2005;15:257–264.

39 Kasa-Vubu JZ, Barkan A, Olton P, Meckmongkol T, Carlson NE, Foster CM: Incomplete modified fast in obese early pubertal girls leads to an increase in 24-hour growth hormone concentration and a lessening of the circadian pattern in leptin. J Clin Endocrinol Metab 2002;87:1885–1893.

40 Maghnie M, Valtorta A, Moretta A, Larizza D, Preti P, Palladini G, Calcante S, Severi F: Diagnosing growth hormone deficiency: the value of short-term hypocaloric diet. J Clin Endocrinol Metab 1993;77:1372–1378.

41 Rose SR, Burstein S, Burghen GA, Pitukcheewanont P, Shope S, Hodnicak V: Caloric restriction for 24 hours increases mean night growth hormone. J Pediatr Endocrinol Metab 1999;12: 175–183.

42 Aimaretti G, Ambrosio MR, Di Somma C, Gasperi M, Cannavo S, Scaroni C, De Marinis L, Baldelli R, Bona G, Giordano G, Ghigo E: Hypopituitarism induced by traumatic brain injury in the transition phase. J Endocrinol Invest 2005;28:984–989.

43 Agha A, Phillips J, O'Kelly P, Tormey W, Thompson CJ: The natural history of post-traumatic hypopituitarism: implications for assessment and treatment. Am J Med 2005;118:1416.

44 Reifschneider K, Blum SD, Weiss M, Rose SR: Endocrinopathies after head injury in children. Abstr, 88th Annu Meet Endocr Soc, Boston, 2006.

45 Rose SR: Endocrinopathies in childhood cancer survivors. Endocrinologist 2003;13:488–495.
46 Gleeson HK, Stoeter R, Ogilvy-Stuart AL, Gattamaneni HR, Brennan BM, Shalet SM: Improvements in final height over 25 years in growth hormone (GH)-deficient childhood survivors of brain tumors receiving GH replacement. J Clin Endocrinol Metab 2003;88:3682–3689.
47 Adan L, Trivin C, Sainte-Rose C, Zucker JM, Hartmann O, Brauner R: GH deficiency caused by cranial irradiation during childhood: factors and markers in young adults. J Clin Endocrinol Metab 2001;86:5245–5251.
48 Rose SR, Lustig RH, Pitukcheewanont P, Broome DC, Burghen GA, Li H, Hudson MM, Kun L, Heideman RL: Diagnosis of hidden central hypothyroidism in survivors of childhood cancer. J Clin Endocrinol Metab 1999;84:4472–4479.
49 Rose SR, Danish RK, Kearney NS, Schreiber RE, Lustig RH, Burghen GA, Hudson MM: ACTH deficiency in childhood cancer survivors. Pediatr Blood Cancer 2005;45:808–813.
50 Merchant TE, Williams T, Smith JM, Rose SR, Danish RK, Burghen GA, Kun LE, Lustig RH: Preirradiation endocrinopathies in pediatric brain tumor patients determined by dynamic tests of endocrine function. Int J Radiat Oncol Biol Phys 2002;54:45–50.
51 Darzy KH, Pezzoli SS, Thorner MO, Shalet SM: The dynamics of growth hormone (GH) secretion in adult cancer survivors with severe GH deficiency acquired after brain irradiation in childhood for nonpituitary brain tumors: evidence for preserved pulsatility and diurnal variation with increased secretory disorderliness. J Clin Endocrinol Metab 2005;90:2794–2803.
52 GH Research Society: Consensus guidelines for the diagnosis and treatment of growth hormone (GH) deficiency in childhood and adolescence: summary statement of the GH Research Society. J Clin Endocrinol Metab 2000;85:3990–3993.
53 Gleeson HK, Gattamaneni HR, Smethurst L, Brennan BM, Shalet SM: Reassessment of growth hormone status is required at final height in children treated with growth hormone replacement after radiation therapy. J Clin Endocrinol Metab 2004;89:662–666.
54 Darzy KH, Aimaretti G, Wieringa G, Rao Gattamaneni H, Ghigo E, Shalet SM: The usefulness of the combined growth hormone (GH)-releasing hormone and arginine stimulation test in the diagnosis of radiation-induced GH deficiency is dependent on the post-irradiation time interval. J Clin Endocrinol Metab 2003;88:95–102.
55 Lissett CA, Saleem S, Rahim A, Brennan BM, Shalet SM: The impact of irradiation on growth hormone responsiveness to provocative agents is stimulus dependent: results in 161 individuals with radiation damage to the somatotropic axis. J Clin Endocrinol Metab 2001;86:663–668.
56 Leung W, Rose SR, Zhou Y, Hancock ML, Burstein S, Schriock EA, Lustig R, Danish RK, Evans WE, Hudson MM, Pui CH: Outcomes of growth hormone replacement therapy in survivors of childhood acute lymphoblastic leukemia. J Clin Oncol 2002;20:2959–2964.
57 Sklar CA, Mertens AC, Mitby P, Occhiogrosso G, Qin J, Heller G, Yasui Y, Robison LL: Risk of disease recurrence and second neoplasms in survivors of childhood cancer treated with growth hormone: a report from the Childhood Cancer Survivor Study. J Clin Endocrinol Metab 2002;87:3136–3141.
58 Swerdlow AJ, Reddingius RE, Higgins CD, Spoudeas HA, Phipps K, Qiao Z, Ryder WD, Brada M, Hayward RD, Brook CG, Hindmarsh PC, Shalet SM: Growth hormone treatment of children with brain tumours and risk of tumour recurrence. J Clin Endocrinol Metab 2000;85:4444–4449.
59 Ergun-Longmire B, Mertens AC, Mitby P, Qin J, Heller G, Shi W, Yasui Y, Robison LL, Sklar CA: Growth hormone treatment and risk of second neoplasms in the childhood cancer survivor. J Clin Endocrinol Metab 2006;91:3494–3498.

Growth Hormone Testing in KIGS

Maïthé Tauber

Pharmacological tests, though extremely variable among different centers, remain the gold standard for evaluating growth hormone (GH) secretion. Two tests are needed in most countries to allow the prescription of GH treatment for GH deficiency (GHD). In other situations of short stature, GH testing is also performed to eliminate GHD. For more than 20 years, types of tests have been discussed, regarding their secretagogue power, their tolerance, the advantage of doing a single versus a combined test, or a physiological versus a pharmacological test, as well as evaluating the value of the study of spontaneous 24-hour – or sleep – GH secretion.

Another issue is the cutoff value arbitrarily chosen without any adjustment for age, pubertal stage or type of test. The methods of GH measurement differed among the centers, and finally, the lack of reproducibility of all methods has been pointed out as well [1, 2].

Nevertheless, knowing all these pitfalls, we have not reached consensus in clinical practice about how to explore GH secretion. Insulin-like growth factor 1 (IGF-1) measurement is probably a good alternative in prepubertal patients, but it can be altered by other factors than GH secretion, mainly nutrition. Free IGF-1 is no better tool in this respect than IGF-binding protein 3, whose measurement remains difficult in plasma. A combination of all approaches – GH, IGF-1 and IGF-binding protein 3 – has been shown to be the most sensitive tool to properly evaluate GH status [3–11].

Keeping that in mind, it is interesting to revisit the clinical practice of GH testing comparing KIGS data in the 10-year analysis with those of the 20-year analysis [12].

Patients and Methods

We used the same method to divide the 87,061 provocative tests according to the major stimulus used. Thus, if a test was conducted using both insulin and a β-blocker, it was identified as an insulin test. A combined insulin-arginine test was represented in both the insulin and arginine tests as clonidine + betaxolol, propranolol + exercise, arginine + clonidine, insulin + L-dopa, clonidine + L-dopa, clonidine + glucagon, arginine + glucagon, insulin + clonidine, insulin + ornithine, insulin + GH-releasing hormone, arginine + ornithine, insulin + propranolol, and clonidine + exercise. The distribution of the 94,180 tests is mentioned in table 1 and table 5.

Most of the analyses were performed in GHD children. Standard parametric and nonparametric tests of significance were used as appropriate.

Department of Endocrinology, Hôpital des Enfants
330 avenue de Grande-Bretagne, TSA 70034
FR–31059 Toulouse Cedex 9 (France)

Table 1. Number of tests (all diagnoses)

	KIGS 10 years		KIGS 20 years	
	n	%	n	%
Arginine	11,491	26	23,594	25.1
Insulin	12,145	27.5	22,688	24.1
Clonidine	5,027	11.4	12,495	13.3
L-Dopa	2,663	6	8,958	9.5
GH-releasing hormone	–	–	4,268	4.5
Glucagon	–	–	3,709	3.9
Ornithine	1,253	2.8	2,806	3.0
Propranolol + glucagon	–	–	2,360	2.5
Exercise	–	–	1,977	2.1
Others	3,719	8.4	1,960	2.1
Spontaneous	7,925	17.9	9,365	9.9

Table 2. Percentage of tests and median GH peak according to test and country in IGHD

	Sweden		UK		Germany		France		Japan		USA	
	%	median GH peak µg/l	%	median GH peak µg/l	%	median GH peak µg/l	%	median GH peak µg/l	%	median GH peak µg/l	%	median GH peak µg/l
Arginine	28.9	4.4	19.4	3.5	42.1	4.7	19.6	5.4	32.3	6.0	26.2	4.8
Insulin	29.4	4.9	49.1	4.2	31.9	4.4	32.6	5.5	23.5	6.0	11.8	4.7
Clonidine	2.0	5.0	24.7	3.9	13.7	4.9	3.2	6.4	14.6	6.1	35.5	5.5
L-Dopa	2.9	2.9	0.3	3.6	0.2	2.3	28.5	6.7	13.6	6.3	24.9	5.0
Spontaneous secretion	36.8	8.1	6.5	1.8	12.2	6.5	16.2	7.7	16.0	9.3	1.6	7.3

Results

Pharmacological and Physiological Stimuli Used in GH Tests

The top 3 tests have not changed during the last decade. Whereas spontaneous GH secretion was used less, i.e. in 9.9 versus 17.9% of tests, the most common pair of stimuli used in a single child was insulin + arginine, accounting for 49% of all combinations of tests.

Analysis of Tests Used in Different Countries in Idiopathic GHD Children (IGHD)

We chose to compare the prevalence and peak GH values of the first 4 tests used, i.e. arginine, insulin, clonidine and L-dopa, and of spontaneous GH secretion in 4 European countries (Sweden, the UK, Germany, France), Japan and the USA. Data are presented in table 2. Insulin was the most frequently used pharmacological test in Sweden, the UK and France, while arginine was the most frequent test in Germany and Japan, and clonidine the most frequent test in the USA. The median maximum GH peak for each test was different between the countries (p < 0.0001). The maximum GH peak occurred in spontaneous GH secretion studies in 5 of 6 countries. In each country, the first test used represented 32.3–49.1% of the tests. Spontaneous GH secretion represents 36.8% of GH testing in Sweden, compared with 1.6% in the USA.

Clonidine was poorly used in Sweden (2%) and France (3.2%), whereas L-dopa was poorly used in Sweden (2.9%), the UK (0.3%) and Germany (0.2%). The secretagogue power of each test was difficult to assess, as the methods of measurement varied from country to country and center to center; however, it seems that L-dopa has the lowest secretagogue power, while clonidine has the highest.

Evolution of the Tests Used before and after 1996 in Idiopathic GHD Children (IGHD)

Clonidine and L-dopa were more frequently used after 1996, as shown in table 3. There was a tendency of increase in GH peak for all tests. Conversely, spontaneous GH secretion was less performed after 1996 (decrease from 16 to 6.7%). Figure 1 shows the trend for the decrease in the use of insulin and 24-hour spontaneous GH study.

Results of Tests According to Sex and Age

Figure 2 shows that there is no sex ratio in response to insulin and arginine. The maximum GH peak is lowest in children under 5 years of age.

Auxological and Biological Characteristics of Idiopathic GHD Children at the Start of GH Treatment from 1987

Figure 3 shows that we have been treating older GHD children since 1987, without any further change in practice since 1997. Nevertheless, the height standard deviation score (SDS) decreased from –3.3 in 1987 to –2.8 after 2002, suggesting that GHD was less severe, a trend which continued since 1997. Mean peak GH levels also increased from <3 µg/l before 1987 to >5 µg/l after 2002.

Tests Used by Etiologies

Table 4 shows that the percentage of tests used did not differ with the etiologies, i.e. GHD versus idiopathic short stature (ISS), Turner syndrome (TS), small for gestational age (SGA) and Prader-Willi syndrome (PWS). About 24% of ISS children underwent a spontaneous GH secretion evaluation. We could hypothesize that this study was performed in order to search for a neurosecretory dysfunction, i.e. children with low GH secretion with normal tests. Children with TS, SGA and PWS underwent spontaneous GH secretion studies more frequently than GHD children.

Table 3. Tests used before and after 1996 in IGHD

	Before 1996		1996 and after	
	%	median GH peak µg/l	%	median GH peak µg/l
Arginine	28.3	4.8	25.5	5.5
Insulin	31.0	4.7	25.1	5.0
Clonidine	14.2	4.6	24.2	5.4
L-Dopa	10.5	4.5	18.6	5.3
Spontaneous secretion	16.0	7.2	6.7	8.4

Table 4. Percentage of tests by diagnosis

	IGHD	ISS	TS	SGA	PWS
Arginine	26.9	26.7	25.2	30.7	31.0
Insulin	28.0	24.1	27.8	20.3	23.3
Clonidine	19.2	16.4	20.6	21.1	18.8
L-Dopa	14.6	8.7	8.7	8.3	13.3
Spontaneous secretion	11.2	24.1	17.6	19.6	13.6

Table 5. Percentage of patients with at least 2 tests, according to diagnosis

Diagnosis	%
IGHD	87.8
ISS	71.7
TS	25.8
SGA	42.4
PWS	20.4

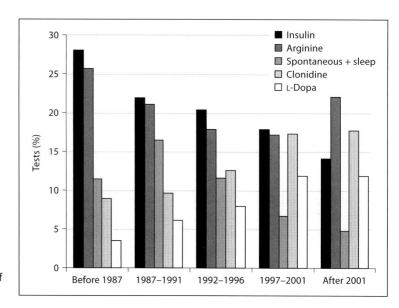

Fig. 1. Tests according to the year of entry (all diagnoses).

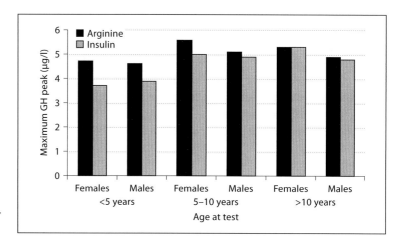

Fig. 2. GH peak according to gender and age in IGHD patients.

Characteristics of the Children

Only 87.8% of GHD children have 2 tests reported, even though most of the countries require 2 tests to confirm the diagnosis. Seventy-two percent of ISS children underwent 2 tests, and in the other groups less than 50% had 2 tests (table 5).

Regarding the combination of the 2 tests, arginine + insulin represented 38 or 39.7%, the second combination being clonidine + insulin (30.3%) or L-dopa + insulin (34.4%). Spontaneous secretion + arginine represented 34.9% (table 6). Eighteen patients were diagnosed with idiopathic GHD (IGHD) without any GH test and 5,096 children with only 1 test, 28% of them with a low IGF-1 value.

Characteristics of the GHD Children at the Start of GH Treatment

Figure 4 shows that the group of children with combined hormonal deficiency started GH treatment earlier, with more severe GHD and a sig-

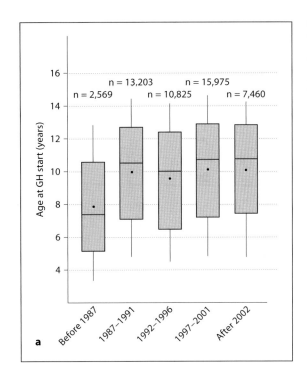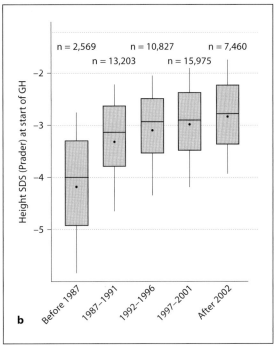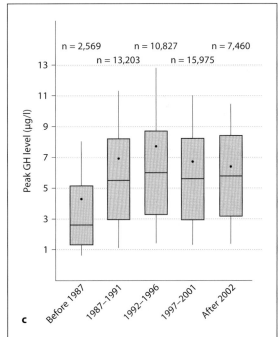

Fig. 3. Age (**a**) and height SDS (**b**) at GH start and peak GH level (**c**) according to the year of entry into KIGS in IGHD patients. Data are given as median and interquartile range (grey box) with the mean indicated as a black dot and the 10th and 90th percentiles as vertical lines.

Table 6. Number of tests and median GH peak levels (all diagnoses)

First test	Second test	n	%	Median GH peak, µg/l	
				first test	second test
Arginine (n = 8,287)	insulin	3,152	38.0	5.5	5.3
	clonidine	1,767	21.3		5.9
	L-dopa	1,387	16.7		5.3
	glucagon	299	3.6		5.5
	spontaneous secretion	957	11.5		8.5
Insulin (n = 6,126)	arginine	2,431	39.7	5.2	5.5
	clonidine	1,238	20.2		5.2
	L-dopa	725	11.8		4.8
	glucagon	315	5.1		5.6
	spontaneous secretion	415	6.8		7.9
Clonidine (n = 4,635)	arginine	1,005	21.7	5.6	5.2
	insulin	1,404	30.3		5.2
	L-dopa	1,123	24.2		5.3
	glucagon	311	6.7		5.1
	spontaneous secretion	264	5.7		8.9
L-Dopa (n = 2,860)	arginine	609	21.3	5.0	5.6
	insulin	985	34.4		4.5
	clonidine	517	18.1		5.6
	glucagon	193	6.7		5.5
	spontaneous secretion	143	5.0		8.7
Spontaneous secretion (n = 3,735)	arginine	1,303	34.9	8.7	6.8
	insulin	749	20.1		6.4
	clonidine	392	10.5		8.0
	L-dopa	163	4.4		6.2
	glucagon	54	1.4		6.8

nificantly higher midparental height. This group also had the best growth velocity during the first year of GH treatment. Children with complete isolated GHD grew better than the other groups but less than the group with multiple pituitary hormonal deficiency. Near adult height (fig. 5) was not significantly different between these two groups, while the group with combined hormonal deficiencies had a significantly better height gain. Complete GHD children also had a higher near adult height compared with partial GHD children.

Discussion

The commonest pharmacological stimuli reported in KIGS continue to be insulin-induced hypoglycemia and arginine. Insulin + arginine accounts for 49% of all the tests. Nevertheless, there is no written consensus explaining this attitude, as it exists in adults. The 20-year analysis also shows a decrease in the study of 24-hour spontaneous GH secretion already noticed in the 10-year KIGS report.

The tests used varied among countries, and the mean GH peak was significantly different.

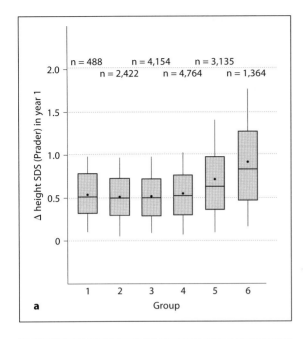
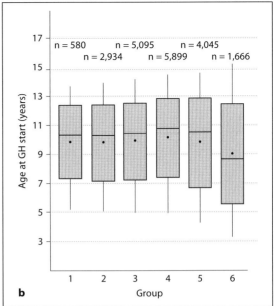
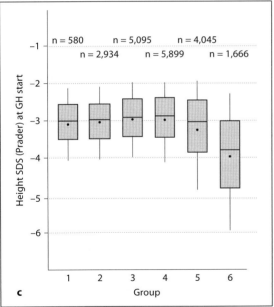
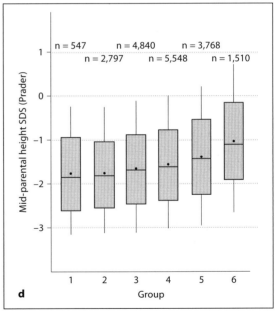

Fig. 4. Δ height SDS (**a**) during the first year of GH treatment, age at GH start (**b**), height SDS at GH start (**c**) and mid-parental height SDS (**d**) in IGHD patients. Group 1: 2 provocation tests, with a peak GH level >10 µg/l; group 2: 2 provocation tests, including 1 test with a peak GH level <10 µg/l and 1 test with a peak GH level >10 µg/l; group 3: 2 tests, with peak GH levels between 5 and 10 µg/l; group 4: 2 tests, including 1 test with a peak GH level between 0 and 5 µg/l and 1 test with a peak GH level between 5 and 10 µg/l; group 5: 2 tests, with peak GH levels between 0 and 5 µg/l in isolated GHD patients; group 6: 2 tests, with peak GH levels between 0 and 5 µg/l in multiple pituitary hormone deficiency patients. Data are given as median and interquartile range (grey box) with the mean indicated as a black dot and the 10th and 90th percentiles as vertical lines.

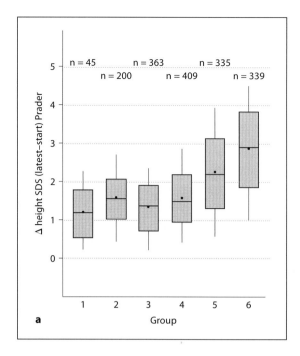
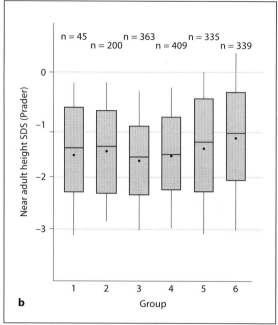

Fig. 5. Δ height SDS (latest – start, Prader) (**a**) and near adult height SDS (Prader) (**b**) in IGHD patients. Group 1: 2 provocation tests, with a peak GH level >10 μg/l; group 2: 2 provocation tests, including 1 test with a peak GH level <10 μg/l and 1 test with a peak GH level >10 μg/l; group 3: 2 tests, with peak GH levels between 5 and 10 μg/l; group 4: 2 tests, including 1 test with a peak GH level between 0 and 5 μg/l and 1 test with a peak GH level between 5 and 10 μg/l; group 5: 2 tests, with peak GH levels between 0 and 5 μg/l in isolated GHD patients; group 6: 2 tests, with peak GH levels between 0 and 5 μg/l in multiple pituitary hormone deficiency patients. Data are given as median and interquartile range (grey box) with the mean indicated as a black dot and the 10th and 90th percentiles as vertical lines.

Only in the UK, the median GH peak on spontaneous GH secretion study is lower, i.e. 1.8 versus 6.5–9.3 μg/l, suggesting it is used in more severe conditions. Spontaneous GH secretion is poorly studied in the USA (1.6%), while it is the first evaluation in Sweden (36.8%). This is partially explained by a specific interest in the 24-hour GH secretion in research and routine practice in Sweden confirmed by several publications. In the USA, the very low use of the spontaneous 24-hour GH secretion study could be due to the higher cost compared with pharmacological studies. Further, these two countries represent quite different health systems, the first being public and the second private. These results prompted us to conclude that the use of tests reflects the practice of a center or a country and is influenced by the health system.

There are differences between the type of test used regarding the etiology, with the exception of a significantly higher prevalence of the 24-hour GH secretion study in the ISS group compared with the GHD, SGA, TS and PWS groups.

The consistent trend of a higher GH peak since 1987 reflects a change in the population treated with GH already reported in the 10-year KIGS book. Age at the start of GH treatment in GHD patients significantly increased since 1987, but the height SDS increased as well, demonstrating that children presented with less severe GHD.

This analysis confirmed that children with complete isolated GHD or multiple pituitary hormonal deficiency were diagnosed earlier, with a more severe height deficit, gained more height during the first year of GH treatment and have a higher near final height than all the other children.

Conclusion

Except for the decreased use of the spontaneous GH secretion study, there were no striking differences from 1996 to 2006 in terms of GH testing in KIGS.

References

1 Rochiccioli P, Enjaume C, Tauber MT, Pienkowski C: Statistical study of 5473 results of nine pharmacological stimulation tests: a proposed weighting index. Acta Paediatr 1993;82:245–248.
2 Ranke MB, Gunnarsson R: Progress in Growth Hormone Therapy – 5 Years of KIGS. Mannheim, J&J Verlag, 1994.
3 Rosenfeld RG, Albertsson-Wikland K, Cassorla F, Frasier SD, Hasegawa Y, Hintz RL, Lafranchi S, Lippe B, Loriaux L, Melmed S, et al: Diagnostic controversy: the diagnosis of childhood growth hormone deficiency revisited. J Clin Endocrinol Metab 1995;80:1532–1540.
4 Growth Hormone Research Society: Consensus guidelines for the diagnosis and treatment of growth hormone (GH) deficiency in childhood and adolescence: summary statement of the GH Research Society. J Clin Endocrinol Metab 2000;85:3990–3993.
5 Sizonenko PC, Clayton PE, Cohen P, Hintz RL, Tanaka T, Laron Z: Diagnosis and management of growth hormone deficiency in childhood and adolescence. 1. Diagnosis of growth hormone deficiency. Growth Horm IGF Res 2001;11:137–165.
6 Drake WM, Howell SJ, Monson JP, Shalet SM: Optimizing GH therapy in adults and children. Endocr Rev 2001;22:425–450.
7 Ranke MB, Schweizer R, Lindberg A, Price DA, Reiter EO, Albertsson-Wikland K, Darendeliler F: Insulin-like growth factors as diagnostic tools in growth hormone deficiency during childhood and adolescence: the KIGS experience. Horm Res 2004;62(suppl 1):17–25 (erratum published in Horm Res 2005;63:210).
8 Jensen RB, Jeppesen KA, Vielwerth S, Michaelsen KF, Main KM, Skakkebaek NE, Juul A: Insulin-like growth factor I (IGF-I) and IGF-binding protein 3 as diagnostic markers of growth hormone deficiency in infancy. Horm Res 2005;63:15–21.
9 Boquete HR, Sobrado PG, Fideleff HL, Sequera AM, Giaccio AV, Suarez MG, Ruibal GF, Miras M: Evaluation of diagnostic accuracy of insulin-like growth factor (IGF)-I and IGF-binding protein-3 in growth hormone-deficient children and adults using ROC plot analysis. J Clin Endocrinol Metab 2003;88:4702–4708.
10 Das U, Whatmore AJ, Khosravi J, Wales JK, Butler G, Kibirige MS, Diamandi A, Jones J, Patel L, Hall CM, Price DA, Clayton PE: IGF-I and IGF-binding protein-3 measurements on filter paper blood spots in children and adolescents on GH treatment: use in monitoring and as markers of growth performance. Eur J Endocrinol 2003;149:179–185.
11 Dattani M, Preece M: Growth hormone deficiency and related disorders: insights into causation, diagnosis, and treatment. Lancet 2004;363:1977–1987.
12 Price DA: GH testing in KIGS: the clinical reality; in Ranke MB, Wilton P (eds): Growth Hormone Therapy in KIGS – 10 Years' Experience. Heidelberg, Johann Ambrosius Barth Verlag, 1999, pp 73–80.

Growth Hormone Deficiency and Modalities of Birth

Angel Ferrández-Longás   Esteban Mayayo
José Ignacio Labarta   Agustin Romo

The association between growth hormone deficiency (GHD) and complicated births was already formulated 50 years ago, mainly by Bierich [1] and Prader and Zachmann [2]. In 1972, Bierich [1] reported a non-cephalic birth presentation in 62% of 45 so-called idiopathic hypopituitary dwarfs, of whom 49% had been delivered after a breech and foot presentation, in contrast to 3–4% of the normal population. In 1978, Prader and Zachmann [2] wrote that many cases of idiopathic GHD (IGHD) combined with multiple pituitary hormonal defects (MPHD) could be due to traumatic births, with a clear predominance of males. In 1979, Ranke et al. [3] reported an incidence of breech delivery of 30% as the major aetiological cause in 36 patients with IGHD. Also at that time, Rona and Tanner [4] published that 42% of children with MPHD were born by breech delivery, and Job [5], in one of his series, found the same in 26 of 27 cases.

Some years later, Bierich [6] reviewed the incidence of non-cephalic presentations in patients with IGHD. From his first publications in 1962, the frequency of 61.5% in 13 cases with IGHD decreased to 29.5% in 44 patients in 1986, which is a reduction of about 50%. A predominance of males to females at 3.5 to 1 was also observed.

Along the years, analysing the data in a non-longitudinal way between 1962 and 1987 including 9 countries and referring to 962 patients with IGHD, Bierich [6] reported an incidence of non-cephalic birth presentations of about 60% in the early 60s to about 30% in the late 80s. In his opinion, this decrease in the incidence of vaginal births by non-cephalic presentations was not due to a decline in the number of such presentations but rather to the sharp increase in caesarean sections (CS) performed in Germany in 72% of breech presentations [6]. In 1992, a collaborative Spanish study, performed in 40 hospitals with a total of 102,038 deliveries, showed a frequency of breech deliveries of 3.8% (11.4% in preterm deliveries) and a frequency of CS of 67.9% in these cases, compared with 14.9% of the total deliveries [7]. A Norwegian study analysing the period between 1968 and 1990 also showed a decrease in

Hospital Infantil Universitario Miguel Servet
Av. Isabel la Católica 3
ES-50009 Zaragoza (Spain)

vaginal birth presentations of about 50% and a parallel increase in CS from 2.0 to 12.6% [8].

In 1994, Albertsson-Wikland et al. [9] studied the frequency of complicated deliveries in 3,721 IGHD and 1,319 organic GHD (OGHD) cases, taken from the KIGS database, up until January 1993 and compared them with 115,282 cases of the Swedish Medical Birth Registry from 1973 to 1986, belonging to 1.4 million newborns and without analysing the tendency along the years. The frequency of breech delivery births was 23% in cases with idiopathic MPHD, 4.6% in cases with isolated GHD, 2.9% in cases with OGHD and 7% in the normal population ($p < 0.001$, MPHD group compared with the others). The instrumental delivery, mainly forceps extraction, was similar in all the groups: IGHD 4%, OGHD 5.5%, normal population 5.5%. The percentage of CS was 9.2% in the IGHD, 6.5% in the OGHD and 11.1% in the normal population [9].

Due to this clear association, breech delivery was assumed to be the most probable principal cause of MPHD related to the mode of birth in the past.

Because of the multiple complications related to breech delivery, not only in respect to pituitary hormonal function, but especially to neurocognitive function and other non-obstetric reasons, the number of CS has greatly increased in the last decades from 3% in the 1960s to 15–21% in the 1990s [10].

In the Miguel Servet Hospital of Zaragoza, the number of instrumental deliveries in the last 14 years (1992–2005) in 88,283 newborns shows an increase from 14.9% in 1992 to 17.9% in 2005, whereas forceps extraction rose from 1.4 to 7% and vacuum extraction decreased from 11.6 to 7.9%, but with a small increase in the latter after the introduction of the almost general epidural analgesia in the last 7 years (71.0% in 2000 vs. 85.9% in 2005).

Nevertheless, the strong decrease in births delivered vaginally in breech presentations has not been the only reason for the increase in CS. A critical review of the published papers in respect to women's reasons to ask for CS was published by Gamble et al. [11] in 2000. In the absence of previous obstetric complications, 1% of women or less request a CS. Other non-obstetric factors like fear of litigation, physician preferences and medical education have played an important role in explaining the major increase in the performance of CS.

Most of the women who demanded a CS had a previous complicated birth or pregnancies with an increased obstetric risk, having been recorded as previous CS or breech deliveries in 8 of the 10 studies analysed [11]. The CS deliveries due to breech presentations rose rapidly in the majority of the hospitals, independently of the country, with percentages around 70–80% in the last years.

One evidence-based medicine publication of a term breech trial [12], a Cochrane review [13] among others, showed a clear decrease in perinatal-neonatal mortality and morbidity by CS. Nevertheless, there is no consensus to choose CS as the unique option for breech presentation. The Swedish Breech Study Group analysing the major increase in CS not only in Sweden but also in Denmark and Norway, found a discrepancy between Swedish Hospitals, with some of them applying a non-selective general CS in more than 95% of the cases, whereas others deliver 30% of the term breech newborns vaginally [14].

A recent British study showed that a planned vaginal delivery of term breech babies is associated with a small but unequivocally increased risk of perinatal death and short-term morbidity, but the long-term outcome is not affected by the method of delivery [15]. The authors referred to 1,433 singleton term breech infants, including 38.5% born by prelabour CS, 29.1% delivered vaginally and 32.4% by CS in labour. In the long-term outcome including deaths, cerebral palsy and the need for special education, they did not observe statistical differences considering the route of delivery. No information about GHD cases can be obtained from this study.

On behalf of the Swedish Collaborative Breech Study Group and the Perinatal Working Group Swedish Society of Obstetrics and Gynecology, Herbst et al. [16] recently published an original article regarding breech delivery at term in Sweden, analysing the mortality relative to fetal presentation and the planned mode of delivery. For this purpose, the authors analysed two cohort studies: (1) data collected from the Swedish Medical Birth Register from 1991 to 2001 analysing, among others, fetal presentation, mode of delivery, mortality (intrauterine, intrapartum, between birth and the 6th day, and death within 1 year), Apgar score at 5 min, birth weight and paediatric diagnosis, having excluded those newborns born before 38 weeks of pregnancy, and (2) data from a study used as matched case control including all deaths (perinatal period to 1 year) among babies delivered by breech presentation from 1991 to 1999. After exclusion of confounding factors and with a well-established selection criterion, the main results of the two studies were similar; nevertheless, the risk of perinatal or infant death was significantly higher in planned vaginal delivery compared with the elective cesarean delivery. The risk in breech deliveries born vaginally is 2- to 3-fold greater, resulting in a less vigorous or dead newborn. On the other hand, to avoid 1 case of low Apgar score, 70 CS were needed, and to avoid 1 death, 400 CS [16].

As mentioned before, another new circumstance has modified the situation: the increase in the frequency of epidural anaesthesia in the last years, especially after the introduction of new techniques and new drugs that provide a pain-free spontaneous vaginal delivery with or without minimal obstetric intervention.

Capogna and Camorcia [17] extensively reviewed the published experience related to epidural analgesia, comparing the traditional technique (epidural catheter) with its combination with spinal analgesia, the use of new drugs like ropivacaine and levobupivacaine and the addition of opioids in low concentrations with the local anaesthetics. They conclude that the combination of epidural plus spinal analgesia seems to have no advantages or disadvantages over epidural analgesia alone, considering the neonatal outcome; however, the administration of intrathecal-epidural opioids may provoke transient changes of the fetal heart frequency.

Some more years are needed to analyse the repercussion of the new delivery techniques on the outcome of these children, but in view of the past experience and the new procedures, the hypothalamic-pituitary defects related to the mode of birth will surely decrease.

References

1. Bierich JR: On the aetiology of hypopituitary dwarfism; in Pecile A, Müller EE (eds): Growth and Growth Hormone. Proceedings of the 2nd International Symposium on Growth Hormone. Amsterdam, Excerpta Medica, 1972.
2. Prader A, Zachmann M: Hypophysärer Minderwuchs; in Labart A (ed): Klinik der Inneren Sekretion, ed 3. Berlin, Springer, 1978, pp 96–102.
3. Ranke M, Weber B, Bierich JR: Long-term response to human growth hormone in 36 children with idiopathic growth hormone deficiency. Eur J Pediatr 1979;132:221–238.
4. Rona RJ, Tanner JM: Aetiology of idiopathic growth hormone deficiency in England and Wales. Arch Dis Child 1977;52:197–208.
5. Job JC: Hypophyse; in Job JC, Pierson M (eds): Endocrinologie Pédiatrique et Croissance. Paris, Flammarion Médecine Science, 1978, pp 73–117.
6. Bierich JR: Aetiology and pathogenesis of growth hormone deficiency. Baillieres Clin Endocrinol Metab 1992;6:491–511.
7. Acien P: Breech presentation in Spain, 1992: a collaborative study. Eur J Obstet Gynecol Reprod Biol 1995;62:19–24.
8. Bergsjo P, Borthen I, Daltveit AK: Surgical delivery in Norway during the last 20 years – analysis of great changes. Tidsskr Nor Laegeforen 1993;113:1206–1211.

9 Albertsson-Wikland K, Wilton P, Ranke M: Growth hormone deficiency: relationship to parental size and mode of birth; in Ranke M, Gunnarsson R (eds): Progress in Growth Hormone Therapy – 5 Years of KIGS. Mannheim, J&J Verlag, 1994, pp 77–87.
10 Ventura SJ, Martin JA, Curtin SC, et al: Births: final data for 1998. Natl Vital Stat Rep 2000;48:13–14.
11 Gamble JA, Health M, Creedy D: Women's request for a cesarean section: a critique of the literature. Birth 2000;27: 256–263.
12 Hannah ME, Hannah WJ, Hewson SA, Hodnett ED, Saigal S, Willan AR: Planned caesarean section versus planned vaginal birth for breech presentation at term: a randomised multicentre trial. Term Breech Trial Collaborative Group. Lancet 2000;356: 1375–1383.
13 Hofmeyr GJ, Hannah ME: Planned caesarean section for term breech delivery (Cochrane methodology review). Oxford, The Cochrane Library, 2003, update software.
14 Alexandersson O, Bixo M, Högberg U: Evidence-based changes in term breech delivery practice in Sweden. Acta Obstet Gynecol Scand 2005;84:584–587.
15 Pradhan P, Mohajer M, Deshpande S: Outcome of term breech births: 10-year experience at a district general hospital. BJOG 2005;112:218–222.
16 Herbst A, et al: Term breech delivery in Sweden: mortality relative to fetal presentation and planned mode of delivery. Acta Obstet Gynecol Scand 2005; 84:593–601.
17 Capogna G, Camorcia M: Epidural analgesia for childbirth. Effects of newer techniques on neonatal outcome. Paediatr Drugs 2004;6:375–386.

7 KIGS

Ranke MB, Price DA, Reiter EO (eds): Growth Hormone Therapy in Pediatrics – 20 Years of KIGS.
Basel, Karger, 2007, pp 60–69

Modalities and Characteristics at Birth: Commentaries Based on KIGS Data

Michael B. Ranke

In general, the interpretation of KIGS data from patients treated with growth hormone (GH) for various reasons in relation to the mode of delivery and parental size is difficult because of the scarcity of published (longitudinal) data. In the World Health Organisation Multicentre Growth Reference Study [1], the mode of delivery (vaginal versus caesarean section), Apgar scores, parental size and size at birth are reported from Brazil, Ghana, India, Norway, Oman and the USA. The data were collected between 1997 and 2003. In order to illustrate the heterogeneity, some data pertinent to the parameters analysed from KIGS are listed in table 1.

There are a few selected items within the KIGS case report forms allowing to collect information at birth such as gestational age (GA) and size (weight, length, head circumference). In addition, there is information about the mode of birth (normal vaginal delivery, vaginal delivery out of breech position, caesarean section and instrumental delivery, e.g., vacuum extraction or forceps). The Apgar index at 1, 5 and 10 min is also documented.

We have analysed some KIGS data based on several hypotheses. (1) The size at birth is related to the underlying diagnosis of short stature, the sex of the individual and the documenting country. (2) The mode of delivery varies according to the country of origin. (3) The size at birth and the mode of delivery are influenced by maternal size.

Hypothesis 1

An analysis was done in all patients (irrespective of the country of origin) with isolated idiopathic GH deficiency (IGHD; code No. 1.1), multiple hormone deficiency (MPHD) in IGHD (code No. 1.1), central nervous system tumour (code No. 2.2.1 ff. and 2.2.2 ff.), small for GA (SGA; code No. 3.4 ff. and 3.5 ff.), idiopathic short stature (ISS; code No. 3.1 ff.) and Turner syndrome (code No. 3.2.1). The data including size at birth, modalities of birth, degree of GH secretion, age and anthropometry at GH start in KIGS are listed in table 2.

Birth weights in relation to GA of IGHD, ISS, MPHD, SGA, Turner syndrome and tumour patients are illustrated in figure 1, and frequencies of caesarean sections and breech deliveries according to the various diagnoses are illustrated in figure 2.

The results can be summarised as follows.

Paediatric Endocrinology Section
University Children's Hospital, University of Tübingen
Hoppe-Seyler-Strasse 1, DE–72076 Tübingen (Germany)

Table 1. Baseline characteristics at birth of a WHO sample [1]

	Brazil	India	Norway	USA
Cross-sectional data				
Patients	487	1,490	1,387	480
Vaginal delivery, %	44.4	63.8	86.7	86.0
Caesarean section, %	55.6	36.2	13.3	14.0
Birth weight, g	3,423 (456)	3,113 (448)	3,636 (455)	3,582 (507)
Height of the mother, cm	160.0 (6.2)	157.6 (5.7)	167.7 (6.5)	164.3 (6.7)
Height of the father, cm	173.2 (7.0)	172.1 (6.0)	181.2 (7.2)	178.0 (7.4)
Longitudinal data				
Patients	310	301	300	208
Apgar score at 5 min	9.7 (0.5)	9.1 (0.6)	9.4 (0.6)	8.9 (0.8)

Values are means with SD in parentheses.

In the groups with GHD (isolated IGHD, MPHD in IGHD), central nervous system tumour children are usually born near term. The size at birth is somewhat lower – half a standard deviation (SD) – in the isolated IGHD and MPHD patients, whereas in those with GHD of tumour origin, the size at birth is near normal. In all diagnoses, there is a small difference in birth size between boys and girls which is typical for the normal population. There is no essential difference between birth sizes in the populations entering KIGS before and after 1995.

Children diagnosed with SGA are born prematurely and – by definition – are too small, having a SD score (SDS) of less than –2.0 at birth. The level of prematurity has increased after 1995.

Children diagnosed with ISS are born at term with a size somewhat below the norm, like in IGHD children. There was no change after 1995.

Girls with Turner syndrome are born near term but with a size of about 1 SDS below the mean. There was no change after 1995.

The parental height is below average (approximately –1.0 SD) in IGHD/MPHD patients, near normal in tumour and Turner syndrome patients, and more pronouncedly decreased (less than –1.0 SDS) in SGA and ISS patients. Furthermore, parental height tended to be lower in the cohorts before 1995.

The patients with organic GHD based on tumour development in childhood are likely to reflect normal frequencies of modalities of birth. Before and after 1995, there was an overall decline in breech and instrument-assisted deliveries from 2.2 to 1.4% and from 8.2 to 6.5%, respectively. At the same time, the frequency of caesarean sections increased from 7.1 to 12.7%. The Apgar score at 5 min averaged 9.6 (0.9 SD). There was no gender difference.

In isolated IGHD children, the frequency of breech deliveries, caesarean sections and the use of instruments was somewhat higher than in the tumour group. The same trends were observed before and after 1995. There were no major differences between males and females.

In MPHD patients, there was a very high frequency of breech deliveries (total 15.9%), particularly before 1995 in boys (25.4%). The frequency, though still increased, was somewhat lower but showed the same male prevalence after 1995. The Apgar score was lower, but did not show a pattern related to gender or year.

In SGA patients, breech deliveries tended to be high before 1995 (6.3%) but were lower (3.3%)

Table 2. Birth characteristics

a Isolated IGHD (code No. 1.1) and MPHD (code No. 1.1)

	Isolated IGHD					MPHD				
n:	all 10,538	females 3,996	males 6,542	<95 4,588	>95 5,950	all 3,767	females 1,128	males 2,639	<95 2,113	>95 1,654
GA, weeks	39.2 (2.1)	39.2	39.2	39.3	39.2	39.0 (2.6)	39.1	38.9	39.0	38.9
Birth weight, g	3,064 (594)	2,981	3,115	3,053	3,073	3,074 (684)	3,018	3,099	3,071	3,079
Birth weight SDS	−0.7 (1.2)	−0.8	−0.7	−0.8	−0.7	−0.6 (1.3)	−0.6	−0.6	−0.6	−0.5
Birth length SDS	−0.5 (1.4)	−0.5	−0.4	−0.6	−0.4	−0.2 (3.6)	−0.2	−0.2	−0.3	−0.2
Breech delivery, %	3.2	3.3	3.1	4.2	2.4	15.9	9.1	18.9	21.4	8.6
Caesarean section, %	14.6	14.5	14.6	11.7	16.8	13.4	13.5	13.4	9.7	18.4
Instrumental delivery, %	5.4	4.4	6.0	6.5	4.7	6.2	5.8	6.3	6.7	5.6
Apgar score at 5 min	9.5 (1.2)	9.6	9.5	9.6	9.5	9.1 (1.6)	9.2	9.0	9.0	9.1
MPH SDS (Prader)	−1.4 (1.2)	−1.5	−1.4	−1.6	−1.3	−1.0 (1.3)	−1.1	−1.0	−1.2	−0.8
Maximum GH, μg/l	6.1 (2.6)	6.2	6.0	6.0	6.1	3.9 (2.9)	3.9	4.0	3.7	4.3
Age, years	11.1 (3.2)	10.6	11.4	10.3	11.7	9.3 (4.6)	8.9	9.5	8.7	10.1
Height SDS (Prader)	−2.9 (1.0)	−3.1	−2.8	−3.2	−2.7	−3.6 (1.5)	−3.9	−3.5	−3.9	−3.2

b Tumours (code No. 2.2.1 ff and No. 2.2.2 ff) and ISS (code No. 3.1 ff)

	Tumours					ISS				
n:	all 4,185	females 1,706	males 2,479	<95 1,981	>95 2,204	all 5,246	females 1,776	males 3,470	<95 2,616	>95 2,630
GA, weeks	39.5 (1.8)	39.5	39.5	39.6	39.4	39.0 (2.3)	39.0	38.9	39.1	38.8
Birth weight, g	3,321 (581)	3,240	3,377	3,314	3,329	3,066 (526)	2,994	3,103	3,068	3,065
Birth weight SDS	−0.2 (1.2)	−0.2	−0.2	−0.3	−0.2	−0.6 (0.9)	−0.6	−0.6	−0.6	−0.5
Birth length SDS	0.2 (1.3)	0.2	0.2	0.2	0.3	−0.3 (1.0)	−0.3	−0.3	−0.4	−0.3
Breech delivery, %	1.8	1.7	1.9	2.2	1.4	3.5	3.8	3.3	4.4	2.6
Caesarean section, %	10	10.1	9.9	7.1	12.7	13.2	12.7	13.5	9.4	17.0
Instrumental delivery, %	7.3	6.5	7.8	8.2	6.5	5.2	4.1	5.8	6.5	4.5
Apgar score at 5 min	9.6 (0.9)	9.6	9.7	9.7	9.6	9.6 (1.0)	9.6	9.5	9.5	9.6
MPH SDS (Prader)	−0.5 (1.2)	−0.5	−0.5	−0.6	−0.3	−1.8 (1.1)	−1.8	−1.7	−2.1	−1.5
Maximum GH, μg/l	4.5 (5.7)	4.4	4.6	4.5	4.6	18.0 (16.9)	17.8	18.1	18.9	17.2
Age, years	10.9 (3.3)	10.4	11.2	10.5	11.2	10.3 (3.3)	10.0	10.5	10.2	10.4
Height SDS (Prader)	−2.1 (1.3)	−2.2	−2.0	−2.2	−1.9	−3.1 (0.8)	−3.3	−2.9	−3.2	−2.9

c SGA (code No. 3.4 ff) and Turner syndrome (code No. 3.2.1)

	SGA					Turner syndrome		
n:	all 2,309	females 838	males 1,471	<95 760	>95 1,549	all 5,829	<95 2,553	>95 3,267
GA, weeks	38.0 (3.1)	38.4	37.9	39.1	37.5	38.9 (2.0)	39.1	38.8
Birth weight, g	2,107 (632)	2,127	2,096	2,277	2,024	2,800 (541)	2,781	2,815
Birth weight SDS	−2.7 (1.1)	−2.6	−2.7	−2.7	−2.6	−1.1 (1.2)	−1.2	−1.0
Birth length SDS	−2.7 (1.3)	−2.7	−2.7	−2.7	−2.7	−0.8 (1.4)	−1.0	−0.7
Breech delivery, %	4.2	5.1	3.7	6.3	3.3	3.3	3.3	3.4
Caesarean section, %	31.7	29.5	33.1	18.9	37.6	13.9	10.0	16.9
Instrumental delivery, %	3.3	2.9	3.6	7.1	2.1	3.8	3.8	3.7
Apgar score at 5 min	9.2 (1.3)	9.2	9.1	9.0	9.2	9.5 (1.1)	9.5	9.4
MPH SDS (Prader)	−1.4 (1.3)	−1.4	−1.5	−1.9	−1.2	−0.6 (1.2)	−0.7	−0.4
Maximum GH, μg/l	18.1 (12.9)	19.2	17.6	17.5	18.6	14.5 (11.6)	14.7	14.2
Age, years	8.7 (3.5)	8.5	8.8	9.2	8.5	9.7 (3.7)	10.2	9.3
Height SDS (Prader)	−3.4 (1.1)	−3.7	−3.3	−3.6	−3.3	−3.4 (1.1)	−3.6	−3.2

Values are means with SD in parentheses. <95 = Before 1995; >95 = after 1995.

thereafter. Caesarean sections were higher after 1995 (37.6%) than before (18.9%), with a trend towards higher frequencies in the male population. Instrument-assisted births declined with the years.

Finally, in the ISS group, the situation regarding the mode of birth resembled that of isolated IGHD children.

Hypothesis 2
We have restricted the analysis to Japan, the USA, the UK, Germany, France and Sweden including isolated IGHD, MPHD and tumour patients. It can be expected that in the tumour groups, the underlying national situation with regard to birth size, parental height and mode of delivery is reflected (table 3). Information about the frequency of breech deliveries and caesarean sections in these countries and the respective diagnoses are illustrated in figure 3.

In all countries, analysed parental height was lower in IGHD and MPHD patients compared with the tumour group. In all countries, the size at birth was lower in IGHD patients. This was also true for MPHD children in Japan, Germany and France. In Japan, caesarean sections were generally of low frequency, whereas the occurrence was highest in the USA. In all countries, except for the USA, there was a markedly increased frequency of breech deliveries in MPHD patients. Also, caesarean sections tended to be slightly higher in MPHD patients in the UK, Germany and France. Apgar scores tended to be lower in the UK and USA for all diagnoses. GHD was generally more severe in the MPHD group, and GH therapy was started at a younger age compared with the IGHD group.

Hypothesis 3
We have assumed that the size at birth and the mode of delivery were influenced by the size of the mother rather than by the size of the father. Therefore, patients with different diagnoses – isolated IGHD, Turner syndrome, tumours, SGA and ISS – were divided into two groups: (A) discrepancies between mothers' (short) and fathers' (tall) height SDS (difference in height SDS ≥ 2), and (B) similarities in height SDS of both parents (± 0.5 SD). Thus, the midparental height was very similar in both groups (table 4, fig. 4).

Differences in the frequency of breech deliveries and caesarean sections according to parental height are illustrated in figure 5.

In the tumour group and in SGA children, the frequency of caesarean sections was similar. However, in the patients with isolated IGHD, Turner syndrome and ISS, the frequency of caesarean sections was higher in the group with smaller mothers. In Turner syndrome and SGA patients, the size at birth was not different between the groups, but differed in isolated IGHD, tumour and ISS patients. Other parameters did not show significant differences.

Conclusions

Birth size and frequencies of modes of delivery vary according to the underlying diagnoses, sex and the country of origin. There are also trends which reflect a change in obstetric practice towards caesarean sections.

In MPHD patients, breech deliveries and caesarean sections tended to be significantly more frequent, particularly in boys. Unfortunately, the causes of caesarean sections are not documented within KIGS. Thus, it remains obscure whether circumstances present in the unborn causing MPHD are also influencing circumstances at birth, which in consequence lead to operative deliveries, or whether the latter (birth trauma) is causative of an insult to the hypothalamus/pituitary. While the latter was assumed in the early days of diagnosis/treatment of GHD, there is currently a trend to favour the former (developmental/genetic) concept. KIGS data give support to both pathogeneses.

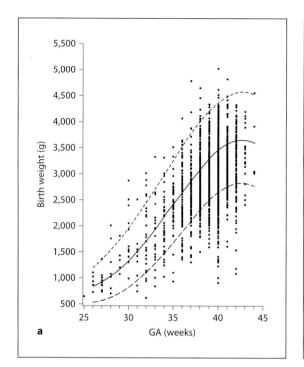
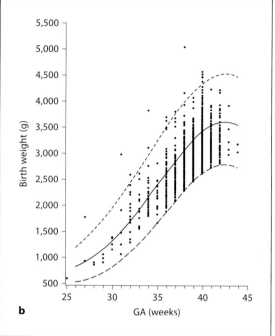
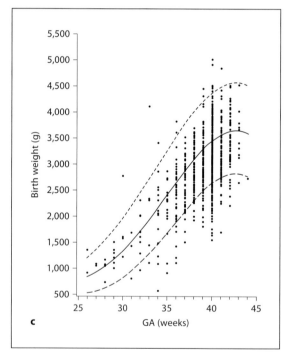
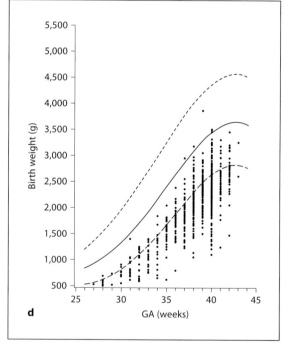

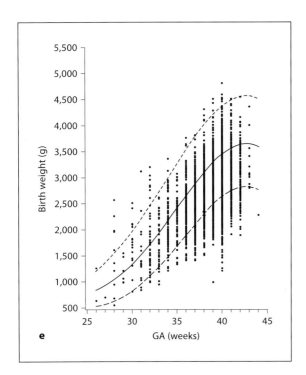
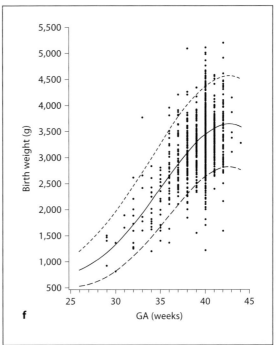

Fig. 1. Birth weight in relation to GA in the IGHD (**a**), ISS (**b**), MPHD (**c**), SGA (**d**), Turner syndrome (**e**) and tumour (**f**) groups. Solid line = 50th centile of normal references; dashed lines = 3rd and 97th centiles of normal referenes.

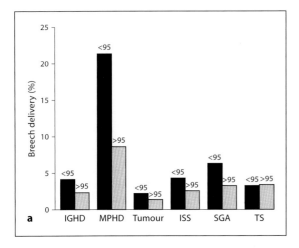
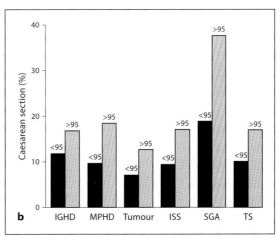

Fig. 2. Frequency of breech deliveries (**a**) and caesarean sections (**b**) before (<95) and after 1995 (>95) according to the various diagnoses. TS = Turner syndrome.

Table 3. Comparison between isolated IGHD (A), MPHD (B) and tumour patients (C) in different countries

a Japan and USA

		Japan			USA		
		A	B	C	A	B	C
	n:	1,633	592	373	1,909	456	502
GA, weeks		39.2 (2.0)	38.9 (2.6)	39.5 (1.7)	39.1 (2.5)	38.9 (3.0)	39.3 (2.0)
Birth weight, g		2,870 (506)	2,910 (561)	3,157 (432)	3,152 (674)	3,147 (737)	3,312 (686)
Birth weight SDS		−1.2 (1.1)	−1.0 (1.1)	−0.6 (0.9)	−0.5 (1.4)	−0.3 (1.3)	−0.1 (1.3)
Birth length SDS		−1.0 (1.2)	−0.8 (1.2)	−0.2 (1.0)	−0.1 (1.7)	0.2 (1.6)	0.4 (1.6)
Breech delivery, %		5.7	31.4	3.4	1.5	1.7	1.5
Caesarean section, %		7.8	4.8	4.2	25.1	26.4	19.9
Instrumental delivery, %		3.4	12.7	0	4.5	6.2	4.5
Apgar score at 5 min		9.3 (0.9)	9.1 (1.2)	9.4 (1.1)	8.5 (1.8)	8.1 (2.1)	8.8 (1.0)
MPH SDS (Prader)		−2.4 (0.8)	−2.2 (0.8)	−1.9 (0.9)	−0.8 (1.1)	−0.5 (1.2)	−0.2 (1.1)
Maximum GH, µg/l		6.9 (2.4)	4.5 (3.0)	3.3 (4.2)	5.9 (2.5)	4.2 (2.9)	4.0 (4.8)
Age, years		10.4 (3.0)	9.5 (4.2)	10.7 (3.6)	12.2 (2.6)	10.2 (4.7)	11.4 (3.5)
Height SDS (Prader)		−3.3 (0.8)	−4.0 (1.2)	−3.0 (1.4)	−2.5 (1.0)	−2.8 (1.5)	−2.1 (1.3)

b UK and Germany

		UK			Germany		
		A	B	C	A	B	C
	n:	663	312	954	1,260	471	477
GA, weeks		39.3 (2.3)	39.0 (2.4)	39.6 (1.8)	39.3 (2.2)	39.1 (2.4)	39.5 (1.7)
Birth weight, g		3,071 (641)	3,181 (719)	3,360 (604)	3,111 (598)	3,096 (688)	3,308 (519)
Birth weight SDS		−0.8 (1.3)	−0.3 (1.3)	−0.2 (1.2)	−0.7 (1.1)	−0.6 (1.2)	−0.3 (1.0)
Birth length SDS		−0.1 (1.7)	0.1 (1.8)	0.9 (2.3)	0.0 (1.3)	0.2 (1.5)	0.6 (1.2)
Breech delivery, %		2.2	6.3	1.9	2.8	10.8	0.9
Caesarean section, %		15.5	18.3	8.5	13.5	17.5	9.9
Instrumental delivery, %		12.7	15.2	12.6	7.9	6.0	6.6
Apgar score at 5 min		8.5 (2.2)	8.5 (1.8)	8.7 (1.6)	9.5 (1.1)	9.1 (1.6)	9.7 (0.8)
MPH SDS (Prader)		−1.2 (1.2)	−0.8 (1.2)	−0.4 (1.1)	−0.8 (1.1)	−0.4 (1.1)	−0.1 (1.0)
Maximum GH, µg/l		4.6 (2.6)	3.1 (2.4)	5.2 (5.8)	5.8 (2.5)	4.0 (2.8)	4.4 (8.7)
Age, years		9.3 (3.7)	7.5 (4.6)	10.3 (3.2)	10.5 (3.4)	8.6 (4.4)	11.3 (3.3)
Height SDS (Prader)		−3.5 (1.1)	−3.8 (1.6)	−1.7 (1.3)	−2.7 (0.9)	−3.3 (1.3)	−1.9 (1.3)

c France

		France		
		A	B	C
	n:	1,478	394	470
GA, weeks		39.2 (1.7)	39.0 (2.3)	39.5 (1.8)
Birth weight, g		3,049 (523)	3,105 (610)	3,232 (514)
Birth weight SDS		−0.7 (1.1)	−0.6 (1.2)	−0.4 (1.0)
Birth length SDS		−0.8 (1.1)	−0.6 (1.1)	−0.3 (1.0)
Breech delivery, %		2.9	10.7	2.2
Caesarean section, %		10.6	11.5	6.4
Instrumental delivery, %		2.7	6.4	5.5
Apgar score at 5 min		9.9 (0.6)	9.6 (1.3)	9.9 (0.4)
MPH SDS (Prader)		−1.5 (0.9)	−1.1 (1.1)	−0.7 (1.0)
Maximum GH, µg/l		7.1 (2.2)	5.1 (3.0)	5.6 (5.2)
Age, years		11.1 (3.1)	9.5 (4.7)	10.7 (3.1)
Height SDS (Prader)		−2.9 (0.8)	−3.3 (1.2)	−2.3 (1.2)

Values are means with SD in parentheses.

Table 4. Comparison between patients with IGHD and MPHD, tumours and ISS, and SGA and Turner syndrome with height discrepancies between father and mother (A) and equal height of father and mother (B)

a IGHD and MPHD

	IGHD			MPHD		
	A	B	p	A	B	p
n:	747	3,207		217	1,062	
GA, weeks	39.0 (2.2)	39.3 (2.0)	<0.001	38.6 (3.1)	39.0 (2.6)	n.s.
Birth weight, g	3,005 (593)	3,086 (578)	<0.001	2,918 (751)	3,069 (668)	<0.01
Birth weight SDS	−0.8 (1.2)	−0.7 (1.2)	n.s.	−0.7 (1.2)	−0.6 (1.2)	<0.05
Birth length SDS	−0.6 (1.4)	−0.4 (1.3)	<0.01	−0.3 (1.4)	−0.2 (1.4)	n.s.
Breech delivery, %	4.0	3.2	n.s.	12.9	18.8	<0.05
Caesarean section, %	24.3	13.5	<0.001	19.8	9.7	<0.001
Instrumental delivery, %	5.3	5.3	n.s.	3.9	5.9	n.s.
Apgar score at 5 min	9.3 (1.5)	9.5 (1.2)	<0.05	8.7 (2.0)	9.1 (1.6)	n.s.
MPH SDS (Prader)	−1.5 (1.3)	−1.4 (1.2)	n.s.	−1.1 (1.2)	−1.1 (1.3)	n.s.
Maximum GH, μg/l	5.9 (2.6)	6.2 (2.5)	<0.01	3.9 (2.8)	4.0 (2.9)	n.s.
Age, years	10.9 (3.2)	11.1 (3.1)	n.s.	9.1 (4.9)	9.3 (4.6)	n.s.
Height SDS (Prader)	−2.9 (1.0)	−2.9 (0.9)	n.s.	−3.7 (1.6)	−3.6 (1.4)	n.s.

b Tumours and ISS

	Tumours			ISS		
	A	B	p	A	B	p
n:	237	1,153		351	1,560	
GA, weeks	39.4 (1.6)	39.5 (1.8)	n.s.	38.8 (2.3)	39.1 (2.1)	n.s.
Birth weight, g	3,252 (588)	3,325 (575)	n.s.	3,049 (520)	3,090 (510)	n.s.
Birth weight SDS	−0.4 (1.3)	−0.2 (1.1)	n.s.	−0.6 (0.9)	−0.6 (0.9)	n.s.
Birth length SDS	0.4 (1.4)	0.2 (1.4)	n.s.	−0.3 (1.0)	−0.4 (1.0)	n.s.
Breech delivery, %	3.2	1.9	n.s.	2.0	3.4	n.s.
Caesarean section, %	16.7	10.2	<0.05	26.3	11.9	<0.001
Instrumental delivery, %	10.7	8.0	n.s.	8.0	5.5	n.s.
Apgar score at 5 min	9.4 (0.9)	9.6 (1.0)	<0.05	9.5 (0.7)	9.6 (1.0)	<0.01
MPH SDS (Prader)	−0.6 (1.2)	−0.5 (1.2)	n.s.	−1.7 (1.1)	−1.8 (1.1)	n.s.
Maximum GH, μg/l	4.6 (4.3)	4.4 (6.2)	<0.05	18.6 (18.1)	17.7 (12.1)	n.s.
Age, years	11.0 (3.1)	10.7 (3.5)	n.s.	10.1 (3.3)	10.3 (3.2)	n.s.
Height SDS (Prader)	−2.0 (1.5)	−2.1 (1.4)	n.s.	−3.1 (0.9)	−3.1 (0.8)	n.s.

c SGA and Turner syndrome

	SGA			Turner syndrome		
	A	B	p	A	B	p
n:	216	609		336	1,709	
GA, weeks	38.0 (3.2)	38.1 (3.1)	n.s.	38.8 (2.0)	38.9 (2.0)	n.s.
Birth weight, g	2,133 (614)	2,118 (639)	n.s.	2,776 (530)	2,792 (529)	n.s.
Birth weight SDS	−2.5 (1.1)	−2.6 (1.1)	n.s.	−1.1 (1.1)	−1.1 (1.2)	n.s.
Birth length SDS	−2.4 (1.2)	−2.8 (1.3)	<0.01	−0.9 (1.4)	−0.8 (1.4)	n.s.
Breech delivery, %	5.2	4.0	n.s.	2.5	3.0	n.s.
Caesarean section, %	36.3	32.8	n.s.	20.1	14.6	<0.05
Instrumental delivery, %	2.7	3.9	n.s.	3.3	3.8	n.s.
Apgar score at 5 min	8.8 (1.5)	9.2 (1.3)	n.s.	9.5 (0.8)	9.4 (1.2)	n.s.
MPH SDS (Prader)	−1.6 (1.3)	−1.4 (1.3)	n.s.	−0.7 (1.2)	−0.6 (1.2)	n.s.
Maximum GH, μg/l	18.1 (10.3)	19.1 (14.1)	n.s.	16.6 (15.8)	14.1 (10.5)	n.s.
Age, years	9.0 (3.4)	8.9 (3.5)	n.s.	9.4 (3.7)	9.7 (3.5)	n.s.
Height SDS (Prader)	−3.4 (1.0)	−3.3 (1.0)	n.s.	−3.4 (1.0)	−3.4 (1.0)	n.s.

Values are means with SD in parentheses. n.s. = Not significant.

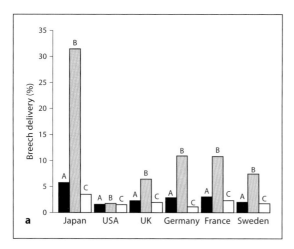
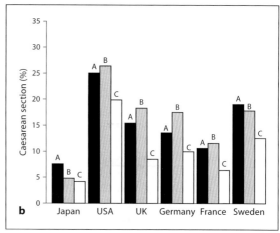

Fig. 3. Frequency of breech deliveries (**a**) and caesarean sections (**b**) according to the countries studied. A = IGHD; B = MPHD; C = tumours.

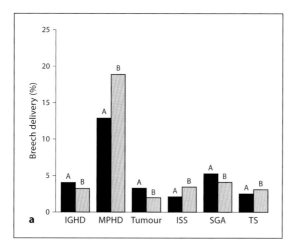
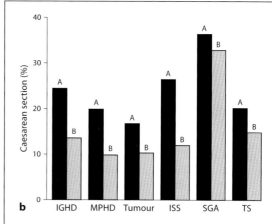

Fig. 4. Frequency of breech deliveries (**a**) and caesarean sections (**b**) in boys and girls according to the various diagnoses. A = Height discrepancies between father and mother; B = equal height of father and mother; TS = Turner syndrome.

In smaller mothers, there is obviously a higher risk of term babies having to be delivered by caesarean section, although these babies are a bit smaller. These data do not favour that caesarean sections per se cause GHD.

This complex situation requires studies in GH-treated children focusing in more detail on the modalities of birth including true control groups in different medical environments.

Our analysis also suggests that data related to the mode of delivery have to be interpreted in context with the national medical praxis.

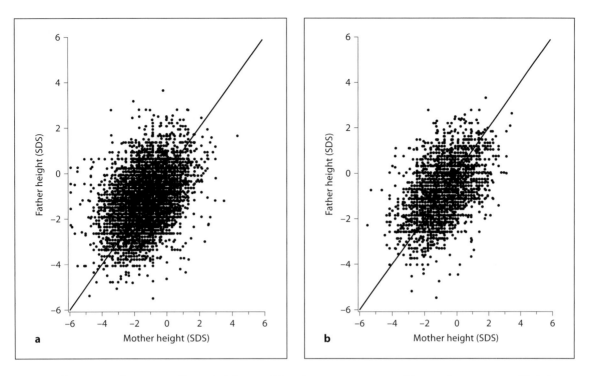

Fig. 5. Differences in frequency of breech deliveries (**a**) and caesarean sections (**b**) according to parental height.

Reference

1 WHO Multicentre Growth Reference Study Group. Enrolment and baseline characteristics in the WHO Multicentre Growth Reference Study. Acta Paediatr Suppl 2006;450:7–15.

The Role of Insulin-Like Growth Factors in Growth Hormone Deficiency

Anders Juul

The insulin-like growth factor (IGF) family of growth factors consists of 3 ligands – insulin, IGF-1 and IGF-2 – that share peptide sequence identity with each other (approximately 50% of their amino acids). All ligand precursors are similar in structure, i.e. carry A, B and C domains. In contrast to insulin, where the C domain is removed during processing, fully processed IGFs are single-chain polypeptides which contain all 3 domains. In addition, IGFs contain a carboxyterminal D domain which does not occur in insulin. IGF-1 and IGF-2 are 70- and 67-amino acid polypeptides with molecular weights of 7,650 and 7,479 Da, respectively. Whereas insulin is generally thought to have metabolic actions, IGF-1 and IGF-2 have metabolic as well as mitogenic actions regulating cellular proliferation. The effects of insulin are mediated after binding to its own specific receptor (IR), whereas the mitogenic effects of IGF-1 and IGF-2 are primarily mediated after binding to the IGF-1 receptor (IGF1R). Both the IR and the IGF1R are cell surface glycoproteins and members of the tyrosine kinase receptors [1]. The IGF1R gene is located on chromosome 15 (15q26.3), and terminal 15q deletions result in decreased IGF receptor binding and intrauterine growth retardation [2], similar to what is found in African pygmies [3], suggesting a possible role of IGF1R gene defects in intrauterine growth retardation. IGF-2 has its own specific receptor (IGF-2/mannose-6-phosphate receptor), which is not a tyrosine kinase receptor and is thought to function as a clearance factor for IGF-2 by internalizing and degrading cell surface-attached IGF-2 [4]. Each ligand binds to its specific receptor with very high affinity (approximately 10^{-9} M). Due to the homology between the IGFs and insulin, and the homology between IR and IGF1R, IGFs can interact with the IR although with a lower affinity than that of insulin. IGF-2 binds the IR with higher affinity than that of IGF-1, but with similar affinity to the IGF1R compared with IGF-1 [5]. In plasma, insulin circulates in picomolar concentrations, whereas IGFs circulate in nanomolar concentrations. Despite the fact that the insulin-like activity of IGFs is

University Department of Growth and Reproduction
Rigshospitalet, Section 5064
Blegdamsvej 9
DK–2100 Copenhagen (Denmark)

only 5% of that of insulin, in theory, the IGFs could be 50 times more glucose lowering than insulin alone because of their abundance. However, this does not occur because the activity of IGFs is inhibited by binding to specific IGF binding proteins (IGFBPs) in the circulation. In extracellular fluids, IGF-1 is bound with high affinity (approximate K_d 10^{-10} M) to a family of 6 specific IGFBPs (IGFBP-1 to IGFBP-6) which have been identified and characterized [6]. The IGFBPs are produced in a variety of biological tissues and found in various biological fluids like plasma. All 6 IGFBPs form binary complexes with IGFs (of approximately 40–50 kDa), but only IGFBP-3 (and to some extent IGFBP-5) forms a high-molecular-weight (150-kDa) ternary complex comprised of IGF-1 or IGF-2, IGFBP-3 and an acid-labile subunit (ALS) of approximately 85 kDa [7]. All three members of this trimeric complex are induced by GH and are therefore affected in GH disorders. The high-molecular-weight complex has no capillary permeability, and thus, is not available to the tissues. It is assumed that complex formation occurs in the liver as IGF-1 and ALS are derived from the hepatocyte, whereas IGFBP-3 is produced in the Kupffer cells of the liver [8, 9]. This may serve to ensure ternary complex formation in the blood passing through the hepatic sinusoids. ALS circulates in molar excess (approximately 250 nM) to IGFBP-3 (approximately 100 nM) [7], which in turn circulates in molar excess to IGF-1, but in equimolar concentrations to the sum of IGF-1 and IGF-2 [10]. ALS binds to the binary IGF-1-IGFBP-3 complex with a constant of 2.5×10^8 M [11]. It is likely that dissociation of the weak ALS-IGFBP-3 bond readily occurs at the endothelial surface mediated by cell surface-associated glycosaminoglycans [12], thereby facilitating the IGF transport to the tissues. Thus, in the circulation, IGF-1 is present in 3 different fractions: a small free fraction (7.5 kDa), binary complexes (40–50 kDa) and ternary complexes (150 kDa) in which more than 95% of circulating IGF-1 is bound. The IGFBP-3 gene is located on chromosome 7 and consists of 5 exons with a size of 8.9 kb. The gene product consists of 264 amino acids and has a molecular weight of 28.7 kDa. However, as IGFBP-3 is strongly glycosylated, it appears as a doublet on Western blots with an apparent molecular weight of 40–42 kDa. IGFBP-3 is regulated by GH and exhibits only minor diurnal variation.

Insulin-Like Growth Factor 1 Levels in Normal Subjects

IGF-1 levels rise with increased pubertal maturation, and maximal levels are seen in Tanner stage 3–4 in girls and Tanner stage 4 in boys [13–16]. In addition, a significant variation with age occurs within each Tanner stage of puberty, showing increased IGF-1 levels with age in the early pubertal stages and a decrease in the late pubertal stages [17, 18]. Increasing testicular volume, as a measure of sexual maturation, was associated with increasing IGF-1 levels [17]. Accordingly, the effects of gender, age and puberty on serum IGF-1 levels cannot be separated into simple additive components. IGFBP-3 levels exhibit similar changes [10, 13, 15, 16, 19, 20], although with less pronounced changes in puberty compared with IGF-1. Consequently, the molar ratio between IGF-1 and IGFBP-3, which may reflect free, biologically active IGF-1, increases in puberty [21]. Furthermore, ALS levels increase [22–24], whereas serum levels of IGFBP-1 decrease [10, 25], probably as a result of decreasing insulin sensitivity [13]. IGF-2 and IGFBP-2 levels are unchanged throughout puberty [10, 26]. Altogether, changes in IGFs, IGFBPs and ALS result in rising levels of free IGF-1 [25, 27].

Due to the large variations according to age, gender and pubertal maturation, normative data based on a large number of individuals are needed to optimize the diagnostic value of IGF-1 when evaluating children suspected of GH deficiency (GHD). Published reference ranges in children vary substantially, which may be due to the use of different IGF-1 assays and different control populations [17, 28–35].

Furthermore, models for converting serum IGF-1 concentrations to standard deviation scores (SDS), not only taking into consideration chronological age but also including gender and puberty, have been constructed [17, 18]; however, the diagnostic value of these models has not yet been evaluated .

Diagnostic Use of Insulin-Like Growth Factor 1 in Growth Hormone Deficiency

The diagnostic use of IGF-1 and IGFBP-3 in children suspected of GHD is based on the assumption that a single determination of these parameters reflects the integrated 24-hour GH secretion. This has indeed been demonstrated in healthy children where circulating IGF-1 levels correlate with the spontaneous GH secretion in numerous studies [36–41], although not in all [42, 43]. Like IGF-1, IGFBP-3 correlated significantly with the endogenous 24-hour GH in a study of 114 normal children with varying heights [39].

In adults, some controversy exists. Rudman et al. [44] demonstrated a highly significant correlation between nocturnal GH release and IGF-1 concentrations in 52 young and elderly healthy subjects. Reutens et al. [45] also demonstrated a significant correlation between IGF-1 and spontaneous GH secretion when GH was determined by an ultrasensitive assay, but not when GH was determined by a conventional radioimmunoassay. However, most other studies have failed to demonstrate a correlation between IGF-1 and 24-hour spontaneous GH secretion in healthy normal-weight subjects [46–48].

Diagnosis of GHD in children can be easy in classical cases with genetic etiologies (like GH, Pit-1 or Prop-1 gene mutations). In these cases, a child presents with short stature, growth failure and a typical phenotype (truncal adiposity, frontal bossing, midfacial hypoplasia and small genitalia in the male). Sometimes, symptoms like hypoglycemia or prolonged jaundice already present in the newborn period, but most frequently, growth failure during the childhood period is the common symptom leading to suspicion of GHD. Traditionally, pituitary somatotropic function is evaluated by GH provocative testing using a variety of stimuli (arginine, clonidine, insulin, GH-releasing hormone). The GH response to testing is evaluated in relation to an arbitrarily selected cutoff value that has changed over time (from 5 to 10 ng/ml in most centers). This fixed threshold to define GHD is used at all ages, which seems unphysiological, especially as a pubertal increase in the response to GH testing has been described [49], and as sex steroid priming in adolescents has marked effects on peak GH levels [49, 50]. Furthermore, different provocative stimuli result in different GH responses [51], and different GH assays give very different results when assaying the same serum sample [52]. Therefore, each laboratory must have its own assay- and test-specific cutoff value which should be compared with other laboratories [53] before the use of the provocative test procedure is ethically sound. Due to these inconveniences of GH provocative testing, other estimates of pituitary GH secretion like the IGFs have been searched for over the years. In contrast to peak GH values following GH provocative testing, well-defined age- and sex-related normal ranges certainly exist for IGF-1 and IGFBP-3. IGF-1 levels are low in GHD as demonstrated by several papers [54–56]. In a classical paper, IGF-1 was below the lower limit of the control population in 82% of the children with GHD and above the lower limit in 68% of short normal children [35]. Hereafter, several papers demonstrated that IGF-1 levels are low in GHD children [30, 31], and later detailed diagnostic sensitivities and specificities have been reported. In a study of 203 short-statured children and adolescents in whom GHD was suspected, GH provocative testing was performed in all children. Of these, 61 (30%) were defined as GHD (peak GH value during GH testing below the cutoff value of 15 mU/l), whereas 142 children had a peak GH value above the cutoff value. In the GHD children, IGF-1 levels were below –2 SD in 42 children (69%) [57], resulting in a positive predictive value (PPV) of 57%. In children below 10 years of age, IGF-1 values were highly predictive of a subnormal GH response to provocative testing [57]. Changing the cutoff value in this study demonstrated optimal separation between GHD and idiopathic short stature (ISS) children using a cutoff value of –2.5 SD for IGF-1 [57]. Rikken et al. [29] used advanced analysis with receiver-operating characteristics of baseline data from 96 children who were valuated for possible GHD and found that the optimal cutoff value for IGF-1 was –0.8 SDS, which resulted in a sensitivity of 92% and a specificity of 47%, respectively. Boquete et al. [58] evaluated the diagnostic use of IGF-1 in 34 GHD children. They found that the optimal cutoff value for IGF-1 SDS was –1.7, which resulted in a diagnostic sensitivity of 68% and a specificity of 97%. Nunez et al. [43] studied IGF-1 levels in 104 short children. They suggested that screening use of IGF-1 with a criterion of –1 SD would identify 88% of GHD and 46% of ISS children. An IGF-1 higher than –1 SD would accurately identify 68% of ISS children, not needing GH testing [43]. Other studies found sensitivities between 61 and 91% and specificities between 47 and 80% for IGF-1 using –2 SD as cutoff criterion [20, 32–34, 59–63]. A single study [64] found a significantly lower sensitivity which may be due to the high number of patients with organic etiology. For some unknown reason, IGF-1 and IGFBP-3 are not as reliable in the diagnosis of GHD in children with organic lesions in the brain [65, 66]. One study advocated that the combination of IGF-1 and IGF-2 measurements provide additional diagnostic information, but this has not been documented since [35]. Others have suggested that inclusion of IGFBP-2 in the diagnostic work-up of short children improved the diagnostic accuracy [32, 60]. Based on the opposite influences of body mass index on IGF-1 and GH secretion, Oerter et al. [67] suggested a new diagnostic test (the bivariate S test) in which the S score equals the sum of IGF-1 (SD), and mean nighttime GH levels (SD) were calculated. Interestingly, the S score was independent of body mass index and highly specific in healthy children (97.9%).

Despite the controversies, the majority of physicians include IGF-1 measurements in their routine diagnostic evaluation of children suspected of GHD [68].

Insulin-Like Growth Factor Binding Protein 3 and Diagnosis of Growth Hormone Deficiency in Children

In 1990, Blum et al. [20] suggested that IGFBP-3 was superior to IGF-1 in diagnosing children with GHD. They reported a diagnostic sensitivity of 97% and a specificity of 95% in their large study of 262 short-statured children suspected of GHD compared with a large normative dataset (n = 487 children). These findings have not been reproduced as convincing in subsequent studies [29, 32, 34, 43, 57, 60, 61, 64, 69] in which diagnostic sensitivities were 15–93% and specificities 50–98%, respectively. Boquete et al. [58] evaluated the diagnostic use of IGFBP-3 in 34 GHD children. They found that the optimal cutoff value for the IGFBP-3 SDS was –1.8, which resulted in a diagnostic sensitivity of 90% and a specificity of 60%. Thus, the majority of these studies in which children of all ages have been included conclude that assessment of IGFBP-3 offers no major advantage over IGF-1 in the diagnosis of GHD in children. However, some studies suggest that combined measurement of both parameters improves the diagnostic value. However, from looking at normative ranges and especially the lower limits of normality, it is apparent that the

IGF-1 lower limits in 0- to 6-year-old children are very close to the detection limits of the used assays, whereas this is not the case for IGFBP-3. Thus, theoretically, IGFBP-3 may be superior to IGF-1 in the 0- to 6-year-old children. This hypothesis is supported by the finding of a higher diagnostic value of IGFBP-3 compared with IGF-1 in the youngest prepubertal children compared with older children [32, 57]. Few studies have evaluated the diagnostic value of ALS determination in short children. In a study of 27 patients with severe GHD due to a mutation in the GH-releasing hormone receptor, ALS showed complete separation between GHD and control subjects [70]. In another study of 44 short children, Barrios et al. [71] found a lower sensitivity (67 vs. 88%) but a higher specificity (70 vs. 65%) for ALS compared with IGF-1. The diagnostic value of IGFBP-2 has been evaluated in a few studies. IGFBP-2 was elevated in GHD children, but did not show superior diagnostic performance compared with that of IGF-1 [32]. Thus, ALS or IGFBP-2 determination did not seem to add diagnostic value beyond that obtained from IGF-1 and IGFBP-3. Altogether, these studies have evaluated the ability of IGF-1 and IGFBP-3 to predict the outcome of GH provocative testing which in turn may not necessarily indicate a good growth response following GH therapy.

One practical approach to overcome some of the problems with the interpretation of GH provocative test results has been suggested by Rosenfeld [72]. He suggests the use of the term 'insulin-like growth factor deficiency', instead of GHD, in short, poorly growing children with low IGF-1 levels and to disregard any peak GH value from a pharmacological provocation test. This implies that the biochemical diagnosis supporting GH treatment in short children would be exclusively based on the determination of IGF-1 and/or IGFBP-3. The important issue is not to be able to predict the outcome of an unphysiological test such as the GH provocation test, but to predict which children will benefit from GH therapy.

Diagnosis of Growth Hormone Deficiency in Adults

The beneficial effects of GH replacement therapy in adults with GHD are well established. Unlike poor growth in children, there is no obvious biological endpoint to support the diagnosis in adults suspected of GHD. Therefore, the criteria for referral of adult patients for GH testing must include a high index of suspicion such as previous GH treatment in childhood because of childhood-onset GHD (CO-GHD), and in adults, in case of known or suspected pituitary disease leading to adult-onset GHD (AO-GHD). The role of IGF-1 in the diagnosis of adult GHD has been debated ever since the initial report by Hoffman et al. [73], in which they demonstrated that the majority of patients (16 out of 23) had IGF-1 values within the normal range of normal subjects. However, in that study, only AO-GHD patients with a mean age of 45 years participated, and a small group of 35 healthy subjects with a wide variation in age (17–78 years) served as controls [73]. Soon thereafter, de Boer et al. [74] demonstrated in a larger study of 50 adults with CO-GHD that almost all patients (96%) had subnormal IGF-1 levels. Several authors have subsequently shown that patients with CO-GHD have lower baseline IGF-1 levels compared with AO-GHD patients [75]. In a study of 108 young CO-GHD patients who were reevaluated after completion of linear growth, 29 patients (27%) had normal a response to oral clonidine [76]. Sixty of the 79 patients with persistent GHD (76%) had IGF-1 levels below –2 SD adjusted for age, and IGF-1 SDS significantly decreased with increasing number of additional hormone deficiencies, and below –2 SD in all patients with two or more additional pituitary deficiencies. In 29 of the previously GH-treated patients who had a normal response, IGF-1 levels were within the normal range in 72% of the cases [76]. The percentage of patients with normal GH secretion at reevaluation represents minimal numbers, because the clonidine test is no longer considered useful in the evaluation of adults due to the large number of healthy subjects who have a pathologically low GH response to clonidine [46]. Different provocative agents have varying potency in stimulating GH release in adults [77]. The recommended 'gold standard' GH stimulation test is the insulin tolerance test, which, however, exhibits poor reproducibility [78], is associated with uncomfortable side effects and is even dangerous in patients with coronary heart disease or seizure disorders. In addition, the time between cessation of GH therapy and GH provocative testing may vary among the different studies, but retesting 1–3 months after GH therapy is recommended [79]. Maghnie et al. [80] found a continuous decline in IGF-1 and IGFBP-3 6–12 months after GH withdrawal, suggesting a limited diagnostic value of IGF-1 and IGFBP-3 in the first 6–12 months after stopping GH therapy. The use of age-appropriate normal ranges provided by the assay kit manufacturer should be discouraged, as demonstrated in two studies comparing their own reference ranges with those obtained from kit inserts [47, 81]. The diagnostic sensitivity and specificity of IGF-1 vary between studies of GHD patients with approximate sensitivities of 76–96 and 55% for CO-GHD and AO-GHD patients, respectively [47, 73, 74, 76, 81, 82–97]. Interestingly, Hartman et al. [97] analyzed data from 817 adult GHD patients enrolled in a large register-based study (HypoCCS) and found that IGF-1 levels below a certain cutoff value reliably predicted GHD with a PPV of 95%. If low IGF-1 values were combined with the presence of 3 or 4 additional hormone deficits, the PPV was 100%, as previously suggested [76, 81]. Altogether, it can be concluded that IGF-1 is a useful diagnostic test in identifying young adults with severe CO-GHD, provided that normal ranges are strictly defined with a sufficiently large number of age- and sex-matched controls. Furthermore, the diagnostic value of IGF-1 is higher in younger subjects compared with older subjects [81, 82, 85, 90, 98, 99]. Age stratification of GHD patients resulted in a sensitivity of 82% and a specificity of 100% in 20- to 30-year-old patients, as compared with a sensitivity of 87.5% but a specificity of 41.5% in 50- to 60-year-old patients [90]. In addition, IGF-1 is a better diagnostic marker in females suspected of GHD compared with males [85, 96, 100]. Determination of free IGF-1 [27], IGFBP-3 [73, 76, 96] and ALS [22, 47, 95] does not seem to offer any advantage over IGF-1 in adults suspected of GHD. In adults with AO-GHD, neither of the analyses can be used as single diagnostic tools. In adults suspected of AO-GHD, a low serum level of IGF-1, especially in combination with multiple pituitary hormone deficiency, is highly indicative of GHD, whereas a normal IGF-1 level necessitates GH provocative testing.

A recent study evaluated the diagnostic use of IGF-1 in the transition period between childhood and adulthood [101]. In this specific period (from attainment of final height until 25 years of age), CO-GHD should be confirmed before adult replacement is considered. The authors concluded that 77% of GHD subjects would be correctly identified using an IGF-1 SDS cutoff value of –1.7 [101].

Monitoring of Growth Hormone Treatment

Childhood GH Replacement Therapy
The relevance of IGF-1 and IGFBP-3 measurements during GH therapy in GHD children has not been evaluated in depth. In theory, assessment of serum IGF-1 and IGFBP-3 during GH therapy could potentially aid in predicting the growth response to therapy, identify noncompliance and assure the safety of GH therapy. During the first year of GH treatment, serum IGF-1 levels increase significantly [102], depending on the GH dose [103, 104] and gender of the child [104]. Serum IGF-1 levels in GH-treated individuals demonstrate a wide range of responsiveness. The IGF-1 increase 24 h after GH administration was

positively correlated with total body fat and leptin levels, but not with the pubertal stage and gender of the child [105]. Sex steroid priming with testosterone had no effect on the IGF-1 increase, whereas priming with ethinylestradiol reduced the increase in IGF-1 after short-term GH administration [105]. IGF-1 levels exceeded the 95th centile in 2.3% of prepubertal GHD children during conventional GH treatment (26 μg/kg/day), whereas supranormal IGF-1 levels were observed in 20% of prepubertal non-GHD children receiving GH treatment in higher doses (39 μg/kg/day) [106]. In another study, 27% of GHD children treated with a higher dose of GH (50 μg/kg/day) displayed IGF-1 values above the normal range for age and sex [104]. It is likely that prepubertal children in whom GH therapy is initiated to achieve substantial catch-up growth may need supraphysiological IGF-1 levels (exceeding +2 SD) for a shorter period of time to obtain this effect. However, long-term supraphysiological elevations of IGF-1 levels should be avoided. Titration of GH dose according to age- and sex-adjusted IGF-1 values seem a physiological sound principle and analogous to monitoring replacement therapy for other endocrine deficiencies such as hypothyroidism. Future studies will determine whether IGF-1 monitoring and individual dose optimization taking IGF-1 values into account will lead to better growth responses and fewer long-term side effects.

Adult GH Replacement Therapy
Concern about the long-term consequences of overtreatment with GH has caused attention and introduced a shift towards the use of biochemical indices of GH, like IGF-1, in the monitoring of GH substitution in adults. In healthy subjects, IGF-1 and IGFBP-3 increased during a short-term study in which varying GH doses were administered for 4 days (1.25 up to 20 μg/kg/day) [107]. In this study, no detectable effects were seen after administration of 1.25 μg/kg/day, whereas significant increases following 2.5 μg/kg/day were seen in men but not in women. Another study found small but significant increases in IGF-1 after 1.7 μg/kg/day in healthy subjects [108]. IGFBP-3 levels were not modified by 1.25 or 2.5 μg/kg/day, but at 5.0 μg/kg/day, increases were seen in men but not in women. At higher doses, IGF-1 and IGFBP-3 increased in both sexes [107]. In GHD adults, IGF-1 increased 4–6 h after intravenous administration of GH [109]. Initial studies of metabolic effects of GH in adults with GHD used high doses (2 IU/m^2) which were comparable with the doses used in childhood [110]. These relatively high doses resulted in increased IGF-1 and IGFBP-3 levels into the normal range in all male patients in a 4-month placebo-controlled study of GH replacement in CO-GHD young adults, although with large variation, and 2 out of 13 patients had supranormal IGF-1 levels [111]. Similarly, IGFBP-3 and ALS levels increased following GH administration, although both these parameters did not increase to the same extent as did IGF-1 [111]. These findings are in accordance with the study of de Boer et al. [112] who studied 50 young males with CO-GHD and examined several parameters to estimate the optimal GH dose: IGF-1, IGFBP-3, ALS, tissue hydration, and being free of clinical signs or symptoms indicative of GH excess. They found that IGF-1 was more sensitive and useful than IGFBP-3 and ALS for the purpose of dose monitoring in adults with GHD [112]. IGF-1 levels were supranormal (above 2 SD) in approximately 20% of 448 GHD patients treated with GH using a weight-based dosing regimen (up to a maximum of 11 μg/kg/day) [113]. During treatment with 3–6 μg/kg/day, supranormal IGF-1 levels were seen in 6.0% of males with AO-GHD, whereas 36.6% of males with CO-GHD had supranormal IGF-1 levels (>2 SD) after 6 months of 6–12 μg/kg/day recombinant GH [114]. Patients who develop side effects during GH replacement therapy have significantly higher IGF-1 levels compared with those without GH-related adverse events [115]. The considerable variation in responsive-

ness to GH in adults may depend on body composition and GH-binding protein levels [116], but baseline GH-binding protein did not predict the change in IGF-1 SDS during GH therapy in 20 adults with GHD [117]. Age per se may affect the increase in IGF-1 following physiological GH replacement therapy, as elderly individuals require lower doses compared with younger patients [118]. Furthermore, a significant gender effect has been shown in numerous studies. Men with GHD are more responsive to GH replacement therapy than GHD women, resulting in higher GH-induced IGF-1 serum levels in males compared with females at the same GH dose [119–125]. Finally, pretreatment IGF-1 was found to be a major negative determinant of the GH dosage in adults [126]. The effect of age, gender and age at onset of GHD on the final GH dose may be accounted for by the lower pretreatment IGF-1 SDS in young, female and childhood-onset patients relative to older, male and adult-onset patients [126]. In summary, it is now recommended to commence a patient on a low dose of GH and increase it according to the individual clinical responses and changes in IGF-1 levels to reduce occurrence of short-term as well as long-term side effects.

Concluding Remarks

Serum IGF-1 is now readily determined by commercially available assays, and measurements of IGF-1 have become routine in the evaluation of short children suspected of GHD. Some problems remain with respect to the interpretation of the results. Clearly, the need for proper age-related reference ranges is obvious. Nevertheless, with the availability of such, IGF-1 has proven a valuable tool in the diagnosis of childhood GHD. In adults, the diagnostic use of IGF-1 may be limited to patients with CO-GHD in the transition period or later, whereas its diagnostic use in AO-GHD patients is limited. IGF-1 assessment during GH treatment is considered standard practice during adult GH replacement, whereas this has not yet gained proper attention in the management of childhood GHD.

References

1 LeRoith D, Werner H, Beitner-Johnson D, Roberts CT: Molecular and cellular aspects of the insulin-like growth factor I receptor. Endocr Rev 1995;16:143–163.
2 Siebler T, Lopaczynski W, Terry CL, Casella SJ, Munson P, De Leon DD, Phang L, Blakemore KJ, McEvoy RC, Kelley RI: Insulin-like growth factor I receptor expression and function in fibroblasts from two patients with deletion of the distal long arm of chromosome 15. J Clin Endocrinol Metab 1995; 80:3447–3457.
3 Hattori Y, Vera JC, Rivas CI, Bersch N, Bailey RC, Geffner ME, Golde DW: Decreased insulin-like growth factor I receptor expression and function in immortalized African Pygmy T cells. J Clin Endocrinol Metab 1996;81:2257–2263.
4 Nielsen FC: The molecular and cellular biology of insulin-like growth factor II. Prog Growth Factor Res 1992;4:257–290.
5 Steele-Perkins G, Turner J, Edman JC, Hari J, Pierce SB, Stover C, Rutter WJ, Roth RA: Expression and characterization of a functional human insulin-like growth factor I receptor. J Biol Chem 1988;263:11486–11492.
6 Baxter RC, Binoux MA, Clemmons DR, Conover CA, Drop SL, Holly JM, Mohan S, Oh Y, Rosenfeld RG: Recommendations for nomenclature of the insulin-like growth factor binding protein superfamily. J Clin Endocrinol Metab 1998;83:3213.
7 Baxter RC: Circulating levels and molecular distribution of the acid-labile (alpha) subunit of the high molecular weight insulin-like growth factor-binding protein complex. J Clin Endocrinol Metab 1990;70:1347–1353.
8 Arany E, Afford S, Strain AJ, Winwood PJ, Arthur MJ, Hill DJ: Differential cellular synthesis of insulin-like growth factor binding protein-1 (IGFBP-1) and IGFBP-3 within human liver. J Clin Endocrinol Metab 1994;79:1871–1876.
9 Chin E, Zhou J, Dai J, Baxter RC, Bondy CA: Cellular localization and regulation of gene expression for components of the insulin-like growth factor ternary binding protein complex. Endocrinology 1994;134:2498–2504.

10 Juul A, Dalgaard P, Blum WF, Bang P, Hall K, Michaelsen KF, Muller J, Skakkebaek NE: Serum levels of insulin-like growth factor (IGF)-binding protein-3 (IGFBP-3) in healthy infants, children, and adolescents: the relation to IGF-I, IGF-II, IGFBP-1, IGFBP-2, age, sex, body mass index, and pubertal maturation. J Clin Endocrinol Metab 1995;80: 2534–2542.

11 Holman SR, Baxter RC: Insulin-like growth factor binding protein-3: factors affecting binary and ternary complex formation. Growth Regul 1996;6: 42–47.

12 Baxter RC: Glycosaminoglycans inhibit formation of the 140 kDa insulin-like growth factor-binding protein complex. Biochem J 1990;271:773–777.

13 Cook JS, Hoffman RP, Stene MA, Hansen JR: Effects of maturational stage on insulin sensitivity during puberty. J Clin Endocrinol Metab 1993;77:725–730.

14 Luna AM, Wilson DM, Wibbelsman CJ, Brown RC, Nagashima RJ, Hintz RL, Rosenfeld RG: Somatomedins in adolescence: a cross-sectional study of the effect of puberty on plasma insulin-like growth factor I and II levels. J Clin Endocrinol Metab 1983;57:268–271.

15 Argente J, Barrios V, Pozo J, Munoz MT, Hervas F, Stene M, Hernandez M: Normative data for insulin-like growth factors (IGFs), IGF-binding proteins, and growth hormone-binding protein in a healthy Spanish pediatric population: age- and sex-related changes. J Clin Endocrinol Metab 1993;77:1522–1528.

16 Blumsohn A, Hannon RA, Wrate R, Barton J, al-Dehaimi AW, Colwell A, Eastell R: Biochemical markers of bone turnover in girls during puberty. Clin Endocrinol (Oxf) 1994;40:663–670.

17 Juul A, Bang P, Hertel NT, Main K, Dalgaard P, Jorgensen K, Muller J, Hall K, Skakkebaek NE: Serum insulin-like growth factor-I in 1030 healthy children, adolescents, and adults: relation to age, sex, stage of puberty, testicular size, and body mass index. J Clin Endocrinol Metab 1994;78:744–752.

18 Lofqvist C, Andersson E, Gelander L, Rosberg S, Blum WF, Albertsson WK: Reference values for IGF-I throughout childhood and adolescence: a model that accounts simultaneously for the effect of gender, age, and puberty. J Clin Endocrinol Metab 2001;86:5870–5876.

19 Wilson DM, Stene MA, Killen JD, Hammer LD, Litt IF, Hayward C, Taylor CB: Insulin-like growth factor binding protein-3 in normal pubertal girls. Acta Endocrinol (Copenh) 1992;126:381–386.

20 Blum WF, Ranke MB, Kietzmann K, Gauggel E, Zeisel HJ, Bierich JR: A specific radioimmunoassay for the growth hormone (GH)-dependent somatomedin-binding protein: its use for diagnosis of GH deficiency. J Clin Endocrinol Metab 1990;70:1292–1298.

21 Juul A, Scheike T, Nielsen CT, Krabbe S, Muller J, Skakkebaek NE: Serum insulin-like growth factor I (IGF-I) and IGF-binding protein 3 levels are increased in central precocious puberty: effects of two different treatment regimens with gonadotropin-releasing hormone agonists, without or in combination with an antiandrogen (cyproterone acetate). J Clin Endocrinol Metab 1995; 80:3059–3067.

22 Juul A, Moller S, Mosfeldt-Laursen E, Rasmussen MH, Scheike T, Pedersen SA, Kastrup KW, Yu H, Mistry J, Rasmussen S, Muller J, Henriksen J, Skakkebaek NE: The acid-labile subunit of human ternary insulin-like growth factor binding protein complex in serum: hepatosplanchnic release, diurnal variation, circulating concentrations in healthy subjects, and diagnostic use in patients with growth hormone deficiency. J Clin Endocrinol Metab 1998; 83:4408–4415.

23 Nimura A, Katsumata N, Horikawa R, Tanae A, Tanaka T: Acid-labile subunit (ALS) measurements in children. Endocr J 2000;47(suppl):S111–S114.

24 Barrios V, Pozo J, Munoz MT, Buno M, Argente J: Normative data for total and free acid-labile subunit of the human insulin-like growth factor-binding protein complex in pre- and full-term newborns and healthy boys and girls throughout postnatal development. Horm Res 2000;53:148–153.

25 Juul A, Flyvbjerg A, Frystyk J, Muller J, Skakkebaek NE: Serum concentrations of free and total insulin-like growth factor-I, IGF binding proteins-1 and -3 and IGFBP-3 protease activity in boys with normal or precocious puberty. Clin Endocrinol (Oxf) 1996;44:515–523.

26 Blum WF, Horn N, Kratzsch J, Jorgensen JO, Juul A, Teale D, Mohnike K, Ranke MB: Clinical studies of IGFBP-2 by radioimmunoassay. Growth Regul 1993;3:100–104.

27 Juul A, Holm K, Kastrup KW, Pedersen SA, Michaelsen KF, Scheike T, Rasmussen S, Muller J, Skakkebaek NE: Free insulin-like growth factor I serum levels in 1430 healthy children and adults, and its diagnostic value in patients suspected of growth hormone deficiency. J Clin Endocrinol Metab 1997;82:2497–2502.

28 Giwercman B, Giwercman A, Kastrup KW, Skakkebaek NE: Age- and sex-related variations in the serum concentration of somatomedin C in normal children and adults. Ugeskr Laeger 1987;149:1320–1323.

29 Rikken B, van Doorn J, Ringeling A, van den Brande JL, Massa G, Wit JM: Plasma levels of insulin-like growth factor (IGF)-I, IGF-II and IGF-binding protein-3 in the evaluation of childhood growth hormone deficiency. Horm Res 1998;50:166–176.

30 Rasat R, Livesey JL, Espiner EA, Abbott GD, Donald RA: IGF-1 and IGFBP-3 screening for disorders of growth hormone secretion. N Z Med J 1996;109: 156–159.

31 Suwa S, Katsumata N, Maesaka H, Tokuhiro E, Yokoya S: Serum insulin-like growth factor I (somatomedin-C) level in normal subjects from infancy to adulthood, pituitary dwarfs and normal variant short children. Endocrinol Jpn 1988;35:857–864.

32 Ranke MB, Schweizer R, Elmlinger MW, Weber K, Binder G, Schwarze CP, Wollmann HA: Significance of basal IGF-I, IGFBP-3 and IGFBP-2 measurements in the diagnostics of short stature in children. Horm Res 2000;54:60–68.

33 Hall CM, Gill MS, Foster P, Pennells L, Tillmann V, Jones J, Price DA, Clayton PE: Relationship between serum and urinary insulin-like growth factor-I through childhood and adolescence: their use in the assessment of disordered growth. Clin Endocrinol (Oxf) 1999;50:611–618.

34 Mitchell H, Dattani MT, Nanduri V, Hindmarsh PC, Preece MA, Brook CG: Failure of IGF-I and IGFBP-3 to diagnose growth hormone insufficiency. Arch Dis Child 1999;80:443–447.

35 Rosenfeld RG, Wilson DM, Lee PD, Hintz RL: Insulin-like growth factors I and II in evaluation of growth retardation. J Pediatr 1986;109:428–433.

36 Rose SR, Ross JL, Uriarte M, Barnes KM, Cassorla FG, Cutler GB: The advantage of measuring stimulated as compared with spontaneous growth hormone levels in the diagnosis of growth hormone deficiency. N Engl J Med 1988;319:201–207.

37 Albertsson-Wikland K, Rosberg S, Hall K: Spontaneous secretion of growth hormone and serum levels of insulin-like growth factor I and somatomedin binding protein in children of different growth rates; in Isaksson O, Binder C, Hall K, Hökfelt B (eds): Growth Hormone – Basic and Clinical Aspects. Amsterdam, Elsevier Science Publishers BV (Biomedical Division), 1987, pp 163–175.

38 Saggese G, Cesaretti G, Cioni C, Cinguanta L, Ginanessi N: Relationship between plasma somatomedin C levels and 24-hour spontaneous growth hormone secretion in short children. J Pediatr Endocrinol Metab 1991;4:159–166.

39 Blum WF, Albertsson-Wikland K, Rosberg S, Ranke MB: Serum levels of insulin-like growth factor I (IGF-I) and IGF binding protein 3 reflect spontaneous growth hormone secretion. J Clin Endocrinol Metab 1993;76:1610–1616.

40 Achermann JC, Brook CG, Robinson IC, Matthews DR, Hindmarsh PC: Peak and trough growth hormone (GH) concentrations influence growth and serum insulin like growth factor-1 (IGF-1) concentrations in short children. Clin Endocrinol (Oxf) 1999;50:301–308.

41 Achermann JC, Hindmarsh PC, Brook CG: The relationship between the growth hormone and insulin-like growth factor axis in long-term survivors of childhood brain tumours. Clin Endocrinol (Oxf) 1998;49:639–645.

42 Phillip M, Chalew SA, Kowarski AA, Stene MA: Plasma IGFBP-3 and its relationship with quantitative growth hormone secretion in short children. Clin Endocrinol (Oxf) 1993;39:427–432.

43 Nunez SB, Municchi G, Barnes KM, Rose SR: Insulin-like growth factor I (IGF-I) and IGF-binding protein-3 concentrations compared to stimulated and night growth hormone in the evaluation of short children – a clinical research center study. J Clin Endocrinol Metab 1996;81:1927–1932.

44 Rudman D, Kutner MH, Rogers CM, Lubin MF, Fleming GA, Bain RP: Impaired growth hormone secretion in the adult population: relation to age and adiposity. J Clin Invest 1981;67:1361–1369.

45 Reutens AT, Hoffman DM, Leung KC, Ho KK: Evaluation and application of a highly sensitive assay for serum growth hormone (GH) in the study of adult GH deficiency. J Clin Endocrinol Metab 1995;80:480–485.

46 Vahl N, Jorgensen JO, Jurik AG, Christiansen JS: Abdominal adiposity and physical fitness are major determinants of the age associated decline in stimulated GH secretion in healthy adults. J Clin Endocrinol Metab 1996;81:2209–2215.

47 Baum HB, Biller BM, Katznelson L, Oppenheim DS, Clemmons DR, Cannistraro KB, Schoenfeld DA, Best SA, Klibanski A: Assessment of growth hormone (GH) secretion in men with adult-onset GH deficiency compared with that in normal men – a clinical research center study. J Clin Endocrinol Metab 1996;81:84–92.

48 Corpas E, Harman SM, Blackman MR: Serum IGF-binding protein-3 is related to IGF-I, but not to spontaneous GH release, in healthy old men. Horm Metab Res 1992;24:543–545.

49 Marin G, Domene HM, Barnes KM, Blackwell BJ, Cassorla FG, Cutler GB: The effects of estrogen priming and puberty on the growth hormone response to standardized treadmill exercise and arginine-insulin in normal girls and boys. J Clin Endocrinol Metab 1994;79:537–541.

50 Martinez AS, Domene HM, Ropelato MG, Jasper HG, Pennisi PA, Escobar ME, Heinrich JJ: Estrogen priming effect on growth hormone (GH) provocative test: a useful tool for the diagnosis of GH deficiency. J Clin Endocrinol Metab 2000;85:4168–4172.

51 Ghigo E, Bellone J, Aimaretti G, Bellone S, Loche S, Cappa M, Bartolotta E, Dammacco F, Camanni F: Reliability of provocative tests to assess growth hormone secretory status. Study in 472 normally growing children. J Clin Endocrinol Metab 1996;81:3323–3327.

52 Granada ML, Sanmarti A, Lucas A, Salinas I, Carrascosa A, Foz M, Audi L: Assay-dependent results of immunoassayable spontaneous 24-hour growth hormone secretion in short children. Acta Paediatr Scand Suppl 1990;370:63–70; discussion 71.

53 Andersson AM, Orskov H, Ranke MB, Shalet S, Skakkebaek NE: Interpretation of growth hormone provocative tests: comparison of cut-off values in four European laboratories. Eur J Endocrinol 1995;132:340–343.

54 Zapf J, Walter H, Froesch ER: Radioimmunological determination of insulin-like growth factors I and II in normal subjects and in patients with growth disorders and extrapancreatic tumor hypoglycemia. J Clin Invest 1981;68:1321–1330.

55 Furlanetto RW, Underwood LE, Van Wyk JJ, D'Ercole AJ: Estimation of somatomedin-C levels in normals and patients with pituitary disease by radioimmunoassay. J Clin Invest 1977;60:648–657.

56 Bala RM, Bhaumick B: Radioimmunoassay of a basic somatomedin: comparison of various assay techniques and somatomedin levels in various sera. J Clin Endocrinol Metab 1979;49:770–777.

57 Juul A, Skakkebaek NE: Prediction of the outcome of growth hormone provocative testing in short children by measurement of serum levels of insulin-like growth factor I and insulin-like growth factor binding protein 3. J Pediatr 1997;130:197–204.

58 Boquete HR, Sobrado PG, Fideleff HL, Sequera AM, Giaccio AV, Suarez MG, Ruibal GF, Miras M: Evaluation of diagnostic accuracy of insulin-like growth factor (IGF)-I and IGF-binding protein-3 in growth hormone-deficient children and adults using ROC plot analysis. J Clin Endocrinol Metab 2003;88:4702–4708.

59 Lee PD, Wilson DM, Rountree L, Hintz RL, Rosenfeld RG: Efficacy of insulin-like growth factor I levels in predicting the response to provocative growth hormone testing. Pediatr Res 1990;27: 45–51.

60 Smith WJ, Nam TJ, Underwood LE, Busby WH, Celnicker A, Clemmons DR: Use of insulin-like growth factor-binding protein-2 (IGFBP-2), IGFBP-3, and IGF-I for assessing growth hormone status in short children. J Clin Endocrinol Metab 1993;77:1294–1299.

61 Cianfarani S, Boemi S, Spagnoli A, Cappa M, Argiro G, Vaccaro F, Manca BM, Boscherini B: Is IGF binding protein-3 assessment helpful for the diagnosis of GH deficiency? Clin Endocrinol (Oxf) 1995;43:43–47.

62 Hasegawa Y, Hasegawa T, Takada M, Tsuchiya Y: Plasma free insulin-like growth factor I concentrations in growth hormone deficiency in children and adolescents. Eur J Endocrinol 1996; 134:184–189.

63 Bussieres L, Souberbielle JC, Pinto G, Adan L, Noel M, Brauner R: The use of insulin-like growth factor 1 reference values for the diagnosis of growth hormone deficiency in prepubertal children. Clin Endocrinol (Oxf) 2000;52: 735–739.

64 Tillmann V, Buckler JM, Kibirige MS, Price DA, Shalet SM, Wales JK, Addison MG, Gill MS, Whatmore AJ, Clayton PE: Biochemical tests in the diagnosis of childhood growth hormone deficiency. J Clin Endocrinol Metab 1997;82:531–535.

65 Sklar C, Sarafoglou K, Whittam E: Efficacy of insulin-like growth factor binding protein 3 in predicting the growth hormone response to provocative testing in children treated with cranial irradiation. Acta Endocrinol (Copenh) 1993;129:511–515.

66 Weinzimer SA, Homan SA, Ferry RJ, Moshang T: Serum IGF-I and IGFBP-3 concentrations do not accurately predict growth hormone deficiency in children with brain tumours. Clin Endocrinol (Oxf) 1999;51:339–345.

67 Oerter KE, Sobel AM, Rose SR, Cristiano A, Malley JD, Cutler GB, Baron J: Combining insulin-like growth factor-I and mean spontaneous nighttime growth hormone levels for the diagnosis of growth hormone deficiency. J Clin Endocrinol Metab 1992;75:1413–1420.

68 Ranke MB, Schweizer R, Lindberg A, Price DA, Reiter EO, Albertsson-Wikland K, Darendeliler F: Insulin-like growth factors as diagnostic tools in growth hormone deficiency during childhood and adolescence: the KIGS experience. Horm Res 2004;62(suppl 1):17–25.

69 Hasegawa Y, Hasegawa T, Aso T, Kotoh S, Nose O, Ohyama Y, Araki K, Tanaka T, Saisyo S, Yokoya S: Clinical utility of insulin-like growth factor binding protein-3 in the evaluation and treatment of short children with suspected growth hormone deficiency. Eur J Endocrinol 1994;131:27–32.

70 Aguiar-Oliveira MH, Gill MS, de A Barrett ES, Alcantara MR, Miraki-Moud F, Menezes CA, Souza AH, Martinelli CE, Pereira FA, Salvatori R, Levine MA, Shalet SM, Camacho-Hubner C, Clayton PE: Effect of severe growth hormone (GH) deficiency due to a mutation in the GH-releasing hormone receptor on insulin-like growth factors (IGFs), IGF-binding proteins, and ternary complex formation throughout life. J Clin Endocrinol Metab 1999;84:4118–4126.

71 Barrios V, Argente J, Munoz MT, Pozo J, Chowen JA, Hernandez M: Diagnostic interest of acid-labile subunit measurement in relationship to other components of the IGF system in pediatric patients with growth or eating disorders. Eur J Endocrinol 2001;144:245–250.

72 Rosenfeld RG: Is growth hormone deficiency a viable diagnosis? J Clin Endocrinol Metab 1997;82:349–351.

73 Hoffman DM, O'Sullivan AJ, Baxter RC, Ho KK: Diagnosis of growth-hormone deficiency in adults. Lancet 1994; 343:1064–1068.

74 de Boer H, Blok GJ, Popp-Snijders C, van der Veen EA: Diagnosis of growth hormone deficiency in adults. Lancet 1994;343:1645–1646.

75 Janssen YJ, Frolich M, Roelfsema F: A low starting dose of genotropin in growth hormone-deficient adults. J Clin Endocrinol Metab 1997;82:129–135.

76 Juul A, Kastrup KW, Pedersen SA, Skakkebaek NE: Growth hormone (GH) provocative retesting of 108 young adults with childhood-onset GH deficiency and the diagnostic value of insulin-like growth factor I (IGF-I) and IGF-binding protein-3. J Clin Endocrinol Metab 1997;82:1195–1201.

77 Rahim A, Toogood AA, Shalet SM: The assessment of growth hormone status in normal young adult males using a variety of provocative agents. Clin Endocrinol (Oxf) 1996;45:557–562.

78 Hoeck HC, Vestergaard P, Jakobsen PE, Laurberg P: Test of growth hormone secretion in adults: poor reproducibility of the insulin tolerance test. Eur J Endocrinol 1995;133:305–312.

79 Anonymous: Consensus guidelines for the diagnosis and treatment of growth hormone (GH) deficiency in childhood and adolescence: summary statement of the GH Research Society. GH Research Society. J Clin Endocrinol Metab 2000;85:3990–3993.

80 Maghnie M, Strigazzi C, Tinelli C, Autelli M, Cisternino M, Loche S, Severi F: Growth hormone (GH) deficiency (GHD) of childhood onset: reassessment of GH status and evaluation of the predictive criteria for permanent GHD in young adults. J Clin Endocrinol Metab 1999;84:1324–1328.

81 Granada ML, Murillo J, Lucas A, Salinas I, Llopis MA, Castells I, Foz M, Sanmarti A: Diagnostic efficiency of serum IGF-I, IGF-binding protein-3 (IGFBP-3), IGF-I/IGFBP-3 molar ratio and urinary GH measurements in the diagnosis of adult GH deficiency: importance of an appropriate reference population. Eur J Endocrinol 2000;142: 243–253.

82 Hilding A, Hall K, Wivall-Helleryd IL, Saaf M, Melin AL, Thoren M: Serum levels of insulin-like growth factor I in 152 patients with growth hormone deficiency, aged 19–82 years, in relation to those in healthy subjects. J Clin Endocrinol Metab 1999;84:2013–2019.

83 Aimaretti G, Baffoni C, Bellone S, Di Vito L, Corneli G, Arvat E, Benso L, Camanni F, Ghigo E: Retesting young adults with childhood-onset growth hormone (GH) deficiency with GH-releasing-hormone-plus-arginine test. J Clin Endocrinol Metab 2000;85:3693–3699.

84 Aimaretti G, Corneli G, Razzore P, Bellone S, Baffoni C, Bellone J, Camanni F, Ghigo E: Usefulness of IGF-I assay for the diagnosis of GH deficiency in adults. J Endocrinol Invest 1998;21: 506–511.

85 Svensson J, Johannsson G, Bengtsson BA: Insulin-like growth factor-I in growth hormone-deficient adults: relationship to population-based normal values, body composition and insulin tolerance test. Clin Endocrinol (Oxf) 1997;46:579–586.

86 Cuneo RC, Judd S, Wallace JD, Perry-Keene D, Burger H, Lim-Tio S, Strauss B, Stockigt J, Topliss D, Alford F, Hew L, Bode H, Conway A, Handelsman D, Dunn S, Boyages S, Cheung NW, Hurley D: The Australian multicenter trial of growth hormone (GH) treatment in GH-deficient adults. J Clin Endocrinol Metab 1998;83:107–116.

87 Bates AS, Evans AJ, Jones P, Clayton RN: Assessment of GH status in adults with GH deficiency using serum growth hormone, serum insulin-like growth factor-I and urinary growth hormone excretion. Clin Endocrinol (Oxf) 1995;42:425–430.

88 Roelen CA, Koppeschaar HP, de Vries WR, Zelissen PM, Snel YE, Doerga ME, Thijssen JH, Blankenstein RA: High-affinity growth hormone binding protein, insulin-like growth factor I and insulin-like growth factor binding protein 3 in adults with growth hormone deficiency. Eur J Endocrinol 1996;135:82–86.

89 Andersen M, Hansen TB, Støving K, et al: The pyridostigmine-growth hormone-releasing hormone test in adults. The reference interval and a comparison with the insulin tolerance test. Endocrinol Metab 1996;3:197–206.

90 Span JP, Pieters GF, Sweep CG, Swinkels LM, Smals AG: Plasma IGF-I is a useful marker of growth hormone deficiency in adults. J Endocrinol Invest 1999;22:446–450.

91 Toogood AA, Jones J, O'Neill PA, Thorner MO, Shalet SM: The diagnosis of severe growth hormone deficiency in elderly patients with hypothalamic-pituitary disease. Clin Endocrinol (Oxf) 1998;48:569–576.

92 Sassolas G, Chazot FB, Jaquet P, Bachelot I, Chanson P, Rudelli CC, Tauber JP, Allannic H, Bringer J, Roudaut N, Rohmer V, Roger P, Latapie JL, Reville P, Leutenegger M: GH deficiency in adults: an epidemiological approach. Eur J Endocrinol 1999;141:595–600.

93 Musolino NR, Da Cunha N, Marino JR, Giannella-Neto D, Bronstein MD: Evaluation of free insulin-like growth factor-I measurement on the diagnosis and follow-up treatment of growth hormone-deficient adult patients. Clin Endocrinol (Oxf) 1999;50:441–449.

94 Colao A, Cerbone G, Pivonello R, Aimaretti G, Loche S, Di Somma C, Faggiano A, Corneli G, Ghigo E, Lombardi G: The growth hormone (GH) response to the arginine plus GH-releasing hormone test is correlated to the severity of lipid profile abnormalities in adult patients with GH deficiency. J Clin Endocrinol Metab 1999;84:1277–1282.

95 Marzullo P, Di Somma C, Pratt KL, Khosravi J, Diamandis A, Lombardi G, Colao A, Rosenfeld RG: Usefulness of different biochemical markers of the insulin-like growth factor (IGF) family in diagnosing growth hormone excess and deficiency in adults. J Clin Endocrinol Metab 2001;86:3001–3008.

96 Kim HJ, Kwon SH, Kim SW, Park DJ, Shin CS, Park KS, Kim SY, Cho BY, Lee HK: Diagnostic value of serum IGF-I and IGFBP-3 in growth hormone disorders in adults. Horm Res 2001;56:117–123.

97 Hartman ML, Crowe BJ, Biller BM, Ho KK, Clemmons DR, Chipman JJ: Which patients do not require a GH stimulation test for the diagnosis of adult GH deficiency? J Clin Endocrinol Metab 2002;87:477–485.

98 Ghigo E, Aimaretti G, Gianotti L, Bellone J, Arvat E, Camanni F: New approach to the diagnosis of growth hormone deficiency in adults. Eur J Endocrinol 1996;134:352–356.

99 Attanasio AF, Howell S, Bates PC, Blum WF, Frewer P, Quigley C, Shalet SM: Confirmation of severe GH deficiency after final height in patients diagnosed as GH deficient during childhood. Clin Endocrinol (Oxf) 2002;56:503–507.

100 Fisker S, Jorgensen JO, Vahl N, Orskov H, Christiansen JS: Impact of gender and androgen status on IGF-I levels in normal and GH-deficient adults. Eur J Endocrinol 1999;141:601–608.

101 Maghnie M, Aimaretti G, Bellone S, Bona G, Bellone J, Baldelli R, de Sanctis C, Gargantini L, Gastaldi R, Ghizzoni L, Secco A, Tinelli C, Ghigo E: Diagnosis of GH deficiency in the transition period: accuracy of insulin tolerance test and insulin-like growth factor-I measurement. Eur J Endocrinol 2005;152:589–596.

102 Ono T, Kanzaki S, Seino Y, Baylink DJ, Mohan S: Growth hormone (GH) treatment of GH-deficient children increases serum levels of insulin-like growth factors (IGFs), IGF-binding protein-3 and -5, and bone alkaline phosphatase isoenzyme. J Clin Endocrinol Metab 1996;81:2111–2116.

103 de Muinck K, Rikken B, Wynne HJ, Hokken-Koelega AC, Wit JM, Bot A, Drop SL: Dose-response study of biosynthetic human growth hormone (GH) in GH-deficient children: effects on auxological and biochemical parameters. Dutch Growth Hormone Working Group. J Clin Endocrinol Metab 1992;74:898–905.

104 Cohen P, Bright GM, Rogol AD, Kappelgaard AM, Rosenfeld RG: Effects of dose and gender on the growth and growth factor response to GH in GH-deficient children: implications for efficacy and safety. J Clin Endocrinol Metab 2002;87:90–98.

105 Coutant R, Boux dC, Rouleau S, Douay O, Mathieu E, Audran M, Limal JM: Body composition, fasting leptin, and sex steroid administration determine GH sensitivity in peripubertal short children. J Clin Endocrinol Metab 2001;86:5805–5812.

106 Ranke MB, Schweizer R, Elmlinger MW, Weber K, Binder G, Schwarze CP, Wollmann HA: Relevance of IGF-I, IGFBP-3, and IGFBP-2 measurements during GH treatment of GH-deficient and non-GH-deficient children and adolescents. Horm Res 2001;55:115–124.

107 Ghigo E, Aimaretti G, Maccario M, Fanciulli G, Arvat E, Minuto F, Giordano G, Delitala G, Camanni F: Dose-response study of GH effects on circulating IGF-I and IGFBP-3 levels in healthy young men and women. Am J Physiol 1999;276:E1009–E1013.

108 Yuen K, Ong K, Husbands S, Chatelain P, Fryklund L, Gluckman P, Ranke M, Cook D, Rosenfeld R, Wass J, Dunger D: The effects of short-term administration of two low doses versus the standard GH replacement dose on insulin sensitivity and fasting glucose levels in young healthy adults. J Clin Endocrinol Metab 2002;87: 1989–1995.

109 Jorgensen JO, Blum WF, Moller N, Ranke MB, Christiansen JS: Short-term changes in serum insulin-like growth factors (IGF) and IGF binding protein 3 after different modes of intravenous growth hormone (GH) exposure in GH-deficient patients. J Clin Endocrinol Metab 1991;72:582–587.

110 Jorgensen JO, Pedersen SA, Thuesen L, Jorgensen J, Ingemann-Hansen T, Skakkebaek NE, Christiansen JS: Beneficial effects of growth hormone treatment in GH-deficient adults. Lancet 1989;i:1221–1225.

111 Juul A, Andersson AM, Pedersen SA, Jorgensen JO, Christiansen JS, Groome NP, Skakkebaek NE: Effects of growth hormone replacement therapy on IGF-related parameters and on the pituitary-gonadal axis in GH-deficient males. A double-blind, placebo-controlled crossover study. Horm Res 1998;49:269–278.

112 de Boer H, Blok GJ, Popp-Snijders C, Stuurman L, Baxter RC, van der Veen E: Monitoring of growth hormone replacement therapy in adults, based on measurement of serum markers. J Clin Endocrinol Metab 1996;81:1371–1377.

113 Abs R, Bengtsson BA, Hernberg-Stahl E, Monson JP, Tauber JP, Wilton P, Wuster C: GH replacement in 1034 growth hormone deficient hypopituitary adults: demographic and clinical characteristics, dosing and safety. Clin Endocrinol (Oxf) 1999;50:703–713.

114 Kehely A, Bates PC, Frewer P, Birkett M, Blum WF, Mamessier P, Ezzat S, Ho KK, Lombardi G, Luger A, Marek J, Russell-Jones D, Sonksen P, Attanasio AF: Short-term safety and efficacy of human GH replacement therapy in 595 adults with GH deficiency: a comparison of two dosage algorithms. J Clin Endocrinol Metab 2002;87:1974–1979.

115 Chipman JJ, Attanasio AF, Birkett MA, Bates PC, Webb S, Lamberts SW: The safety profile of GH replacement therapy in adults. Clin Endocrinol (Oxf) 1997;46:473–481.

116 Johannsson G, Bjarnason R, Bramnert M, Carlsson LM, Degerblad M, Manhem P, Rosen T, Thoren M, Bengtsson BA: The individual responsiveness to growth hormone (GH) treatment in GH-deficient adults is dependent on the level of GH-binding protein, body mass index, age, and gender. J Clin Endocrinol Metab 1996;81:1575–1581.

117 Florkowski CM, Barnard R, Livesey JH, Veveris T, Espiner EA, Donald RA: Growth hormone binding protein correlates strongly with leptin and percentage body fat in GH-deficient adults, is increased by GH replacement but does not predict IGF-I response. Growth Horm IGF Res 1999; 9:35–40.

118 Toogood AA, Shalet SM: Growth hormone replacement therapy in the elderly with hypothalamic-pituitary disease: a dose-finding study. J Clin Endocrinol Metab 1999;84:131–136.

119 Juul A, Pedersen SA, Sorensen S, Winkler K, Jorgensen JO, Christiansen JS, Skakkebaek NE: Growth hormone (GH) treatment increases serum insulin-like growth factor binding protein-3, bone isoenzyme alkaline phosphatase and forearm bone mineral content in young adults with GH deficiency of childhood onset. Eur J Endocrinol 1994;131:41–49.

120 Burman P, Johansson AG, Siegbahn A, Vessby B, Karlsson FA: Growth hormone (GH)-deficient men are more responsive to GH replacement therapy than women. J Clin Endocrinol Metab 1997;82:550–555.

121 Johansson AG, Engstrom BE, Ljunghall S, Karlsson FA, Burman P: Gender differences in the effects of long term growth hormone (GH) treatment on bone in adults with GH deficiency. J Clin Endocrinol Metab 1999; 84:2002–2007.

122 Hayes FJ, Fiad TM, McKenna TJ: Gender difference in the response of growth hormone (GH)-deficient adults to GH therapy. Metabolism 1999;48:308–313.

123 Drake WM, Coyte D, Camacho-Hubner C, Jivanji NM, Kaltsas G, Wood DF, Trainer PJ, Grossman AB, Besser GM, Monson JP: Optimizing growth hormone replacement therapy by dose titration in hypopituitary adults. J Clin Endocrinol Metab 1998;83:3913–3919.

124 Bengtsson BA, Abs R, Bennmarker H, Monson JP, Feldt-Rasmussen U, Hernberg-Stahl E, Westberg B, Wilton P, Wuster C: The effects of treatment and the individual responsiveness to growth hormone (GH) replacement therapy in 665 GH-deficient adults. KIMS Study Group and the KIMS International Board. J Clin Endocrinol Metab 1999;84:3929–3935.

125 Ekman B, Lindstrom T, Nystrom F, Olsson AG, Toss G, Arnqvist HJ: A dose titration model for recombinant GH substitution aiming at normal plasma concentrations of IGF-I in hypopituitary adults. Eur J Endocrinol 2002;147:49–57.

126 Murray RD, Howell SJ, Lissett CA, Shalet SM: Pre-treatment IGF-I level is the major determinant of GH dosage in adult GH deficiency. Clin Endocrinol (Oxf) 2000;52:537–542.

Insulin-Like Growth Factor 1 Levels in Patients within the KIGS Database

Michael B. Ranke

Insulin-like growth factor 1 (IGF-1) levels can be used as (1) a diagnostic tool in growth hormone deficiency (GHD), (2) response parameters during GH treatment, and (3) safety parameters during GH treatment. Data from KIGS may support the utility of IGF-1 measurements within these contexts. Currently, there is no centralised IGF-1 assaying in KIGS.

Insulin-Like Growth Factor 1 Measurements within KIGS

We elected to analyse cases before the onset of GH therapy with IGF-1 measurements performed in 1995 and thereafter, since by then, IGF-1 measurements had reached a higher degree of standardisation [1]. In order to exclude cases with extreme (thus improbable) readings, we also analysed the data after excluding the highest 5% and all measurements <5 μg/l.

Prepubertal and pubertal patients at onset of GH treatment with the diagnosis of idiopathic GHD (IGHD; KIGS code No. 1.1), i.e. maximum GH to GH testing <10 μg/l, were included into the analysis. In addition, IGF-1 data before GH treatment from prepubertal patients with other selected diagnoses, such as neurosecretory deficiency (NSD), central malformations, pituitary tumours, central nervous system tumours distant to the pituitary, idiopathic short stature (ISS), Turner syndrome (TS) and small for gestational age (SGA), were analysed, as were prepubertal patients with the diagnosis of IGHD (KIGS code No. 1.1) with IGF-1 measurements available before and during the first year on GH (after 3, 6 or 12 months). Transformation of IGF-1 data into standard deviation scores (SDS) was done, based exclusively on the age-related normative references of Juul et al. [2]. Changes in IGF-1 levels during the first-year GH treatment were expressed in terms of (1) IGF-1 (during GH treatment)/basal IGF-1 (micrograms/litre) or (2) Δ IGF-1 SDS. The transformation of the anthropometrical data into SDS as well as statistical procedures were performed according to the published KIGS procedure.

Paediatric Endocrinology Section
University Children's Hospital, University of Tübingen
Hoppe-Seyler-Strasse 1, DE–72076 Tübingen (Germany)

Table 1. Characteristics of all prepubertal and pubertal patients with IGHD and documented serum IGF-1 levels before GH start

Variables	Prepubertal				Pubertal			
	n	median	10th centile	90th centile	n	median	10th centile	90th centile
Background								
Sex (male), %	64.4				73.3			
Birth weight SDS	3,845	−0.7	−2.3	0.8	1,151	−0.5	−2.0	1.0
MPH SDS (Prader)	4,016	−1.2	−2.7	0.4	1,264	−1.1	−2.6	0.5
Maximum GH, μg/l	4,299	6.4	2.1	9.3	1,333	6.1	2.2	9.2
At GH start								
Age, years	4,299	9.0	4.0	13.0	1,333	13.5	11.6	15.7
Height SDS (Prader)	4,297	−3.0	−4.2	−2.0	1,333	−2.4	−3.5	−1.6
Height velocity, cm/year	1,419	4.6	2.9	6.5	371	4.5	2.0	6.9
BMI SDS	4,299	−0.3	−1.8	1.3	1,333	0.0	−1.8	2.0
IGF-1, μg/l	4,299	88	20	204	1,333	179	85	363
IGF-1 SDS	4,299	−1.9	−3.3	−0.4	1,333	−1.9	−3.4	−0.2

MPH = Midparental height; BMI = body mass index.

Results

Basal Levels in IGHD Patients

The characteristics of the IGHD patients at prepubertal (n = 4,299) and pubertal (n = 1,333) GH start are listed in table 1. Before puberty, the median IGF-1 level was 88 μg/l, corresponding to −1.9 SDS. At puberty onset, the median IGF-1 level was 179 μg/l, also corresponding to −1.9 SDS. In only about 10% of the patients, IGF-1 levels above the mean for chronological age were observed. The IGF-1 levels (micrograms/litre) for prepubertal and pubertal children were also illustrated in comparison with the age-related references of Juul et al. [2] (fig. 1). Basal serum IGF-1 SDS levels in prepubertal children with IGHD in relation to the maximum GH (log) levels in tests are illustrated in figure 2. There was a weak (R = 0.2) but significant (p < 0.001) correlation between these parameters.

Basal IGF-1 Levels in Other Patient Groups

The characteristics (medians) of the prepubertal patients with IGHD and other diagnoses are listed in table 2. The data show an overall positive relationship between the degree of GH secretion and the IGF-1 SDS levels. By definition, the IGF-1 levels were in some discordance with GH levels in NSD. However, it is notable that in all short children, IGF-1 levels tend to be low.

IGF-1 Levels in GHD before and during GH Treatment

Patient characteristics and IGF-1 levels before and during the first year on GH in prepubertal patients with IGHD (n = 770) are listed in table 3. During the first year on GH, almost all IGF-1 levels were within the normal range for chronological age. The levels during GH treatment were on the average 2.5 times as high as basal levels. This corresponds to a median increment of 1.5 SDS. The IGF-1 levels (micrograms/litre) during the first prepubertal year on GH in relation to normal references are also illustrated in figure 3.

Patient characteristics and IGF-1 levels before and during the first year on GH in prepubertal patients with NSD, central malformations, pituitary tumours, cranial tumours distant to the pi-

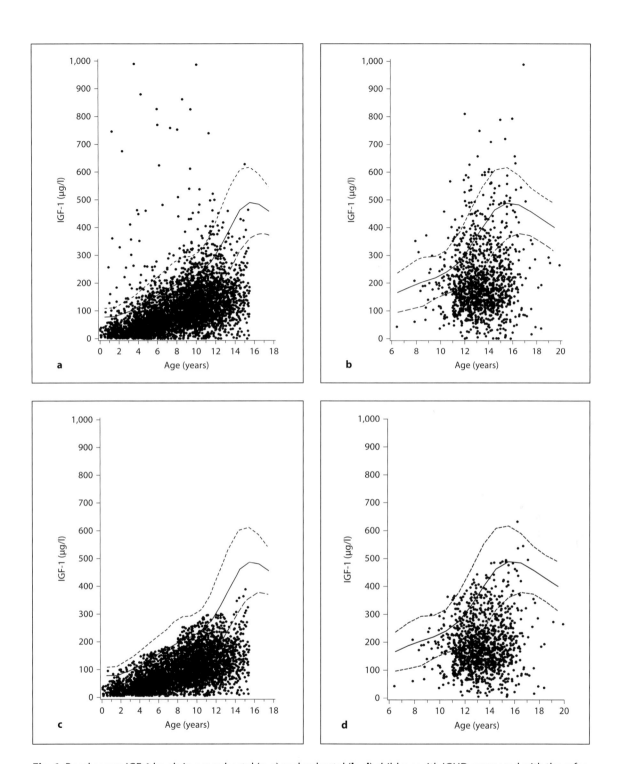

Fig. 1. Basal serum IGF-1 levels in prepubertal (**a**, **c**) and pubertal (**b**, **d**) children with IGHD compared with the references of Juul et al. [2]. **a**, **b** All data analysed; **c**, **d** data analysed excluding the highest 5% and all measurements <5 μg/l. Dashed lines = 3rd and 97th centiles of normal references; solid lines = 50th centile of normal references.

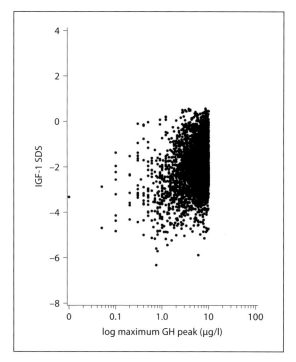
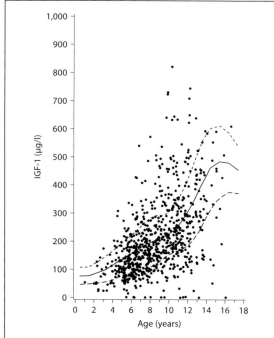

Fig. 2. Basal serum IGF-1 level SDS (excluding the highest 5% and all measurements <5 μg/l) in prepubertal children with IGHD in relation to the maximum GH (log) levels in tests.

Fig. 3. IGF-1 levels during the first year on GH in prepubertal children with IGHD. Dashed lines = 3rd and 97th centiles of normal references; solid line = 50th centile of normal references.

Table 2. Characteristics (medians) of prepubertal patients with various diagnoses and documented serum IGF-1 levels (excluding the highest 5% and all measurements <5 μg/l) before GH treatment

	IGHD	NSD	Central malformations	Pituitary tumours	Cranial tumours distant to the pituitary	ISS	TS	SGA
KIGS code No.	1.1	1.2	2.1.2.+	2.2.1.+	2.2.2.+	3.1.+	3.2.1	3.4+3.5
Patients, n	3,996	371	170	202	170	305	791	566
Sex (male), %	66	69	67	53	67	73	–	67
Maximum GH, μg/l	6.4	13.9	4.4	1.1	4.4	15.5	11.2	15.9
At GH start								
Age, years	9.1	9.6	9.4	10.3	9.4	9.5	9.0	7.7
Height SDS (Prader)	−2.9	−2.9	−2.0	−1.9	−2.0	−3.1	−3.2	−3.2
BMI SDS	−0.4	−0.6	0.4	1.2	0.4	−0.7	0.3	−1.1
IGF-1, μg/l	85	88	76	60	76	92	123	101
IGF-1 SDS	−2.0	−2.0	−2.3	−2.9	−2.3	−1.8	−1.7	−1.3
GH dose, mg/kg/week	0.23	0.21	0.19	0.18	0.20	0.26	0.32	0.31

BMI = Body mass index.

Table 3. Characteristics of prepubertal patients with IGHD with IGF-1 levels documented before and during the first year on GH

Variables	All			
	n	median	10th centile	90th centile
At GH start				
Age, years	770	7.6	4.2	11.5
Height SDS (Prader)	770	−3.0	−3.2	−1.5
BMI SDS	770	−0.4	−1.9	1.2
GH dose, mg/kg/week	770	0.20	0.16	0.27
IGF-1, μg/l	770	72	17	167
IGF-1 SDS	770	−2.0	−3.3	−0.6
During the first year				
Age, years	770	8.6	5.3	12.5
Height SDS (Prader)	770	−2.3	−2.7	−0.8
Height velocity, cm/year	770	8.4	6.1	11.5
Δ height SDS (Prader)	770	0.6	0.2	1.2
Studentised residual (1)−	574	−0.3	−1.5	0.9
Studentised residual (2)+	574	−0.2	−1.7	1.1
Body mass index SDS	769	0.2	−1.0	1.2
IGF-1, μg/l	770	182	76	416
IGF-1 SDS	770	−0.4	−1.9	1.3
IGF-1/basal IGF-1, μg/l	770	2.5	1.4	6.0
Δ IGF-1 SDS	769	1.5	0.3	3.0

Studentised residuals: − = model excluding maximum GH; + = model including maximum GH.

tuitary, ISS, TS and SGA in comparison with IGHD (n = 770) are listed in table 4. The data show that in TS and SGA patients, basal IGF-1 levels are higher compared with those in IGHD patients. Also, GH doses are higher than in the other groups. During the first year, IGF-1 levels are predominantly in the range of the reference, but are above this range in about 10%.

Basal IGF-1 Levels and Changes in IGF-1 Levels in Relation to the First-Year Growth Response in IGHD Patients

Correlation coefficients of simple linear correlations between height response variables (centimetres/year; Δ height SDS) and IGF-1 parameters before and during the first-year GH treatment are listed in table 5. The data show that there is a negative correlation with the response parameters and the basal IGF-1 levels either expressed in micrograms/litre or as SDS. There was no significant correlation between the response parameters and the ratio of IGF-1 during GH treatment to basal IGF-1 expressed in terms of micrograms/litre. However, there was a significant positive correlation with the Δ IGF-1 expressed in terms of SDS.

Furthermore, there was no correlation between basal IGF-1 levels (micrograms/litre or SDS) and the studentised residuals based on the first-year prediction model [3] containing maximum GH levels to tests. However, there was a small but significant negative correlation between the parameters if the model without maximum GH was applied (no data shown). This indicates that the information contained in maximum GH levels to tests and in basal IGF-1 levels is to a certain extent redundant.

The relationship between basal IGF-1 SDS and first-year Δ height SDS during GH treatment in prepubertal children with IGHD is illustrated in

Table 4. Groups of prepubertal children with IGF-1 follow-up during the first year on GH

	IGHD	NSD	CM	PT	CT	ISS	TS	SGA
KIGS Code No.	1.1	1.2	2.1.2.+	2.2.1.+	2.2.2.+	3.1.+	3.2.1	3.4+3.5
Patients, n	770	73	75	35	21	86	206	133
Variables at GH start								
Age, years	7.6	9.0	5.5*	9.1	9.1	7.4	8.6	7.3
Height SDS (Prader)	−3.0	−2.9	−3.3	−2.0*	−1.9*	−3.3	−3.2	−3.3
Body mass index SDS	−0.4	−0.7	−0.3	1.2*	0.6*	−0.7	0.1	−1.2*
GH dose, mg/kg/week	0.20	0.19	0.21	0.17	0.18	0.19	0.31*	0.31*
IGF-1, μg/l	72	78	29*	54	80	91	122*	105*
IGF-1 SDS	−2.0	−2.1	−2.6	−3.0	−2.0	−1.6	−1.6	−1.2*
Variables during the first year								
Age, years	8.6	10.1	6.6*	10.1	10.1	8.5	9.6	8.3
Height SDS (Prader)	−2.3	−2.3	−2.1	−1.4*	−1.4*	−2.8	−2.6	−2.5
Height velocity, cm/year	8.4	7.5	11.1*	9.4	8.6	7.6	7.9	8.9
Δ height SDS (Prader)	0.6	0.5	1.2*	0.7	0.7	0.5	0.6	0.8
Studentised residual (1)−	−0.3	−0.5	0.1	0.1	−0.3	−0.6	−1.2*	−0.2
Studentised residual (2)+	−0.2	0.4	−0.4	−0.8	−0.6	0.5	−0.5	0.5
Δ body mass index SDS	−0.1	0.0	−0.2	−0.4	−0.3	−0.1	0.1	0.2
IGF-1, μg/l	182	193	100*	204	261	193	352*	251*
IGF-1 SDS	−0.4	−0.5	−1.3*	−0.7	0.2	−0.4	0.7*	0.6*
IGF-1/ basal IGF-1, μg/l	2.5	2.5	4.0*	4.0	3.0	2.0	2.8	2.2
Δ IGF-1 SDS	1.5	1.5	1.6	2.4	2.0	1.2	2.3	1.6

Variables are presented as medians. CM = Central malformations; PT = pituitary tumours; CT = cranial tumours distant to the pituitary. Studentised residuals: − = model excluding maximum GH; + = model including maximum GH. * p < 0.01 compared with IGHD.

Table 5. Simple linear correlations between response variables and IGF-1 parameters in IGHD during first-year GH treatment (n = 770)

Parameter	Height velocity, cm/year		Δ height SDS	
	R	p	R	p
Basal IGF-1, μg/l	−0.4	<0.001	−0.3	<0.001
Basal IGF-1 SDS	−0.2	<0.001	−0.1	<0.001
IGF-1 during GH treatment/basal IGF-1, μg/l	−0.0	NS	−0.1	NS
Δ IGF-1 (during GH treatment/basal) SDS	0.2	<0.001	0.2	<0.001

NS = Not significant.

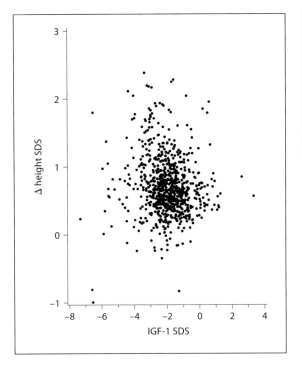 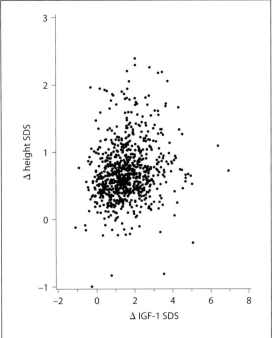

Fig. 4. Relationship between basal IGF-1 SDS and first-year Δ height SDS during GH treatment in prepubertal children with IGHD.

Fig. 5. Relationship between Δ IGF-1 SDS during the first year on GH and first-year Δ height SDS during GH treatment in prepubertal children with IGHD.

figure 4. The relationship between Δ IGF-1 SDS during the first year on GH and first-year Δ height SDS during GH treatment in prepubertal children with IGHD is illustrated in figure 5.

Discussion

IGF-1 in the KIGS Database
While IGF-1 measurements in single centres are commonly done with one assay and the values are compared with assay-specific normative data, the values reported to KIGS are based on a multitude of (commercial or in-house) assays [4]. Thus, the information gathered from KIGS is perhaps not suited to give the highest level of evidence on the diagnostic value of these measurements. However, they may give some valuable information about the general use and robustness of these parameters within the diagnostic process in global practice.

IGF-1 as a Diagnostic Tool in GHD
The confirmation of GHD as the cause of short stature requires (by definition) proof of an impaired/absent GH secretion compared with normality by means of GH measurements [5, 6]. In practice, this is a difficult, invasive and costly task due to the pulsatility of GH secretion and the multitude of biological factors influencing its variability [for a review, see ref. 7]. The diagnostic process proves particularly difficult in cases with idiopathic (no anatomical or genetic abnormality), isolated (no further pituitary hormonal defect) GHD, which is by far the most frequent form of GHD diagnosed in childhood and ado-

lescence. Experience shows that particularly in these instances, GH testing tends to give inaccurate results, both in terms of falsely low and falsely normal readings when compared with the assumed normal range. It is currently accepted that part of the biological effects of GH are (mainly) mediated through IGF-1, whose production and level in blood is GH dependent. It is still not clear whether IGFs in the circulation or IGFs produced at the target site, or both, are the predominant components of the process of bone growth. The somatomedin hypothesis was actually formulated before GH could be measured by observing the absence of a factor in blood (somatomedins = the sum of biologically effective IGFs) in the case of GHD. Therefore, it appears logical that measurements of IGFs are part of the diagnostic process, and it was even suggested that GHD is only a special case of IGF impairment [8].

The performance of IGF-1 measurements in the diagnosis of GHD in short children and adolescents has been extensively studied by a number of authors [for a review, see ref. 2, 9–12]. All these studies follow the same principle. (1) In a varying number of short children, the diagnosis/exclusion of GHD was primarily based on GH stimulation testing. Usually, standard GH stimulation tests were applied. The maximum GH level observed during such tests (commonly two tests) was taken to distinguish between GHD and ISS (non-GHD). The cut-off for this distinction varied between <1 and 10 μg/l. The proportion of individuals with organic causes of GHD varied amongst the groups investigated. (2) In order to define pathological IGF-1 levels, the authors used various normative references and different limits (from below the 10th to below the 0.1st centile). The results in terms of calculated sensitivity (correct diagnosis of GHD) and specificity (correct exclusion of GHD) between the studies varied to a great extent [for a review, see ref. 9]. In general, there was a tendency towards a higher sensitivity over specificity. This means that a low IGF-1 level in a short child is not very likely to be caused by GHD. On the other hand, a normal IGF-1 level is more likely to exclude the possibility of GHD. If the cut-off level of IGF-1 is lowered, then the percentage of sensitivity decreases, while the relative specificity increases. The data also suggest that the diagnostic performance is somewhat better in the older age group of children (>8–10 years). This is probably due to the fact that the limits of normality are low in younger children.

IGF-1 as a Safety Parameter
In adults with GHD, dosing of GH is titrated according to the IGF-1 level [13, 14]. It is assumed that the optimal levels of IGF-1 should be within the upper normal range for sex and age. It has also been shown that levels above the normal range are associated with a higher incidence of side effects. Epidemiological studies in normal adults have shown that the incidence of some malignancies is positively correlated with IGF-1 levels but negatively correlated with IGFBP-3 levels [15–18]. Thus, it is assumed that the relationship between IGF-1 and IGFBP-3 plays an important physiological role. Based on these observations, Park and Cohen [19] have suggested that dosing in children should take IGF-1 levels and their relationship to IGFBP-3 levels into consideration. Even if one accepts that the reasoning based on this suggestion is correct, the realisation appears to be difficult given the limited standardisation of IGF-1 and, in particular, IGFBP-3 measurements. There is no firm empirical basis about the true cut-off of the IGF-1 to IGFBP-3 ratio with regard to safety aspects in children. Intuitively, there is probably no dissension about the assumption that IGF-1 levels – or any other biochemical parameter – should not exceed normal ranges for a long time. However, it is questionable whether a normalisation in height can be achieved with IGF levels always remaining within the normal range in all cases. This is particularly true for disorders with short stature not caused by GHD.

Given the importance of the issue, this area needs to be the subject of structured future research including data collection within KIGS.

IGF-1 as a Response Parameter
It is assumed that longitudinal bone growth is a function of both direct effects of GH and IGF-1-mediated effects at the growth plate. It still remains somewhat obscure which role circulating IGF plays in relation to locally produced IGF. Treatment with IGF-1 in patients with GH resistance has proven that circulating IGF-1 promotes growth in a dose-dependent manner, thus supporting the endocrine role of IGF-1. Based on these facts, it appears reasonable to assume that IGF-1 levels (basal or the changes observed in response to GH treatment) are related to the observed growth response.

The KIGS data analysed in prepubertal patients with IGHD show that growth during the first year is negatively correlated with basal IGF-1 levels. In light of the fact that the degree of GH secretion is positively correlated with IGF-1 levels (fig. 2) and that in prediction models for GHD the maximal GH to stimulation tests is a predictor (negative) of the first-year height response, it is understandable that first-year height velocity is (negatively) correlated to basal IGF-1 levels. Basically, GH and IGF-1 levels contain the same information in disorders with impaired GH secretion.

Our data also show that first-year prepubertal height velocity is positively correlated with the change in IGF-1 levels. This has been described for patients with GHD and other growth disorders [20–22]. In the future, it needs to be investigated whether the change in IGF-1 levels can be utilised to design GH treatment more optimally.

Conclusion

Data from KIGS support the view that IGF-1 levels can be used as a diagnostic tool in GHD, as response parameters during GH treatment, and probably, also as safety parameters during GH treatment [23]. In the future, IGF-1 measurements need to be a mandatory part of GH treatment in children and documented within KIGS.

References

1 Ranke MB, Schweizer R, Lindberg A, Price DA, Reiter EO, Albertsson-Wikland K, Darendeliler F: Insulin-like growth factors as diagnostic tools in growth hormone deficiency during childhood and adolescence: the KIGS experience. Horm Res 2004;62(suppl 1):17–25.

2 Juul A, Dalgaard P, Blum WF, Bang P, Hall K, Michaelsen KF, Muller J, Skakkebaek NE: Serum levels of insulin-like growth factor (IGF)-binding protein-3 (IGFBP-3) in healthy infants, children, and adolescents: the relation to IGF-I, IGF-II, IGFBP-1, IGFBP-2, age, sex, body mass index, and pubertal maturation. J Clin Endocrinol Metab 1995;80:2534–2542.

3 Ranke MB, Lindberg A, Chatelain P, Wilton P, Cutfield W, Albertsson W, Price DA: Derivation and validation of a mathematical model for predicting the response to exogenous recombinant human growth hormone (GH) in prepubertal children with idiopathic GH deficiency. KIGS International Board. Kabi Pharmacia International Growth Study. J Clin Endocrinol Metab 1999; 84:1174–1183.

4 Sensitivity to growth hormone, standardisation of IGF-I measurements. 5th KIGS/KIMS Expert Meeting on Growth Hormone and Growth Disorders. Horm Res 2001;55(suppl 2).

5 GH Research Society: Consensus guidelines for the diagnosis and treatment of growth hormone (GH) deficiency in childhood and adolescence: summary statement of the GH Research Society. GH Research Society. J Clin Endocrinol Metab 2000;85:3990–3993.

6 Shalet SM, Toogood A, Rahim A, Brennan BM: The diagnosis of growth hormone deficiency in children and adults. Endocr Rev 1998;19:203–223.

7 Ranke MB: Diagnosis of growth hormone deficiency and growth hormone stimulation tests; in Ranke MB (ed): Diagnostics of Endocrine Fuction in Children and Adolescents. Karger, Basel, 2003, pp 107–128.

8 Rosenfeld RG, Albertsson-Wikland K, Cassorla F, Frazier SD, Hasegawa Y, Hintz RL, Lafranchi S, Lippe B, Loriaux L, Melmed S, Preece MA, Ranke MB, Reiter EO, Rogol AD, Underwood LE, Werther GA: Diagnostic controversy: The diagnosis of childhood growth hormone deficiency revisited. J Clin Endocrinol Metab 1995;80:1532–1540.

9 Clayton P: The role of insulin-like growth factors in the diagnosis of growth hormone deficiency; in Ranke MB, Wilton P (eds): Growth Hormone Therapy in KIGS – Ten Years of Experience. Barth Verlag, Heidelberg, 1999, pp 53–64.
10 Blum WF, Schweizer R: Insulin-like growth factors and their binding proteins; in Ranke MB (ed): Diagnostics of Endocrine Function in Children and Adolescents. Karger, Basel, 2003, pp 166–199.
11 Mitchell H, Dattani MT, Nanduri V, Hindmarsh PC, Preece MA, Brook CGD: Failure of IGF-I and IGFBP-3 to diagnose growth hormone insufficiency. Arch Dis Child 1999;80:443–447.
12 Ranke MB, Schweizer R, Elmlinger MW, Weber K, Binder G, Schwarze CP, Wollmann HA: Significance of basal IGF-I, IGFBP-3 and IGFBP-2 measurements in the diagnostics of short stature in children. Horm Res 2000;54:60–68.
13 de Boer H, van der Veen E: Guidelines for optimizing growth hormone replacement therapy in adults. Horm Res 1997;48:21–30.
14 Growth Hormone Research Society: Consensus guidelines for the diagnosis and treatment of adults with growth hormone deficiency: summary statement of the Growth Hormone Research Society Workshop on Adult Growth Hormone Deficiency. J Clin Endocrinol Metab 1998;83:379–381.
15 Chan JM, Stampfer MJ, Giovannucci E, Gann PH, Ma J, Wilkinson P, et al: Plasma insulin-like growth factor-I and prostate cancer risk: a prospective study. Science 1998;279:563–566.
16 Burroughs KD, Dunn SE, Barrett JC, Taylor JA: Insulin-like growth factor-I: a key regulator of human cancer risk? J Natl Cancer Inst 1999;91:579–581.
17 Hankinson SE, Willett WC, Colditz GA, Hunter DJ, Michaud DS, Deroo B, et al: Circulating concentrations of insulin-like growth factor-I and risk of breast cancer. Lancet 1998;351:1393–1396.
18 Ma J, Pollak MN, Giovannucci E, Chan JM, Tao Y, Hennekens CH, et al: Prospective study of colorectal cancer risk in men and plasma levels of insulin-like growth factor (IGF)-I and IGF-binding protein-3. J Natl Cancer Inst 1999;91:620–625.
19 Park P, Cohen P: The role of insulin-like growth factor I monitoring in growth-hormone treated children. Horm Res 2004;62(suppl 1):59–65.
20 Ranke MB, Schweizer R, Elmlinger MW, Weber K, Binder G, Schwarze CP, Wollman HA: Relevance of IGF-I, IGFBP-3, and IGFBP-2 measurements during GH treatment of GH-deficient and non-GH-deficient children and adolescents. Horm Res 2001;55:115–124.
21 Ranke MB, Feldt-Rasmussen U, Bang P, Baxter RC, Camacho-Hübner C, Clemmons DR, Juul A, Ørskov H, Strasburger CJ: How should insulin-like growth factor be measured? Horm Res 2001;55(suppl 2):106–109.
22 Boguszewski M, Jansson C, Rosberg S, Albertsson-Wikland K: Changes in serum insulin-like growth factor I (IGF-I) and IGF-binding protein-3 levels during growth hormone treatment in prepubertal short children born small for gestational age. J Clin Endocrinol Metab 1996;81:3902–3908.
23 The role of IGF parameters in the management of growth disorders and acromegaly – diagnosis, efficacy and safety. 7th KIGS/KIMS Expert Meeting on Growth Hormone and Growth Disorders. Horm Res 2004;62(suppl 2).

… Review

Neuroimaging in Growth Hormone Deficiency

Mohamad Maghnie[a]   Natascia di Iorgi[a]   Andrea Rossi[b]
Roberto Gastaldi[a]   Paolo Tortori-Donati[b]   Renata Lorini[a]

Magnetic resonance imaging (MRI) allows a detailed and precise anatomical study of the pituitary gland by differentiating between the anterior and posterior pituitary lobes. The MRI identification of pituitary hyperintensity in the posterior part of the sella, now considered a marker of neurohypophyseal functional integrity, has been the most striking recent finding contributing to the diagnosis and understanding of some forms of 'idiopathic' and permanent growth hormone deficiency (GHD). Indeed, the advent of molecular biology and MRI has led to significant progress in the understanding of the pathogenesis of disorders affecting the hypothalamic-pituitary area. This article reviews the impact of MRI findings in the current management of diseases associated with GHD.

Short Note on the Principle and Technical Requirement

MRI is the imaging modality of first choice in the evaluation of the hypothalamic-pituitary and parasellar regions thanks to its multiplanar capability, noninvasiveness and tissue characterization capabilities. The goal is to obtain high quality images with elevated spatial resolution in a reasonable amount of time. Special considerations in children include incomplete collaboration or need for sedation/anesthesia which may have a significant impact on scanning time and eventual imaging quality. MRI has contraindications, including those represented by pacemakers, vascular clips or other metallic devices, foreign bodies and cochlear implants. Safety issues must be carefully evaluated in individual cases before admitting the patient to the MRI suite.

The maximum information is obtained by acquiring <3-mm-thick, high-resolution T_1- and T_2-weighted images in the sagittal and coronal planes. The coronal plane allows for visualization of the pituitary gland, stalk, chiasm and parasellar regions. Sagittal images are best suited for an evaluation of the midline plane. Ideally, T_1-weighted images should be obtained both before and after intravenous gadolinium chelate ad-

Departments of
[a]Pediatrics and [b]Neuroradiology
IRCCS Giannina Gaslini, University of Genova
Largo Gerolamo Gaslini 5
IT–16147 Genova (Italy)

ministration. The amount of contrast used for the investigation of pituitary adenomas is half the usual dose (i.e. 0.05 mmol/kg) in order to better appreciate the lack of enhancement of the adenoma in contrast to the normally enhancing pituitary gland parenchyma. Other conditions, including diabetes insipidus and precocious puberty, are more conveniently studied with a full-dose contrast material administration in order to improve detection of abnormal enhancing lesions in the pituitary stalk, hypothalamus and pineal gland. Postcontrast imaging can be safely dropped only in patients with isolated GHD, in whom an anatomic characterization of the pituitary gland and stalk is usually sufficient. Axial T_2-weighted images covering the entire brain should also be obtained in all cases in order to screen for possible associated abnormalities.

When MRI is unavailable or contraindicated, computerized tomography remains a viable alternative for imaging the sellar and parasellar regions. The hazards of ionizing radiations, while minimal, should not be overlooked, especially in infants and small children. The coronal plane is the optimal imaging plane, but direct coronal imaging requires hyperextension of the neck which is difficult to obtain in sedated or uncooperative patients. Helical computerized tomography acquisitions offer the opportunity to obtain high-quality coronal (and sagittal) reformatted images from axial acquisitions. Helical imaging is also useful to minimize imaging time and radiation dose administration. Examinations should be performed using 1.5- to 2-mm contiguous slices both before and after intravenous administration of iodized contrast agent.

Normal Anatomy and Magnetic Resonance Imaging Appearance and Size

Normal Anatomy
The pituitary gland consists of two major parts, differing in their origin, structure and function: the neurohypophysis is a diencephalic downgrowth connected with the hypothalamus, whereas the adenohypophysis is an ectodermal derivative of the stomodeum. Both portions include part of the infundibulum, which has a central infundibular stem, called the 'pituitary stalk', and is continuous with the median eminence of the hypothalamus. Surrounding the infundibular stem is the pars tuberalis or infundibularis, a component of the adenohypophysis. The latter can be divided into the pars anterior or distalis and pars intermedia, separated from one another in fetal and early postnatal life by the so-called hypophyseal cleft, a vestige of Rathke's pouch from which the adenohypophysis develops. Usually obliterated in childhood, the hypophyseal cleft may sometimes persist as a variably sized cystic cavitation. In brief, the neurohypophysis includes the pars posterior, the infundibulum or pituitary stalk, and the median eminence, while the adenohypophysis, which makes up about 75% of the gland, includes the pars anterior, pars intermedia and pars tuberalis [1].

MRI Appearance
The pituitary gland undergoes dynamic changes in size and shape throughout life, reflecting its complex hormonal environment (fig. 1). In newborns, the gland is typically convex, sometimes pear shaped, with very high signal intensity on T_1-weighted images. This appearance persists for the first month, but changes during the second month as it progresses towards adult appearance, i.e. with a flat superior surface and isointensity of the anterior lobe on T_1- and T_2-weighted images. In addition, in preterm babies, a bright anterior pituitary gland has recently been reported during the first age-corrected 2 months [2]. By the second month of life, the posterior neural lobe of the gland becomes progressively recognizable next to the dorsum sellae as the 'bright spot', because of its marked hyperintensity on T_1-weighted images. Regardless of its chemical origin, the bright spot serves as an important marker of

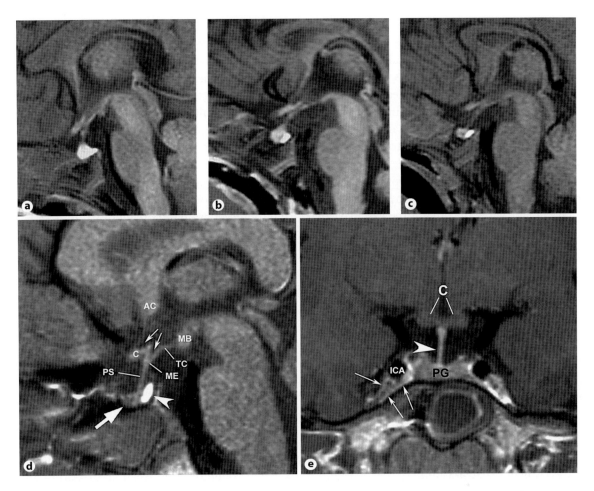

Fig. 1. Normal sellar region. Normal pituitary gland appearance on sagittal T_1-weighted images at different ages. **a** Neonate: typical spontaneous hyperintensity and pear-shaped appearance. **b** At the end of the first month of life: the signal intensity of the anterior pituitary lobe decreases with respect to the posterior bright spot. **c** At 2 months of age: the pituitary gland shows a typical adult pattern. **d** Sagittal T_1-weighted image. The posterior pituitary bright spot (arrowhead), anterior pituitary lobe (thick arrow), pituitary stalk (PS), median eminence (ME), chiasm (C), tuber cinereum (TC) and mammillary bodies (MB) are clearly visible. The chiasmatic and infundibular recesses of the third ventricle are also recognizable (thin arrows). AC = Anterior commissure. **e** Gadolinium-enhanced coronal T_1-weighted image. Following gadolinium injection, the pituitary gland (PG) and cavernous sinuses (thin arrows) are enhanced. The internal carotid arteries (ICA) are recognizable within the cavernous sinuses. The pituitary stalk is clearly visible (arrowhead) in its midline position, generating a T shape together with the overlying optic chiasm (C).

neurohypophyseal function and, when present, documents integrity of the hypothalamic-neurohypophyseal tract. However, it is important to point out that the bright spot may be absent in 10% of normal individuals. The posterior pituitary does not undergo physiological variations in either size or signal intensity during childhood [1].

Following gadopentetate dimeglumine (Gd-DTPA) administration, marked enhancement of the adenohypophysis, due to its high capillary density, and the infundibulo-tuberal region is clearly evident. The appearance of the posterior lobe blends with the anterior lobe due to its spontaneous hyperintensity. A normal pituitary stalk usually tapers smoothly along its course. It is approximately 3 mm in diameter near the optic chiasm and 2 mm where it inserts into the gland; it should not exceed the basilar artery diameter. The pituitary stalk is divided into two parts: one is the neuronal component made up of the track of axons extending from the hypothalamic nuclei down to the axon terminals in the posterior pituitary pouch, while the other is the vascular component that provides blood supply to the anterior pituitary gland from the superior hypophyseal arteries through the pituitary portal system [1].

Normal Pituitary Size

The pituitary gland may have a slightly concave superior margin throughout childhood and is not expected to reach a height of less than 3 mm or greater than 6 mm prior to puberty. During puberty, the pituitary gland undergoes profound changes in size and shape, basically represented by marked enlargement. In girls, the gland may swell symmetrically to a height of 10 mm, appearing nearly spherical, whereas in pubertal boys, it may reach 7–8 mm [1]. The maximum height of the anterior pituitary is measured (sagittal image) on a plane perpendicular to the sella turcica floor, whereas the volume is calculated using the Di Chiro formula [2]: $V = 1/2$ length $\times$ height $\times$ width (underestimated) or, alternatively, V = area $\times$ width (overestimated). Most data on pituitary size and volume come from 1- or 2-dimensional indirect measurements [3], whereas a 3-dimensional (3D) age-related reference range for pituitary volume is currently lacking. Recently, estimated pituitary volumes obtained from 3D MRI sequences were calculated showing a wide variation in pituitary morphology and shape, as well as in the distribution of the signal intensity of both the anterior and posterior pituitary, independent of the subject's age [4]. The overall information provided by this study of the 3D assessment of pituitary volume represents a significant advance over currently used methods. However, the weak correlation between pituitary height and directly measured pituitary volume, as well as between estimated pituitary calculation and measured pituitary volume, make the simple evaluation of pituitary height unreliable. This technique cannot be used with children over 10 years of age or in adolescents. The relative discrepancy between the results of this study and two earlier reports [5, 6], as well as the absence of interobserver evaluation render its results rather incomplete.

Value of Magnetic Resonance Imaging in the Clinical Setting

Idiopathic GHD

Idiopathic GHD (IGHD) is the most common sporadic form of hypopituitarism, and its incidence is estimated to be between 1/4,000 and 1/10,000 among live births. It is a heterogeneous condition whose pathophysiology remains largely unknown. The diagnosis of GHD in childhood can be straightforward when short stature and persistent growth failure are consistently associated with frontal bossing, midfacial hypoplasia, truncal adiposity, small genitalia in the male, and/or hypoglycemia and cholestatic jaundice. However, this presentation tends to be the exception rather than the rule, and thus, the clinical phenotype may not be particularly notable.

Patients with IGHD can present with a variety of pituitary MRI features including normal pituitary gland size, isolated anterior pituitary hypoplasia (congenital) or small pituitary (acquired), empty sella (these 3 conditions present with normal location of the posterior pituitary gland and normal pituitary stalk connecting the hypothalamus to the pituitary gland), as well as moderate (height 2–3 mm) to severe (height <2 mm) pituitary hypoplasia and sella turcica associated with

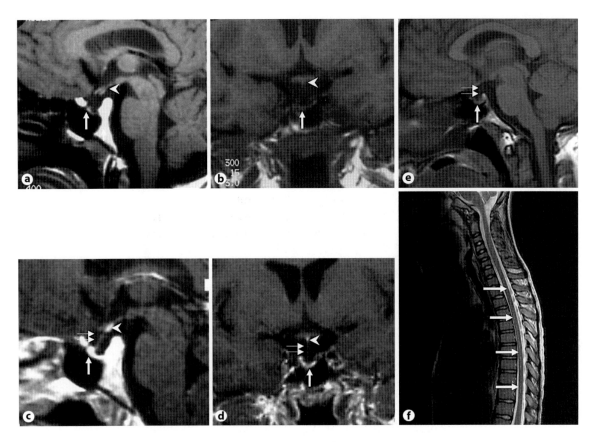

Fig. 2. Patients with CPHD (**a–d, f**) and isolated GHD (**e**). Sagittal (**a, c, e**) and coronal (**b, d**) T$_1$-weighted images before (**a, b, e**) and after (**c, d**) gadolinium injection showing pituitary hypoplasia (white arrows) and ectopic posterior pituitary lobe (white arrowheads). The thin vascular pituitary stalk is identified after contrast medium administration (**c, d**; double white arrows); MRI of the spine showed syringomyelia (**f**; white arrows). **e** Patient with isolated GH, anterior pituitary hypoplasia (white arrow) and normal pituitary stalk (double white arrows).

ectopic posterior pituitary gland at the level of the median eminence or along the stalk projection up to its distal extremity with partial or complete pituitary stalk agenesis (fig. 2). All of these features have been reported with or without additional malformations of the central nervous system [3, 7–20].

In most cases, patients with isolated IGHD show an anterior pituitary gland that is of normal size or 'reduced' at MRI examination of the hypothalamic-pituitary region; ectopic posterior pituitary and anterior pituitary hypoplasia are also common features. A finding of empty sella has been reported in 9% of patients with IGHD [21]. On the contrary, in cases of idiopathic multiple pituitary hormone deficiency (MPHD), the most frequent MRI findings included: (1) moderate to severe anterior pituitary hypoplasia or anterior pituitary aplasia, frequently associated with a sella turcica of reduced size or flattened sella; (2) ectopic posterior pituitary at the median eminence or along the stalk projection up to its distal extremity, the hypoplastic stalk (the maintenance of neurohypophyseal function in these types of patients is demonstrated by the presence, albeit in the ectopic site, of an area of hyperin-

Table 1. Reports from the literature on MRI features in subjects with IGHD (n ≥ 35)

Reference	Year	Patients	MRI			Presenting pituitary functions	
			EPP	HA	NA	IGHD (EPP)	CPHD (EPP)
Bressani et al. [7]	1990	57	34 (59)	23 (40)	0	36 (37)	21 (95)
Maghnie et al. [8]	1991	45	20 (44)	13 (29)	12 (26)	33 (24)	8 (100)
Abrahams et al. [9]	1991	35	15 (43)	20 (57)	15 (43)	2 (10)	13 (87)
Argyropoulou et al. [10]	1992	46	29 (63)	10 (21)	7 (15)	26 (38)	20 (95)
Triulzi et al. [11]	1993	101	59 (48)	ND	ND	67 (44)	34 (85)
Pinto et al. [12]	1997	51	51 (100)	41 (83)	6 (13)	16 (100)	35 (100)
Nagel et al. [13]	1997	56	24 (42)	11 (19)	17 (30)	43 (27)	13 (92)
Kornreich et al. [14]	1997	51	41 (80)	0	10 (20)	23 (56)	28 (100)
Hamilton [15]	1998	35	25 (71)	3 (<1)	2 (<1)	20 (70)	15 (73)
Arifa et al. [16]	1999	100	20 (20)	28 (28)	41 (41)	79 (ND)	19 (ND)
Bozzola et al. [17]	2000	93	30 (32)	69 (65)	24 (35)	5 (8)	25 (76)
Osorio et al. [18]	2002	76	54 (71)	36 (84)	ND	33 (55)[a]	43 (57)[b]
Arends et al. [19]	2002	39	24 (61)	22 (56)	17 (44)	11 (44)	13 (87)

Figures in parentheses are percentages. EPP = Ectopic posterior pituitary; HA = hypoplastic anterior pituitary with normal located posterior pituitary; NA = normal anatomy; ND = not determined.
[a] One patient with GH-1 deletion; [b] 5 Prop1 and 1 Pit1 defects.

tense signal and by a lack of clinical signs suggestive of water metabolism dysfunction); (3) complete agenesis of the pituitary stalk (both nervous and vascular components), and (4) cerebral malformations like Arnold-Chiari I, Arnold-Chiari II, agenesis of the septum pellucidum, septo-optic dysplasia, vermis dysplasia, syringomyelia (fig. 2), absence of the internal carotid artery, dysgenesis of the corpus callosum, arachnoid cysts, and tentorium anomalies with basilar impression [3, 7–20]. The frequency of these radiological findings and their distribution between isolated GHD and combined pituitary hormone deficiency (CPHD) varies among reports. In particular, MPHD has been shown to be associated with ectopic posterior pituitary and anterior pituitary hypoplasia with high frequency, ranging between 57 and 100% of cases; on the other hand, isolated GHD is associated with these particular MRI pituitary features at a lesser rate, ranging between 8 and 100% of cases observed (table 1). The variability between different studies could be attributed to the degree of restriction in diagnostic criteria, the diagnostic limits of GHD (transitory deficits, recovery, false positives) and/or the lack of a convincing standard normal size of the pituitary gland among the prepubertal pediatric population. Idiopathic MPHD has been reported less frequently in association with anterior pituitary hypoplasia and more frequently with normal posterior pituitary and pituitary stalk; under such conditions, the search for gene involvement becomes mandatory. It is worth pointing out that the high frequency of sporadic forms of IGHD associated with ectopic posterior pituitary in the absence of genetic identification remains intriguing, suggesting that other factors may play a role as well.

A detailed study of the pituitary stalk should be carried out following the administration of Gd-DTPA. The finding of a vascular component of the stalk has a great deal of prognostic significance, since patients with agenesis of the pituitary stalk run a greater risk of developing MPHD than

Table 2. Endocrine/pituitary phenotypes and genotypes in genes involved in anterior pituitary development and pituitary dysfunction

Genes	Hormone deficiencies					Pituitary phenotypes	Associated abnormalities
GH-N	GH					normal, EPP	none
GH-1 (IGHD II)	GH		TSH		ACTH	normal to small	none
GHRH-R	GH	PRL (?)				small	none
POU1F1	GH	PRL	TSH			small to normal	none
PROP1	GH	PRL	TSH	LH/FSH	± ACTH	all sizes	none
HESX1	GH	± PRL	± TSH	± LH/FSH	± ACTH	normal, aplasia, APH + EPP, APH	SOD, SOD variants coloboma
LHX3	GH	PRL	TSH	LH/FSH		APH to large	stubby neck, limited rotation
LHX4	GH		TSH	LH/FSH (?)	ACTH	APH, EPP	Chiari I
GLI2	GH	PRL (?)	TSH (?)	LH/FSH (?)	ACTH (?)	APH to aplasia	holoprosencephaly-like
SOX3	GH	PRL (?)	TSH	LH/FSH	ACTH	APH, EPP	mental retardation (?)
SOX2	± GH		± TSH	LH/FSH	± ACTH	normal, APH, EPP	microphthalmia, anophthalmia, CNS abnormalities

EPP = Ectopic posterior pituitary; TSH = thyroid-stimulating hormone; PRL = prolactin; LH = luteinizing hormone; FSH = follicle-stimulating hormone; APH = anterior pituitary hypoplasia; SOD = septo-optic dysplasia; CNS = central nervous system.

those who show a vascular residue of the stalk (fig. 2). Patients in whom a pituitary stalk cannot be identified after Gd-DTPA have, in fact, a risk factor for developing CPHD evolving to panhypopituitarism that is 27 times greater than those with a residual vascular pituitary stalk [22, 23].

Genetic Forms of GHD

The endocrine/pituitary phenotypes and genotypes in genes involved in anterior pituitary development and pituitary dysfunction are summarized in table 2.

Familial Type of IGHD
Four distinct familial types of isolated GHD have been defined on the basis of inheritance and other hormone deficiencies. This classification includes IGHD type IA (autosomal recessive with absent endogenous GH), type IB (autosomal recessive with diminished GH), type II (autosomal dominant with diminished GH), and type III (X-linked with diminished GH) [24].

The MRI appearance in GH-N deletion has been reported in association with normal pituitary anatomy in the few patients in whom MRI scanning has been performed. There have been a few cases reported of pituitary hypoplasia with or without ectopic posterior pituitary [18, 25]. The former association is not suggestive of a causal link, but rather, could simply be a chance occurrence. Conversely, evolving pituitary hormone deficits and pituitary hypoplasia have recently been reported in patients with isolated GHD type II caused by a P89L GH missense mutation [26–28]. This suggests that misfolded proteins may have an adverse impact on the anterior pituitary secretory pathways leading to a local toxic effect with consequent 'acquired' disease.

In the type IB form of familial IGHD caused by GH-releasing hormone receptor (GHRH-R) mutation, MRI findings provide evidence of significantly small anterior pituitary. The great majority of patients (children older than 8 years and adults) with GHRH mutations who have had MRI have a pituitary height that is 2 standard deviations lower than the average for their age [29]. In cases of GHRH-R mutations, the volume of the bony sella turcica, contrasting with small pituitary size, is relatively normal, while the posterior pituitary is in its normal site and the pituitary stalk is connecting the hypothalamus to the pituitary gland. It is noteworthy that anterior pituitary height has recently been reported to be normal in patients with GHRH-R mutation [29], although long-term MR follow-up may add additional information regarding a possible evolution towards a reduction in pituitary size over time. In GH insensitivity, normal pituitary gland size has been reported, despite the fact that one would expect an increased anterior pituitary size due to the absence of insulin-like growth factor 1 feedback and the large amount of GH secretion [30].

Pituitary Hormone Deficiencies and Transcription Factors

POU1F1 Mutation. Since the first report by Tatsumi et al. [31], POU1F1 mutations have been described in a large number of patients from 34 families originating in 17 different countries, all of whom have been associated with a broadly similar endocrine phenotype [32]. Anterior pituitary size in these cases, as assessed by MRI, is commonly small, though sometimes normal. It appears that there is no relationship between the size of the pituitary and the age of the patient or the type of mutation. However, an analysis of the type of mutation and the age at the time of the MRI study, if available, indicates that in the most common A/C→T sporadic mutations, changing an arginine to a tryptophan in codon 271 (R271W) in one allele of the POU1F1 gene is associated with normal pituitary size under the age of 2 years [33]. A lack of longitudinal studies presently impedes a final conclusion, though sequential MRI may potentially be valuable for better understanding the role of the POU1F1 gene in anterior pituitary cell survival. Normally, the pituitary stalk is connecting the hypothalamus to the pituitary gland, and the posterior pituitary hyperintensity is located in its normal site.

PROP1 Mutation. In humans, the clinical picture and hormone phenotype partially resemble those of POU1F1 mutation with low basal and stimulated GH, thyroid-stimulating hormone, prolactin and follicle-stimulating hormone/luteinizing hormone. The clinical phenotype of CPHD in the PROP1 defect varies considerably, especially depending on the time of onset and the severity of the pituitary-derived hormone deficiencies. Adrenocorticotropic hormone (ACTH) deficiency is a striking and unexpected associated feature because PROP1 is not expressed in corticotrophs; it is not linked to a given mutation and has been reported in as many as one third of these patients. The mechanism of ACTH deficiency remains unclear, and longitudinal analysis shows that the frequency of cortisol deficiency may be even higher than generally supposed [34].

The most frequently observed MRI pituitary feature is of small anterior pituitary size [35, 36]. There have been reports of families with PROP1 mutations and enlargement of the anterior pituitary [37]. In some cases, there has been progression from a large and full sella turcica to suprasellar extension of a pituitary mass, followed by areas of cystic change, loss of contrast enhancement of the mass and eventual regression to large empty sella [18, 38, 39]. The mass can even wax and wane before involuting [40].

The phenomenon of pituitary hyperplasia followed by shrinkage of the pituitary gland has not been observed in Ames mice and is still puzzling in humans. Several hypotheses have been proposed, including an abnormal proliferation of pituitary undifferentiated cells leading to a 'pseudotumor' mass. Recently, it has been shown that patients with anterior pituitary enlargement can have spontaneous regression of the mass lesion that seems to originate from the intermediate lobe [41]. Indeed, the study by the Sally Camper group [42] provides insight into our understanding of the mechanism of PROP1 action and provides an explanation for the intriguing transition from pituitary hyperplasia to hypoplasia in humans with such a mutation. Specifically, with loss of function, progenitors are trapped and cause a hyperplastic overgrowth; they can subsequently undergo apoptosis and disappear [42]. In PROP1 mutation, the pituitary stalk is connecting the hypothalamus to the pituitary gland, and posterior pituitary hyperintensity is in its normal location.

HESX1 Mutation. Hesx1 is necessary in mice for normal development of the forebrain, eyes, olfactory placodes and anterior pituitary gland; a lack of hesx1 also interferes with the formation of forebrain commissures, but does not affect regions caudal to the forebrain [43]. The array of defects including the variability and occasional laterality of phenotype is reminiscent of the characteristics of septo-optic dysplasia in humans. Eight mutations of the HESX1 gene have been reported in the familial form of septo-optic dysplasia and in some other GHD-related conditions. Hesx1 is the transcription factor most clearly identified as a repressor in pituitary organogenesis, and, in fact, Prop1-dependent regulation of pituitary development occurs during the attenuation of Hesx1 expression. Furthermore, premature expression of Prop1 leads to pituitary abnormalities, as does prolonged expression of Hesx1 and transducin-like enhancer of split-1, suggesting that the switch from hesx1 to Prop1 must be carefully timed for normal development to take place. Although repressors are known to play a crucial role in the development of many tissues, their role in pituitary development has not yet been fully defined [44, 45].

Various pituitary phenotypes have been reported in association with HESX1 mutation, and interestingly, HESX1 was the first gene mutation described with ectopic posterior pituitary (a common finding in IGHD). However, the majority of a cohort of over 500 patients with a variety of pituitary disorders (of whom approximately 200 were candidates for variants of septo-optic dysplasia) showed no mutation when screened [43]. The pituitary phenotype in HESX1 mutations has been reported to be associated with agenesis of the corpus callosum, hypoplasia of the optic nerves, pituitary hypoplasia and ectopic posterior pituitary; in other cases, MRI examination has evidenced unilateral hypoplasia of the optic nerve associated with the normal or hypoplasic pituitary gland in patients with isolated GHD or with panhypopituitarism [32, 43]. Aplasia of the anterior pituitary and optic nerve coloboma, as well as anterior pituitary aplasia in the absence of optic nerve abnormalities, have recently been reported [46, 47]; this suggests that the pituitary phenotype in HESX1 mutations is rather complex and reflects the heterogeneity of multiple conditions with different interacting pathways affecting forebrain/midbrain development.

LHX3/LHX4 Mutation. LHX3 maps to human chromosome 9q, and mutations in the gene have been identified in two families [48]. These patients displayed growth retardation, GH, thyroid-stimulating hormone, prolactin and follicle-stimulating hormone/luteinizing hormone defects and stubby neck associated with a severe restriction of neck rotation without any evidence of vertebral malformations or gross abnormalities of the surrounding soft tissue; the pituitary stalk was connecting the hypothalamus to the pituitary gland, and the posterior pituitary hyperintensity was in its normal location [48]. Anterior pituitary hypoplasia or an enlarged anterior pituitary have both been documented in these cases, while anterior pituitary aplasia has been reported in mice generated with disruption of Lhx-3. Recently, among 235 patients with CPHD from 23 countries, additional Lhx-3 gene defects were found in 4 patients (1.7%) with early-onset severe signs of CPHD [49]. Recently, 1 additional case with an LHX3 mutation and an MRI picture of hypointense lesion within the pituitary gland has been reported [50].

There has only been 1 published report of a mutation in LHX4. The patient with LHX4 germline splice mutation displayed CPHD, anterior pituitary hypoplasia, ectopic posterior pituitary and extrapituitary manifestations that included a poorly formed sella turcica, a persistent craniopharyngeal canal and pointed cerebellar tonsils suggestive of Chiari malformation [51].

GLI2 Mutation. The Sonic hedgehog signaling pathway has been implicated in more complex disorders of pituitary development. Seven heterozygous sequence variations in GLI2 have been identified. In particular, four pedigrees segregating GLI2 loss-of-function mutations have been characterized [52]. Although phenotypic penetrance with craniofacial abnormalities varied, the principal common feature among the patients of the study was the development of the pituitary gland from hypoplasia to absent pituitary and that of anterior pituitary function. The association of GLI2 mutation with defects of pituitary development and function supports growing evidence that many other unknown transcription factors are involved in pituitary organogenesis.

SOX3 Mutation. Recent studies implicate SOX3, a single exon gene closely related to SRY, in the etiology of X-linked hypopituitarism in both humans and mice. The phenotype of SOX3 mutant mice is variable and complex, with abnormalities throughout the hypothalamic-pituitary-gonadal axis [53]. Indeed, in humans, mutations of SOX3 and duplications at Xq26–27 are implicated in a syndrome of X-linked hypopituitarism and mental retardation [54, 55]. A submicroscopic duplication at Xq27.1 containing SOX3 and two other transcripts of unknown function were found in 2 siblings with variable endocrine phenotype without evidence of mental retardation [56]. Both SOX3 overdosage and underdosage cause clinical and endocrine hypopituitarism-related conditions associated with posterior pituitary ectopia, anterior pituitary hypoplasia and abnormality of both the infundibulum and corpus callosum. This suggests that SOX3 is involved in the development of midline forebrain structures. Although the full contribution of the genetic background to the variability of the SOX3 mutant (duplication, expansion, polymorphysm) or the phenotype has yet to be explored, there is a good chance that SOX3 mutations in humans may account not only for familial forms of hypopituitarism, but also for sporadic conditions of GHD. Indeed, as in HESX1 and LHX4 mutations, both of which are associated with a variable MRI picture including posterior pituitary ectopia, SOX3 seems to be critically involved in hypothalamic-pituitary development. This implies that selection of some IGHD patients for molecular analysis could be worthwhile. The absence of mental retardation suggests that SOX3 is the candidate gene most likely to be implicated in male hypopituitarism, in agreement with the reported male to female preponderance of this condition.

SOX2 Mutation. The transcription factor SOX2 is expressed in the developing central nervous system and placodes, where it plays a critical role in embryogenesis. Recent study data show that SOX2 mutations in humans are associated with defects of eye development, such as anophthalmia, microphthalmia and/or optic nerve hypoplasia, as well as with variable central nervous system abnormalities including small hippocampus, partial agenesis of the corpus callosum, absence of septum pellucidum, porencephalic cyst, bilateral schizencephaly, hypothalamic hamartoma and reduction of white matter bulk. While gonadotropin deficiency is the most common endocrine dysfunction, GH, ACTH and thyroid-stimulating hormone deficiencies are reported in one case and GHD in another; cryptorchidism and micropenis are described in affected males. Normal anterior pituitary gland or structural hypothalamic-pituitary abnormalities such as anterior pituitary hypoplasia, ectopic posterior pituitary and absent infundibulum have been reported [57].

Implications of Magnetic Resonance Imaging Pituitary Morphology after Adult Height Achievement

The diagnosis of GHD in young adults is not straightforward and presents a major clinical challenge. The key predictors of persistent GHD are based on the severity of the original GHD, the presence of additional pituitary hormone deficits, severely low insulin-like growth factor 1 concentration and structural hypothalamic-pituitary abnormalities [58, 59]. We have shown that patients with GHD and congenital hypothalamic-pituitary abnormalities might not require re-evaluation of GH secretion, whereas patients with isolated GHD and a normal or small pituitary gland should be retested well before the attainment of adult height [58]. MRI findings of the hypothalamic-pituitary area in patients with GHD may be the most important criterion upon which the decision to re-evaluate the patient should be based, rather than the response to pharmacological stimulation.

In a recent study, a subgroup of subjects with IGHD of childhood onset presenting with congenital structural hypothalamic-pituitary abnormalities confirmed that GHD patients – defined as those with a GH response <5 μg/l and with anterior pituitary hypoplasia, pituitary stalk agenesis and posterior pituitary ectopia at the level of the median eminence – are clearly candidates for permanent GHD in adult life [60], while those with less severe MRI features have an uncertain diagnosis or a likelihood of normal GH response after stimulation tests. These findings have important clinical implications in the diagnosis and prognosis of GHD after adult height achievement. However, by applying the criteria of peak GH values <3 or 5 μg/l, several misdiagnosed GHD subjects would be wrongly excluded from a potentially beneficial renewal of GH replacement treatment [61]. On the other hand, the diagnostic cut-off value of peak GH that should be adopted in young adults after combined arginine insulin or propranolol glucagon (used by the authors) has yet to be established; the role of sex hormones following the onset of puberty should not be underestimated. It is worth noting that pituitary function should be periodically assessed in subjects with pituitary stalk agenesis and IGHD or CPHD, as they may develop additional pituitary hormone deficiencies. In our recent study, ACTH deficiency characterized a subset of patients with IGHD and pituitary stalk abnormalities showing that several of them had undiagnosed subclinical ACTH deficiency [62]. The relationship between pituitary MRI features and final outcome has also been studied, showing that structural hypothalamic-pituitary abnormalities are determinant parameters in the prediction of growth response and adult height [3, 63].

Conclusion

MRI is advisable in all patients with GHD, although hypothalamic-pituitary abnormalities are more common in severe GHD. MRI pituitary morphology has important clinical implications, both in terms of diagnostic accuracy and long-term prognosis; indeed, when MR findings are appropriately interpreted, they clearly represent a gold standard in the work-up of children with GHD. Undoubtedly, MRI is the technique of choice in the diagnosis of children with 'idiopathic' hypopituitarism: their MR findings show marked differences in pituitary morphology, which suggests different etiologies of GHD and different prognoses. Establishing endocrine and MRI phenotypes is extremely helpful in the selection and management of patients with hypopituitarism, both in terms of possible genetic counseling and early diagnosis of evolving anterior pituitary hormone deficiencies.

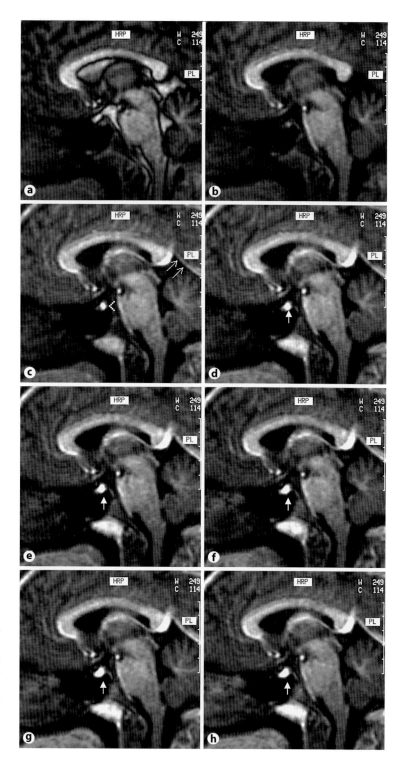

Fig. 3. Sagittal dynamic MRIs in a normal subject showing simultaneous enhancement of the straight sinus (**c**; double white arrows) and the posterior pituitary (white arrowhead). **d–h** Progressive enhancement of the anterior pituitary (white arrows) is compatible with a normal superior hypophyseal artery system.

Future Development

MRI is the 'new' gold standard for the diagnosis of pituitary-related diseases. It is essential in the evaluation of patients with suspected hypothalamic-pituitary pathology. Physicians involved in the care of such patients have a valuable tool that can assist in the characterization of a pituitary phenotype which will further elucidate the pathogenesis of these complex conditions. Although MRI allows for a clear selection of affected patients with structural hypothalamic-pituitary abnormalities, to date, no genetic etiology has been established in most patients with 'idiopathic' hypopituitarism. However, the future accumulation of detailed MRI information and the consequent classification of patients into specific categories will lead us towards a greater understanding of the disorder in the future, as well as helping to unravel the processes involved in pituitary organogenesis. The use of magnetization transfer techniques that measure the magnetization transfer ratio offer additional information on the functional status of the pituitary gland, while dynamic contrast-enhanced studies will be helpful in the assessment of the vascularization of the hypothalamic-pituitary region (fig. 3).

However, MRI evaluation of anterior pituitary size still has to overcome the hurdle of technique assessment. The recent information furnished by the 3D estimation of pituitary volume represents a significant advance over currently used methods; indeed, once more data and extended adoption of the technique with measurements of 3D pituitary volume become available, the current simple evaluation of pituitary height will no longer be adequate. The major challenge remains to accurately analyze structural hypothalamic-pituitary abnormalities and to better define normal standards for anterior pituitary size.

Neuroimaging techniques are expected to progressively expand and improve our knowledge and understanding of pituitary diseases. New imaging techniques that evaluate blood perfusion and metabolism by using various tracers that can be trapped within the pituitary tissues will provide additional important and complementary information.

References

1 Tortori-Donati P, Rossi A, Biancheri R: Sellar and suprasellar disorders; in Tortori-Donati P (ed): Pediatric Neuroradiology. Berlin, Springer, 2005, pp 855–891.
2 Argyropoulou MI, Xydis V, Kiortsis DN, Pantou K, Zikou A, Efremidis SC, Andronikou S: Pituitary gland signal in pre-term infants during the first year of life: an MRI study. Neuroradiology 2004;46:1031–1035.
3 Maghnie M, Ghirardello S, Genovese E: Magnetic resonance imaging of the hypothalamus-pituitary unit in children suspected of hypopituitarism: who, how and when to investigate. J Endocrinol Invest 2004;27:496–509.
4 Fink AM, Vidmar S, Kumbla S, Pedreira CC, Kanumakala S, Williams C, Carlin JB, Cameron FJ: Age-related pituitary volumes in prepubertal children with normal endocrine function: volumetric magnetic resonance data. J Clin Endocrinol Metab 2005;90:3274–3278.
5 Takano K, Utsunomiya H, Ono H, Ohfu M, Okazaki M: Normal development of the pituitary gland: assessment with three-dimensional MR volumetry. AJNR Am J Neuroradiol 1999;20:312–315.
6 Marziali S, Gaudiello F, Bozzao A, Scire G, Ferone E, Colangelo V, Simonetti A, Boscherini B, Floris R, Simonetti G: Evaluation of anterior pituitary gland volume in childhood using three-dimensional MRI. Pediatr Radiol 2004;34:547–551.
7 Bressani N, di Natale B, Pellini C, Triulzi F, Scotti G, Chiumello G: Evidence of morphological and functional abnormalities in the hypothalamus of growth-hormone-deficient children: a combined magnetic resonance imaging and endocrine study. Horm Res 1990;34:189–192.
8 Maghnie M, Triulzi F, Larizza D, Preti P, Priora C, Scotti G, Severi F: Hypothalamic-pituitary dysfunction in growth hormone-deficient patients with pituitary abnormalities. J Clin Endocrinol Metab 1991;73:79–83.
9 Abrahams JJ, Trefelner E, Boulware SD: Idiopathic growth hormone deficiency: MR findings in 35 patients. AJNR Am J Neuroradiol 1991;12:155–160.

10 Argyropoulou M, Perignon F, Brauner R, Brunelle F: Magnetic resonance imaging in the diagnosis of growth hormone deficiency. J Pediatr 1992;120:886–891.

11 Triulzi F, Scotti G, di Natale B, Pellini C, Lukezic M, Scognamiglio M, Chiumello G: Evidence of a congenital midline brain anomaly in pituitary dwarfs: a magnetic resonance imaging study in 101 patients. Pediatrics 1993;93:409–416.

12 Pinto G, Netchine I, Sobrier ML, Brunelle F, Souberbielle JC, Brauner R: Pituitary stalk interruption syndrome: a clinical-biological-genetic assessment of its pathogenesis. J Clin Endocrinol Metab 1997;82:3450–3454.

13 Nagel BHP, Palmbach M, Petersen D, Ranke MB: Magnetic resonance images of 91 children with different causes of short stature: pituitary size reflects growth hormone secretion. Eur J Pediatr 1997;156:758–763.

14 Kornreich L, Horev G, Lazar L, Josefsberg Z, Pertzelan A: MR findings in hereditary isolated growth hormone deficiency. AJNR Am J Neuroradiol 1997;18:1743–1747.

15 Hamilton J, Chitayat D, Blaser S, Cohen LE, Phillips JA, Daneman D: Familial growth hormone deficiency associated with MRI abnormalities. Am J Med Genet 1998;80:128–132.

16 Arifa N, Léger J, Garel C, Czernichow P, Hassan M: Cerebral anomalies associated with growth hormone insufficiency in children: major markers for diagnosis? Arch Pediatr 1999;6:14–21.

17 Bozzola M, Mengarda F, Sartirana P, Tato L, Chaussain JL: Long-term follow-up evaluation of magnetic resonance imaging in the prognosis of permanent GH deficiency. Eur J Endocrinol 2000;143:493–496.

18 Osorio MG, Marui S, Jorge AA, Latronico AC, Lo LS, Leite CC, Estefan V, Mendonca BB, Arnhold IJ: Pituitary magnetic resonance imaging and function in patients with growth hormone deficiency with and without mutations in GHRH-R, GH-1, or Prop-1 genes. J Clin Endocrinol Metab 2002;87:5076–5084.

19 Arends NJT, V d Lip W, Robben SGF, Hokken-Koelega ACS: MRI findings of the pituitary gland in short children born small for gestational age (SGA) in comparison with growth hormone-deficient (GHD) children and children with normal stature. Clin Endocrinol (Oxf) 2002;57:719–724.

20 Maghnie M, Loche S, Cappa M: Pituitary magnetic resonance imaging in idiopathic and genetic growth hormone deficiency. J Clin Endocrinol Metab 2003;88:1911–1912.

21 Cacciari E, Zucchini S, Ambrosetto P, Tani G, Carla G, Cicognani A, Pirazzoli P, Sganga T, Balsamo A, Cassio A, Zappulla F: Empty sella in children and adolescents with possible hypothalamic-pituitary disorders. J Clin Enocrinol Metab 1994;780:767–771.

22 Maghnie M, Genovese E, Villa A, Spagnolo L, Campani R, Severi F: Dynamic MRI in the congenital agenesis of the neural pituitary stalk syndrome: the role of the vascular pituitary stalk in predicting residual anterior pituitary function. Clin Endocrinol (Oxf) 1996;45:281–290.

23 Genovese E, Maghnie M, Beluffi G, Villa A, Sammarchi L, Severi F, Campani R: Hypothalamic-pituitary vascularization in the pituitary stalk transection syndrome: is the pituitary stalk really transected? The role of gadolinium-DTPA with spin-echo T_1 imaging and turbo-FLASH technique. Pediatr Radiol 1997;27:48–53.

24 Mullis PE: Genetic control of growth. Eur J Endocrinol 2005;52:11–31.

25 Binder G, Nagel BH, Ranke MB, Mullis PE: Isolated GH deficiency (IGHD) type II: imaging of the pituitary gland by magnetic resonance reveals characteristic differences in comparison with severe IGHD of unknown origin. Eur J Endocrinol 2002;147:755–760.

26 Besson A, Salemi S, Deladoey J, et al: Short stature caused by a biologically inactive mutant growth hormone (GH-C53S). J Clin Endocrinol Metab 2005;90:2493–2499.

27 Mullis PE, Robinson IC, Salemi S, Eble A, Besson A, Vuissoz JM, Deladoey J, Simon D, Czernichow P, Binder G: Isolated autosomal dominant growth hormone deficiency: an evolving pituitary deficit? A multicenter follow-up study. J Clin Endocrinol Metab 2005;90:2089–2096.

28 Salemi S, Yousefi S, Baltensperger K, Robinson IC, Eble A, Simon D, Czernichow P, Binder G, Sonnet E, Mullis PE: Variability of isolated autosomal dominant GH deficiency (IGHD II): impact of the P89L GH mutation on clinical follow-up and GH secretion. Eur J Endocrinol 2005;153:791–802.

29 Oliveira HA, Salvatori R, Krauss MP, Oliveira CR, Silva PR, Aguiar-Oliveira MH: Magnetic resonance imaging study of pituitary morphology in subjects homozygous for a null mutation of the growth hormone releasing hormone receptor gene. Eur J Endocrinol 2003;148:427–432.

30 Kornreich L, Horev G, Schwarz M, Karmazyn B, Laron Z: Pituitary size in patients with Laron syndrome (primary GH insensitivity). Eur J Endocrinol 2003;148:339–341.

31 Tatsumi K, Miyai K, Notomi T, Kaibe K, Amino N, Mizuno Y, Kohno H: Cretinism with combined hormone deficiency caused by a mutation in the PIT1 gene. Nat Genet 1992;1:56–58.

32 Dattani MT: Growth hormone deficiency and combined pituitary hormone deficiency: does the genotype matter? Clin Endocrinol (Oxf) 2005;63:121–130.

33 Cohen LE, Radovick S: Molecular basis of combined pituitary hormone deficiencies. Endocr Rev 2002;23:431–442.

34 Bottner A, Keller E, Kratzsch J, Stobbe H, Weigel JF, Keller A, Hirsch W, Kiess W, Blum WF, Pfaffle RW: PROP1 mutations cause progressive deterioration of anterior pituitary function including adrenal insufficiency: a longitudinal analysis. J Clin Endocrinol Metab 2004;89:5256–5265.

35 Pfäffle R, Blankenstein O, Wüller S, Heimann K, Heimann G: Pituitary transcription factors, POU1F1 and Prop-1 defects; in Rappaport R, Amselem S (eds): Hypothalamic-pituitary development. Karger, Basel, 2001, pp 61–67.

36 Fofanova O, Takamura N, Kinoshita E, Vorontsov A, Vladımırova V, Dedov I, Peterkova V, Yamashita S: MR imaging of the pituitary gland in children and young adults with congenital combined pituitary hormone deficiency associated with Prop-1 mutations. Am J Roentgenol 2000;174:555–559.

37 Riepe FG, Partsch CJ, Blankenstein O, Mönig H, Pfäffle RW, Sippell WG: Longitudinal imaging reveals pituitary enlargement preceding hypoplasia in two brothers with combined pituitary hormone deficiency attributable to Prop-1 mutation. J Clin Endocrinol Metab 2001;86:4353–4357.

38 Teinturier C, Vallette S, Adamsbaum C, Bendaoud M, Brue T, Bougnères PF: Pseudotumor of the pituitary due to Prop-1 deletion. J Ped Endocrinol Metab 2002;15:95–101.

39 Vallette-Kasic S, Barlier A, Teinturier C, Diaz A, Manavela M, Berthezene F, Bouchard P, Chaussain JL, Brauner R, Pellegrini-Bouiller I, Jaquet P, Enjalbert A, Brue T: Prop-1 gene screening in patients with multiple pituitary hormone deficiency reveals two sites of hypermutability and a high incidence of corticotroph deficiency. J Clin Endocrinol Metab 2001;86:4529–4535.

40 Turton JP, Mehta A, Raza J, Woods KS, Tiulpakov A, Cassar J, Chong K, Thomas PQ, Eunice M, Ammini AC, Bouloux PM, Starzyk J, Hindmarsh PC, Dattani MT: Mutations within the transcription factor PROP1 are rare in a cohort of patients with sporadic combined pituitary hormone deficiency (CPHD). Clin Endocrinol (Oxf) 2005;63:10–18.

41 Voutetakis A, Argyropoulou M, Sertedaki A, Livadas S, Xekouki P, Maniati-Christidi M, Bossis I, Thalassinos N, Patronas N, Dacou-Voutetakis C: Pituitary magnetic resonance imaging in 15 patients with Prop1 gene mutations: pituitary enlargement may originate from the intermediate lobe. J Clin Endocrinol Metab 2004;89:2200–2206.

42 Ward RD, Raetzman LT, Suh H, Stone BM, Nasonkin IO, Camper SA: Role of PROP1 in pituitary gland growth. Mol Endocrinol 2005;19:698–710.

43 Dattani MT, Robinson IC: Hesx1 and septo-optic dysplasia. Rev Endocrinol Metab Disord 2002;3:289–300.

44 Carvalho LR, Woods KS, Mendonca BB, Marcal N, Zamparini AL, Stifani S, Brickman JM, Arnhold IJ, Dattani MT: A homozygous mutation in HESX1 is associated with evolving hypopituitarism due to impaired repressor-corepressor interaction. J Clin Invest 2003; 112:1192–1201.

45 Cohen RN, Cohen LE, Botero D, Yu C, Sagar A, Jurkiewicz M, Radovick S: Enhanced repression by HESX1 as a cause of hypopituitarism and septo-optic dysplasia. J Clin Endocrinol Metab 2003;88:4832–4839.

46 Sobrier ML, Netchine I, Heinrichs C, Thibaud N, Vie-Luton MP, Van Vliet G, Amselem S: Alu-element insertion in the homeodomain of HESX1 and aplasia of the anterior pituitary. Hum Mutat 2005;25:503–511.

47 Sobrier ML, Maghnie M, Vié-Luton MP, Secco A, Di Iorgi N, Amselem S: Novel HESX1 mutations are associated with life-threatening neonatal phenotype, anterior pituitary aplasia, normally located posterior pituitary and developmental defects in the absence of optic nerve abnormalities. Proc ESPE 7th Joint Meet, Lyon, 2005, p 2751.

48 Netchine I, Sobrier ML, Krude H, Schnabel D, Maghnie M, Marcos E, Duriez B, Cacheux V, Moers A, Goossens M, Gruters A, Amselem S: Mutations in Lhx3 result in a new syndrome revealed by combined pituitary hormone deficiency. Nat Genet 2000;25:182–186.

49 Palme C, Bellone F, Schonau E, et al: Frequency and phenotype of panhypopituitarism due to LHX-3 gene defects. Proc 42nd ESPE Meet, Ljubljana, 2003, p 1137.

50 Bhangoo AP, Hunter CS, Savage JJ, Anhalt H, Pavlakis S, Walvoord EC, Ten S, Rhodes SJ: Clinical case seminar: a novel LHX3 mutation presenting as combined pituitary hormonal deficiency. J Clin Endocrinol Metab 2006;91: 747–753.

51 Machinis K, Pantel J, Netchine I, Leger J, Camand OJ, Sobrier ML, Dastot-Le Moal F, Duquesnoy P, Abitbol M, Czernichow P, Amselem S: Syndromic short stature in patients with a germline mutation in the LIM homeobox. Am J Hum Genet 2001;69:961–968.

52 Roessler E, Du YZ, Mullor JL, Casas E, Allen WP, Gillessen-Kaesbach G, Roeder ER, Ming JE, Ruiz i Altaba A, Muenke M: Loss-of-function mutations in the human GLI2 gene are associated with pituitary anomalies and holoprosencephaly-like features. Proc Natl Acad Sci USA 2003;100:13424–13429.

53 Rizzoti K, Brunelli S, Carmignac D, Thomas PQ, Robinson IC, Lovell-Badge R: SOX3 is required during the formation of the hypothalamo-pituitary axis. Nat Genet 2004;36:247–255.

54 Laumonnier F, Ronce N, Hamel BC, Thomas P, Lespinasse J, Raynaud M, Paringaux C, Van Bokhoven H, Kalscheuer V, Fryns JP, Chelly J, Moraine C, Briault S: Transcription factor SOX3 is involved in X-linked mental retardation with growth hormone deficiency. Am J Hum Genet 2002;71:1450–1455.

55 Solomon NM, Nouri S, Warne GL, Lagerstrom-Fermer M, Forrest SM, Thomas PQ: Increased gene dosage at Xq26-q27 is associated with X-linked hypopituitarism. Genomics 2002;79: 553–559.

56 Woods KS, Cundall M, Turton J, Rizzoti K, Mehta A, Palmer R, Wong J, Chong WK, Al-Zyoud M, El-Ali M, Otonkoski T, Martinez-Barbera JP, Thomas PQ, Robinson IC, Lovell-Badge R, Woodward KJ, Dattani MT: Over- and underdosage of SOX3 is associated with infundibular hypoplasia and hypopituitarism. Am J Hum Genet 2005;76:833–849.

57 Kelberman D, Rizzoti K, Avilion A, Bitner-Glindzicz M, Cianfarani S, Collins J, Chong WK, Kirk JM, Achermann JC, Ross R, Carmignac D, Lovell-Badge R, Robinson IC, Dattani MT: Mutations within Sox2/SOX2 are associated with abnormalities in the hypothalamo-pituitary-gonadal axis in mice and humans. J Clin Invest 2006;116:2442–2455.

58 Maghnie M, Strigazzi C, Tinelli C, Autelli M, Cisternino M, Loche S, Severi F: Growth hormone (GH) deficiency (GHD) of childhood onset: reassessment of GH status and evaluation of the predictive criteria for permanent GHD in young adults. J Clin Endocrinol Metab 1999;84:1324–1328.

59 Adan L, Souberbielle JC, Brauner R: Diagnostic markers of permanent idiopathic growth hormone deficiency. J Clin Endocrinol Metab 1994;78:353–358.

60 Leger J, Danner S, Simon D, Garel C, Czernichow P: Do all patients with childhood-onset growth hormone deficiency (GHD) and ectopic neurohypophysis have persistent GHD in adulthood? J Clin Endocrinol Metab 2005; 90:650–656.

61 Maghnie M, Aimaretti G, Bellone S, Bona G, Bellone J, Baldelli R, de Sanctis C, Gargantini L, Gastaldi R, Ghizzoni L, Secco A, Tinelli C, Ghigo E: Diagnosis of GH deficiency in the transition period: accuracy of insulin tolerance test and insulin-like growth factor-I measurement. Eur J Endocrinol 2005; 152:589–596.

62 Maghnie M, Uga E, Temporini F, Di Iorgi N, Secco A, Tinelli C, Papalia A, Casini MR, Loche S: Evaluation of adrenal function in patients with growth hormone deficiency and hypothalamic-pituitary disorders: comparison between insulin-induced hypoglycemia, low-dose ACTH, standard ACTH and CRH stimulation tests. Eur J Endocrinol 2005;152:735–741.

63 Coutant R, Rouleau S, Despert F, Magontier N, Loisel D, Limal JM: Growth and adult height in GH-treated children with non-acquired GH deficiency and idiopathic short stature: the influence of pituitary magnetic resonance imaging findings. J Clin Endocrinol Metab 2001;86:4649–4654.

Characteristics of Idiopathic Growth Hormone Deficiency at the Start of Growth Hormone Therapy and the Response to Growth Hormone

Herwig Frisch

Diagnosis of growth hormone deficiency (GHD) in children includes careful evaluation of anamnestic data and the clinical phenotype, as well as endocrine tests and imaging procedures. Patients may present with variable degrees of GHD and it is generally accepted that GHD comprises a continuum from absent to subnormal secretory capacity. In agreement with this concept is the variable clinical picture of a more characteristic phenotype, especially if not only GH but also other pituitary hormones are affected, to a normal appearance, except for short stature.

Although continuous monitoring of growth and development in children is part of our welfare services, the diagnosis and consequent initiation of treatment are still considerably delayed. This is of importance as it is well known that the success of GH treatment to reach normal adult height depends to a considerable extent on a timely initiation of GH substitution.

Endocrinological Features

There is a wide spectrum of underlying pathology causing GHD which has an impact on the clinical picture at presentation and diagnosis (see KIGS classification) [1]. Because of its characteristics and the consequences for the future development, special attention should be paid to the neonatal and infancy period.

During prenatal life, insulin-like growth factor 1 (IGF-1) and IGF-2 are the most important growth factors [2], shown by the relationship between birth size and IGF-1 levels of the newborn [3]. In the newborn child, IGF-1 serum levels are low and start to increase only after 12–18 months of life. Similarly, the levels of IGF-binding protein 3 are very low during this period. However, despite the difficulties in discriminating pathologically decreased IGF-1 concentrations at this age, a high sensitivity for IGF-1 in detecting GHD has been demonstrated [4]. It is interesting to see that during this period, the molar concentration of IGF-1 plus IGF-2 is still higher than that of its major binding protein, IGF-binding protein 3; thereby, a high bioavail-

St. Anna Children's Hospital
Kinderspitalgasse 6
AT–1090 Vienna (Austria)

ability of IGF-1 facilitates rapid growth during infancy.

High GH levels are detectable in the fetus, but do not seem to play a major role in growth regulation. At birth, GH levels are around 30 ng/ml and decline rapidly during the following weeks [5]. At the same time, the GH receptor, as reflected by serum GH-binding protein levels, is upregulated and the maturation of the hypothalamo-pituitary axis is responsible for the development of the characteristic pulsatile pattern of GH secretion with high levels during sleep. Because of this changing pattern of GH secretion in the neonatal and infancy period, no clear reference values for diagnosis of GHD are available. Random GH samples of <10 ng/ml are suspicious of GHD. GH stimulation tests will be a difficult task in very young infants.

Table 1. Complications in patients with idiopathic GHD (n = 47) [6]

a During pregnancy

Imminent abortion, bleeding	12%
Renal diseases, hypertension	6%
Hyperemesis	4%
Diabetes mellitus	2%
Pregnancy concealed	2%
Infection	2%
Total	28%

b At delivery

Delivery at home, complications	4%
Prolonged delivery, asphyxia	10%
Vacuum extraction	4%
Caesarean section	2%
Footling presentation	4%
Breech delivery	24%
Total	48%

Characteristics in the Neonatal Period

In children with congenital GHD, a high incidence of perinatal morbidities has been documented. We found complications during pregnancy such as imminent abortion, renal disorders with hypertension, hyperemesis and others in approximately one third of our patients (table 1) [6]. These complications may represent a problematic period during intrauterine life when a damage to the hypothalamic-pituitary axis occurs, resulting in the clinical picture of congenital GHD (see below) [7–9].

Likewise, complications at delivery are frequently observed in children with 'idiopathic' GHD (table 1). Abnormal presentation or asphyxia in complicated delivery was found to be more frequent in children with hypopituitarism than in reference populations, suggesting perinatal injury as a causal factor [9–13]. It is not clear whether such a birth trauma may cause pituitary stalk interruption with the characteristic findings of hypoplastic anterior pituitary gland and ectopic neurohypophysis, which can be visualized by sensitive magnetic resonance imaging methods in a high percentage of GHD patients [14, 15]. On the other hand, from the clinical presentation of GHD in infancy and because abnormalities of the pituitary are also found without a birth trauma, it is suggested that congenital developmental anomalies in the hypothalamic-pituitary region may not be the consequence but rather the cause of birth complications and congenital hypopituitarism [16, 17].

In the neonatal period, prolonged jaundice (conjugated hyperbilirubinaemia) and severe hypoglycaemia which may present as cerebral convulsions are characteristic symptoms of GHD [6, 8, 18]. Children with this spectrum of symptoms represent a severe form of pituitary insufficiency, most of them suffering from multiple pituitary hormone deficiency (MPHD). In boys, micropenis may be an additional indicator.

There is some controversy about length and weight data at birth. In 48 unselected patients

Table 3. Characteristics of patients with congenital GHD with an early diagnosis and treatment

	Gluckman [11] 1994	De Luca et al. [7] 1995	Huet et al. [10] 1999	Pena-Almazan et al. [18], 2001	Ranke et al. [20] 2005
Patients, n	130	16	59	46	265
Age	1.2 ± 0.6 years	1.2 ± 0.6 years	5.8 ± 3.8 months	5.3 ± 3.8 years	1.9 ± 0.7 years
Height SDS	–3.6 ± 1.8	–3.8 ± 1.5	–3.5 ± 1.9	(1.0)^a (–1.8 ± 1.2)^a	–3.1 ± 1.4
Birth length SDS	–0.9 ± 1.8	–2.1 ± 1.1	–0.9 ± 1.4	0.4 ± 1.6	–0.8 ± 1.5
GH peak	<1 mU/ml	2.4 ± 1.7 ng/ml	2.2 ± 2.8 ng/ml	2.9 ± 2.5 ng/ml	4.2 ± 2.8 ng/ml
MPHD, %	n.d.	44	76	85	38
Follow-up, years	5	n.d.	8	5.8	n.d.

n.d. = No data.
^{a} Height was analysed only in a subset of patients at 1 year of age.

with complete GHD (24 isolated GHD (IGHD) and 24 MPHD children), the birth length of boys and girls was reduced when compared with standards allowing for gestational age (table 2). There was no difference between the birth length of IGHD and MPHD children, i.e. –0.9 ± 1.3 versus –0.8 ± 1.2 standard deviation score (SDS), which is not significant. These data indicate that children with idiopathic GHD were short already at birth and had relative overweight, which may be explained by the lack of the lipolytic effect of GH. The reduced birth length indicates that GH may also play a role in prenatal growth regulation. This assumption is supported by observations of reduced birth length in children with GH gene deletion [19]. However, data from the literature are conflicting and report either reduced [6, 8, 12] or normal [18] birth data.

The number of children diagnosed in the infancy period is limited (table 3), but the most striking feature is a very rapid growth deceleration during the first year of life [7, 8, 10, 18, 20]. In these patients, a loss of more than 3 SDS during the first year of life was found. In agreement with this observation of GH being essential for early postnatal growth is the very good response to GH treatment in this age period. In a group of patients who started treatment at a mean age of 1.3 years, the growth response during the first year of treatment was 1.6 SDS/year which is much better than the first-year response of 0.5 SDS/year in a control group in which treatment was started only at 7.5 years [11]. In the same order of magnitude was the response in 59 children who started therapy at 5.8 ± 3.8 months (1.7 SDS) [10]. This catch-up growth was inversely related with the height SDS at the onset of treatment. After a mean treatment period of 8 years, this group of patients had reached a height greater than their respective target height, emphasizing the importance of an early onset of therapy. The 265 patients from the KIGS group who started treatment at 1.9 years showed the same response [20].

Table 2. Birth length and birth weight SDS of 48 children with congenital GHD compared with standards allowing for gestational age

	Birth length	p	Birth weight	p
Boys	–1.0 ± 1.3	<0.01	–0.8 ± 1.2	<0.05
Girls	–0.4 ± 1.0	n.s.	0.1 ± 1.3	n.s.

No difference in length and weight between children with IGHD and MPHD was found [22]. n.s. = Not significant.

Table 4. Chronological age (CA), bone age (BA) and height SDS for CA and BA in patients with IGHD and MPHD at onset of treatment, as analysed in 1983 [22]

	CA, years	BA, years	BA SDS	Height SDS for CA	Height SDS for BA
IGHD (n = 25)	8.9 ± 0.9	6.1 ± 0.8	–3.7 ± 0.3	–3.8	–0.6
MPHD (n = 25)	9.2 ± 0.8	4.6 ± 0.5	–5.4 ± 0.3	–4.1	0.7

Clinical Presentation

The main reason for presenting a child who is later diagnosed as having GHD is short stature and low growth velocity; in addition, clinical features like moderate obesity with fat deposits at the trunk and a round, immature face may be seen. There is acromicria and the skin appears pale and smooth. If the diagnosis is delayed to a greater extent and children become aware of being different, the immature physical appearance or even lack of pubertal development will provoke psychological problems with an impact on well-being, social integration and school performance [21].

It is essential to put growth data from a longer observation period into an appropriate growth and velocity reference curve created for the respective population. This should be taken into consideration, especially today, when immigrants from countries with shorter populations compare their offspring with the standards of another country. The height deficit should be expressed as SDS which allows the evaluation of individual development and the comparison with reference data.

The degree of growth retardation will depend on the age of the child at presentation and the degree of pituitary insufficiency, whether only GH or various other hormones are affected as well. If additional pituitary hormones are lacking, the clinical picture may show features of hypothyroidism, gonadotropin deficiency (at puberty) or the relatively rare adrenocorticotropic hormone deficiency. In a previous analysis, we found a relatively advanced age of approximately 9 years at diagnosis and a significant growth retardation of about 4 SDS which was even more pronounced in patients with MPHD (table 4). Bone age was severely retarded, and patients with multiple deficiencies demonstrated a higher degree of retardation which is clearly shown when the data are expressed as SDS. If the growth retardation is related to bone age, patients with IGHD are 'short for their bone age', as shown by a negative SDS for bone age value; however, MPHD patients are 'tall for their bone age', which is explained by the more pronounced bone age retardation. Patients with MPHD are more affected with respect to their growth retardation, they grow even slower, and bone age is more retarded.

Growth velocity before treatment was –2.8 SDS in children with IGHD and –3.7 SDS in MPHD patients [22]. This demonstrates that the synergistic effect of thyroid hormone and GH is essential for adequate growth.

Several reports that have been published in the 1980s show similar characteristics of patients at the onset of therapy; in general, chronological age at diagnosis was considerably advanced with pronounced retardation of bone age and final height data below –2 SDS [23–28].

However, in the 1990s, the mean age at diagnosis of GHD was generally below 10 years, children were not so short at diagnosis, and the outcome has improved [29–32] (table 5).

Bone Age

IGF-1 has a direct effect on the growth plate, thereby stimulating the growth of the bone. However, circulating IGF-1 which is produced pre-

Table 5. Data from GHD patients at the start of GH therapy

Reference	Patients	CA at GH start years	Height SDS at GH start	Maximum GH ng/ml	Multiple/ isolated	HV before therapy cm/years	Bone age
Goodman et al. [24], 1968	16 (8 males)	n.d.	−5.7	1.2	isolated	n.d.	n.d.
	19 (14 males)		−5.4	1.3	multiple		
Burns et al. [25], 1981	11 males	11.3	−4.7	<3	isolated	n.d.	7.8
	6 females	11.0	−5.0		isolated		8.0
	5 males	11.2	−5.4		multiple		8.5
	1 female	14.6	−2.9		multiple		12.2
Lenko et al. [26], 1982	41 (32 males)	10.9	−4.8	<7	17/24	3.2	6.7
Joss et al. [27], 1983	18	12.2	−5.8	<2	2/16	2.4	7.7
Hibi et al. [28], 1989	91 males	12.4	−4.1	<5	isolated	n.d.	8.6
	17 females	11.0	−4.9		isolated		8.5
	23 males	12.3	−4.0		multiple		7.4
	6 females	11.0	−4.5		multiple		7.4
Frisch and Birnbacher [29], 1995	10 (5 males)	9.9	−4.2	<3.3	isolated	2.9	6.4
	23 (14 males)	10.2	−4.7		multiple	3.0	5.9
Rikken et al. [30], 1995	91	12.2	−4.4	<10	42/49	n.d.	n.d.
Yokoya et al. [31], 1999	15 males	6.6	−3.3	<10	isolated	4.8	n.d.
Cutfield et al. [32], 1999	369 (246 males)	9.8	−3.1	3.3	185/184	n.d.	n.d.

CA = Chronological age; HV = height velocity; n.d. = no data.

dominantly in the liver plays only a minor role in the pathogenesis of hypopituitarism. It has been shown that GH has a direct effect on differentiation of the stem cells in the growth plate, and the proliferating chondrocytes produce local IGF-1 which acts in an autocrine manner to stimulate proliferation [33]. Retardation of osseous development is a main characteristic of GHD. Therefore, analysis of bone age or bone maturation is one of the primary investigations in short children. Generally, an X-ray of the left hand is compared with the atlas of Greulich and Pyle or Tanner; in newborns and very young children, the bone development of the knee will be evaluated. Depending on the age at diagnosis (and thereby the duration of the hormone deficit), there will be a considerable retardation of the bone age. In children with MPHD, bone age retardation will be more pronounced, especially at the time of puberty. Patients with pathologically retarded bone age may show inhomogeneous degrees of maturation of individual bones resulting in a 'dissociated bone age' which makes the analysis more difficult. This problem is partly overcome when the atlas of Tanner is used where individual bones are evaluated.

During treatment with GH, the progress of bone age development should be analysed in yearly intervals. During the first year of therapy, the progression of bone age was 1 year, although there is some individual variation. Bone age progression was not correlated with chronological age, bone age, height or the dosage of GH (in the therapeutic range) at the onset of therapy [34].

Table 6. Data on GH-deficient children during the first year of treatment

Reference	Patients	CA at GH start, years	Height SDS at GH start	GH dose IU/kg/week	Δ height SDS	HV cm/year
Ranke and Guilbaud [35], 1991	289 (202)	7.0	−2.8	0.5	0.7	8.8
De Muink Keizer-Schrama et al. [36], 1992	21 (16)	6.8 6.9	−3.6 −3.2	0.46 0.93	1.16 1.56	11.0 13.3
Boersma et al. [37], 1995	26 (16)	1.6 1.4	−4.5 −4.1	8 IU/week 0.46	0.7 1.3	n.d.
Karavanaki et al. [38], 2001	100 (64)	10.1	−2.9	0.5	0.5	8.8
Ranke et al. [20], 2005	265 (180) 509 (331)	1.9 7.5	−3.1 −2.5	0.83 0.66	1.7 0.6	13.3 8.6

Figures in parentheses are numbers of male patients. CA = Chronological age; HV = height velocity.

Growth Response

An important parameter is the evaluation of the initial response and analysis of height velocity during the first year of GH substitution which is mainly governed by the catch-up phenomenon (table 6). It does not predict the final outcome, but a good initial response is reassuring and encouraging for further therapeutic procedure. Today, it is general praxis to give GH in daily injections; less frequent application is not acceptable as it has been shown that the growth response is better when the same total GH dose is given in daily instead of less frequent injections [39]. However, as GHD is not a uniform diagnosis, patients will respond in different ways and may require distinct treatment modalities. Usually, an initial dose of 25 μg/kg body weight/day is given which should be adapted accordingly. Data from the literature show a considerable inter-individual variability in GH treatment response. Therefore, models for prediction of the response to GH using anamnestic and diagnostic variables were developed to calculate the expected growth response and to optimize therapy [40]. However, this prediction model was derived from a large international database from prepubertal children. In patients with profound GHD, allowance for the severity of the disease should be made and the result of the GH stimulation test should be included [41]. Very young children under the age of 3 years showed an increased response to GH and the prediction model was adapted accordingly for this age group [21].

In conclusion, children with an early diagnosis have a more profound form of pituitary insufficiency which probably has its onset during intrauterine life; this disorder is accompanied in a higher percentage by the characteristic clinical symptoms of GHD and a more pronounced growth retardation. This is in agreement with the current view of GHD representing a continuum from the severe congenital form of GHD to more moderate forms which are diagnosed in midchildhood with the main symptom being growth retardation.

References

1 Ranke, MB: The KIGS aetiology classification system; in Ranke MB, Wilton P (eds): Growth Hormone Therapy in KIGS – 10 Years Experience. Leipzig, Johann Ambrosius Barth Verlag, 1999, pp 389–401.
2 Baker J, Liu JP, Robertson EJ, Efstratiadis A: Role of insulin-like growth factors in embryonic and postnatal life. Cell 1993;75:73–82.
3 Ogilvy-Stuart AL, Hands SJ, Adcock CJ, Holly JM, Matthews DR, Mohammed-Ali V, Yudkin JS, Wilkinson AR, Dunger DB: Insulin, insulin-like growth factor-I (IGF-I), IGF-binding protein-1, growth hormone, and feeding in the newborn. J Clin Endocrinol Metab 1998;83:3550–3557.
4 Jensen RB, Jeppesen KA, Vielwerth S, Michaelsen KF, Main KM, Skakkebaek NE, Juul A: Insulin-like growth factor I (IGF-I) and binding protein 3 as diagnostic markers of growth hormone deficiency in infancy. Horm Res 2005;63:15–21.
5 Leger J, Noel M, Limal JM, Czernichow P: Growth factors and intrauterine growth retardation. 2. Serum growth hormone, insulin-like growth factor (IGF) I, and IGF-binding protein 3 levels in children with intrauterine growth retardation compared with normal control subjects: prospective study from birth to two years of age. Pediatr Res 1996;40:101–107.
6 Burda G, Frisch H, Schober E: Birth Data of Patients with Growth Hormone Deficiency. San Francisco, LWPES/ESPE, 1993.
7 De Luca F, Bernasconi S, Blandino A, Cavallo L, Cisternino M: Auxological, clinical and neuroradiological findings in infants with early onset growth hormone deficiency. Acta Paediatr 1995;84:561–565.
8 Gluckman PD, Gunn AJ, Wray A, Cutfield W, Chatelain PG, Guilbaud O, Ambler GR, Wilton P, Albertsson-Wikland K: Congenital idiopathic growth hormone deficiency is associated with prenatal and early postnatal growth failure. J Pediatr 1992;121:920–923.
9 Craft WH, Underwood LE, Van Wyk JJ: High incidence of perinatal insult in children with idiopathic hypopituitarism. J Pediatr 1980;96:397–402.
10 Huet F, Carel JC, Nivelon JL, Chaussain JL: Long-term results of GH therapy in GH-deficient children treated before 1 year of age. Eur J Endocrinol 1999;140:29–34.
11 Gluckman PD: Growth hormone deficiency diagnosed and treated in the first 2 years of life: evidence of the role of growth hormone in human perinatal growth; in Ranke MB, Gunnarsson R (eds): Progress in Growth Hormone Therapy – 5 Years of KIGS. Mannheim, J&J Verlag, 1994, pp 88–96.
12 Albertsson-Wikland K, Niklasson A, Karlberg P: Birth data for patients who later develop growth hormone deficiency: preliminary analysis of a national register. Acta Paediatr Scand Suppl 1990;370:115–120.
13 Wit JM, van Unen H: Growth of infants with neonatal growth hormone deficiency. Arch Dis Child 1992;67:920–924.
14 Leger J, Danner S, Simon D, Garel C, Czernichow P: Do all patients with childhood-onset growth hormone deficiency (GHD) and ectopic neurohypophysis have persistent GHD in adulthood? J Clin Endocrinol Metab 2005;90:650–656.
15 Meszaros F, Vergesslich K, Riedl S, Haeusler G, Frisch H: Posterior pituitary ectopy in children with idiopathic growth hormone deficiency. J Pediatr Endocrinol Metab 2000;13:629–635.
16 Triulzi F, Scotti G, di Natale B, Pellini C, Lukezic M, Scognamiglio M, Chiumello G: Evidence of a congenital midline brain anomaly in pituitary dwarfs: a magnetic resonance imaging study in 101 patients. Pediatrics 1994;93:409–416.
17 Nagel BHP, Palmbach M, Ranke MB: Magnetic resonance imaging in growth hormone deficiency; in Ranke MB, Wilton P (eds): Growth Hormone Therapy in KIGS – 10 Years Experience. Leipzig, Johann Ambrosius Barth Verlag, 1999, pp 65–71.
18 Pena-Almazan S, Buchlis J, Miller S, Shine B, MacGillivray M: Linear growth characteristics of congenitally GH-deficient infants from birth to one year of age. J Clin Endocrinol Metab 2001;86:5691–5694.
19 Riedl S, Frisch H: Effects of growth hormone (GH) and insulin-like growth factor-I therapy in patients with gene defects in the GH axis. J Pediatr Endocrinol Metab 2006;19:229–236.
20 Ranke MB, Lindberg A, Albertsson-Wikland K, Wilton P, Price DA, Reiter EO, on behalf of the KIGS International Board: Increased response, but lower responsiveness, to growth hormone (GH) in very young children (aged 0–3 years) with idiopathic GH deficiency: analysis of data from KIGS. J Clin Endocrinol Metab 2005;90:1966–1971.
21 Sartorio A, Conti A, Molinari E, Riva G, Morabito F, Faglia G: Growth, growth hormone and cognitive function. Horm Res 1996;45:23–29.
22 Frisch H: Wachstumshormonmangel bei Kindern. Beurteilung hypophysärer Funktionstests, Therapie und Verlaufsbeobachtung. Wien, Facultas Verlag, 1983.
23 Wit JM, Kamp G, Rikken B: Spontaneous growth and response to GH treatment in children with GHD or with idiopathic short stature. Pediatrics 1996;39:295–302.
24 Goodman HG, Grumbach MM, Kaplan SL: Growth and growth hormone. N Engl J Med 1968;278:57–68.
25 Burns EC, Tanner JM, Preece MA, Cameron N: Final height and pubertal development in 55 children with idiopathic growth hormone deficiency, treated for between 2 and 15 years with human growth hormone. Eur J Pediatr 1981;137:155–164.
26 Lenko HL, Leisti S, Perheentupa J: The efficacy of growth hormone in different types of growth failure. Eur J Pediatr 1982;138:241–249.
27 Joss E, Zuppinger K, Schwarz HP, Roten H: Final height of patients with pituitary growth failure and changes in growth variables after long-term hormonal therapy. Pediatr Res 983;17:676–679.
28 Hibi I, Tanaka T, Tanae A, Kagawa J, Hashimoto N, Yoshizawa A, Shizume K: The influence of gonadal function and the effect of gonadal suppression treatment on final height in growth hormone (GH)-treated GH-deficient children. J Clin Endocrinol Metab 1989;69:221–226.

29 Frisch H, Birnbacher R: Final height and pubertal development in children with growth hormone deficiency after long-term treatment. Horm Res 1995; 43:132–134.
30 Rikken B, Massa C, Wit JM, on behalf of the Dutch Growth Hormone Working Group: Final height in a large cohort of Dutch patients with growth hormone deficiency treated with growth hormone. Horm Res 1995;43: 135–137.
31 Yokoya S, Araki K, Igarashi Y, Kohno H, Hasegawa Y, Fujita K, Iwatani N, Tachibana K, Ohyama Y, Seino Y, Satoh M, Fujieda K, Tanaka T: High-dose growth hormone (GH) treatment in prepubertal GH-deficient children. Acta Paediatr Suppl 1999;428:76–79
32 Cutfield WS, Lindberg A, Chatelain P, Price DA, Albertsson-Wikland K, Wilton P, Ranke MB, on behalf of the KIGS International Board: Final height following growth hormone treatment of idiopathic growth hormone deficiency in KIGS; in Ranke MB, Wilton P (eds): Growth Hormone Therapy in KIGS – 10 Years Experience. Leipzig, Johann Ambrosius Barth Verlag, 1999, pp 65–71.
33 Sjogren K, Liu LJ, Blad K, Skrtic S, Vidal O, Wallenius V, LeRoith D, Tornell J, Isaksson OG, Jansson JO, Ohlsson C: Liver derived insulin-like growth factor I (IGF-I) is the principal source of IGF-I in blood but is not required for postnatal body growth in mice. Proc Natl Acad Sci USA 1999;96:7088–7092.
34 Darendeliler F, Ranke MB, Bakker B, Lindberg A, Cowell CT, Albertsson-Wikland K, Reiter EO, Price DA: Bone age progression during the first year of growth hormone therapy in pre-pubertal children with idiopathic growth hormone deficiency, Turner syndrome or idiopathic short stature, and in short children born small for gestational age: analysis of data from KIGS (Pfizer International Growth Database). Horm Res 2005;63:40–47.
35 Ranke MB, Guilbaud O: Growth response in prepubertal children with idiopathic growth hormone deficiency during the first two years of treatment with human growth hormone. Analysis of the Kabi Pharmacia International Growth Study. Acta Paediatr Scand Suppl 1991;379:109–115.
36 De Muinck Keizer-Schrama SMPF, Rikken B, Wynne HJ, Hokken-Koelega ACS, Wit JM, Bot A, Drop SLS: Dose-response study of biosynthetic human growth hormone (GH) in GH-deficient children: effects on auxological and biochemical parameters. J Clin Endocrinol Metab 1992;74:898–905.
37 Boersma B, Rikken B, Wit JM, Dutch Growth Hormone Working Group: Catch-up growth in early treated patients with growth hormone deficiency. Arch Dis Child 1995;72:427–431.
38 Karavanaki K, Kontaxaki C, Maniati-Chriatidi M, Petrou V, Dacou-Voutetakis C: Growth response, pubertal growth and final height in Greek children with growth hormone (GH) deficiency and long-term GH therapy and factors affecting outcome. J Pediatr Endocrinol Metab 2001;14:397–405.
39 Kastrup KW, Christiansen JS, Andersen JK, Orskov H: Increased growth rate following transfer to daily sc administration from three weekly im injection of hGH in growth hormone deficient children. Acta Endocrinol (Copenh) 1983;104:148–152.
40 Ranke MB, Lindberg A, Chatelain P, Wilton P, Cutfield W, Albertsson-Wikland K, Price DA: Derivation and validation of a mathematical model for predicting the response to exogenous recombinant human growth hormone (GH) in prepubertal children with idiopathic GH deficiency. J Clin Endocrinol Metab 1999;84:1174–1183.
41 Vosahlo J, Zidek T, Lebl J, Riedl S, Frisch H: Validation of a mathematical model predicting the response to growth hormone treatment in prepubertal children with idiopathic growth hormone deficiency. Horm Res 2004; 61:143–147.

10 KIGS

Ranke MB, Price DA, Reiter EO (eds): Growth Hormone Therapy in Pediatrics – 20 Years of KIGS.
Basel, Karger, 2007, pp 116–135

Idiopathic Growth Hormone Deficiency in KIGS: Selected Aspects

Michael B. Ranke[a]   Edward O. Reiter[b]   David A. Price[c]

Patients with idiopathic growth hormone deficiency (IGHD) are the largest group within KIGS (code No. 1.1). Although these patients have been treated with GH (with pituitary human GH from 1957 and with recombinant human GH from about 1981), the literature on many aspects of this disorder and its development during treatment is comparatively small. Many publications are based on small cohorts, even if including data from several centres or from an entire country. Some aspects which appear to be simplistic and are assumed to be common knowledge have not even found their way into reviewed journals. When we analysed the KIGS database for the publication of the 10 years KIGS book, we also neglected to document the great variety of aspects within this group of patients. The information which can be derived from this group is extensive and could almost be documented in a separate volume to this book. Therefore, we have selected to describe and comment on only a few aspects.

Data analyses were done according to common KIGS principles. Anthropometrical data are compared with the references of Prader, if not indicated otherwise.

Development of Some Characteristics at the Start of Growth Hormone Treatment over Time and in Various Countries

Context
It may be assumed that even disorders such as GHD which are based on complex analyses (anthropometrical, biochemical) are diagnosed in a more standardised mode, since with information being universally available, there is potential for a global standardisation. On the other hand, medical traditions, public health systems, diagnostic strategies, health economics and other factors may affect the diagnostic process, its timing and the decisions on initiation and modalities of treatment. Changes may also have manifested themselves.

Methods
The analysis was stratified according to the years of initiation of GH treatment, divided into three groups: before 1995, 1995–1999, and 2000–2005.

[a]Paediatric Endocrinology Section
University Children's Hospital, University of Tübingen
Hoppe-Seyler-Strasse 1, DE–72076 Tübingen (Germany)
[b]Baystate Children's Hospital, Tufts University School of Medicine
759 Chestnut Street, Springfield, MA 01199 (USA)
[c]Royal Manchester Children's Hospital, Hospital Road
Pendlebury, Swinton, Manchester M27 4HA (UK)

Table 1. Characteristics at GH start

Country	Years	n	Males %	Age years	Height SDS (Tanner)	Height SDS (Prader)	Ht – MPH SDS (Tanner and Prader)	Maximum GH peak μg/l	GH dose mg/kg/week
ROW	<1995	9,376	70	10.0	–2.6	–3.2	–1.5	5.9	0.18
	95–99	6,069	68	10.4	–2.4	–2.9	–1.7	6.1	0.22
	00–05	6,823	66	10.9	–2.3	–2.8	–1.6	6.2	0.23
Japan	<1995	3,161	70	10.1	–2.7	–3.3	–0.8	6.7	0.17
	95–99	657	65	8.2	–2.5	–3.2	–0.8	7.5	0.18
	00–05	1,085	63	9.2	–2.6	–3.3	–0.9	7.5	0.18
USA	<1995	–	–	–	–	–	–	–	–
	95–99	1,639	73	11.0	–2.3	–2.8	–2.1	5.9	0.30
	00–05	2,468	73	11.7	–2.1	–2.5	–1.8	5.9	0.30
UK	<1995	821	69	8.0	–3.0	–3.6	–2.4	3.9	0.22
	95–99	255	71	8.3	–2.7	–3.3	–2.4	4.7	0.21
	00–05	132	63	9.6	–2.4	–3.0	–2.1	4.5	0.20
Sweden	<1995	745	75	10.5	–2.2	–2.7	–2.0	6.0	0.24
	95–99	279	74	9.9	–2.0	–2.5	–1.6	6.5	0.24
	00–05	110	66	10.1	–1.9	–2.4	–1.9	6.5	0.24
Germany	<1995	763	71	8.2	–2.5	–3.1	–2.2	4.7	0.18
	95–99	677	71	9.4	–2.2	–2.8	–2.0	5.6	0.18
	00–05	924	69	10.0	–2.0	–2.5	–1.9	6.0	0.19
France	<1995	1,376	66	11.0	–2.4	–2.9	–1.4	7.2	0.14
	95–99	853	64	10.8	–2.3	–2.9	–1.5	7.4	0.22
	00–05	678	59	11.1	–2.2	–2.7	–1.5	7.5	0.24

Data are given as medians. MPH = Midparental height.

The analysis included all patients in the founding countries of KIGS (Sweden, France, UK, Germany), the USA (no data before 1995) and Japan, and all minus these specific countries (rest of the world).

The selected characteristics are listed in table 1.

Results
The development of the numbers of IGHD patients entering KIGS has been steady over the years but varies in different countries.

Age at GH start varies (earliest in the UK, latest in France), but shows no clear trend over time.

The calculated height standard deviation score (SDS) at entry varies among countries, based on the difference between the height references and the height within the respective populations. There is a global tendency to include less tall individuals, which is probably not only the result of a secular growth trend.

The difference between the height SDS and the target height SDS varies among countries (greatest in the UK, smallest in Japan), without a clear trend over time.

Maximum GH levels to tests differ significantly (smallest in the UK, greatest in France). There is no general trend over time.

GH doses are similar in most countries except for the USA (highest) and Japan (lowest).

There has been an overall increase of about 20% in dosing from before 1995 to after 2000.

Commentary

The results document the variability and regionality of the medical world, which provides the opportunity to learn many aspects from different points of view. The results show that changes have been occurring in different medical environments. More standardisation is probably needed in GH measurements in order to create more homogeneity within heterogeneity.

Characteristics before and during 3 Prepubertal Years in all Patients with Idiopathic Growth Hormone Deficiency

Context

We believe that the first few prepubertal years of catch-up growth are the most important in terms of achievement of normal adult height. Knowledge of the variability may help to understand and aid individual treatment.

Methods

1 Groups of patients treated longitudinally for 3 prepubertal years were analysed.
2 The analysis was stratified according to the years of initiation of GH treatment, divided into three groups: before 1995, 1995–1999, and 2000–2005.
3 The analysis included all patients in the founding countries of KIGS (Sweden, France, UK, Germany), the USA (no data before 1995) and Japan, and all minus these specific countries (rest of the world).

Results

Results of characteristics at the start of GH treatment and changes of growth response parameters in all of these patients (irrespective of year of initiation) are listed in table 2.

Some results of groups analysed according to the year of GH start and the country of origin are listed in table 3.

Summary

1 Children treated with GH over a period of 3 prepubertal years are on average 6.7 years old at the initiation of treatment, have a bone age which is delayed by 2.4 years, have a height SDS of –3.3 and receive GH at a dose of 0.21 mg/kg/week.
2 Before GH initiation, the bone age progression is 0.5 year/year, Δ height is –0.1, height velocity is 4.7 cm/year, and Δ body mass index (BMI) is 0.0 SDS.
3 Height velocity during the first, second and third year ranges between 6.2 and 12.7, between 5.1 and 9.6, and between 4.5 and 8.6 cm/year, respectively. In terms of the Δ height SDS, this corresponds to 0.5–0.9, 0.3–0.5 and 0.2–0.4 SDS, respectively.

Studentised residuals scatter narrowly around 0.0 in all years.

Commentary

Given the heterogeneity of patient characteristics and treatment modalities, the responses to GH are rather homogenous, even if the progression of time is considered. The KIGS prediction models for GH are very robust.

First-Year Growth Response in Patients with Extreme Weights

Context

Generally, patients with GHD have more fat mass and less muscle mass, a fact which is not always expressed by the BMI. In KIGS prediction models, weight has been observed to be a factor positively related to the response to GH (the heavier, the better). Nutrition and the glucose-insulin system may play a major part in the response to GH.

Table 2. Characteristics before and during 3 prepubertal years in all IGHD patients

	n	Median	10th percentile	90th percentile	Mean ± SD
At GH start					
Age, years	4,802	6.7	3.3	11.8	7.1 ± 3.3
Bone age, years	1,913	4.3	2.0	9.5	5.1 ± 3.0
Δ bone age, years	264	0.5	0.0	1.2	0.6 ± 0.6
Height SDS	4,802	−3.3	−4.9	−2.3	−3.5 ± 1.1
Δ height SDS	2,111	−0.1	−0.6	0.3	−0.1 ± 0.6
Height velocity, cm/year	2,111	4.7	2.9	7.0	4.9 ± 2.0
BMI SDS	4,802	−0.3	−1.8	1.2	−0.3 ± 1.3
Δ BMI SDS	1,881	0.0	−0.7	0.9	0.1 ± 0.8
1st year on GH					
Height SDS	4,802	−2.5	−3.9	−1.4	−2.6 ± 1.1
Δ bone age, years	1,132	1.0	0.2	2.0	1.1 ± 0.9
Δ height SDS	4,802	0.7	0.2	1.6	0.8 ± 0.7
Height velocity, cm/year	4,802	8.6	6.2	12.7	9.1 ± 2.7
Δ BMI SDS	4,780	−0.1	−0.9	0.6	−0.1 ± 0.7
2nd year on GH					
Height SDS	4,802	−2.1	−3.5	−0.8	−2.2 ± 1.1
Δ bone age, years	1,315	1.0	0.3	2.1	1.2 ± 0.9
Δ height SDS	4,802	0.4	−0.2	0.8	0.3 ± 0.5
Height velocity, cm/year	4,700	7.1	5.1	9.6	7.2 ± 1.8
Δ BMI SDS	4,765	0.1	−0.5	0.8	0.1 ± 0.6
3rd year on GH					
Height SDS	4,802	−1.8	−3.2	−0.4	−1.8 ± 1.2
Δ bone age, years	1,246	1.0	0.3	2.2	1.2 ± 0.9
Δ height SDS	4,802	0.2	−0.5	0.6	0.1 ± 0.5
Height velocity, cm/year	4,669	6.3	4.5	8.6	6.5 ± 1.7
Δ BMI SDS	4,770	0.1	−0.5	0.6	0.1 ± 0.5

Methods

Of all prepubertal patients (at the start and end of the first year on GH), those 20% with the lowest and those 20% with the highest BMI SDS were grouped and compared with each other.

Results

The results of the 1,680 and 1,670 patients in the groups are listed in table 4. The relationship between the Δ height SDS and the Δ BMI SDS is illustrated in figure 1.

Commentary

The comparison shows a multitude of interesting results, which are mostly self-explanatory. The data during the first treatment year show greater height velocity and gain in height SDS in the overweight group. However, in terms of studentised residuals [(observed − predicted height velocity)/error SD], there is no difference, which is in support of the prediction model. Interestingly, the lean group gains in terms of the BMI SDS, while the overweight group loses. Thus, in the overweight group, there is probably a higher loss in fat mass compared with the gain in lean body mass.

Table 3. Characteristics after 3 years of prepubertal longitudinal growth

Country	Years	Before GH treatment				1st year on GH			2nd year on GH			3rd year on GH		
		n	age years	height SDS	height velocity cm/year	dose mg/kg/week	height velocity cm/year	Δ height SDS (Prader)	studentised residual	height velocity cm/year	Δ height SDS (Prader)	studentised residual	height velocity cm/year	Δ height SDS (Prader)	studentised residual
All	<1995	2,585	6.7	–3.4	4.6	0.18	8.5	0.7	–0.1	7.0	0.3	0.0	6.2	0.2	0.0
	95–99	1,544	6.4	–3.2	4.8	0.21	8.9	0.7	–0.1	7.3	0.4	0.0	6.5	0.2	–0.2
	00–05	673	6.9	–3.2	5.1	0.20	8.5	0.7	–0.3	7.2	0.4	0.1	6.5	0.2	0.1
Japan	<1995	846	6.5	–3.3	4.3	0.18	7.5	0.5	–0.4	6.5	0.3	0.0	6.0	0.2	–0.1
	95–99	301	6.6	–3.3	4.8	0.18	7.6	0.5	–0.2	6.4	0.3	–0.1	6.1	0.2	–0.1
	00–05	237	7.3	–3.5	4.9	0.18	7.7	0.6	–0.3	6.5	0.3	0.1	6.0	0.2	0.2
USA	<1995	–	–	–	–	–	–	–	–	–	–	–	–	–	–
	95–99	374	6.2	–3.1	4.8	0.30	9.8	0.9	–0.2	7.9	0.4	0.1	6.9	0.2	–0.3
	00–05	164	7.7	–2.9	4.5	0.30	9.5	0.7	–0.4	7.9	0.4	–0.2	6.7	0.2	–0.1
UK	<1995	283	6.1	–3.9	4.6	0.24	9.5	0.9	–0.2	7.4	0.4	–0.1	6.3	0.3	–0.2
	95–99	87	4.2	–3.7	5.0	0.21	10.1	1.1	0.1	7.8	0.5	0.1	6.6	0.2	–0.4
	00–05	13	4.6	–3.7	6.1	0.21	8.9	0.8	–	7.6	0.5	–0.1	7.0	0.4	0.0
Sweden	<1995	178	6.5	–3.1	5.3	0.24	9.4	0.9	0.2	7.4	0.4	–0.1	6.6	0.3	0.0
	95–99	91	6.8	–2.7	5.5	0.24	9.2	0.8	0.0	7.1	0.4	–0.1	6.4	0.3	–0.2
	00–05	23	6.9	–2.6	5.3	0.24	9.3	0.8	–0.7	7.9	0.6	0.4	6.9	0.3	0.1
Germany	<1995	242	5.9	–3.4	4.7	0.19	9.7	0.9	–0.2	7.5	0.4	0.0	6.5	0.3	–0.1
	95–99	198	6.1	–3.1	4.6	0.19	9.2	0.8	–0.1	7.5	0.4	0.2	6.7	0.3	–0.1
	00–05	114	6.4	–3.0	5.0	0.19	8.9	0.7	–0.2	7.2	0.4	0.0	6.7	0.3	0.3
France	<1995	397	7.6	–3.1	4.7	0.15	7.7	0.5	0.0	6.5	0.3	0.1	5.9	0.1	0.1
	95–99	287	7.6	–3.0	4.7	0.23	8.7	0.7	–0.2	7.2	0.3	–0.2	6.5	0.2	–0.2
	00–05	66	7.4	–2.9	5.5	0.24	10.0	0.8	–0.1	7.7	0.4	0.3	6.9	0.2	–0.4

Data are given as medians.

Table 4. First-year response in IGHD patients with extreme weights

	Lowest BMI				Highest BMI				p
	n	median	10th percentile	90th percentile	n	median	10th percentile	90th percentile	
Background									
Birth weight SDS	1,680	−1.1	−2.7	0.4	1,670	−0.5	−2.0	1.1	<0.0001
MPH SDS (Prader)	1,707	−1.2	−2.7	0.4	1,743	−1.2	−2.8	0.4	n.s.
Maximum GH peak, μg/l	1,867	6.4	1.8	9.4	1,867	5.0	1.1	8.8	<0.0001
At start of GH treatment									
Age, years	1,867	9.4	3.4	13.8	1,867	8.7	3.7	13.6	<0.05
Height SDS (Prader)	1,867	−3.0	−4.7	−2.0	1,867	−2.9	−4.3	−1.6	<0.0001
Height − MPH SDS (Prader)	1,707	−1.8	−4.0	−0.1	1,743	−1.6	−3.9	0.2	<0.0001
Height velocity, cm/year	710	4.5	2.7	7.2	727	4.4	2.4	6.5	n.s.
Δ height SDS (before GH start)	710	0.0	−0.4	0.6	727	0.0	−0.6	0.4	<0.0001
Weight SDS	1,867	−3.4	−5.1	−2.4	1,867	−0.6	−2.0	0.8	<0.0001
BMI SDS	1,867	−1.8	−3.0	−1.4	1,867	1.3	0.8	2.4	<0.0001
Δ BMI SDS (before GH start)	649	−0.2	−0.9	0.8	662	0.2	−0.4	1.2	<0.0001
GH dose, mg/kg/week	1,867	0.22	0.16	0.32	1,867	0.20	0.14	0.30	<0.0001
After first year on GH									
Height SDS (Prader)	1,867	−2.4	−3.8	−1.3	1,867	−2.0	−3.4	−0.8	<0.0001
Height velocity, cm/year	1,867	8.0	5.7	11.7	1,867	9.2	6.4	13.0	<0.0001
Δ height SDS (Prader)	1,867	0.5	−0.5	1.3	1,867	0.7	−0.2	1.4	<0.0001
Studentised residual SDS (GHD with maximum peak)	400	−0.2	−1.7	1.2	593	−0.3	−2.0	1.4	n.s.
Δ BMI SDS	1,861	0.2	−0.5	1.1	1,860	−0.3	−1.1	0.3	<0.0001

MPH = Midparental height; n.s. = not significant.

Near-Adult Height in Patients with Extreme Weights

Context

Response to GH during the first year is positively correlated with weight. When weight is considered, the response to GH is not different. The effect of weight on long-term GH treatment is unknown.

Methods

The near adult height (NAH) values of those 20% of patients with the lowest and those 20% with the highest BMI SDS were grouped and compared with each other. The patients were treated for at least 1 prepubertal year and had reached NAH (NAH = height velocity <2 cm/year and asymptotic nearing of the growth curve towards final height; bone age >16 years in boys and >14 years in girls).

Results

The results of the 477 lean and 477 obese patients are listed in table 5.

The two groups are different in respect to pretreatment variables such as birth weight and maximum GH to tests. The overweight patients tend to receive about 3% less GH.

At puberty onset, the lean group is shorter and marginally older. Both groups do not gain in height SDS during puberty.

Commentary
In the long run, obesity does not appear to have a major effect on height outcomes in adult life. The data also pose the question whether dosing according to weight is necessary in overweight (obese) children.

Sitting Height – First Year on Growth Hormone

Context
Leg and trunk length differ in adult males and females and show a characteristic pattern of development in childhood and adolescence. There is hardly any investigation into the first-year effect of GH on sitting height in relation to height in prepubertal boys and girls.

Methods
Three hundred and ninety-nine girls and 1,042 boys, who were investigated during the first year of treatment in terms of height and sitting height, were compared.

Results
The results are listed in table 6.

Before GH treatment, height and sitting height show the same degree (SDS) of deviation from normal in boys and girls. Likewise, the gain in the height SDS and sitting height SDS is the same in both sexes.

Commentary
GH treatment during the prepubertal phase induces proportional growth in both sexes.

Head Circumference – First Year on Growth Hormone

Context
A disproportional, large neurocranium compared with body size gives children with GHD a commonly cited 'doll-like' appearance. The degree to which changes in head circumference is part of the catch-up process in IGHD is largely unknown.

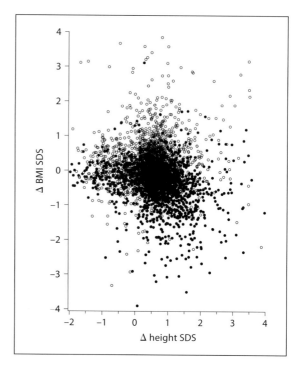

Fig. 1. The correlation between the Δ height SDS and Δ BMI SDS during the first year on GH in IGHD patients suggests a higher gain in height if the reduction in BMI is greater. ○ = Low BMI; ● = high BMI.

Methods
One hundred and eleven girls and 243 boys, who were investigated during the first year of treatment in terms of height and head circumference, were compared.

Results
The results are listed in table 7.

Before treatment, the height was about –3.0 SDS in the cohorts, while the head circumference was about –1.0 SDS. The degree of variability of the head circumference was smaller than that for height.

Change in height was in the order of 0.7 SDS, while change in head circumference was in the order of 0.3 SDS.

Table 5. NAH in IGHD patients with extreme weights

	Lowest BMI				Highest BMI				p
	n	median	10th percentile	90th percentile	n	median	10th percentile	90th percentile	
Patients (total)	477				477				<0.01
Background									
Birth weight SDS	432	−1.1	−2.6	0.5	427	−0.5	−1.7	1.1	<0.001
MPH SDS (Prader)	444	−1.3	−2.9	0.2	442	−1.2	−2.7	0.4	n.s.
Maximum GH peak, μg/l	477	5.5	1.0	9.2	477	3.8	0.8	8.4	<0.001
Males, %	60				69				
At start of GH treatment									
Age, years	477	10.0	4.2	13.2	477	9.3	4.3	12.6	<0.05
Height SDS (Prader)	477	−3.4	−5.3	−2.1	477	−3.2	−4.9	−2.0	<0.01
Height – MPH SDS (Prader)	444	−2.0	−4.5	−0.3	442	−2.0	−4.2	−0.2	n.s.
Height velocity, cm/year	211	4.4	2.4	6.4	228	4.3	2.0	6.3	
Δ height SDS (before GH start)	211	0.1	−0.4	0.6	228	0.0	−0.6	0.4	<0.05
Weight SDS	477	−3.6	−5.9	−2.5	477	−0.8	−2.2	0.6	<0.001
BMI SDS	477	−1.8	−2.9	−1.3	477	1.2	0.8	2.3	<0.001
Δ BMI SDS (before GH start)	190	−0.2	−0.7	0.6	214	0.1	−0.5	0.9	<0.001
GH dose, mg/kg/week	477	0.20	0.15	0.32	477	0.17	0.11	0.27	<0.001
At start of puberty									
Age, years	199	13.3	11.1	15.9	172	12.9	11.1	15.3	
Height SDS (Prader)	199	−1.7	−2.8	−0.3	172	−1.3	−2.4	0.3	<0.001
Height – MPH SDS (Prader)	182	−0.4	−2.0	1.0	163	−0.1	−1.6	1.2	n.s.
Δ height SDS (puberty – start, Prader)	199	1.7	0.7	3.7	172	1.8	0.7	4.1	n.s.
BMI SDS	197	−1.6	−2.9	0.0	172	1.1	−0.2	2.1	<0.001
Δ BMI SDS (puberty – start)	197	0.2	−0.7	2.2	172	−0.3	−1.3	0.5	<0.001
Mean prepuberty GH dose, mg/kg/week	199	0.20	0.15	0.27	173	0.17	0.11	0.24	<0.001
NAH									
Age, years	477	17.7	15.6	20.0	477	17.4	15.4	19.8	
Height SDS (Prader)	477	−1.6	−3.3	−0.2	477	−1.4	−3.0	0.3	<0.01
Δ height SDS (latest – puberty, Prader)	199	0.1	−0.9	1.0	172	0.0	−1.0	0.9	n.s.
Δ height SDS (latest – start, Prader)	477	1.8	0.5	3.5	477	1.7	0.2	3.8	n.s.
Studentised residual SDS (TPG)	119	−0.2	−1.5	1.1	110	−0.1	−1.5	1.2	n.s.
BMI SDS	466	−1.1	−2.7	0.5	467	1.0	−0.3	2.5	<0.001
Δ BMI SDS (latest – puberty)	193	0.5	−0.8	1.5	169	0.2	−0.8	1.0	<0.001
Δ BMI SDS (latest – start)	466	0.8	−0.6	2.6	467	−0.3	−1.5	1.0	<0.001
Years on GH treatment	477	7.3	4.7	12.4	477	7.5	4.5	12.8	n.s.

MPH = Midparental height; TPG = total pubertal growth.

Commentary

Since the head circumference reflects not only soft tissue and bone growth but also brain growth, it must be assumed that GH treatment affects the growth of brain size during the first year on GH. Little is known about the dose dependence of this effect and the functional consequences of it. More sophisticated morphometric analyses (e.g., magnetic resonance tomography) and neurocognitive analyses should be conducted in selected cohorts.

Table 6. Development of height and sitting height

	Females				Males				p
	n	median	10th percentile	90th percentile	n	median	10th percentile	90th percentile	
At start of GH treatment									
Age, years	399	7.9	4.1	11.6	1,042	8.2	4.3	11.8	
Height SDS (Prader)	399	−3.3	−5.0	−2.1	1,042	−2.8	−4.0	−2.0	<0.001
Height − MPH SDS (Prader)	376	−2.3	−4.3	−0.7	996	−1.8	−3.5	−0.4	<0.001
Sitting height SDS (Prader)	399	−3.2	−4.9	−2.0	1,042	−2.7	−4.0	−1.6	<0.001
Sitting height, %	399	55	52	58	1,042	55	52	58	
Sitting height ratio SDS	300	0.6	−1.3	2.1	1,042	0.4	−1.3	1.7	
Mean GH dose, mg/kg/week	399	0.21	0.16	0.28	1,042	0.22	0.16	0.28	
After first year on GH									
Age, years	399	8.8	5.1	12.5	1,042	9.3	5.3	12.8	
Height SDS (Prader)	399	−2.4	−3.8	−1.3	1,042	−2.1	−3.3	−1.2	<0.001
Height − MPH SDS (Prader)	376	−1.4	−3.2	0.1	996	−1.1	−2.6	0.2	<0.001
Δ height SDS (Prader)	399	0.7	−0.1	1.6	1,042	0.7	0.3	1.3	
Sitting height SDS (Prader)	399	−2.4	−4.1	−1.0	1,042	−1.9	−3.3	−0.8	<0.001
Δ sitting height SDS (Prader)	399	0.8	−0.1	1.8	1,042	0.7	0.0	1.5	
Sitting height, %	399	55	52	57	1,042	54	52	57	
Sitting height ratio SDS	399	0.7	−1.3	2.2	1,042	0.4	−1.1	1.7	
Mean GH dose, mg/kg/week	399	0.21	0.16	0.28	1,042	0.22	0.16	0.27	

MPH = Midparental height.

Table 7. Development of height and head circumference

	Females				Males				p
	n	median	10th percentile	90th percentile	n	median	10th percentile	90th percentile	
At start of GH treatment									
Age, years	111	7.6	3.4	10.9	243	6.4	3.5	11.1	
Height SDS (Prader)	111	−3.3	−5.1	−2.1	243	−2.8	−4.1	−2.0	<0.001
Height − MPH SDS (Prader)	107	−2.1	−4.2	−0.5	232	−1.8	−3.4	−0.6	
Head circumference SDS (Prader)	111	−1.0	−3.0	0.6	243	−1.3	−3.0	0.5	
GH dose, mg/kg/week	111	0.20	0.15	0.29	243	0.22	0.16	0.31	
After first year on GH									
Age, years	111	8.6	4.2	11.9	243	7.5	4.4	12.0	
Height SDS (Prader)	111	−2.5	−4.1	−1.3	243	−2.1	−3.1	−1.2	<0.001
Height − MPH SDS (Prader)	107	−1.3	−3.0	0.1	232	−1.1	−2.3	0.1	
Head circumference SDS (Prader)	111	−0.5	−2.5	0.9	243	−0.9	−2.5	0.8	
Δ head circumference SDS (Prader)	111	0.3	−0.3	1.0	243	0.3	−0.3	1.1	

MPH = Midparental height.

Table 8. GH dosing during prepuberty

	Before 1995			1995–1999			2000–2005		
	median	10th percentile	90th percentile	median	10th percentile	90th percentile	median	10th percentile	90th percentile
Patients	2,585			1,544			673		
Age, years	6.7	3.2	11.8	6.4	3.3	11.6	6.9	3.5	12.1
Height SDS	–3.4	–5.1	–2.4	–3.2	–4.5	–2.2	–3.2	–4.5	–2.1
GH dose, mg/kg/week	0.18	0.13	0.27	0.21	0.16	0.31	0.20	0.17	0.31

Growth Hormone Dosing during Prepuberty

Context
The principle of GH dosing has changed over time. Initially, GH was injected 2–3 times per week and given in fixed dosages in international units. With the introduction of recombinant human GH with a specific potency of 3 IU/mg and daily injections, a dosing according to IU/kilogram body weight/week – or recently, milligrams/kilogram body weight/day – was commonly used.

Method
Groups of patients treated longitudinally for 3 prepubertal years were analysed with regard to the dose given at start of treatment. The analysis was stratified according to the years of initiation of GH treatment, divided into three groups: before 1995, 1995–1999, and 2000–2005.

Results
The results are listed in table 8. The overall median dose and the range of dosing increased slightly, but significantly after 1995. This is probably not only a result of the generally higher dose level approved in the USA.

The relationship between weight and GH dose in the three cohorts is illustrated in figure 2. There was a pronounced inverse relationship between weight and GH dose before 1995 and (less so) in 1995–1999. After 2000, this trend was not significant.

Commentary
It must be assumed that dosing was previously fixed. Thus, small children received a relatively higher dose and large children a smaller dose. During recent years, the dose is calculated according to weight (or body surface area) considering the circumstance of the individual.

Growth Hormone Dosing at Puberty

Context
During puberty, there is an increase in GH secretion and an increase in insulin-like growth factors. Whether this plays a role in height development is not completely clear. KIGS analyses and few studies on dosing suggest that there is a positive but relatively small effect of the GH dose on total pubertal growth in patients with GHD.

Method
Patients with a defined onset of treatment were analysed. The analysis was stratified according to the years of treatment, divided into three groups: before 1995, 1995–1999, and 2000–2005.

Results
The results at puberty onset are listed in table 9. The overall median dose and the range of dosing increased significantly over the years.

The relationship between weight and GH dose in the three cohorts is illustrated in figure 3.

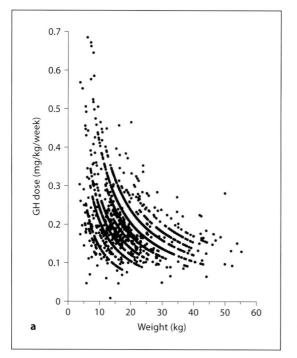
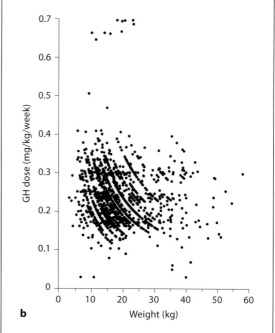
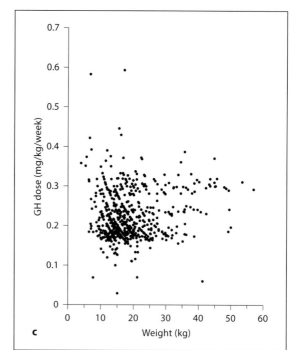

Fig. 2. Relationship between weight and GH dose in prepubertal children with GHD before 1995 (**a**), in 1995–1999 (**b**), and in 2000–2005 (**c**).

Table 9. GH dosing during puberty

	Before 1995			1995–1999			2000–2005		
	median	10th percentile	90th percentile	median	10th percentile	90th percentile	median	10th percentile	90th percentile
Patients	954			1,011			1,454		
Age, years	13.6	11.3	16.0	13.7	11.4	15.9	13.4	11.2	15.7
Height SDS	–2.7	–3.8	–1.8	–2.6	–3.8	–1.6	–2.4	–3.5	–1.4
GH dose, mg/kg/week	0.18	0.12	0.26	0.22	0.15	0.30	0.24	0.17	0.33

There was a pronounced inverse relationship between weight and GH dose before 1995 and (less so) in 1995–1999. After 2000, this correlation was no longer present.

Commentary
It must be assumed that dosing, like during prepubertal years, used to be fixed during puberty. This means that a certain daily dose in units/milligram was injected. As a consequence, smaller children received a relatively higher dose and heavier children a smaller dose. During recent years, the dose tends to be calculated – and adapted – according to weight (or body surface area) considering the circumstance of the individual.

Prepubertal Height Velocity (Height Gain) before and during 3 Years on Growth Hormone

Context
It can be assumed that in prepubertal IGHD patients, both pretreatment growth and growth during the first 3 years on GH depend on the degree of GHD.

Method
Prepubertal patients treated longitudinally for 3 prepubertal years and with height velocity data before treatment were analysed. The patients were stratified according to the maximum GH levels observed to testing: <5, 5–7 and 7–10 μg/l.

Results
Data are listed in table 10.

Growth in terms of centimetres/year before and during the first 3 pubertal years and related to the degree of GHD is illustrated in figure 4.

Growth in terms of the Δ height SDS before and during the first 3 pubertal years and related to the degree of GHD is illustrated in figure 5.

Individual growth in boys in terms of centimetres/year in relation to age at treatment start is plotted within the height velocity references before (fig. 6a, c, e) and during the first year on GH (fig. 6b, d, f). The plots are grouped according to the degree of GHD.

Comments
Height velocity before GH treatment is not much dependent on the documented degree of GHD. A height velocity below the 50th percentile for age is probably compatible with the diagnosis (in boys and girls; data not shown).

During the first year on GH, children with severe maximum GH (<5 ng/ml) have significantly higher height responses (in terms of centimetres/year or Δ height SDS) compared with the other groups. These differences are less pronounced in subsequent years.

During the first year on GH, a height velocity >97th percentile for age (or a Δ height SDS >0.5) should be considered an appropriate response.

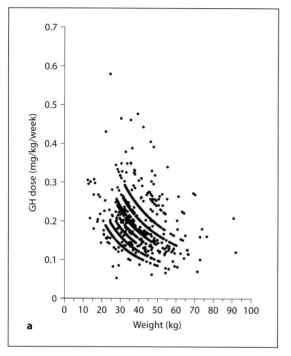
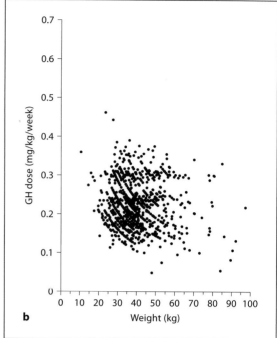
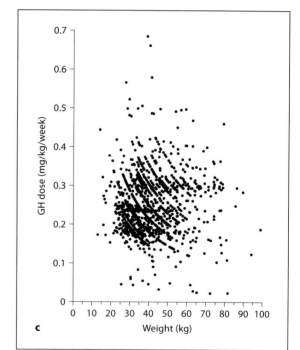

Fig. 3. Relationship between weight and GH dose in pubertal children with GHD before 1995 (**a**), in 1995–1999 (**b**), and in 2000–2005 (**c**).

Table 10. Prepubertal height velocity/height gain during 3 years on GH related to maximum GH to tests

	Maximum GH								
	<5 ng/ml (n = 828)			5–7 ng/ml (n = 421)			7–10 ng/ml (n = 759)		
	median	10th percentile	90 percentile	median	10th percentile	90th percentile	median	10th percentile	90th percentile
At GH start									
Age, years	6.2	2.6	11.2	6.3	3.6	10.9	6.9	3.7	11.7
Height SDS[1]	–3.7	–5.5	–2.5	–3.2	–4.6	–2.3	–3.2	–4.3	–2.3
Height velocity, cm/year	4.6	2.5	7.5	4.8	3.0	6.7	4.8	3.2	6.8
Δ height SDS[1]	–0.1	–0.9	0.4	0.0	–0.5	0.3	0.0	–0.4	0.3
GH dose, mg/kg/week	0.19	0.14	0.30	0.19	0.15	0.29	0.19	0.15	0.29
1st year on GH									
Height velocity, cm/year	9.6	6.7	13.8	8.2	6.2	11.0	8.0	6.1	11.0
Δ height SDS[1]	0.9	0.3	1.9	0.6	0.2	1.3	0.6	0.2	1.1
2nd year on GH									
Height velocity, cm/year	7.5	5.2	10.0	6.9	5.1	8.9	6.6	5.0	8.9
Δ height SDS[1]	0.4	0.0	0.9	0.3	–0.1	0.7	0.3	–0.1	0.6
3rd year on GH									
Height velocity, cm/year	6.5	4.6	8.7	6.1	4.6	8.4	6.2	4.4	8.1
Δ height SDS[1]	0.3	–0.4	0.6	0.2	–0.4	0.6	0.2	–0.6	0.5

[1] Prader reference values.

Effects of Thyroxin and Cortisol on Growth during the First Prepubertal Year in Patients with Idiopathic Growth Hormone Deficiency

Context
Prepubertal children with combined (multiple) pituitary hormone deficiencies (MPHD) receive additional replacement therapy with thyroid hormone (mostly thyroxin) or glucocorticoids (mostly hydrocortisone), or a combination of both. There is still some controversy about the appropriate glucocorticoid replacement in MPHD patients.

Methods
Prepubertal children with IGHD – either with isolated or combined pituitary deficiencies (excluding diabetes insipidus) – who were treated for a full first year were analysed. Only patients receiving thyroxin or cortisol (hydrocortisone) were analysed, even if the doses were not available in all of the patients. The parameters of the groups were compared.

Results
The results are summarised in table 11. There were a total of 7,831 children with isolated GHD and 1,504 patients with MPHD. Of the children with MPHD, 779 received thyroid hormone alone, 119 received glucocorticoids alone and 286 received a combination. The remaining (not analysed) received a combination of other medication. As a whole group, children with MPHD had taller parents, a higher degree of GH insufficiency and were slightly younger and shorter. However, both groups received the same dose of GH.

Thyroxin was given at a median dose of 50 μg/day which amounted to 2.0 μg/kg/day in the

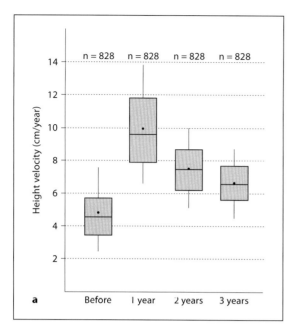
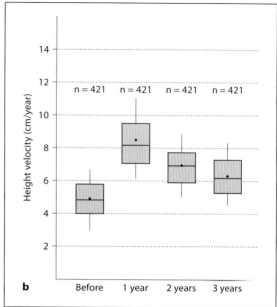
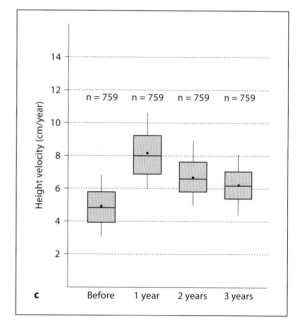

Fig. 4. Height velocity during the first 3 prepubertal years in IGHD patients in relation to the maximum GH levels observed in response to GH testing: maximum GH <5.0 μg/l (**a**), 5–7 μg/l (**b**), and 7–10 μg/l (**c**).

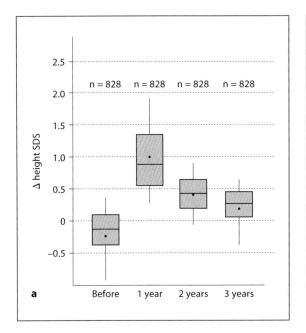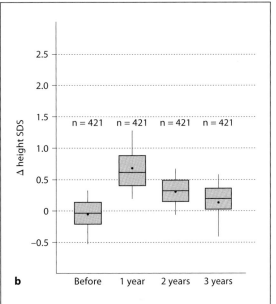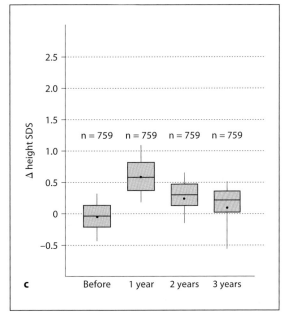

Fig. 5. Δ height SDS during the first 3 prepubertal years in IGHD patients in relation to the maximum GH levels observed in response to GH testing: maximum GH <5.0 μg/l (**a**), 5–7 μg/l (**b**), and 7–10 μg/l (**c**).

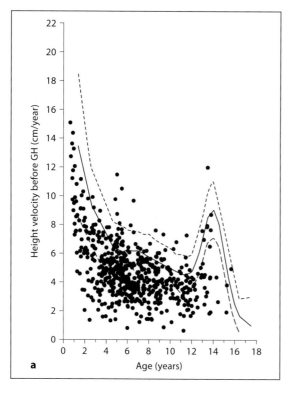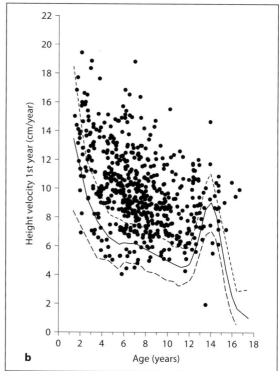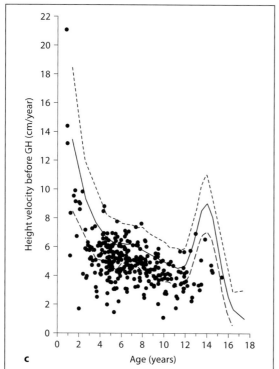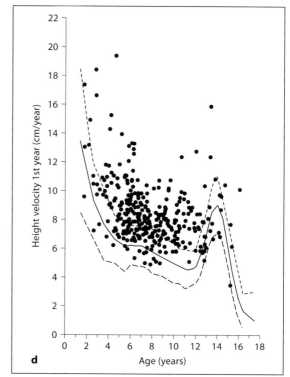

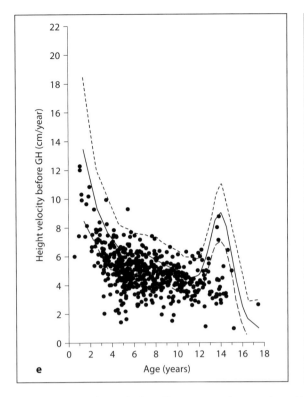
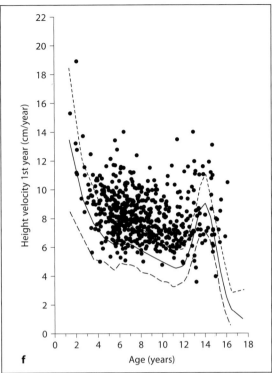

Fig. 6. Height velocity before GH treatment in prepubertal boys with IGHD and during the first year on GH in relation to chronological age and the degree of GHD (maximum GH to tests). Before GH treatment: maximum GH <5.0 μg/l (**a**), 5–7 μg/l (**c**), and GH 7–10 μg/l (**e**). First year on GH: maximum GH <5.0 μg/l (**b**), GH 5–7 μg/l (**d**), and GH 7–10 μg/l (**f**). Dashed lines = 3rd and 97th centiles; solid line = 50th centile.

group with thyroid hormone alone and at a median dose of 2.9 μg/kg/day ($p < 0.01$) in the combination group.

Hydrocortisone was given at a median dose of 20 mg/day which amounted to 1.5 mg/kg/day in the group with glucocorticoids alone and at a median dose of 10 mg/day which amounted to 0.5 mg/kg/day in the combination group.

Of the three groups receiving additional treatment, those in the combination group had the tallest parents and were most severely GH insufficient. In this group, the patients were the youngest and shortest, but the GH doses were not different.

When the first-year growth in the total groups (isolated vs. MPHD) was compared, a significantly higher height velocity (centimetres/year) and gain in height SDS was observed, but the studentised residuals (based on the prediction model including maximum GH) were only marginally lower in children with isolated GHD. The first-year growth response in terms of centimetres/year and Δ height SDS and the studentised residuals did not differ between the groups receiving one additional hormone. However, in the group with combined replacement, not only the height velocity and Δ height SDS were greater but also the studentised residuals.

Comments

It is obviously difficult to establish additional pituitary hormone deficiencies in prepubertal chil-

Table 11. IGHD and MPHD with and without thyroxin and glucocorticoids

	Isolated IGHD	Idiopathic MPHD				p < 0.001
Treatment:	GH	GH	GH + thyroxin	GH + gluco-corticoids	GH + thyroxin + gluco-corticoids	
	A	B	C	D	E	
Background						
Patients	7,831	1,504	779	119	286	
Males, %	72	73	71	82	72	
Birth weight SDS	–0.8	–0.6	–0.6	–0.5	–0.4	
MPH SDS (Prader)	–1.4	–0.8	–1.0	–1.0	–0.4	
Maximum GH peak, µg/l	6.5	3.5	3.8	6.0	1.7	B/D, B/E, C/D, D/E
At start of GH treatment						
Age, years	8.9	8.0	7.9	8.7	5.3	B/E, D/E
Height SDS (Prader)	–2.9	–3.3	–3.4	–2.9	–3.5	B/C, B/D, C/D, D/E
Height – MPH SDS (Prader)	–1.5	–2.4	–2.5	–1.8	–3.1	B/D, B/E, C/D, D/E
Weight SDS	–2.1	–2.3	–2.3	–1.7	–2.4	B/D, C/D, D/E
BMI SDS	–0.3	–0.2	–0.2	0.0	–0.2	
GH dose, mg/kg/week	0.20	0.21	0.20	0.23	0.21	B/C, B/D, C/D
Thyroxin dose, µg/day			50.0		50.0	
Thyroxin dose, µg/kg/day			2.0		2.9	
Cortisol dose, mg/day				20.0	10.0	
Cortisol dose, mg/kg/day				1.5	0.5	
1st year of GH therapy						
Age, years	9.9	9.0	8.9	9.8	6.3	B/E, D/E
Height SDS (Prader)	–2.2	–2.3	–2.4	–2.1	–2.2	B/C
Height – MPH SDS (Prader)	–0.8	–1.5	–1.5	–1.1	–1.8	B/E, D/E, D/E
Height velocity, cm/year	8.4	9.7	9.7	8.7	11.9	B/D, B/E, D/E
Δ height SDS (Prader)	0.6	0.8	0.8	0.6	1.2	B/E
Studentised residual SDS (GHD with maximum peak)	–0.2	0.0	0.0	–0.1	0.4	
Weight SDS	–1.7	–1.7	–1.7	–1.2	–1.5	B/D
BMI SDS	–0.4	–0.3	–0.3	–0.2	–0.4	
Mean GH dose, mg/kg/week	0.2	0.20	0.19	0.22	0.20	B/C

Data are given as medians. MPH = Midparental height.

dren with IGHD. Often only severe deficits of thyroid hormones and/or glucocorticoids will be recognised.

The dose levels of thyroxin applied in MPHD patients are lower (about one third in the group receiving thyroid hormone alone) than if primary hypothyroidism is treated. On the other hand, hydrocortisone replacement appears to be relatively high compared with replacement in primary hypocortisolism.

When GH is combined with thyroxin and hydrocortisone, the greatest first-year response is observed. Whether this is the result of the doses of the additional hormones given or due to the fact that in the groups with one additional hormone replaced the other hormone should also be

Table 12. Clinical chemistry parameters before and during the first year on GH

	n	Basal	First year on GH	Increase %	p
Haemoglobin, g/dl	259	12.4	12.6	1.7	<0.001
Glucose, mg/dl	192	82.4	86.5	3.9	<0.05
Haemoglobin A_{1c}, %	144	4.7	4.9	1.8	n.s.
Calcium, mg/dl	229	9.6	9.6	0.0	n.s.
Phosphate, mg/dl	197	4.6	5.1	6.3	<0.001
Triglycerides, mg/dl	130	69.9	77.5	10.9	<0.05
Cholesterol, mg/dl	227	174	172	−2.9	n.s.
ALT, U/l	126	13.0	13.0	0.0	n.s.
AST, U/l	127	29.0	26.0	−7.7	<0.001
Alkaline phosphatase, U/l	294	438	583	22.1	<0.001

ALT = Alanine aminotransferase; AST = aspartate aminotransferase; n.s. = not significant.

given, remains unclear. Certainly, more efforts should be undertaken to disclose the full extent of pituitary deficits in order to replace all components appropriately.

Changes of Common Biochemical Parameters in the Blood of Prepubertal Children with Idiopathic Growth Hormone Deficiency

Context
Usually, a number of biochemical parameters are documented during routine follow-up in children treated with GH. This is probably done as part of general paediatric care and as part of monitoring for safety reasons. KIGS case report forms allow for the documentation of these parameters with respect to the various methods and units used in different centres. So far, these parameters have never been analysed.

Methods
We have restricted the analysis to prepubertal patients with IGHD (code No. 1.1) where biochemical parameters were documented before and during the first year on GH (n >50) and when the method applied allowed the combined analysis of data.

Results
The parameters investigated, the number of cases, the median levels before and during the first year, the percentage of change and the level of significance of the change are listed in table 12. There was a large increment in alkaline phosphatase, a small increment in haemoglobin and phosphate and a small decrease in aspartate aminotransferase. There were marginal changes in glucose and triglycerides, but no changes in haemoglobin A_{1c}, calcium, cholesterol and alanine aminotransferase.

Commentary
Obviously GH replacement in IGHD patients does not have major effects on common parameters of blood chemistry. Changes in alkaline phosphatase are the expression of an augmented growth process induced by GH. Perhaps, quantitative changes in alkaline phosphatase (bone specific) may be utilised for the evaluation of the efficacy of GH treatment in various growth disorders.

Growth Hormone Deficiency: Puberty and Final Height

Edward O. Reiter[a]   Wayne S. Cutfield[b]

As untreated patients with growth hormone deficiency (GDH) have profound short stature, averaging nearly –5 standard deviation score (SDS) [1–4], a clinical urgency existed to utilize GH therapy as soon as it was available [5]. GH action is species specific, and humans do not respond to animal-derived GH [6–11]. Human cadaver pituitary glands were for many years the only practical source of primate GH for treatment of GHD, and more than 27,000 children with GHD worldwide were treated with pituitary-derived GH (pit-GH) [12]. The limited supplies of pit-GH, low doses and interrupted treatment regimens resulted in incomplete growth increments; usually, therapy was discontinued in boys who reached 166 cm and in girls who reached 152 cm. Nonetheless, this treatment did increase linear growth and in many patients enhanced final adult height. The dose-response relationship and the relation of age to GH response were recognized during this period [13].

Distribution of pit-GH was halted in the United States and most of Europe in 1985 because of concern about a causal relationship with Creutzfeldt-Jakob disease, a rare and fatal spongiform encephalopathy that had been previously reported to be capable of iatrogenic transmission through human tissue [14, 15]. When the risks of pit-GH were discovered, biosynthetic recombinant GH was already being tested for safety and efficacy [16–18] and now has universally replaced pit-GH as the treatment for children with GHD.

Treatment Regimens
The recommended therapy starting dose of GH in GHD patients is 0.18–0.35 mg/kg body weight/week, administered in 7 daily doses. In general, the growth response to GH is a function of the log dose given, so that increasing dosages further enhance growth velocities [12, 13, 19], but daily dosing may be the more important treatment parameter [20]. The importance of dosage frequency is emphasized by data from an assessment of growth responses of prepubertal GHD children randomly assigned to receive thrice-weekly or daily GH at the same total weekly dose (0.30 mg/kg/week). The mean total height gain during this period was 9.7 cm greater in the daily-treated pa-

[a]Baystate Children's Hospital, Tufts University School of Medicine
759 Chestnut Street, Springfield, MA 01199 (USA)
[b]Liggins Institute, University of Auckland
2–6 Park Avenue, Grafton, Auckland (New Zealand)

Table 1. Adult height in children with GHD treated with biosynthetic GH

Study	Sex	Patients	Dose, mg/kg/week	Duration years	Age years	Height SDS	Δ height SDS	Height vs. MPH
KIGS [39]	M	792	0.18	8.1	18.5	–1.0	+1.7	–0.2
	F	466	0.18	7.9	16.9	–1.3	+1.6	–0.5
NCGS [36, 93]	M	2,095	0.28	5.2	18.2	–1.1	+1.4	–0.7
	F	1,116	0.29	5.0	16.7	–1.3	+1.6	–0.9

MPH = Midparental target height.

tients (38.4 vs. 28.7 cm; p < 0.0002) with similar increments in skeletal maturation and no acceleration of the onset of puberty. Mean height SDS at the end of 4 years was +0.2, or at the midpoint of normal for age.

Growth responses to exogenous GH vary, in addition to the frequency of administration and dosage, according to age (greater absolute gain in a younger child, though not necessarily of growth velocity SDS), weight and GH receptor type and amount, as assessed by serum GH binding protein levels, and perhaps seasonality [21–25]. Nonetheless, on the general regimen of daily GH at the recommended doses, the typical GHD child accelerates growth from a pretreatment rate of 3–4 cm/year to 10–12 cm/year in year 1 of therapy and 7–9 cm/year in years 2 and 3. Progressive waning of GH efficacy then occurs but is poorly understood. Newer studies utilizing variable dosing of GH based on gender, growth responsivity and growth factor concentrations suggest the need for greater individualization of current treatment regimens [26, 27].

Longer-Term/Final Height Results
Final height data in patients treated with pituitary GH have been reported elsewhere [28]. Patients treated largely with biosynthetic GH [5, 29–39] have had a gradually improving actual or near-final adult height SDS, with an average final height in more than 1,400 patients approximating –1.3 SD below the mean. Data from the two largest databases [36–39], representing the North American and European experiences, are shown in table 1. The KIGS data are reviewed in detail in the accompanying chapter. Despite availability of GH therapy, long-term studies still show that most patients fail to reach their genetic target heights. Evaluation of adult heights in 121 patients with childhood GHD treated in Genentech GH research trials indicate a mean adult height in both male and female patients of –0.7 SDS, with 106 patients being within 2 SDS for normal adult Americans [32]. Even in these closely followed patients, a –0.4 to –0.6 SDS difference from midparental targeted height occurred. However, the achievement of the genetic target is possible, as a Swedish subgroup (in the KIGS database) of consistently treated patients reached a median final height SDS of –0.3 which was equivalent to the midparental target height [38]. By multiple regression analysis, factors found to correlate with enhanced adult height were baseline height, younger age at onset of treatment, longer treatment duration, especially during prepubertal years, and a greater growth velocity during the first year of treatment [39]. Increased height velocity and subsequent superior adult height outcome, though with considerable overlap, were demonstrated in children with GHD who carried one or both GH receptor alleles with an exon 3 deletion [25, 40]. While the development of recombinant GH has solved the problem of supply experienced in the pituitary GH era, delays in di-

agnosis and initiation of therapy have still compromised adult height.

Sophisticated mathematical models [19, 41] have examined many laboratory and auxologic parameters that influence response to GH therapy. As age at onset of treatment is inversely correlated with growth responses and the smaller, lighter child requires less GH (with marked economic benefit), growth data in early-treated children are important to assess. In short-term studies of 134 patients [42–44], treated prior to age 3, marked early catch-up occurred with a mean height gain of around 3 SDS by 4 years of therapy allowing most children to reach the normal height range by midchildhood. Mean height in one study [44] reached –0.4 SDS after 8 years of treatment. Near adult height data in 13 patients treated before 5 years of age [33] did not differ from the midparental target height (–0.9 vs. –0.7 SDS). In a group of 25 children treated prior to 12 months of age [45], adult height also matched the target height despite low dosage and less frequent administration. In an analysis of KIGS data for the development of a growth prediction model, a greater height gain per GH amount occurred in the very young children, but a seemingly lowered sensitivity to endogenous GH in early infancy adds complexity to the interpretation of these data [46]. Nonetheless, as long-term outcome studies continue to show excellent growth responses with achievement of genetic target height and if there is adherence to treatment regimens in very young children, strong recommendations for early treatment seem appropriate [47].

Ethnic and Gender Factors

The KIGS database provides contrasting information on near adult height in Caucasians and Japanese patients, along with some assessment of gender-based outcomes in GH-treated children [39]. Caucasian patients with isolated, idiopathic GHD (IGHD) achieved a near adult height of –0.8 and –1.0 SDS in males and females, respectively; in the patients with multiple pituitary hormone deficiency, near adult heights were –0.7 and –1.1 SDS in males and females, respectively. In contrast, Japanese patients with IGHD achieved a much lower near adult height (–1.6 SDS in males and –2.1 SDS in females), although still within the normal range for the population. The multiple pituitary hormone deficiency patients reached heights of –1.3 and –1.8 SDS for males and females. As has been shown in earlier studies [4], patients with gonadotropin deficiency generally have a slightly better adult height outcome than those with endogenous presence of normal sex steroid levels.

The difference between the near adult height SDS and the midparental target height SDS is perhaps the best indication of whether an individual has achieved genetic height potential. This difference was –0.2 to –0.4 in male and –0.4 to –0.5 in female Caucasian patients and +0.1 to +0.2 in male and –0.3 to –0.6 in female Japanese patients. Both ethnic groups seem to have reached heights close to genetic potential. However, in Japanese patients, interpretation of the data is complicated by the current secular trend in height of the Japanese population, with parental heights not necessarily representing the true genetic potential of the current generation [48, 49].

Modulating Growth at Puberty

As final height correlates with height at the onset of puberty in GHD patients [23, 30, 50–53], every effort must be made to achieve a height within the normal range at the onset of puberty by optimizing growth velocity during prepuberty. Nonetheless, as pubertal growth represents about 12–20% of final adult height [28, 54], attempts at modulating this growth period seemed reasonable in short GHD peripubertal patients [54, 55]. In data from the two large international data registries, the total height gained during puberty in patients with GHD was generally comparable with that in healthy children with delayed bone ages [36, 56]. The pubertal height gain is negatively correlated with the age of pubertal onset, both in normal and in GH-treated children [54, 57].

Increased GH Dosage at Puberty
In an effort to increase the final height of GHD patients, the use of high-dose GH during puberty has been studied, based on the rationale that GH secretion normally rises 2- to 4-fold during the pubertal growth spurt with dramatic concomitant increases in serum insulin-like growth factor 1 (IGF-1) levels. Earlier studies by Stanhope at al. [58, 59] indicated that little difference in height gain could be observed when adolescent patients were treated with 30 versus 15 IU GH/m^2/week (approximately 0.04 vs. 0.02 mg/kg/day). However, Mauras et al. [60] evaluated higher pubertal GH doses (0.1 vs. 0.043 mg/kg/day) and found that the higher dosage resulted in a 4.6-cm increase in near final height. The mean height SDS achieved in the 0.043-mg/kg/day group, as in the earlier report [32], was -0.7 ± 0.9, but 0.0 ± 1.2 in the 0.1-mg/kg/day group. The higher GH dosage did not result in more rapid acceleration of skeletal maturation, nor in any appreciable increase in adverse events. IGF-1 levels were quite high in some of the adolescents, and the cost of such GH dosing would be substantial.

Decrease in Estrogen Action: Gonadotropin-Releasing Hormone Agonist Therapy
The use of higher doses of GH, the ability to treat until growth cessation, early initiation of treatment, progressive weight-related dose increments, attention to compliance with daily administration, and appropriate thyroid hormone and glucocorticoid replacement therapy are important factors in these improved adult height outcomes. However, when these considerations did not yield fully satisfactory results, attempts at modulating puberty and the nature of its growth spurt were made. The earlier the age of pubertal onset, the lower the final height outcome [36, 56], while GHD patients with delayed puberty or hypogonadotropic hypogonadism have a taller adult height [4, 23, 61]. Such findings suggest that the rate and timing of the pubertal process of growth plate senescence ultimately determine the cessation of growth. When precocious puberty or normal puberty with rapid tempo threatens to limit the response to GH, delaying pubertal progression, and thus, the rate of skeletal maturation, by the use of gonadotropin-releasing hormone agonists (GnRH-Ag) seems reasonable [54, 62]. Treatment of children with central precocious puberty with GnRH-Ag yields much improved final adult height [63–67]. The concept is to prolong the growth process by attenuating puberty and achieving greater long-term growth despite a slowing of the actual growth velocity [55]. Use of this strategy in pubertal GHD patient groups, though theoretically inviting, especially with central precocious puberty, has not yet been clearly documented to enhance final height in patients with generally normal puberty [54, 55, 68–75].

Small, controlled studies in adolescents with GHD [72, 76] have shown that achievement of the midparental target height is possible with addition of GnRH-Ag to the treatment regimen. American data were recently reassessed [77]. Mericq et al. [72] studied teenagers with late-diagnosed GHD (mean age 14 years, skeletal age 11 years) by treating one group with GnRH-Ag and GH for a 3-year period and another with GH alone. Despite starting at an extremely short stature of –4.0 SDS below the mean, the GH + GnRH-Ag treated adolescents gained 2.7 SDS and 12 cm of predicted adult height, in contrast to 1.3 SDS and 3 cm of predicted adult height in the group given GH alone. Height outcomes in the dual drug-treated group equaled the midparental target height, while the GH alone group remained –0.7 SDS distant from the midparental goal. The 3-year duration of agonist treatment in early teenagers was substantial, while GH dosage (around 0.23 mg/kg/week) was lower than the usual American levels. The final height designation was not clearly specified, and patients were certainly a group of late-treated children, probably including some with constitutional delay of pubertal maturation. Contrasting data were reported by Lee [55]. He showed that adult height outcomes in the GH alone treatment group exceeded those of the combined treatment group (173.7 vs. 170.7 cm, with the GH alone group 2 cm greater than the target, and the dual drug group falling 3.6 cm below the target). He also found that children who showed 'catch-up' in height before the onset of puberty had greater final heights than those who did not (174.2 vs. 169.2 cm, with the former group exceeding the target by 3.9 cm, in contrast to the latter being 5.8 cm below the target). These latter data support the notion that growth prior to the onset of puberty is most critical in predicting final height [53].

Information regarding the value of adding GnRH-Ag to the GH treatment regimen in children with IGHD is also found in the large databases KIGS and the National Cooperative Growth Study (NCGS) [36, 78–80]. Clinical and neuroimaging assessments largely excluded structural abnormalities of the hypothalamic-pituitary area so that the populations studied are not likely to have concomitant lesions that could cause sexual precocity. Details of the regimens utilized by the investigators to suppress the hypothalamic-pituitary-gonadal axis to delay the onset and/or progression of puberty are not readily available in the database files. The girls are younger, but have comparable height deficits with the boys; the GH alone and GnRH-Ag-treated children are generally similar. However, the bone age delays are less in the patients treated with GnRH-Ag, thus yielding smaller predicted final heights. Near adult height data show that the children treated with GH + GnRH-Ag actually achieved shorter height outcomes and growth increments, though they gain comparably in predicted adult height. Both groups do not approximate the midparental target heights. In another group (from NCGS) selected for the combination of precocious puberty and GHD, the bone age was more advanced, yielding an even smaller predicted height in the latter group despite the taller height at initiation of therapy. The near adult height outcome in these more compromised girls was short (–2.4 SDS) and farther from the midparental target. They lost height relative to the predicted height during the course of treatment [77].

The ratio of males to females at near final height in both databases, without GnRH-Ag treatment, was around 2.2:1. In striking contrast, the male to female ratio in the agonist-treated children at near final height was only 0.8 [78, 80]. A recent assessment of the NCGS database [February 2005, B. Lippe, pers. commun.] revealed a ratio (males/females) of 3.0 in non-GnRH-Ag-treated children in contrast to 1.2 in agonist-treated patients. Clearly, females are more likely to receive agonist treatment in the American experience with GHD therapy. Additionally, the male/female ratio was 6.0 in patients with organic etiologies for GHD, presumably accounted for by the greater incidence of precocious puberty in such children.

Taken together, these data, along with the review of Carel [54], affirm the notion that the use of GnRH-Ag to enhance final height outcome in patients with GHD is not likely to be successful. Careful selection of patients for GnRH-Ag treatment in whom pubertal tempo is accelerated might be a reasonable consideration, though evidence is lacking.

Decrease in Estrogen Action: Aromatase Inhibition or Receptor Blockade
The role of estrogen in the maturation (or senescence) of the epiphyseal growth plates, and its presumed central role in the cessation of growth, has encouraged consideration of blocking estrogen production or action [81]. Utilization of aromatase inhibition [81–85] may be an effective regimen in boys with GHD in whom skeletal age

is inordinately advancing, as they would get growth benefit from continued androgen presence, while the elimination of estrogen would slow bone age advancement. The potent aromatase inhibitor, letrozole, has been used to slow the rate of skeletal maturation in boys with short stature and delayed puberty, while also receiving testosterone, in a double-blinded, placebo-controlled trial. Predicted adult heights were significantly enhanced by this regimen (182.1 vs. 175.2 cm in placebo-treated boys) [82, 86]. In a group of prepubertal boys with idiopathic short stature treated for 2 years with letrozole in a double-blinded, randomized, placebo-controlled trial, Hero et al. [87] demonstrated a mean increase in predicted adult height of 5.9 cm and a 0.7 SDS in height for bone age. Generally, similar efficacy of aromatase inhibition was reported by a retrospective study of a mixed group of children with short stature [88]. Trials utilizing aromatase inhibitors plus GH in children with IGHD are ongoing.

Short-term treatment has not impaired skeletal mineralization [89] nor altered spermatogenesis [90]. Attempts at altering aromatase activity in girls have not been reported. The long-term safety of the plan to alter aromatase activity remains to be demonstrated. In an uncontrolled study, the selective estrogen receptor modulator, tamoxifen, slowed skeletal maturation and increased height prediction when used in conjunction with GH in pubertal males [91].

Taken in aggregate, current recommendations regarding attempts to enhance growth outcomes must thus center upon initiation of GH treatment in an early, aggressive and closely optimized manner, rather than upon attempts at gaining substantial SDS increments during the pubertal process. Taken together, these findings suggest that the pubertal period is not the best time to attempt to enhance final height outcomes in IGHD patients. Earlier diagnosis of GHD with concomitant initiation of GH treatment, progressive weight-related dose increments, as well as strict attention to compliance with daily administration and perhaps to titration of GH doses based on frequent measurements of IGF levels (or other GH-modulated peptides) might yield heights in the target range for families. The treatment program of the addition of GnRH-Ag to GH in peripubertal children with IGHD should, potentially, still be considered experimental, and trials to address efficacy should be reinitiated. Whether GnRH-Ag therapy could be more successful if its use were related to the tempo of puberty in the specific child is not known, though the slightly greater success in children with GHD and precocious puberty suggests further evaluation of this consideration. The use of aromatase inhibition, certainly theoretically attractive and orally administered, awaits proof of safety and value.

For the Caucasian patients in this study (n = 980), the near adult height outcomes were slightly better than those reported 5 years previously in the KIGS database (n = 269, final height = –0.9 to –1.2 SDS, males and females) [37, 38] and in the NCGS in the USA (n = 258, final height = –1.3 to –1.9 SDS, males and females) [36]. However, the present results for the European patients are generally similar to those of GH-treated children reported in the early Genentech trials (n = 121, final height = –0.7 SDS, males and females) [32] and of Belgian children (n = 61, final height = –0.8, males and females) reported by Thomas et al. [92]. However, in these children with GHD, near adult height remained below the midparental height, except for data reported by Hintz et al. [17], suggesting a failure to achieve full genetic height potential. The GH dose in all of the European trials was approximately 0.18 mg/kg/week, while the Genentech data from the United States were based on a GH dose of 0.3 mg/kg/week. The general similarity of height outcomes suggests that the GH dose has a finite impact, though earlier treatment with the higher dosing may lead to improved responses with greater catch-up growth. Total GH exposure during prepubertal years may be a significant factor.

References

1. Rimoin DL, Merimee TJ, Rabinowitz D, McKusick VA: Genetic aspects of clinical endocrinology. Recent Prog Horm Res 1968;24:365–437.
2. Ranke MB: A note on adults with growth hormone deficiency. Acta Paediatr Scand Suppl 1987;331:80–82.
3. Van der Werff ten Bosch JJ, Bot A: Growth of males with idiopathic hypopituitarism without growth hormone treatment. Clin Endocrinol 1990;32:707–717.
4. Wit JM, Kamp G, Rikken B: Spontaneous growth and response to growth hormone treatment in children with growth hormone deficiency and idiopathic short stature. Pediatr Res 1996;39:295–302.
5. Grumbach MM, Bin-Abbas BS, Kaplan SL: The growth hormone cascade: progress and long-term results of growth hormone treatment in growth hormone deficiency. Horm Res 1998;49(suppl 2):41–57.
6. Bennett LL: Failure of hypophyseal growth hormone to produce nitrogen storage in a girl with hypophyseal dwarfism. J Clin Endocrinol 1950;10:492–495.
7. Shelton EK, Cavanaugh RA, Evans HM: Hypophyseal infantilism: treatment with anterior hypophyseal extract; final report. Am J Dis Child 1936;52:100–113.
8. Shelton EK, Cavanaugh RA, Long ML: Studies on effects of human blood serum upon growth of rat. Endocrinology 1936;19:543–548.
9. Wilhelmi AE: Camparative biochemistry of growth hormone from ox, sheep, pig, horse and fish pituitaries; in Smith RW Jr, Gaebler OH, Long CNH (eds): The Hypophyseal Growth Hormone: Nature and Actions. New York, McGraw-Hill, 1955, pp 59–69.
10. Knobil E, Greep RO: Physiological effects of growth hormone of primate origin in the hypophysectomized monkey. Fed Proc 1956;15:111–112.
11. Knobil E, Wolf RC, Greep RO: Some physiologic effects of primate pituitary growth-hormone preparations in the hypophysectomized rhesus monkey. J Clin Endocrinol 1956;16:916.
12. Frasier SD: Human pituitary growth hormone (hGH) therapy in growth hormone deficiency. Endocr Rev 1983;4:155–170.
13. Frasier SD, Costin G, Lippe BM, Aceto H, Bunger PF: A dose-response curve for human growth hormone. J Clin Endocrinol Metab 1981;53:1213–1217.
14. Fradkin JE: Creutzfeldt-Jakob disease in pituitary growth hormone recipients. Endocrinologist 1993;3:108–114.
15. Buchanan CR, Preece MA, Milner RDG: Mortality, neoplasia, and Creutzfeldt-Jakob disease in patients treated with human pituitary growth hormone in the United States. Br Med J 1991;302:824–828.
16. Rosenfeld RG, Aggarwal BB, Hintz RL, Dollar LA: Recombinant DNA-derived methionyl growth hormone is similar in membrane binding properties to human pituitary growth hormone. Biochem Biophys Res Commun 1982;106:202–209.
17. Hintz RL, Rosenfeld RG, Wilson DM, Bennett A, Finno J, McClellan B, Swift R: Biosynthetic methionyl-human growth hormone is biologically active in adult humans. Lancet 1982;i:1276–1279.
18. Kaplan SL, Underwood LE, August GP, Bell JJ, Blethen SL, Blizzard RM, Brown DR, Foley TP, Hintz RL, Hopwood NJ: Clinical studies with recombinant-DNA-derived methionyl human growth hormone in growth hormone deficient children. Lancet 1986;i:697–700.
19. Ranke MB, Lindberg A, Chatelain P, Wilton P, Cutfield W, Albertsson-Wikland K, Price DA, on behalf of the KIGS International Board: Derivation and validation of a mathematical model for predicting the response to exogenous recombinant human growth hormone (GH) in prepubertal children with idiopathic GH deficiency. J Clin Endocrinol Metab 1999;84:1174–1183.
20. MacGillivray MH, Baptista J, Johanson A, Genentech Study Group: Outcome of a four-year randomized study of daily versus three times weekly somatropin treatment in prepubertal naive growth hormone-deficient children. J Clin Endocrinol Metab 1996;81:1806–1809.
21. Martha PM, Reiter EO, Davila N, Shaw MA, Holcombe JH, Baumann G: Serum growth hormone (GH)-binding protein/receptor: an important determinant of GH responsiveness. J Clin Endocrinol Metab 1992;75:1464–1469.
22. Martha PM, Reiter EO, Davila N, Shaw MA, Holcombe JH, Baumann G: The role of body mass in the response to growth hormone therapy. J Clin Endocrinol Metab 1992;75:1470–1473.
23. Price DA, Ranke MB: Final height following growth hormone treatment; in Ranke MB, Gunnarsson R (eds): Progress in Growth Hormone Therapy – 5 Years of KIGS. Mannheim, J&J Verlag, 1994, pp 129–144.
24. Land C, Blum WF, Stabrey A, Schoenau E: Seasonality of growth response to GH therapy in prepubertal children with idiopathic growth hormone deficiency. Eur J Endocrinol 2005;152:727–733.
25. Jorge AA, Marchisotti FG, Montenegro LR, Carvalho LR, Mendonca BB, Arnhold IJ: Growth hormone (GH) pharmacogenetics: influence of GH receptor exon 3 retention or deletion on first-year growth response and final height in patients with severe GH deficiency. J Clin Endocrinol Metab 2006;91:1076–1080.
26. Cohen P, Bright GM, Rogol AD, Kappelgaard AM, Rosenfeld RG: Effects of dose and gender on the growth and growth factor response to GH in GH-deficient children: implications for efficacy and safety. J Clin Endocrinol Metab 2002;87:90–98.
27. Cohen P, Rogol AD, Howard C, Kappelgaard AM, Rosenfeld RG: IGF-based dosing of growth hormone accelerates the growth velocity of children with growth hormone deficiency (GHD) and idiopathic short stature. Horm Res 2005;64(suppl 1):48.
28. Reiter EO, Rosenfeld RG: Normal and aberrant growth; in Larsen PR, Kronenberg HM, Melmed S, Polonsky KS (eds): Williams Textbook of Endocrinology. Philadelphia, Saunders, 2002, pp 1003–1114.
29. Bramswig JH, Schlosser H, Kiese K: Final height in children with growth hormone deficiency. Horm Res 1995;43:126–128.
30. Severi F: Final height in children with growth hormone deficiency. Horm Res 1995;43:138–140.
31. Birnbacher R, Riedl S, Frisch H: Long-term treatment in children with hypopituitarism: pubertal development and final height. Horm Res 1998;49:80–85.
32. Blethen SL, Baptista J, Kuntze J, Foley T, LaFranchi S, Johanson A, Genentech Growth Study Group: Adult height in growth hormone (GH)-deficient children treated with biosynthetic GH. J Clin Endocrinol Metab 1997;82:418–420.

33 de Luca F, Maghnie M, Arrigo T, Lombardo F, Messina MF, Berasconi S: Final height outcome of growth hormone-deficient patients treated since less than five years of age. Acta Paediatr 1996;85:1167–1171.

34 MacGillivray MH, Blethen SL, Buchlis JG, Clopper RR, Sandberg DE, Conboy TA: Current dosing of growth hormone in children with growth hormone deficiency: how physiologic? Pediatrics 1998;102:527–530.

35 Bernasconi S, Arrigo T, Wasniewsk M, Ghizzoni L, Ruggeri C, Di Pasquale G, Vottero A, de Luca F: Long-term results with growth hormone therapy in idiopathic hypopituitarism. Horm Res 2000;53:55–59.

36 August GP, Julius JR, Blethen SL: Adult height in children with growth hormone deficiency who are treated with biosynthetic growth hormone: the National Cooperative Growth Study experience. Pediatrics 1998;102:512–516.

37 Cutfield WS, Lindberg A, Chatelain P, Price DA, Albertsson-Wikland K, Wilton P, Ranke MB: Final height following growth hormone treatment of idiopathic growth hormone deficiency in KIGS; in Ranke MB, Wilton P (eds): Growth Hormone Therapy in KIGS – 10 Years' Experience. Heidelberg-Leipzig, Johann Ambrosius Barth Verlag, 1999, pp 93–110.

38 Cutfield W, Lindberg A, Albertsson-Wikland K, Chatelain P, Ranke MB, Wilton P, KIGS International Board: Final height in idiopathic growth hormone deficiency: the KIGS experience. Acta Paediatr Suppl 1999;428:72–75.

39 Reiter EO, Price DA, Wilton P, Albertsson-Wikland K, Ranke MB: Effect of growth hormone (GH) treatment on the final height of 1258 patients with idiopathic GH deficiency: analysis of a large international database. J Clin Endocrinol Metab 2006;91:2047–2054.

40 Rosenfeld RG: Editorial: the pharmacogenomics of human growth. J Clin Endocrinol Metab 2006;91:795–796.

41 Albertsson-Wikland K, Kristrom B, Rosber S, Svensson B, Nierop AFM: Validated multivariate models predicting the growth response to GH treatment in individual short children with a broad range in GH secretion capacities. Pediatr Res 2000;48:475–484.

42 Boersma B, Rikken B, Wit JM: Catch-up growth in early treated patients with growth hormone deficiency. Arch Dis Child 1995;72:427–431.

43 Rappaport R, Mugnier E, Limoni C, Crosnier H, Czernichow P, Leger J, Limal JM, Rochiccioli P, Soskin S, French Serono Study Group: A 5-year prospective study of growth hormone (GH)-deficient children treated with GH before the age of 3 years. J Clin Endocrinol Metab 1997;82:452–456.

44 Huet F, Carel JC, Nivelon JL, Chaussain JL: Long-term results of GH therapy in GH-deficient children treated before 1 year of age. Eur J Endocrinol 1999;140:29–34.

45 Carel JC, Huet F, Chaussain JL: Treatment of growth hormone deficiency in very young children. Horm Res 2003;60:10–17.

46 Ranke MB, Lindberg A, Albertsson-Wikland K, Wilton P, Price DA, Reiter EO: Increased response, but lower responsiveness, to growth hormone (GH) in very young children (aged 0–3 years) with idiopathic GH deficiency: analysis of data from KIGS. J Clin Endocrinol Metab 2005;90:1966–1971.

47 Saenger P: Growth hormone in growth hormone deficiency. BMJ 2002;325:58–59.

48 Matsumoto K: Secular acceleration of growth in height in Japanese and its social background. Ann Hum Biol 1982;9:399–410.

49 Takahashi BE: Secular trend in milk consumption and growth in Japan. Hum Biol 1984;56:427–437.

50 Frisch H, Birnbacher R: Final height and pubertal development in children with growth hormone deficiency after long-term treatment. Horm Res 1995;43:132–134.

51 Burns EC, Tanner JM, Preece MA, Cameron N: Final height and pubertal development in 55 children with idiopathic growth hormone deficiency, treated for between 2 and 15 years with human growth hormone. Eur J Pediatr 1981;137:155–164.

52 Bourguignon JP, Vandeweghe M, Vanderschuren-Lodeweyckx M, Malvaux P, Wolter R, Du Caju M, Ernould C: Pubertal growth and final height in hypopituitary boys: a minor role of bone age at onset of puberty. J Clin Endocrinol Metab 1986;63:376–382.

53 Ranke MB, Lindberg A, Martin DD, Bakker B, Wilton P, Albertsson-Wikland K, Cowell CT, Price DA, Reiter EO: The mathematical model for total pubertal growth in idiopathic growth hormone (GH) deficiency suggests a moderate role of GH dose. J Clin Endocrinol Metab 2003;88:4748–4753.

54 Carel JC: Can we increase adolescent growth? Eur J Endocrinol 2004;151(suppl 3):U101–U108.

55 Lee PA: The effects of manipulation of puberty on growth. Horm Res 2003;60:60–67.

56 Ranke MB, Price DA, Albertsson-Wikland K, Maes M, Lindberg A: Factors determining pubertal growth and final height in growth hormone treatment of idiopathic growth hormone deficiency. Horm Res 1997;48:62–71.

57 Ranke MB, Martin DD, Lindberg A: Prediction model of total pubertal growth in idiopathic growth hormone deficiency: analysis of data from KIGS. Horm Res 2003;60:58–59.

58 Stanhope R, Urena M, Hindmarsh P, Brook CGD: Management of growth hormone deficiency through puberty. Acta Paediatr Scand Suppl 1991;372:47–52.

59 Stanhope R, Albanese A, Hindmarsh P, Brook CGD: The effects of growth hormone therapy on spontaneous sexual development. Horm Res 1992;38:9–13.

60 Mauras N, Attie KM, Reiter EO, Saenger P, Baptista J, Genentech, Inc, Cooperative Study Group: High dose recombinant human growth hormone (GH) treatment of GH-deficient patients in puberty increases near-final height: a randomized, multicenter trial. J Clin Endocrinol Metab 2000;85:3653–3660.

61 Hibi I, Tanaka T, Tanae A, Kagawa J, Hashimoto N, Yoshizawa A, Shizume K: The influence of gonadal function and the effect of gonadal suppression treatment on final height in growth hormone (GH)-treated GH-deficient children. J Clin Endocrinol Metab 1989;69:221–226.

62 Wit JM, Balen HV, Kamp GA, Oostdijk W: Benefit of postponing normal puberty for improving final height. Eur J Endocrinol 2004;151(suppl 1):S41–S45.

63 Conn PM, Crowley WF Jr: Gonadotropin-releasing hormone and its analogs. Annu Rev Med 1994;45:391–405.

64 Partsch C-J, Heger S, Sippell WG: Management and outcome of central precocious puberty. Clin Endocrinol (Oxf) 2002;56:129–148.

65 Klein KO, Barnes KM, Jones JV, Feuillan PP, Cutler GB Jr: Increased final height in precocious puberty after long-term treatment with LHRH agonists: the National Institutes of Health experience. J Clin Endocrinol Metab 2001;86:4711–4716.

66 Paul D, Conte FA, Grumbach MM, Kaplan SL: Long-term effect of gonadotropin-releasing hormone agonist therapy on final and near-final height in 26 children with true precocious puberty treated at a median age of less than 5 years. J Clin Endocrinol Metab 1995; 80:546–551.
67 Carel JC, Lahlou N, Roger M, Chaussain JL: Precocious puberty and statural growth. Hum Reprod Update 2004; 10:135–147.
68 Balducci R, Toscano V, Mangiantini A, Municchi G, Vaccaro F, Picone S: Adult height in short normal adolescent girls treated with gonadotropin-releasing hormone analog and growth hormone. J Clin Endocrinol Metab 1995;80:3596–3600.
69 Saggese G, Pasquino AM, Bertelloni S, Baroncelli GI, Battinin R, Pucarelli I, Segni M, Franchi G: Effect of combined treatment with gonadotropin releasing hormone analogue and growth hormone in patients with central precocious puberty who had subnormal growth velocity and impaired height prognosis. Acta Paediatr 1995;84:299–304.
70 Pasquino AM, Municchi G, Pucarelli I, Segni M, Mancini MA, Troiani S: Combined treatment with gonadotropin-releasing hormone analog and growth hormone in central precocious puberty. J Clin Endocrinol Metab 1996;81:948–951.
71 Job JC, Toublanc JE, Landier F: Growth of short normal children in puberty treated for three years with growth hormone alone or in association with gonadotropin-releasing hormone agonist. Horm Res 1994;41:177–184.
72 Mericq MV, Eggers M, Avila A, Cutler GBJ, Cassorla F: Near final height in pubertal growth hormone (GH)-deficient patients treated with GH alone or in combination with luteinzing hormone-releasing hormone analog: results of a prospective, randomized trial. J Clin Endocrinol Metab 2000;85:569–573.
73 Walvoord EC, Pescovitz OH: Combined use of growth hormone and gonadotropin-releasing hormone analogues in precocious puberty: theoretic and practical considerations. Pediatrics 1999; 104:1010–1014.
74 Codner E, Mericq V, Cassorla F: Optimizing growth hormone therapy during puberty. Horm Res 1997;48:16–20.
75 Yanovski JA, Rose SR, Municchi G, Pescovitz OH, Hill SC, Cassorla FG, Cutler GB Jr: Treatment with a luteinizing hormone-releasing hormone agonist in adolescents with short stature. N Engl J Med 2003;348:908–917.
76 Mul D, Wit JM, Oostdijk W, Van den Broeck J, Dutch Advisory Group on Growth Hormone: The effect of pubertal delay by GnRH agonist in GH-deficient children on final height. J Clin Endocrinol Metab 2001;86:4655–4656.
77 Reiter EO: A brief review of the addition of gonadotropin-releasing hormone agonists (GnRH-Ag) to growth hormone (GH) treatment of children with idiopathic growth hormone deficiency: previously published studies from America. Mol Cell Endocrinol 2006;254/255:221–225.
78 Kohn B, Julius JR, Blethen SL: Combined use of growth hormone and gonadotropin-releasing hormone analogues: the National Cooperative Growth Study Experience. Pediatrics 1999;104:1014–1017.
79 Wyatt D: Lessons from the national cooperative growth study. Eur J Endocrinol 2004;151(suppl 1):S55–S59.
80 Ranke MB, Lindberg A: Early-onset idiopathic growth hormone deficiency within KIGS. Horm Res 2003;60:18–21.
81 Grumbach MM: Estrogen, bone, growth and sex: a sea change in conventional wisdom. J Pediatr Endocrinol Metab 2000;13:1439–1455.
82 Dunkel L, Wickman S: Novel treatment of short stature with aromatase inhibitors. J Steroid Biochem Mol Biol 2003; 86:345–356.
83 Zhou P, Shah B, Prasad K, David R: Letrozole significantly improves growth potential in a pubertal boy with growth hormone deficiency. Pediatrics 2005; 115:e245–e248.
84 Eugster EA: Aromatase inhibitors in procoocious puberty: rationale and experience to date. Treat Endocrinol 2004;3:141–151.
85 Mauras N, Welch S, Rini A, Klein KO: An open label 12-month pilot trial on the effects of the aromatase inhibitor anastrozole in growth hormone (GH)-treated GH-deficient adolescent boys. J Pediatr Endocrinol Metab 2004;17:1597–1606.
86 Wickman S, Sipila I, Ankarberg-Lindgren C, Norjavaara E, Dunkel L: A specific aromatase inhibitor and potential increase in adult height in boys with delayed puberty: a randomised controlled trial. The Lancet 2001;357:1743–1748.
87 Hero M, Norjavaara E, Dunkel L: Inhibition of estrogen biosynthesis with a potent aromatase inhibitor increases predicted adult height in boys with idiopathic short stature: a randomized controlled trial. J Clin Endocrinol Metab 2005;90:6396–6402.
88 Turpin AL, Jacobson JD, Karmazin HM, Moore WV, Popovic J: Effect of letrozole treatment on skeletal maturation in females. Horm Res 2004; 62(suppl 2):149–155.
89 Wickman S, Kajantie E, Dunkel L: Effects of suppression of estrogen action by the p450 aromatase inhibitor letrozole on bone mineral density and bone turnover in pubertal boys. J Clin Endocrinol Metab 2003;88:3785–3793.
90 Mauras N, Bell J, Snow BG, Winslow KL: Sperm analysis in growth hormone-deficient adolescents previously treated with an aromatase inhibitor: comparison with normal controls. Fertil Steril 2005;84:239–242.
91 Kreher NC, Eugster EA, Shankar RR: The use of tamoxifen to improve height potential in short pubertal boys. Pediatrics 2005;116:1513–1515.
92 Thomas M, Massa G, Bourguignon JP, Craen M, De Schepper J, de Zegher F, Dooms L, Du Caju M, Francois I, Heinrichs C, et al: Final height in children with idiopathic growth hormone deficiency treated with recombinant human growth hormone: the Belgian experience. Horm Res 2001;55:88–94.
93 Dana K, Baptista J, Blethen SL: Updated NCGS data. Personal communication, 2001.

Growth Hormone Treatment to Final Height in Idiopathic Growth Hormone Deficiency: The KIGS Experience

Wayne S. Cutfield[a] Georgios Karagiannis[b] Edward O. Reiter[c]

The principal goals of growth hormone (GH) treatment of children with GH deficiency (GHD) are first to accelerate growth during childhood to create a height more comparable with peers, and ultimately and more importantly, to achieve a normal adult height. Assessment in young adults of the psychological benefits of childhood GH therapy for GHD is very limited [1, 2]. Those adults who remained very short felt disadvantaged in terms of obtaining employment, with a greater likelihood of psychological problems [1, 2]. In more recent years, body composition, skeletal mineralisation and metabolism have begun to be assessed in GHD children, and improvements in these parameters are expected and are increasingly being monitored [3–6]. Thus, justification to treat GHD children with GH extends across the range of actions of GH to include growth, body composition, metabolism and cardiovascular function.

Several small studies of childhood-onset GHD not treated with GH have reported extreme short stature in adults with adult height standard deviation scores (SDS) of –3.1 to –4.2 [7–9]. Between 1958 and 1985, very limited amounts of cadaveric human GH were available to treat children with severe GHD. Given the constrained availability of cadaveric GH, treatment regimens consisted of fixed low doses administered thrice weekly [10–12]. Early final height studies included small numbers of GH-treated GHD children who demonstrated appreciable improvements in final height; however, the majority of patients did not achieve a normal adult height [12, 13]. Since 1985, large quantities of synthetic recombinant human GH have been produced to allow treatment of a broad range of childhood growth disorders including GHD. With greater availability of GH therapy, the definition of GHD broadened during the 1990s from a peak stimulated GH level of ≤ 7 to ≤ 10 µg/l that has led to a change in clinical characteristics of children with idiopathic GHD [14, 15].

[a]Liggins Institute, University of Auckland
2–6 Park Avenue, Grafton, Auckland (New Zealand)
[b]Pfizer Endocrine Care
KIGS/KIMS/ACROSTUDY Medical Outcomes
Vetenskapsvägen 10, SE-191 90 Sollentuna (Sweden)
[c]Baystate Children's Hospital, Tufts University School of Medicine
759 Chestnut Street, Springfield, MA 01199 (USA)

KIGS, a large pharmacoepidemiological database, has now accrued final height data on 3,966 GHD patients which allows separation of idiopathic from organic GHD patients. Children with idiopathic GHD have quite distinct clinical characteristics to those with organic GHD. Patients in the latter group have more severe GHD and have often undergone surgery, chemotherapy and radiotherapy to treat central nervous system tumours, all of which serve to constrain growth response to GH independently of GH secretory status. In this chapter, cumulative final height in children with idiopathic GHD treated with GH and enrolled into KIGS will be examined. The large number of these children allows a logical further division of idiopathic GHD into isolated GHD (IGHD) and multiple pituitary hormone deficiency (MPHD) groups. The different clinical characteristics and height outcomes of these two groups are examined. In addition, variables that influence final height are assessed. Recently, a detailed analysis of approximately 1260 idiopathic GHD patients was published [16]. Since that time there have been considerably more children with idiopathic GHD that have reached final height.

Patients and Methods

Patients enrolled within KIGS with idiopathic GHD classified by the investigators according to the KIGS Aetiology Classification List were included in this analysis. The two subgroups of children within this group were IGHD and MPHD, which included GHD and deficiency of at least one other pituitary hormone. All of the following characteristics were met.
1 A peak stimulated GH level of <10 µg/l in response to at least one stimulus. The majority of patients (81%) had testing performed with two stimuli. The most commonly used stimuli were arginine and/or insulin (50%), followed by clonidine (15%), L-Dopa (11%) and spontaneous GH secretion (9%).
2 Near final height was defined as a height velocity of <2 cm/year over at least 9 months and is within 0.3 SD of the actual final height. In addition, males had reached a chronological age of >16 years and/or a bone age of >14 years and females a chronological age of >14 years and/or a bone age of >13 years.
3 Demonstration of pubertal development at final height to ensure that older prepubertal adolescents with marked slowing in height velocity are not included.
4 Minimum requirements for selection were 1 year of GH treatment before puberty and at least 4 years total treatment to ensure that subjects included have received a reasonably long and therefore meaningful course of treatment.
5 Auxological data were available at the start of GH treatment, after the first year and at final height.

Prader height standards were applied to all except Japanese patients in whom national reference standards were used [17, 18]. Although there is considerable racial diversity within KIGS, country-specific growth charts were not used for all countries represented, as they are misleading and not comparable. Across country-specific height standards, the centimetre sizes of an SDS are highly variable and the periods in which the charts were constructed vary by as much as 30 years; thus, secular growth trends would be very different. Country-specific growth charts do not exist for many countries. Bone age estimation was excluded from the variables that could influence response to GH therapy as it was not centrally reported nor assessed by a single set of standards and not consistently performed immediately prior to the commencement of therapy.

Assessment of the growth response to GH therapy was made at three time points: at the start of GH therapy, at the start of puberty and at near final height. At each of these, response to GH therapy was calculated and expressed by three different but complementary techniques: (1) final height in centimetres or expressed as an SDS, (2) the amount of height gained expressed as height SDS – initial height SDS, and (3) the influence of genetic height potential on height expressed as height SDS – midparental height SDS (MPH SDS).

Simple linear correlations were used to identify pretreatment and treatment variables that could influence final height. Multiple regression analysis was conducted using the R^2 selection method and Mallow's C(p) as the criteria for choosing parameters predictive of final height as initially identified by simple linear correlations. All statistical analyses were conducted with the program package SAS version 8. Values are expressed as medians with 10th and 90th percentiles. Standard non-parametric statistical tests (Wilcoxon rank test and Kruskal-Wallis test) were used for comparisons of outcome measures due to the non-linear distribution of data. P values were determined for two-sided tests, with a value <0.05 indicating a significant difference.

Table 1. Evaluation of the baseline characteristics of patients with idiopathic IGHD who have achieved final height

Variable	Males	Females	p value
Total patients	741	480	
Caucasians	652	384	
Japanese	73	87	
Chronological age, years	9.8 (5.2, 12.5)	8.7 (4.5, 11.4)	<0.001
Birth weight SDS	−0.6 (−2.1, 0.9)	−0.7 (−2.2, 0.7)	
MPH SDS	−1.3 (−2.7, 0.1)	−1.4 (−3.0, 0.3)	
Caucasians	−1.2 (−2.4, 0.2)	−1.2 (−2.5, 0.5)	
Japanese	−2.6 (−3.8, −1.5)	−2.7 (−3.7, −1.8)	
Maximum GH peak, μg/l	6.0 (1.9, 9.0)	6.0 (1.6, 9.4)	
IGF-1 SDS	−1.8 (−3.3, −0.5)	−1.8 (−4.7, −0.2)	
Height SDS	−2.9 (−4.3, −2.0)	−3.2 (−5.0, −2.1)	<0.001
Caucasians	−2.9 (−4.2, −2.1)	−3.2 (−5.0, −2.1)	<0.001
Japanese	−2.9 (−4.8, −2.1)	−3.1 (−4.5, −2.4)	
Body mass index SDS	−0.3 (−1.8, 1.2)	−0.5 (−1.9, 0.8)	<0.01
Induced puberty, %	0	0	

Values in parentheses are 10th and 90th percentiles.

Results

Pretreatment Auxological Characteristics

The analyses were conducted on data that were collected up to January 2006 from patients with idiopathic GHD who were in the KIGS Aetiology Classification List group No. 1.1. The entire patient population within the KIGS database consisted of 56,123 patients from 50 countries amassing a total of 164,558 GH treatment years. Just 4 countries contributed two thirds of all idiopathic GHD patients: Japan, the USA, France and Germany. The idiopathic GHD group is the largest group within the KIGS database. At the start of GH therapy, there were 21,473 idiopathic GHD patients comprising 38.3% of all patients enrolled, treated with GH for 82,950 years. The idiopathic GHD group includes 17,366 patients with isolated GHD of whom 68% were males and 21% were Japanese patients.

Further analyses were only conducted on the 1,907 idiopathic GHD patients who had reached final height. The pre-treatment characteristics of the IGHD and MPHD groups are shown in tables 1 and 2. The IGHD females were younger and shorter than the males, with the remaining pre-treatment characteristics between sexes in the IGHD group being remarkably similar. Similarly, the MPHD girls were younger and shorter than the males without any differences in the other pre-treatment clinical characteristics. When the IGHD group is compared with the MPHD group, there are obvious differences between the groups, i.e. the MPHD patients were younger ($p < 0.001$), shorter ($p < 0.001$) and had more severe GHD, as reflected in lower peak stimulated serum GH ($p < 0.001$) and baseline insulin-like growth factor (IGF) levels ($p < 0.001$).

First-Year Response to GH

At the end of the first year of GH treatment, there was an increase in height SDS of 0.6 in the IGHD group, which is similar to a value of 0.7 in the MPHD group. In both of these groups, the actual first-year height velocity achieved was very close to that predicted from the idiopathic GHD model without the maximum GH peak for both the IGHD and MPHD groups (8.6 vs. 8.9 and 10.3 vs. 9.8 cm/year, respectively).

Table 2. Evaluation of the baseline characteristics of patients with idiopathic MPHD who have achieved final height

Variable	Males	Females	p value
Total patients	427	259	
Caucasians	365	222	
Japanese	51	31	
Chronological age, years	8.2 (3.5, 12.8)	7.6 (2.9, 11.8)	<0.01
Birth weight SDS	–0.7 (–2.2, 0.7)	–0.5 (–2.1, 1.2)	<0.05
MPH SDS	–1.1 (–2.5, 0.5)	–0.8 (–2.6, 0.7)	
Caucasians	–0.9 (–2.3, 0.6)	–0.7 (–2.4, 0.7)	
Japanese	–2.2 (–2.9, –1.0)	–2.1 (–3.1, –1.4)	
Maximum GH peak, μg/l	3.0 (0.6, 7.8)	2.5 (0.5, 8.0)	
IGF-1 SDS	–1.9 (–4.4, 0.4)	–2.4 (–5.3, –1.4)	
Height SDS	–3.5 (–5.2, –2.2)	–3.9 (–6.0, –2.5)	<0.001
Caucasians	–3.5 (–5.2, –2.2)	–3.9 (–6.2, –2.5)	<0.001
Japanese	–3.5 (–4.8, –2.5)	–3.5 (–5.3, –2.7)	
Body mass index SDS	–0.2 (–1.7, 1.5)	–0.2 (–1.9, 1.4)	
Induced puberty, %	54	47	

Values in parentheses are 10th and 90th percentiles.

Final Height

The GH treatment regimen which included dose and duration of treatment is summarised in tables 3 and 4 for the IGHD and MPHD groups, respectively. The GH doses used varied by as much as 100% and were likely to reflect different dosing practices and funding allowances across countries with doses as low as 0.14 mg/kg/week used in at least 10% of patients. There was no difference between the IGHD and the MPHD doses when the sexes were combined at GH start, but the mean total IGHD dose during treatment was higher than the MPHD dose (p < 0.001). GH doses have increased over time: doses of 0.16 mg/kg/week were reported in the KIGS 10 Year Book [19]; current doses are about 25% higher. KIGS is a cumulative database, and thus, the first 10 years of data that included lower GH doses are incorporated in this analysis.

Final height achieved following GH therapy is shown in centimetres for patients with IGHD in figure 1 and for patients with MPHD in figure 2. In addition, final height is also expressed as SDS for IGHD and MPHD groups in tables 3 and 4, respectively. Healthy untreated Japanese adolescents are shorter than Caucasian adolescents. The Japanese adolescents contributed 13% of the total idiopathic GHD final height group and are therefore separately shown in figures 1 and 2, as well as in tables 3 and 4. Both IGHD and MPHD males and females were shorter than normal untreated males and females. Nevertheless, it was encouraging to see that 78% of IGHD and 76% of MPHD males achieved a height within the normal range. Unfortunately, females faired less well, with 69% of the IGHD and 71% of the MPHD group achieving a height within the normal range. Arguably, one of the most important assessments of final height is in relation to parents' heights (final height – MPH SDS) as an index of genetic height potential. Both Caucasian and Japanese adolescent males with IGHD or MPHD virtually achieve genetic height potential, whereas females in both of these groups fall considerably short of genetic height potential. The Japanese female patients with MPHD achieved the poorest final height relative to MPH falling 0.8 SD below the MPH SDS. The obvious explanation for the poorer final height achieved in IGHD and MPHD females is that they had more severe

Table 3. GH treatment regimens and auxological features of IGHD patients who have achieved near final height

Variable	Males	Females	p value
Age, years	17.7 (16.5, 19.6)	15.8 (14.5, 17.9)	<0.001
Mean GH dose, mg/kg/week	0.20 (0.14, 0.28)	0.19 (0.14, 0.26)	<0.01
Mean GH injection frequency per week	6.8 (5.0, 7.0)	6.2 (4.0, 7.0)	<0.001
GH treatment duration, years	7.5 (5.2, 11.7)	6.7 (4.5, 10.7)	<0.001
Height SDS	−1.3 (−2.7, 0.0)	−1.5 (−2.8, −0.1)	<0.001
Caucasians	−1.2 (−2.5, 0.0)	−1.4 (−2.7, 0.0)	<0.05
Japanese	−1.8 (−3.1, −0.5)	−2.1 (−3.4, −1.0)	
Final height − initial height SDS	1.7 (0.6, 3.2)	1.7 (0.5, 3.5)	
Caucasians	1.7 (0.7, 3.2)	1.9 (0.5, 3.7)	<0.05
Japanese	1.3 (0.1, 3.2)	1.2 (0.1, 2.4)	
Final height − MPH SDS	0.0 (−1.6, 1.1)	−0.3 (−1.7, 1.0)	<0.01
Caucasians	0.0 (−1.5, 1.1)	−0.3 (−1.6, 1.0)	<0.01
Japanese	−0.1 (−2.0, 1.0)	−0.3 (−2.0, 1.1)	

Values in parentheses are 10th and 90th percentiles.

Table 4. GH treatment regimens and auxological features of MPHD patients who have achieved near final height

Variable	Males	Females	p value
Age, years	18.5 (16.8, 21.0)	17.0 (15.0, 19.9)	<0.001
Mean GH dose, mg/kg/week	0.18 (0.12, 0.25)	0.18 (0.14, 0.25)	
Mean GH injection frequency per week	6.0 (3.8, 7.0)	6.2 (4.1, 7.0)	
GH treatment duration, years	9.3 (5.4, 14.8)	8.9 (4.9, 13.6)	<0.05
Height SDS	−1.1 (−2.8, 0.3)	−1.2 (−3.0, 0.4)	
Caucasians	−1.1 (−2.8, 0.3)	−1.2 (−3.0, 0.5)	
Japanese	−1.3 (−3.2, 0.2)	−1.7 (−3.6, −0.3)	
Final height − initial height SDS	2.3 (0.9, 4.1)	2.7 (0.7, 5.0)	<0.01
Caucasians	2.3 (1.0, 4.0)	2.9 (0.8, 5.0)	<0.001
Japanese	2.3 (0.4, 4.1)	2.0 (0.0, 3.8)	
Final height − MPH SDS	−0.2 (−1.9, 1.2)	−0.4 (−2.5, 1.3)	
Caucasians	−0.2 (−1.9, 1.2)	−0.4 (−2.4, 1.3)	
Japanese	−0.2 (−1.9, 1.0)	−0.8 (−3.5, 0.9)	

Values in parentheses are 10th and 90th percentiles.

short stature prior to GH treatment. Interestingly, Caucasian females experience a greater gain in height over the course of GH treatment (expressed as final height − initial height SDS) than males (p < 0.05 for both groups), which was not seen with the IGHD group.

To evaluate the impact of GHD on the outcome and to define the clinical characteristics associated with the severity of GHD patients, severe GHD patients (stimulated peak GH ≤3 μg/l) were compared with those with partial GHD (stimulated peak GH 7–10 μg/l), as shown

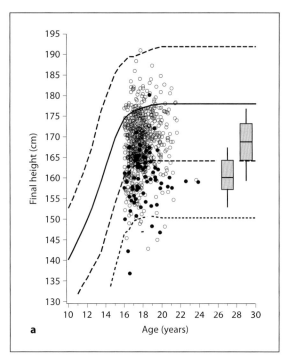 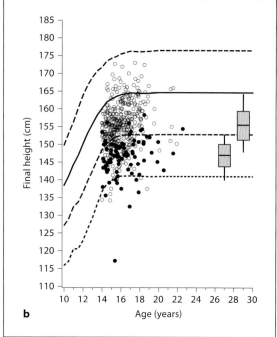

Fig. 1. a Final height achieved for males with idiopathic IGHD. Closed circles represent Japanese and open circles Caucasian adolescent males. The box plots shown display medians with 25th and 75th percentiles with whiskers at the 10th and 90th percentiles for Japanese (left) and Caucasian patients (right). Solid line (—) = Means; dashed lines (- - -) = ±2 SD; lower dashed curve (-----) = –4 SD (Prader). **b** Final height achieved for females with idiopathic IGHD. Closed circles represent Japanese and open circles Caucasian adolescent females. The box plots shown display medians with 25th and 75th percentiles with whiskers at the 10th and 90th percentiles for Japanese (left) and Caucasian patients (right). Solid line (—) = Means; dashed lines (- - -) = ±2 SD; lower dashed curve (-----) = –4 SD (Prader).

in table 5. Striking differences are seen between the groups, with severe GHD children being younger and having taller parents as well as a taller final height.

Puberty
A subgroup of 851 idiopathic GHD children also had auxological assessments performed at the start of puberty, which allows assessment of the phases of prepubertal and pubertal growth as well as total growth. The patients with spontaneous puberty had slightly later puberty than normal children, which was less delayed than reported in the KIGS analysis of this group 10 years ago (12.8 vs. 13.8 years in males and 11.8 vs. 12.9 years in females, respectively) [19]. Table 6 compares and contrasts the growth patterns of those with spontaneous versus those with induced puberty. Subjects with induced puberty were younger ($p < 0.01$), shorter ($p < 0.001$) and had more severe GHD ($p < 0.001$). The gain in height during the prepubertal years was far greater in the induced puberty group and could largely be explained by the 3.5–4.0 years of additional prepubertal growth due to the younger age at the start of treatment and the older age at which puberty was induced when compared with the spontaneous puberty group. Conversely, the induced puberty group had a shorter period of pubertal growth ($p < 0.001$) and less total pubertal growth (TPG;

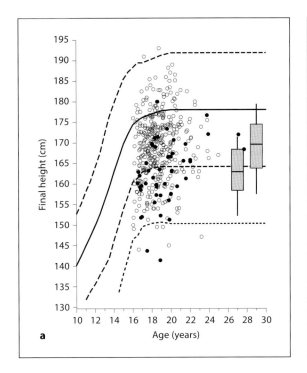 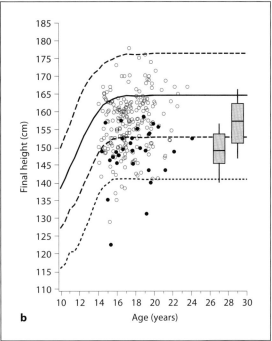

Fig. 2. a Final height achieved for males with idiopathic MPHD. Closed circles represent Japanese and open circles Caucasian adolescent males. The box plots shown display medians with 25th and 75th percentiles with whiskers at the 10th and 90th percentiles for Japanese (left) and Caucasian patients (right). Solid line (——) = Means; dashed lines (– – –) = ±2 SD; lower dashed curve (-----) = –4 SD (Prader). **b** Final height achieved for females with idiopathic MPHD. Closed circles represent Japanese and open circles Caucasian adolescent females. The box plots shown display medians with 25th and 75th percentiles with whiskers at the 10th and 90th percentiles for Japanese (left) and Caucasian patients (right). Solid line (——) = Means; dashed lines (– – –) = ±2 SD; lower dashed curve (-----) = –4 SD (Prader).

$p < 0.001$), setting off some of the apparent gains in height during the prepubertal years. However, the two groups achieved similar final heights as reflected in the height SDS and the height relative to MPH. The better overall growth response of the induced group is likely due to shorter pretreatment height, creating the opportunity for greater capacity to grow together with the presence of more severe GHD.

Comparing the two extremes of responders illustrates the markedly different clinical characteristics of the two groups that could influence response to treatment. Table 7 compares the top 10% of responders (favourable responders) to GH therapy as measured by the gain in height (final height – initial height SDS) with the lowest 10% of responders (unfavourable responders). The favourable responders are much younger, with more severe GHD, more marked short stature with taller parents and receive a higher GH dose than the unfavourable responders. All of these factors are likely to influence the first-year growth response of the favourable responders with a 4-fold increase in the height velocity SDS. The greatest gains in growth of the favourable responders compared with the poor responders occur during the prepubertal years. Whilst the favourable responders still achieve a height gain during puberty, although modest, the unfavourable responders have a poor height gain during

Table 5. Comparison of clinical characteristics and final heights of patients with severe GHD (maximum peak GH ≤3 μg/l) with those with partial GHD (maximum peak GH 7–10 μg/l) for patients with idiopathic IGHD and idiopathic MPHD

Variable	IGHD		MPHD		p value
	severe GHD (n = 240)	partial GHD (n = 471)	severe GHD (n = 370)	partial GHD (n = 120)	
At the start of GH therapy					
Chronological age, years	7.7 (3.9, 11.8)	9.8 (5.8, 12.3)	7.1 (2.5, 11.9)	9.6 (5.4, 12.6)	<0.001
Maximum peak GH, μg/l	1.8 (0.6, 2.9)	8.5 (7.2, 9.7)	1.4 (0.4, 2.7)	8.0 (7.1, 9.6)	<0.001
MPH SDS	–1.0 (–2.5, 0.7)	–1.5 (–3.0, –0.1)	–0.7 (–2.3, 0.8)	–1.5 (–3.0, –0.0)	<0.001
Height SDS	–3.6 (–5.4, –2.5)	–2.9 (–4.0, –2.0)	–4.1 (–6.0, –2.5)	–3.1 (–4.3, –2.3)	<0.001
Birth weight SDS	–0.6 (–2.1, 1.0)	–0.8 (–2.4, 0.6)	–0.4 (–2.0, 1.2)	–1.0 (–2.5, 0.4)	<0.001
First year on GH					
Height velocity SDS	4.6 (0.5, 9.6)	3.0 (–0.5, 6.6)	4.4 (–0.0, 9.6)	2.8 (–1.0, 6.6)	<0.001
At the start of puberty					
Height SDS	–1.3 (–2.7, 0.4)	–1.5 (–2.6, –0.6)	–1.3 (–2.8, 0.5)	–1.6 (–2.9, –0.1)	0.021[a]
Puberty height – initial height SDS	2.8 (1.0, 5.0)	1.3 (0.6, 2.3)	2.9 (1.2, 4.8)	1.5 (0.7, 2.9)	<0.001
At final height					
Mean GH dose, mg/kg/week	0.19 (0.13, 0.25)	0.20 (0.14, 0.29)	0.18 (0.12, 0.23)	0.20 (0.14, 0.27)	<0.01
Height SDS	–1.3 (–2.9, 0.3)	–1.5 (–2.8, –0.2)	–1.0 (–2.8, 0.6)	–1.6 (–3.0, –0.2)	<0.01
Height – MPH SDS	–0.3 (–1.9, 1.1)	–0.1 (–1.6, 1.2)	–0.3 (–2.2, 1.2)	–0.3 (–2.0, 1.2)	<0.05[a]
Final height– puberty height SDS	0.1 (–0.7, 1.1)	0.3 (–0.5, 1.0)	0.2 (–1.0, 1.4)	0.2 (–1.0, 1.4)	n.s.

Values in parentheses are 10th and 90th percentiles. n.s. = Not significant.
[a] Data of MPHD patients were not significant.

puberty with a pronounced fall in height SDS during this period.

Correlations

The final height SDS was selected as the outcome to determine which pre-treatment and treatment variables could influence final height. The reason why the final height SDS was selected rather than the magnitude of growth response (final height – initial height SDS) is that the critical outcome in patients is the actual height achieved rather than growth development during treatment. Data for the sexes were combined and a comparison made between the IGHD and MPHD groups for both simple linear correlations and multiple regression analysis which are ranked in tables 8 and 9. Some of the simple linear correlations listed in table 8 are not independent and are obviously linked to other variables listed, e.g., the total dose is linked to the duration of GH treatment and age. There are also less obvious associations created by clusters of clinical characteristics. For example, MPH was associated with the duration of treatment (r = 0.14, p < 0.001) and the severity of GHD (r = –0.17 for peak GH levels, p < 0.0001). In other words, some short children had short parents and less severe GHD that was treated with GH for a longer time period.

The simple linear correlations with final height are similar between the IGHD and MPHD groups as shown in table 8. Not surprisingly, the starting height SDS was most strongly correlated with final height, as a taller child would be expected to achieve a taller final height following GH treatment. Genetic height potential is not only a critical determinant of final height in nor-

Table 6. Comparison of patients with spontaneous onset of puberty versus those with induced puberty in whom auxological data were available at the start of GH treatment, at the onset of puberty and at final height

Variable	Males		Females		p value
	spontaneous puberty (n = 375)	induced puberty (n = 135)	spontaneous puberty (n = 268)	induced puberty (n = 73)	
At the start of GH therapy					
Chronological age, years	9.3 (4.9, 12.2)	7.4 (2.8, 13.5)	8.6 (4.2, 11.3)	7.1 (2.4, 12.0)	<0.01
Maximum peak GH, μg/l	5.8 (1.8, 8.8)	2.2 (0.5, 6.0)	6.0 (1.5, 9.3)	1.6 (0.5, 4.5)	<0.001
MPH SDS	–1.1 (–2.3, 0.3)	–1.0 (–2.5, 0.6)	–1.2 (–2.7, 0.6)	–0.6 (–2.0, 0.8)	<0.01[a]
Height SDS	–2.9 (–4.5, –2.1)	–3.7 (–5.3, 2.4)	–3.3 (–5.0, –2.1)	–4.4 (–6.7, –2.7)	<0.001
At the start of puberty					
Chronological age, years	12.8 (11.4, 14.6)	14.8 (12.6, 17.5)	11.8 (10.3, 13.5)	13.6 (11.7, 16.8)	<0.001
Height SDS	–1.5 (–2.6, –0.4)	–1.4 (–3.0, 0.3)	–1.3 (–2.6, –0.2)	–1.2 (–2.8, 0.4)	n.s.
Pubertal height – initial height SDS	1.4 (0.7, 3.0)	2.5 (1.0, 4.0)	1.9 (0.9, 4.0)	3.3 (1.1, 5.1)	<0.001
Height – MPH SDS	–0.3 (–1.7, 0.8)	–0.3 (–1.6, 1.2)	–0.0 (–1.7, 1.1)	–0.5 (–2.5, 0.9)	<0.01[a]
At final height					
Chronological age, years	17.9 (16.5, 19.8)	19.0 (17.0, 21.4)	15.7 (14.5, 18.3)	17.3 (15.9, 20.2)	<0.001
Puberty duration, years	5.0 (3.4, 7.0)	4.1 (2.0, 6.6)	4.0 (2.5, 6.6)	3.6 (1.7, 7.5)	<0.001
Total pubertal growth, cm	26.5 (19.0, 35.0)	18.8 (8.5, 31.1)	17.5 (9.5, 25.4)	11.2 (3.6, 19.9)	<0.001
Height SDS	–1.0 (–2.3, 0.1)	–1.2 (–2.6, 0.4)	–1.3 (–2.5, 0.1)	–1.1 (–2.7, 0.7)	n.s.
Final height – initial height SDS	1.9 (0.9, 3.4)	2.7 (1.1, 4.3)	1.9 (0.6, 4.1)	3.6 (1.2, 5.2)	<0.001
Final height – MPH SDS	0.1 (–1.4, 1.3)	–0.2 (–1.9, 1.3)	–0.2 (–1.7, 1.0)	–0.4 (2.3, 1.2)	n.s.

Values in parentheses are 10th and 90th percentiles. n.s. = Not significant.
[a] Data of males were not significant.

mal children but also determines responsiveness to GH therapy across a range of growth disorders including idiopathic GHD. A clear difference between the IGHD and MPHD groups was seen with the GH dose-related parameters (total dose and mean dose) in which there were correlations with final height in the IGHD group (albeit small) but no relationships with final height in the MPHD group.

Correlations identified between variables and final height from simple linear correlations were selected for multiple regression analysis to determine variables that will predict the variability in final height. Inevitably, variables are associated in a way that when included in multiple regression analysis, the apparent influence on final height diminishes. This is particularly evident with the GH dosing regimen for the IGHD group in that duration of treatment becomes the most important variable and total dose and mean dose become less influential variables. Conversely, it is only the total GH dose in MPHD that influences final height in multiple regression analysis. From multiple regression analysis, multiple regression models have been determined to account for the variability in final height for both IGHD and MPHD patients and are detailed below.

IGHD final height SDS = –0.90 + (0.72 × starting height SDS) + (0.24 × MPH SDS) + (0.94 × first-year change in height SDS) + (0.16 × years of GH treatment) + (0.08 × birth weight SDS) + (0.03 × chronological age at GH start).

This model is based upon 1,091 patients with an R^2 of 0.61 and an error SD of 0.7.

MPHD final height SDS = –0.34 + (0.53 × starting height SDS) + (0.28 × MPH SDS) + (0.52 × first-year change in height SDS) + (0.10 × years of GH treatment) + (0.09 × birth weight SDS).

Table 7. Comparison of the clinical characteristics and final heights of the lowest and the highest 10% of GH responders as measured by the improvement in height SDS during GH treatment for patients with idiopathic IGHD and idiopathic MPHD

	IGHD		MPHD		p value
	lowest 10% (n = 123)	highest 10% (n = 122)	lowest 10% (n = 69)	highest 10% (n = 69)	
At the start of GH therapy					
Chronological age, years	11.0	5.3	10.9	4.1	<0.001
Maximum peak GH, μg/l	7.0	2.6	5.5	1.3	<0.001
MPH SDS	−2.3	−0.4	−1.9	0.3	<0.001
Height SDS	−2.9	−4.4	−3.1	−5.5	<0.001
Birth weight SDS	−1.0	−0.1	−1.1	−0.2	<0.001
First year on GH					
Height velocity SDS	1.2	5.5	1.2	4.4	<0.001
At start of puberty					
Height SDS	−2.0	−0.8	−2.1	−0.9	<0.001
Puberty height – initial height SDS	0.6	3.8	0.8	4.9	<0.001
At final height					
Mean GH dose, mg/kg/week	0.17	0.20	0.17	0.20	<0.05
Height SDS	−2.8	−0.5	−2.8	−0.3	<0.001
Height – MPH SDS	−0.6	0.1	−1.2	−0.1	<0.001
Final height– puberty height SDS	−0.5	0.3	−0.5	0.4	<0.001

This model is based upon 604 patients with an R^2 of 0.47 and an error SD of 1.0.

Discussion

Final Height

This is the largest reported analysis of children with idiopathic GHD treated with GH to final height, consisting of longitudinal data for more than 1,900 patients. We have found that approximately 75% of those with IGHD or MPHD achieved heights within the normal height range with most reaching a height above the 10th percentile for normal adult height. Importantly, this is the first large study to report that GH therapy has led to final height that matches genetic height potential in a large subgroup of GHD patients, i.e. IGHD males. IGHD females and MPHD males achieved final heights that fall just below MPH (final height – MPH SDS −0.3 and −0.2). However, actual final height is likely to be higher than near final height reported for these KIGS patients. Near final height is up to 0.3 SD lower than actual final height, and thus, IGHD males and females will achieve actual final heights at or above MPH.

The first reports of GH treatment to final height in GHD patients appeared during the 1980s and principally encompassed treatment with fixed, low-dose cadaveric GH administered 3 times weekly [10, 11, 13, 20]. In these studies, mean final heights were well below the normal height range with height SDS values of −3.3 to −2.1. Most of these studies consisted of a mixture of idiopathic and organic GHD, with better responses seen with organic than with idiopathic GHD [10, 11, 13, 20]. The availability of recombinant human GH in the mid 1980s allowed larger GH doses and an increase in dose frequency to be

Table 8. Relationship between pre-treatment and treatment parameters and final height based upon simple linear correlations in GH-treated children with idiopathic GHD, comparing children with IGHD with those with MPHD

	IGHD		MPHD	
	Pearson correlation coefficient	p value	Pearson correlation coefficient	p value
Starting height SDS	0.53	<0.0001	0.43	<0.0001
MPH SDS	0.50	<0.0001	0.46	<0.0001
Total GH dose	0.38	<0.0001	0.35	<0.0001
First-year change in height SDS	0.27	<0.0001	0.19	<0.0001
Birth weight SDS	0.26	<0.0001	0.21	<0.0001
Mean GH dose	0.17	<0.0001	0.00	0.99
Prepubertal change in height SDS	0.15	0.0008	0.22	<0.0001
Duration of GH treatment	0.15	<0.0001	0.20	<0.0001
Age	–0.1	0.0008	–0.15	<0.0001
Maximum GH peak	–0.09	0.0023	–0.13	0.0008
GH dose at start	0.11	<0.0001	–0.04	0.30

Table 9. Relationship between pre-treatment and treatment parameters and final height based upon multivariate analysis of correlations in GH-treated children with idiopathic GHD, comparing children with IGHD with those with MPHD

	IGHD		MPHD	
	Spearman partial correlation coefficient	p value	Spearman partial correlation coefficient	p value
Starting height SDS	0.59	<0.0001	0.63	<0.0001
Duration of GH treatment	0.15	<0.002	0.07	0.27
Age	0.17	0.0002	0.16	0.008
Maximum GH peak	–0.04	0.41	–0.05	0.44
Birth weight SDS	0.12	0.0075	0.06	0.33
MPH SDS	0.34	<0.0001	0.14	0.01
Total GH dose	0.11	0.014	0.21	0.0005
First-year change in height SDS	0.27	<0.0001	0.19	<0.0001
Prepubertal change in height SDS	0.32	<0.0001	0.50	<0.0001
GH dose at start	–0.03	0.59	–0.10	0.09
Mean GH dose	–0.14	0.0018	–0.14	0.0151

assessed in GHD children. Most published final height studies in GHD children that followed were audits of local, national or international databases and contained children with very heterogeneous clinical characteristics treated with changing GH doses during treatment making direct comparison across studies difficult. These studies showed that increases in GH dose, and perhaps more importantly dose frequency, were associated with better final heights, which were in the lower half of the normal height range [21–27]. However, many of these children did not achieve final heights in the normal height range and fell well short of genetic height potential with final heights of 0.6–1.0 SD below MPH [23, 27]. In the only other study in which MPH was approximated, 13 GHD children were treated with GH before the age of 5 years [24], highlighting the importance of beginning treatment at a young age.

Comparison of extremes of final heights achieved provides extreme and illuminating differences in clinical characteristics. Those who had a good final height response (top 10% of final heights achieved) had severe GHD, were unlikely to be small for gestational age (SGA) and had parents that were close to average height. Conversely, poor responders (lowest 10% of final heights achieved) had partial GHD, and almost 20% were SGA and had short parents. It is very likely that an appreciable portion of the IGHD poor responders had familial short stature and/or SGA rather than GHD. There is considerable overlap in stimulated peak GH levels between those defined as having partial GHD and normal children with normal height velocities [26]. Up to 50% of normal children had peak GH levels of <10 μg/l to a single test and 10% had peak GH levels of <10 μg/l to two tests [26]. The good responders group received a GH dose that was almost 20% higher and, despite being considerably shorter before treatment started, were more than 1 SD taller at the start of puberty. Although the good responders only showed modest further improvement in the height SDS during puberty, the poor responders lost 0.8 SD in height. Recognition of differing clinical characteristics that lead to different growth responses to GH treatment has led to the development of individualisation of GH treatment schedules such as the Ranke prediction model for idiopathic GHD [27, 28]. Individualised GH treatment strategies are likely to be far more efficacious for those with a predicted poor response than simply applying GH doses adjusted only for weight.

The KIGS database is celebrating 20 years of GH treatment outcome data for many growth disorders including idiopathic GHD and straddles the evolution in clinical characteristics and GH treatment with this group. To date, data analyses have been cumulative, and thus, comparisons between different time periods will dilute any real changes that have occurred. In 1998, there were 369 GH-treated patients with IGHD that had achieved final height compared with 1,907 patients in this 2006 analysis which of course includes the 1998 patients. During this 8-year interval, GH dose increased by 18% in males with an additional weekly GH dose in both sexes. Although in 1998 the final height SDS was greater by approximately 0.3 SD, this difference could be explained by a change in growth standards from Tanner et al. [31, 32] to Prader et al. [17].

Across the idiopathic GHD group, the Japanese patients achieved a slightly lower final height and final height – MPH than Caucasian patients. This was most evident in Japanese females with IGHD in whom the majority of patients did not achieve a final height within the normal height range (final height SDS of –2.1). In Japanese patients, final height in relation to MPH may be overestimated given the more pronounced secular trend of increasing height in the Japanese population [33]. One of the obvious differences between the two groups that could account for the slightly different height outcomes was in the GH treatment regimen. The Japanese patients received a GH dose that was 25% lower than in Caucasian patients and 1–2 fewer GH doses per week.

In this analysis, females achieved a slightly lower final height SDS than males, which became more apparent when final height was corrected for MPH. We found that IGHD and MPHD females were 0.3 and 0.4 SD shorter than males prior to GH treatment and achieved the same increase in height as males. Thus, the most likely explanation is that more severe short stature prior to treatment has led to shorter final height. This finding serves as a salutary reminder that delay in presentation or diagnosis of GHD will lead to more severe short stature which will compromise final height following GH treatment. The reported final height in GHD females has been lower than in males in some but not in all studies [12, 13, 23, 27, 34, 35]. In studies in which females achieved a poorer final height, the pretreatment height SDS was much lower than in males as we observed [13, 23].

There are two key factors which limit final height in idiopathic GHD children: firstly, cessation of GH treatment before final height is reached, and secondly and potentially more important, non-compliance with GH administration. It is impossible to quantify the effect that these factors have had in diminishing final height across the IGHD and MPHD groups; however, it is likely to be meaningful. Practices across countries vary widely as to when GH therapy is stopped in GHD adolescents. These practices range from cessation of GH treatment once the height falls within the normal height range to treatment right to the final height and then continuation at lower adult replacement doses. KIGS analysis performed 11 years ago [36] found that 22% of children enrolled within KIGS have had their GH therapy stopped before final height was reached. More recent analysis has not yet been performed to determine whether the practice of premature cessation of GH therapy continues. Only a single study has assessed compliance with GH treatment in largely GHD patients and found that 50% of subjects did not comply with all aspects of treatment [37]. Frequently missed GH doses will contribute to a poorer final height and create the illusion that the particular dose used is less efficacious.

Growth in Puberty

When GH therapy is started in mid- to late childhood, the majority of height gain occurs prior to the onset of puberty in IGHD and MPH children, as shown in figure 3. In KIGS, idiopathic GHD males with spontaneous puberty experienced 75% of their height gain prior to puberty, whereas in females with spontaneous puberty, all of the height gain occurred prior to puberty. The induced puberty group had an increase in prepubertal height gain that was 1.5-fold greater than in the spontaneous group which could be largely attributed to the additional 3–4 years of prepubertal growth for the induced puberty group. An additional minor contributing factor may have been more severe GHD which was weakly correlated with final height in the induced puberty group. Thus, the induced pubertal group achieved a similar prepubertal height to the spontaneous puberty group but patients were 2 years older at the start of puberty. Height gains during puberty were small at best and were really only evident in males in the spontaneous puberty group (0.4 SDS). Even the top 10% of GH responders (table 7) only had height gains in puberty that were small in the IGHD and MPHD groups (0.3 and 0.4 SDS, respectively). Conversely, the poorest 10% of GH responders had a fall in height SDS during puberty, losing some of the benefits of prepubertal height gain.

The TPG phase was shorter in the induced than in the spontaneous puberty group with the difference more evident in males than in females. Later onset of puberty has been shown to be associated with a shorter pubertal growth period and less TPG in those with GHD treated with GH who undergo spontaneous puberty [13]. The median TPG of 26.5 cm in males with spontaneous puberty matches the TPG of 26.7 cm seen in normal adolescent males with delayed onset of puberty [38]. Similarly, the TPG in females of 17.5 cm with spontaneous puberty falls just below the 18.2 cm seen in adolescent females with delayed onset of puberty [38]. Adolescents with induced puberty have considerably less TPG, achieving only 71% of that seen in males with spontaneous puberty and 64% of that in females. The primary reason for diminished pubertal growth in those with induced puberty is the later age of onset of puberty rather than a shorter pubertal growth period. Females with induced puberty had a pu-

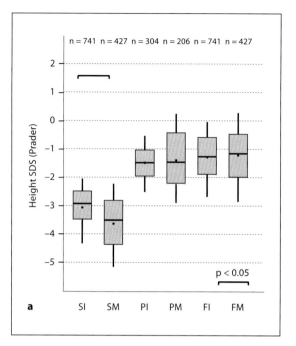 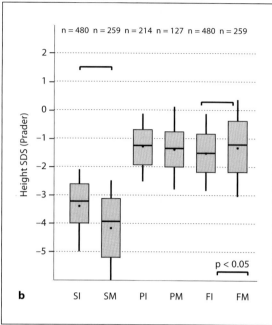

Fig. 3. Comparison of height SDS at the start of GH treatment, at the onset of puberty and at final height in males (**a**) and females (**b**) with idiopathic IGHD with those with MPHD. SI = IGHD at GH start; SM = MPHD at GH start; PI = IGHD at puberty start; PM = MPHD at puberty start; FI = IGHD at near adult height; FM = MPHD at near adult height.

bertal growth period that was only 0.4 years shorter, yet they only achieved two thirds of the TPG of females with spontaneous puberty.

Not surprisingly, final height correlates with prepubertal height [10, 13, 22, 23, 30]. This finding is consistent with our finding that prepubertal height gain correlated with final height in IGHD and MPHD patients. To achieve a meaningful improvement in final height, GH therapy needs to be initiated as early in the prepubertal period as possible using an optimal treatment regimen to achieve a maximal height at the onset of puberty. From KIGS analysis, expectation of an appreciable gain in height during puberty with conventional prepubertal GH doses in adolescents with idiopathic GHD is unrealistic. In both the IGHD and MPHD groups, the GH dose did not increase during puberty. A doubling in GH dose during puberty to approximately 0.28 mg/kg/week has not been shown to further improve final height in GHD adolescents [39]. It is only with extremely high GH doses administered during puberty (0.7 mg/kg/week) that an appreciable improvement in pubertal height gain has been shown with an increase in height SDS of 0.7 [40]. However, serum IGF-1 levels were above the normal range for pubertal controls in about 25% of this high-dose treatment group [40]. GH secretion during puberty doubles with maximum GH secretion reached at peak pubertal height velocity [41, 42]. Interestingly, when GH doses are increased to 0.3 mg/kg/week, which is 50% higher than the prepubertal GH doses used in KIGS idiopathic GHD patients, mean serum IGF-1 levels were still below the mean levels seen in healthy untreated adolescents in puberty [40]. Collectively, these observations suggest that when GH therapy is started late in the prepubertal period, greater reliance is placed on height gain during puberty due to the very short period of prepubertal growth. In such a situation, optimisation of pubertal growth is essential, and high-dose therapy at 0.5–0.7 mg/kg/week with serum IGF-1 monitoring would improve final height, but the financial cost of such a height gain is likely to be considerable.

Factors Influencing Final Height
The variables associated with final height from univariate and multivariate analysis were remarkably similar between the IGHD and MPHD groups. Height at the start of GH therapy was most strongly correlated with final height in IGHD and MPHD patients and contributes to the multiple regression equation of variables that collectively account for 61% of variability in IGHD and 47% in MPHD. It is intuitively obvious that a child who is less short at the start of GH therapy will have less height to gain to reach a normal adult height than a child that is extremely short at the start of treatment. Whilst some studies have found that the pre-treatment height SDS is correlated with final height in GHD children [22, 23], others have not, but they may not have included this variable in univariate or multiple regression analysis [27].

Genetic height potential is the major determining influence on adult height in normal children and is predictably a major influence on growth response to GH. Children with idiopathic GHD grow better during GH therapy and reach taller adult heights. Multiple regression analysis identified MPH as a major influence on final height in IGHD but less so in MPHD patients; however, it is not clear why this discrepancy occurred. Most studies have found that MPH is one of the most influential factors on final height in GHD children [21, 22, 34, 43]. Furthermore, MPH has been shown to influence the amount of height gain during puberty [44].

Age, GH treatment duration and total GH dose are all very closely linked variables that influence final height as shown in table 9. A younger child will receive a longer course of GH treatment and ultimately receive a greater amount of GH over time. GH treatment from an earlier age enables more treatment years during the more efficacious prepubertal growth period. This is most graphically illustrated when GH treatment is started very early in childhood. In extremely short GHD children aged <3 years who were treated with GH for 4 years, an increase in the height SDS of 2.4–2.7 occurred [45, 46]. Short GHD children that started GH treatment aged <5 years achieved their MPH following an impressive gain in height of almost 4 SD [24]. One of the striking differences between the good and the poor GH responder groups is the age at which GH treatment is started, i.e. 5 and 11 years, respectively.

Surprisingly, GH dose was not associated with final height. The improvement in final height in GHD children from early final height studies has been attributed to an increase in dose frequency and to a lesser extent in dose. Since that time, GH doses of 0.18–0.3 mg/kg/day have yielded similar final heights which have fallen short of genetic height potential [21–25, 27]. All of these studies are audits of routine clinical management and contain enormous heterogeneity in clinical characteristics. Consequently, it is much more difficult to evaluate the effect of GH dose than in a randomised study in which the only variable that is different between groups is the GH dose. Within KIGS, the GH dose is likely to be increased in a child with an initial poor growth response which creates the illusion that higher doses in these patients are associated with poor response. In a cohort of Swedish KIGS patients where all were treated with 0.22 mg/kg/week from midchildhood throughout the treatment period, final height approximated the 50th percentile and MPH was reached [43]. Furthermore, when GH treatment was started just before puberty, high-dose GH therapy at 0.7 mg/kg/week was needed to achieve a final height that was 0.8 SD greater than with a dose of 0.3 mg/kg/week [40]. In the ideal situation when GH treatment is started at a young age in children with idiopathic GHD, more conventional GH doses of 0.2–0.3 mg/kg/week administered daily are likely to achieve a normal final height that approximates MPH. However, all too often clinicians are faced with a very short, older child in whom an individualised regimen with much higher doses of GH would be needed in an attempt to achieve a height within the normal height range [30, 47].

Stimulated peak GH levels, an index of severity of GHD, did not appear to be associated with final height. Many of the variables that could contribute to final height are quite closely associated. Comparing extremes of outcomes or extremes of pre-treatment variables can help to highlight the clinical profile and impact that a variable could have on final height. When patients with severe GHD are compared with those with partial GHD (table 5), very different final heights are achieved with very different clinical profiles. Patients in the severely GHD group were diagnosed at a younger age, treated with longer courses of GH therapy and achieved much greater prepubertal height gain, reaching greater final heights. Patients in the partial GHD group were taller at the start of GH therapy, had shorter parents, were less likely to have multiple hormone deficiency and achieved poorer final heights.

Conclusion

Most KIGS patients with idiopathic GHD manifested as IGHD or MPHD and treated with GH achieved a final height within the normal height range. Encouragingly, males with IGHD reached genetic height potential. Females with IGHD and patients with MPHD achieved heights that fall just short of MPH. The most important message from this data analysis is that a normal adult height and genetic height potential can be reached with conventional GH doses administered to children with idiopathic GHD from an early age. However, if adverse clinical characteristics are present prior to starting GH treatment, such as late childhood, short parents or extreme short stature, a more aggressive individualised treatment regimen will be needed if a normal adult height is to be achieved.

References

1 Busschbach JJV, Rikken B, Grobbe DE, De Charro FT, Wit JM: Quality of life in short adults. Horm Res 1998;49:32–38.
2 Takano K, Tanaka T, Saito T, Committee for the Study Group of Adult GH Deficiency: Psychological adjustment in a large cohort of adults with growth hormone deficiency treated with growth hormone in childhood: summary of a questionnaire survey. Acta Paediatr Suppl 1994;399:16–19.
3 Cutfield WS, Wilton P, Bennmarker H, et al: Incidence of diabetes mellitus and impaired glucose tolerance in children and adolescents receiving growth-hormone treatment. Lancet 2000;355:610–613.
4 Hogler W, Briody J, Moore B, Lu PW, Cowell CT: Effect of growth hormone therapy and puberty on bone and body composition in children with idiopathic short stature and growth hormone deficiency. Bone 2005;37:642–650.
5 Radetti G, D'Addato G, Gatti D, Bozzola M, Adami S: Influence of two different GH dosage regimens on final height, bone geometry and bone strength in GH-deficient children. Eur J Endocrinol 2006;154:479–482.
6 Salerno M, Esposito V, Farina V, et al: Improvement of cardiac performance and cardiovascular risk factors in children with GH deficiency after two years of GH replacement therapy: an observational, open, prospective, case-control study. J Clin Endocrinol Metab 2006;91:1288–1295.
7 Wit JM, Kamp GA, Rikken B: Spontaneous growth and response to growth hormone treatment in children with growth hormone deficiency and idiopathic short stature. Pediatr Res 1996;39:295–302.
8 van der Werff ten Bosch JJ, Bot A: Growth of males with idiopathic hypopituitarism without growth hormone treatment. Clin Endocrinol 1990;32:707–717.

9 Ranke MB: A note on adults with growth hormone deficiency. Acta Paediatr Scand Suppl 1987;331:80–82.
10 Burns EC, Tanner JM, Preece MA, Cameron N: Final height and pubertal development in 55 children with idiopathic growth hormone deficiency, treated for between 2 and 15 years with human growth hormone. Eur J Pediatr 1981;137:155–164.
11 Joss E, Zuppinger K, Schwarz HP, Roten H: Final height of patients with pituitary growth failure and changes in growth variables after long-term hormonal therapy. Pediatr Res 1983;17:676–679.
12 Libber SM, Plotnick LP, Johanson AJ, Blizzard RM, Kwiterovich PO, Migeon CJ: Long-term follow-up of hypopituitary patients treated with human growth hormone. Medicine 1990;69:46–55.
13 Bourguignon JP, Vandeweghe M, Vanderschueren-Lodeweyckx M, et al: Pubertal growth and final height in hypopituitary boys: a minor role of bone age at onset of puberty. J Clin Endocrinol Metab 1986;63:376–382.
14 Furlanetto R, Drug A: Guidelines for the use of growth hormone in children with short stature. A report by the Drug and Therapeutics Committee of the Lawson and Wilkins Pediatric Endocrine Society. J Pediatr 1995;127:857–867.
15 Rosenfeld RG, Albertsson-Wikland K, Cassorla F, et al: Diagnostic controversy: the diagnosis of childhood growth hormone deficiency revisited. J Clin Endocrinol Metab 1995;80:1532–1540.
16 Reiter EO, Price DA, Wilton P, Albertsson-Wikland K, Ranke MB: Effect of growth hormone treatment on the near-final height of 1258 patients with idiopathic GH deficiency: analysis of a large international database. J Clin Endocrinol Metab 2006;91:2047–2054.
17 Prader A, Largo RH, Molinari L, Issler C: Physical growth of Swiss children from birth to 20 years of age. First Zurich longitudinal study of growth and development. Helv Paediatr Acta Suppl 1989;52:1–125.
18 Tachibana K, Suwa S: Standard growth charts for height and weight of Japanese children from cross-sectional data. Tokyo, the Ministry of Health, Labor and Welfare and the Ministry of Education, Culture, Sports, Science and Technology, 2000.

19 Cutfield WS, Lindberg A, Chatelain P, et al: Final height following growth hormone treatment of idiopathic growth hormone deficiency in KIGS; in Ranke MB, Wilton P (eds): Growth Hormone Therapy in KIGS – 10 Years' Experience. Heidelberg, Johann Ambrosius Barth Verlag, 1999, pp 93–110.
20 Hibi I, Tanaka T: Final height of patients with idiopathic growth hormone deficiency after long-term growth hormone treatment. Committee for Treatment of Growth Hormone Deficient Children, Growth Science Foundation, Japan. Acta Endocrinol 1989;120:409–415.
21 Rikken B, Massa GG, Wit JM: Final height in a large cohort of Dutch patients with growth hormone deficiency treated with growth hormone. Dutch Growth Hormone Working Group. Horm Res 1995;43:135–137.
22 Severi F: Final height in children with growth hormone deficiency. Horm Res 1995;43:138–140.
23 Frisch H, Birnbacher R: Final height and pubertal development in children with growth hormone deficiency after long-term treatment. Horm Res 1995;43:132–134.
24 De Luca F, Maghnie M, Arrigo T, Lombardo F, Messina MF, Bernasconi S: Final height outcome of growth hormone-deficient patients treated since less than five years of age. Acta Paediatr 1996;85:1167–1171.
25 Coste J, Letrait M, Carel JC, et al: Long-term results of growth hormone treatment in France in children of short stature: population, register based study. BMJ 1997;315:708–713.
26 Birnbacher R, Riedl S, Frisch H: Long-term treatment in children with hypopituitarism: pubertal development and final height. Horm Res 1998;49:80–85.
27 Blethen SL, Baptista J, Kuntze J, Foley T, LaFranchi S, Johanson A: Adult height in growth hormone (GH)-deficient children treated with biosynthetic GH. The Genentech Growth Study Group. J Clin Endocrinol Metab 1997;82:418–420.
28 Ghigo E, Aimaretti G, Bellone S, et al: Reliability of provocative tests to assess growth hormone secretory status. Study in 472 normally growing children. J Clin Endocrinol Metab 1996;81:3323–3327.

29 Ranke MB, Schweizer R, Wollmann HA, Schwarze P: Dosing of growth hormone in growth hormone deficiency. Horm Res 1999;3:70–74.
30 Ranke MB, Lindberg A, Martin DD, et al: The mathematical model for total pubertal growth in idiopathic growth hormone (GH) deficiency suggests a moderate role of GH dose. J Clin Endocrinol Metab 2003;88:4748–4753.
31 Tanner JM, Whitehouse RH, Takaishi M: Standards from birth to maturity for height, weight, height velocity and weight velocity: British children. Arch Dis Child 1965;41:613–635.
32 Tanner JM, Whitehouse RH, Takaishi M: Standards from birth to maturity for height, weight, height velocity and weight velocity: British children. Arch Dis Child 1965;41:454–471.
33 Matsumoto K: Secular acceleration of growth in height in Japanese and its social background. Ann Hum Biol 1982;9:427–437.
34 Thomas M, Massa G, Bourguignon JP, et al: Final height in children with idiopathic growth hormone deficiency treated with recombinant human growth hormone: the Belgian experience. Horm Res 2001;55:88–94.
35 Bramswig JH, Schlosser H, Kiese K: Final height in children with growth hormone deficiency. Horm Res 1995;43:126–128.
36 Ranke MB, Jonsson P: Who stops growth hormone therapy in KIGS – the International Kabi Growth Study – and why? KIGS Biannual Report 1995;12:33–40.
37 Smith SL, Hindmarsh PC, Brook CG: Compliance with growth hormone treatment – are they getting it? Arch Dis Child 1993;68:91–93.
38 Buckler J: A Longitudinal Study of Adolescent Growth. London, Springer, 1990.
39 Stanhope R, Urena M, Hindmarsh P, Brook C: Management of growth hormone deficiency through puberty. Acta Paediatr Scand Suppl 1991;372:47–52.
40 Mauras N, Attie KM, Reiter EO, Saenger P, Baptista J: High dose recombinant human growth hormone (GH) treatment of GH-deficient patients in puberty increases near-final height: a randomized, multicenter trial. J Clin Endocrinol Metab 2000;85:3653–3660.

41 Rose SR, Municchi G, Barnes KM: Spontaneous growth hormone secretion increases during puberty in normal boys and girls. J Clin Endocrinol Metab 1991;64:596–601.
42 Martha PMJ, Rogol AD, Veldhius JD, Keerigan JR, Godman DW, Blizzard RM: Alterations in the pulsatile properties of circulating growth hormone concentrations during puberty in boys. J Clin Endocrinol Metab 1989;69:563–570.
43 Cutfield W, Lindberg A, Albertsson-Wikland K, Chatelain P, Ranke MB, Wilton P: Final height in idiopathic growth hormone deficiency: the KIGS experience. KIGS International Board. Acta Paediatr Suppl 1999;88:72–75.
44 Ranke MB, Price DA, Albertsson-Wikland K, Maes M, Lindberg A: Factors determining pubertal growth and final height in growth hormone treatment of idiopathic growth hormone deficiency. Analysis of 195 Patients of the Kabi Pharmacia International Growth Study. Horm Res 1997;48:62–71.
45 Rappaport R, Mugnier E, Limoni C, et al: A 5-year prospective study of growth hormone (GH)-deficient children treated with GH before the age of 3 years. J Clin Endocrinol Metab 1997;82:452–456.
46 Boersma B, Rikken B, Wit JM: Catch-up growth in early treated patients with growth hormone deficiency. Dutch Growth Hormone Working Group. Arch Dis Child 1995;72:427–431.
47 Ranke MB, Lindberg A, Chatelain P, et al: Derivation and validation of a mathematical model for predicting the response to exogenous recombinant human growth hormone (GH) in prepubertal children with idiopathic GH deficiency. KIGS International Board. Kabi Pharmacia International Growth Study. J Clin Endocrinol Metab 1999;84:1174–1183.

The Transition from Childhood to Adulthood: Managing Those with Growth Hormone Deficiency

Helena Gleeson[a] Peter E. Clayton[b]

Adolescence represents a time of change physically and psychologically. Physically, the adolescent completes puberty in parallel with the cessation of linear growth, and in the years following the attainment of final height, peak bone mass (PBM) and peak muscle mass are achieved resulting in mature somatic development. Psychosocially, the adolescent reduces dependence on carers to achieve relative independence as an adult. This period encompasses the years from the mid- to late teens to the mid-twenties.

For endocrinologists, the management of adolescents with growth hormone deficiency (GHD) in the years spanning adolescence into young adulthood, popularly called the 'transition period', poses a challenge. It is now recognized that discontinuation of GH replacement therapy (GHRT) at the completion of linear growth may have detrimental consequences for somatic development in those with persistent GHD. The consensus is that GHRT should be continued into young adulthood [1]. The attainment of final height provides an opportunity for reassessment of GH status and management of the underlying condition. However, there is a need to establish which young people with GHD should be treated, what dose of GHRT should be used and how the response to GHRT should be monitored. Paediatric and adult endocrinologists need to organize and deliver care during this period so that the transition from childhood to adulthood is achieved both physically and psychologically.

The following topics are discussed, pertinent to the development of an optimal transitional care plan: (1) achievement of adult somatic development; (2) childhood-onset (CO-GHD) versus adult-onset GHD (AO-GHD); (3) reassessment of GH status at final height, and (4) impact of continuation of GHRT in the transition period compared with discontinuation.

[a]Department of Endocrinology
Christie Hospital NHS Trust, Wilmslow Road
Withington, Manchester M20 4BX (UK)
[b]Department of Child Health and Paediatric Endocrinology
University of Manchester
Oxford Road, Manchester M13 9PT (UK)

Normal Somatic Development and the Role of Growth Hormone

PBM is defined as the highest level of bone mass achieved as a result of normal growth, which, together with subsequent age-related loss, is an important determinant of an individual's risk of osteoporosis-related fracture in later life. Adolescence is a crucial time for the acquisition of bone mass.

During pubertal maturation, areal bone mineral content (BMC) and bone mineral density (BMD) at the lumbar spine and femur increase by 4- to 6-fold over 3 years (11–14 years of age in girls and 13–16 years of age in boys), such that approximately 37% of skeletal mass is accrued between pubertal stages 2 and 5. Bone mineral accretion continues after this time although the precise timing of the achievement of PBM is not certain. Areal BMD at the femur peaks around the age of 20 years, whereas maximum total skeletal mass occurs 6–10 years later [2].

The development of an adult level of lean body mass (LBM) is necessary to achieve PBM. LBM increases in children with age, with the maximal increase around the age of 13 years in girls and 15 years in boys [3]. However, complete muscle maturation is reached at a later stage, at 22–25 years of age in the healthy population [4]. The ratio of LBM/height increases particularly in males until 20 years of age and in females up to 14 years and beyond.

The increase in gonadal steroid secretion around the time of puberty is the most important hormonal regulator of both bone mass and LBM, but GH has also been shown to be an important factor. Firstly, GH and insulin-like growth factor 1 (IGF-1) are both mitogens for osteoblasts (in vitro), and secondly, GHRT in adults and children with GHD is associated with a stimulation of bone remodelling and sustained increases in BMD as well as increases in LBM [for a review, see ref. 5].

Comparison of Childhood-Onset and Adult-Onset Growth Hormone Deficiency

GHD in adulthood is associated with metabolic consequences including altered body composition (increased fat mass (FM) and reduced LBM), osteopaenia, increased cardiovascular risk factors (adverse lipid profile, premature atherosclerosis and cardiac dysfunction) and reduced quality of life (QoL), all of which can be improved with GHRT [6]. The long-term goals of GHRT in adulthood include reduction in the increase in cardiovascular morbidity and improvement in QoL.

The metabolic effects of GHD, the focus of attention in adulthood, are also present in children with untreated GHD, including altered body composition, osteopaenia and increased cardiovascular risk [7]. However, these are not routinely monitored on GHRT, nor is their improvement considered to be a treatment goal. Even at final height, GHD children who have received conventional GHRT have been reported as having metabolic abnormalities compared with controls [8].

The clinical presentation of adults with CO-GHD differs from that of AO-GHD patients. CO-GHD patients have significantly lower levels of IGF-1, less reduction in QoL and less marked derangement of lipid profile than AO-GHD patients. Attanasio et al. [9] compared body composition in 92 CO-GHD patients with 35 age-matched untreated AO-GHD patients; the mean age of those with severe GHD was 21 years and they had been off GHRT for a mean of 1.6 years. Compared with AO-GHD, CO-GHD patients were shorter [height standard deviation score (SDS) –1.2 vs. –0.4] and had a lower body mass index (23 vs. 29). Corrected for height, CO-GHD compared with AO-GHD patients had a lower BMC (2.1 vs. 2.4 kg; $p < 0.001$), LBM (38.5 vs. 50 kg; $p < 0.001$) and FM (22.3 vs. 30.1 kg; $p < 0.001$) [9]. The closer the CO-GHD patients were to achieving their genetic target height, the higher the BMC and LBM [9]. Therefore, there is a significant maturational deficit (16–20% less compared with AO-GHD patients) in somatic development in CO-GHD patients treated with GHRT during childhood [9]. Although a causal relationship has not been clearly identified, failure to reach PBM, due in part to not reaching peak muscle mass, may be an important determinant of the risk of fractures later in life in GHD patients. These deficits in body composition could be due to inadequate GHRT in childhood, in particular during the pubertal years. They are also likely to be due to the absence of GHRT for 18 months following discontinuation at final height.

Defining Growth Hormone Deficiency in the Transition Period

Reassessment of GHD in the Transition Period
The attainment of final height provides an appropriate time to re-evaluate pituitary function including GH status and the underlying diagnosis. All patients require reassessment of GH status with the exception of those with severe congenital or acquired panhypopituitarism with four or five pituitary hormone deficiencies. Reassessment is essential for the following reasons: (1) poor reproducibility of GH provocative tests; (2) criteria for the diagnosis of GHD differ between childhood and adulthood, with GHRT being considered only in severe GHD (<3 μg/l) in adulthood, but in all degrees of GHD (<10 μg/l) in childhood; (3) GHD may evolve, and therefore, reassessment will identify those children who have become more severely GH deficient; (4) many children (25–75%) with idiopathic or isolated GHD will have a normal GH status on retesting at final height. The presence of an abnormal hypothalamic-pituitary axis on magnetic resonance imaging, for instance an ectopic posterior pituitary and/or an absent stalk, should not be taken as clear evidence of continued GHD into adulthood, as a proportion (22%) will retest as having normal GH status [10]. These data emphasize the importance of re-evaluation of pituitary function at the end of growth. It is proposed that reassessment of GH status should occur at least 1 month after GHRT to avoid potential treatment-induced suppression of endogenous GH secretion.

Biochemical Criteria for the Definition of GHD
The diagnosis of GHD is reliant on baseline IGF-1 levels and GH levels in response to provocative testing. When considering IGF-1 as a diagnostic tool, robust normative data are required. The latter demonstrate the influence of gender, age and pubertal status, with IGF-1 reaching a maximum at mid- to late puberty, and subsequently, declining rapidly until the mid-twenties. A normal IGF-1 level does not exclude a diagnosis of GHD, as evidenced by a third of GHD adults who have IGF-1 levels within the normal range. However, a low IGF-1 level in the transition period would support a diagnosis of GHD.

The peak GH response to provocative testing (≤ 3 μg/l) below which severe GHD is diagnosed in an adult is based on a cohort of 45-year-old patients with hypopituitarism. Therefore, adopting the adult criteria for severe GHD in adolescence is inappropriate. Spontaneous 24-hour GH secretion peaks during late puberty and begins to decrease only after the second decade of life [11]. Peak GH levels during provocative testing follow a similar pattern. An appropriate peak GH cut-off level in the transitional period has been examined. Leger et al. [10] found that on retesting children with CO-GHD and an ectopic posterior pituitary treated with GHRT to final height, a peak GH <5 μg/l was most likely in the presence of multiple pituitary deficiencies and if the ectopic posterior pituitary was located in the median eminence and the stalk was absent. Similarly, Maghnie et al. [12] studied the GH responses to an insulin tolerance test and IGF-1 retest data in 26 patients with multiple pituitary hormone deficiencies or a significant magnetic resonance imaging abnormality of the hypothalamic-pitui-

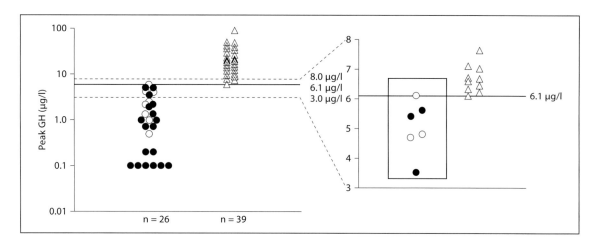

Fig. 1. Peak GH response to an insulin tolerance test in 26 adolescents with multiple pituitary hormone deficiencies or a significant structural hypothalamic pituitary lesion compared with 39 normal controls [12]. Black circles = multiple pituitary hormone deficiencies; white circles = isolated GHD; white triangles = normal controls.

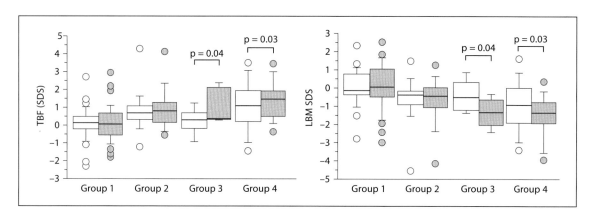

Fig. 2. Change in body composition [total body fat (TBF) SDS and LBM SDS] 1 year after GHRT completion at final height in adolescents with normal GH secretion (>11.8 μg/l) (group 1) compared with partial GHD (3–11.8 μg/l) to two tests (group 4) at two testing time points [13]. Group 1: 2 tests normal at completion of growth and 1 year later; group 2: first test partial, second test normal; group 3: vice versa; group 4: both tests partial.

tary axis at the end of growth compared with age-matched normal controls. A peak GH of 6.1 μg/l to insulin tolerance test gave a sensitivity of 66% and a specificity of 100% (fig. 1), similarly an IGF-1 SDS of –1.7 gave a sensitivity of 77% and a specificity of 100% for the diagnosis of GHD [12].

The majority of studies of GHRT in the transition period demonstrating benefit have used a peak GH level of <5 μg/l on provocative testing to diagnose severe GHD. However, Tauber et al. [13] have examined the outcome over 1 year in adolescents who retested with partial/moderate GHD (peak GH 3–11.8 μg/l) or normal GH status either at completion of growth or 1 year after discontinuing GHRT. At baseline, body composition was adverse in adolescents with partial

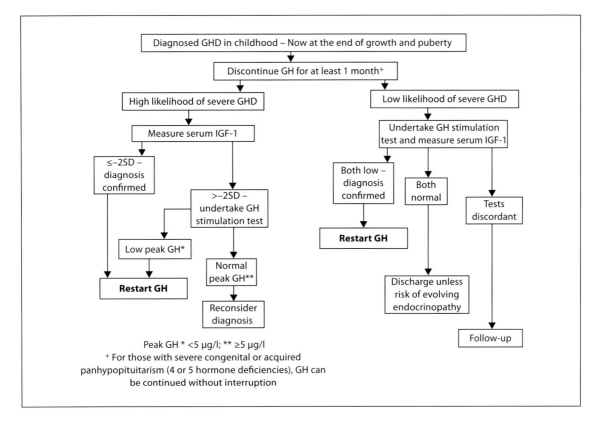

Fig. 3. Schematic for the reassessment of GH status in adolescents in the transition period [1].

GHD (higher FM, reduced LBM) compared with those with normal GH status, and this deteriorated over the year of the study with no change in the adolescents with normal GH status (fig. 2). There was no difference in BMD or alteration in lipid profile or insulin levels. This study has important implications for selecting patients for ongoing treatment. Those with moderate GHD may benefit from intervention in the transition period.

The current consensus on reassessment of GHD in the transition period depends on the likelihood of severe GHD (fig. 3): for patients with a high likelihood of severe GHD, a single test is required to diagnose severe GHD, i.e. either an IGF-1 SDS of less than –2 or a peak GH response to provocative testing <5 μg/l; for patients with a low likelihood of persistent GHD, two tests (IGF-1 and a GH provocative test) are recommended to confirm GH status.

GHRT in the Transition Period
To answer whether continuation of GHRT after final height in the transition period in GHD adolescents is necessary to achieve normal somatic development and to maintain a reduced cardiovascular risk, studies have examined the consequence of discontinuation of GHRT stratified by GH status [8, 14, 15], the consequence of discontinuation compared with seamless continuation of GHRT [5, 16–19], and the reintroduction of GHRT after a treatment break [16, 17, 20–25]. In

Table 1. Effect of discontinuation, continuation and recommencement of GHRT on bone health and body composition in studies of GHD patients in the transition period

Reference	GHD subjects n	Mean age ± SD years	Duration years	Treatment	Change from baseline, %				
					TB BMC	LS BMD	LBM	FM	FM%
8, 14, 15	21	19 ± 2	2	off GHRT	+5	+4	–8		+7
5, 18	24	17 ± 1	1	off GHRT	+2	+3	–2	+10	+3
			1	continued GHRT (17)	+6	+5	+4	–7	–1
19	45	16 ± 2	2	off GHRT	↓	↓	–6		+6
			2	continued GHRT (20)	↓	↓	–5		+5
16, 17	19	20 ± 1	1	off GHRT			+2	+17	
			2	continued GHRT (18)			+6	–6	
			1	recommenced GHRT (20)			+14	–25	
22, 24	149	20 ± 3	2	off GHRT	+6	+3	+2	+13	
				recommenced GHRT					
			2	paediatric dose (25)	+8	+5	+14	–6	
			2	adult dose (12.5)	+10	+6	+13	–7	
23	64	24 ± 4	2	off GHRT		+1	+3	+11	
				recommenced GHRT					
			2	paediatric dose (25)		+5	+13	–18	
			2	adult dose (12.5)		+3	+13	–1	
	Average change/year			off GHRT	+2.5	+1.7	–0.8	+9.7	+3.3
				continued GHRT	+6.0	+5.0	+1.5	–5.0	+0.8
				recommenced GHRT	+4.5	+2.4	+8.1	–8.2	

Figures in parentheses indicate treatment doses in micrograms/kilogram/day. TB = Total body; LS = lumbar spine; FM% = percent fat mass; ↓ = direction of change, numerical data not available.

addition, efficacy of a paediatric versus an adult dose has been assessed [22–25].

Effect on Somatic Development

Bone
The goals of GHRT through childhood should not only include attainment of height within a genetic target range but also the acquisition of normal BMD for age. As PBM is achieved in the early twenties, and this is in part GH dependent, continuation of GHRT is a logical proposal.

The effect of discontinuation of GHRT on bone mass in severe GHD subjects has been quantified by a number of studies (table 1). Total body BMC increases at a rate of 2.5%/year and lumbar spine BMD at a rate of 2%/year [5, 14, 22]. Underwood et al. [23] demonstrated that the lowest increase in lumbar spine BMD over 2 years (1%) was probably related to the older age of the young people when BMD was being assessed and hence a longer period since prior GHRT. Other studies comparing the effect of discontinuation of GHRT at final height in adolescents retesting with severe GHD with those retesting GH sufficient (GHS) demonstrated no differences at baseline or after 2 years of observation. Both studies used relatively high doses of GHRT in childhood (>30 μg/kg/day) [14, 19].

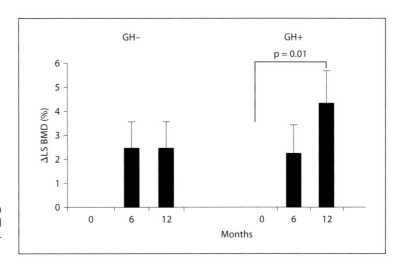

Fig. 4. Continuation compared with discontinuation of GHRT at final height: percentage change in lumbar spine (LS) BMD over 1 year [5].

In studies comparing the effect of 'seamless' continuation with discontinuation, there were contrasting results. In a 1-year study, Drake et al. [5] reported a greater increase in total body BMC (6%) and lumbar spine BMD (5%) in GHD subjects on GHRT compared with those off GHRT (fig. 4). The increase in BMC of 6% is similar to the increase in healthy adolescents over a similar time period. In a similar design of a study over 2 years, Mauras et al. [19] found no effect of GHRT on total or lumbar spine BMD. When considering the results of these studies, one needs to take into consideration that the patients in the study by Mauras et al. [19] had less severe GHD (GH <5 μg/l) and were treated with higher doses of GHRT (42 μg/kg/day) up to final height resulting in suprapysiological IGF-1 levels, while the patients in the study by Drake et al. [5] had more severe GHD (GH <3 μg/l) and received a lower dose of GHRT (25 μg/kg/day) up to final height as evidenced by an IGF-1 SDS of –1 at final height. The higher dose of GHRT may have resulted in increased accrual of bone mass during growth.

Studies examining the effect of recommencement of GHRT demonstrated improvement in total body and lumbar spine BMC and BMD [22, 23]. However, the increase in total body BMC and lumbar spine BMD after 2 years of GHRT [22, 23] was of similar magnitude to the increase seen after 1 year of 'seamless' continuation [5]. This supports the notion that a period of discontinuation of GHRT in adolescent GHD patients limits progression towards PBM. This is partly due to an initial reduction in BMC and BMD when GHRT is restarted after a period of discontinuation with bone resorption being at first greater than bone mineralization in both recommencement studies [22, 23].

Two studies have examined the effect of a paediatric (25 μg/kg/day) versus an adult dose (12.5 μg/kg/day) of GHRT on bone mass accrual [22, 23]. Shalet et al. [22] found no dose effect on BMC or BMD, while Underwood et al. [23], in a similarly designed study, identified a dose effect on improvement in lumbar spine BMD. Underwood et al. [23] only showed a trend in improvement in total body BMD. The older mean age of subjects in the latter study (4 years older, recruitment age <35 years of age) and the longer duration of time off GHRT (5.6 ± 3.2 vs. 1.3 ± 1.1 years) may have affected bone mass accrual.

Studies examining biochemical markers of bone formation and resorption have found a decrease when GHRT is discontinued and an increase when GHRT is recommenced, indicating that bone remodelling activity is reduced after

GHRT [14, 22]. In addition, there was a negative correlation between markers of bone turnover and time off paediatric GHRT [22].

Summary

The majority of studies demonstrate that discontinuation of GHRT results in a reduced accrual of bone mass, while continuation or recommencement of GHRT results in significant accrual of bone mass towards PBM. The longer a patient is off GHRT, the less efficient bone accrual appears to be, and the opportunity to achieve PBM may be lost. A clear GHRT dose effect is not apparent.

Body Composition

LBM at final height should be normal for age and height if puberty is complete and hormone replacements including GHRT are adequate in childhood GHD. If GHRT is discontinued at final height, one would expect deterioration with increasing FM and either static or reducing levels of LBM due to the loss of the lipolytic and anabolic effects of GHRT.

Discontinuation of GHRT in GHD subjects results in minimal change (±2%) in LBM over 1–2 years but a marked increase in FM (+10–17%) [17, 18, 23, 24] (table 1). One study demonstrated a more marked reduction in LBM (–8%) in comparison with no change in GHS patients [15] and a large increase in truncal body fat in both GHD and GHS subjects (34%) compared with normal controls (12%) [8]. The dramatic effects observed in this latter study may be more related to the withdrawal of high doses of GHRT which had induced suprapholysiological levels of IGF-1 than the effect of untreated GHD.

In the 'seamless' placebo-controlled continuation studies, there were contrasting results. Two studies demonstrated a modest improvement in body composition with a 4–6% increase in LBM and a 6–8% decrease in FM over 1–2 years consistent with normal changes in body composition [17, 18]. Mauras et al. [19] demonstrated an increase in percent FM and a decrease in percent

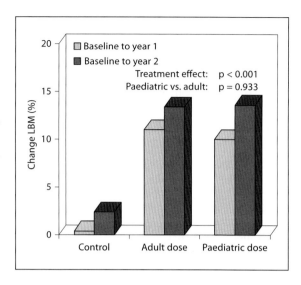

Fig. 5. Recommencement of GHRT with paediatric and adult doses of GHRT compared with untreated controls: percentage change in LBM over 2 years [24].

LBM in all three groups (GHD treated with GHRT, GHD off GHRT, and children retesting GHS) but no significant differences between the groups. The adolescents continuing on GHRT studied by Carroll et al. [18] and Vahl et al. [17] had no significant change in IGF-1 compared with a reduction in IGF-1 in the study by Mauras et al. [19], consistent with the reduction in GHRT dosage (from 42 to 20 μg/kg/day). The fall in IGF-1 levels may have influenced the apparent lack of effect of continued GHRT on body composition [19].

Recommencement of GHRT results in a marked improvement in body composition with an increase in LBM (13–14%) regardless of the duration off GHRT (fig. 5) [17, 23, 24]. This increase in LBM equates to 65–85% of the deficit observed in young adults with CO-GHD compared with age-matched AO-GHD subjects [9]. A less consistent effect was seen for FM reduction (1–25%) [17, 23, 24]. Differences in FM response may be related in part to GHRT dose and in part to a gender effect. Underwood et al. [23] demonstrated a dose effect on FM reduction, while in the study of Attanasio et al. [24], females in the first year of GHRT had a greater increase in LBM and a decrease in FM on the higher paediatric GHRT dose.

Several studies have examined whether the alteration in LBM translates to improved muscle strength, with conflicting results. Hulthen et al. [15] showed an increase in isometric knee flexion and handgrip strength (7–15%) in GHS patients and normal controls, while GHD patients off GHRT demonstrated no such improvement over the 2 years. However, other studies have shown no difference in grip or isometric quadriceps strength on or off GHRT [17, 19].

Summary
The majority of studies demonstrate that discontinuation of GHRT results in a worsening of body composition, whereas continuation results in maintenance and recommencement of GHRT results in improvement in body composition. There appears to be a gender and dose response relating in particular to reduction in FM.

Effect on Cardiovascular Risk

Lipid Profile
Some studies have reported an adverse lipid profile (elevated total and low-density lipoprotein cholesterol, triglycerides and apoliporotein B, and reduced high-density lipoprotein cholesterol) at final height despite conventional GHRT [8, 20, 21]. Colao et al. [20, 21] also observed elevated fibrinogen. On discontinuation of GHRT, the lipid profile deteriorates [8, 20, 21, 24] and fibrinogen increases further [20, 21]. In contrast, some studies comparing discontinuation with continuation of GHRT have shown no difference in lipid profile changes [18, 19], while another study demonstrated an increase in high-density lipoprotein cholesterol on GHRT [17]. Similarly, recommencement of GHRT resulted in improvements in total cholesterol/high-density lipoprotein cholesterol ratio, triglycerides and fibrinogen levels in some studies [20, 21, 24], but not all [17, 23].

Cardiac and Common Carotid Artery Morphology and Function
The studies of Colao et al. [20, 21] have assessed cardiac and common carotid artery function during discontinuation of GHRT for 6 months before recommencement of GHRT for 6 months in GHD subjects compared with normal controls.

Cardiac structure and function were assessed by echocardiography. At baseline, GHD subjects had a lower early-to-late mitral flow velocity ratio (E/A; marker of diastolic function) but a normal left ventricular (LV) mass index and ejection fraction compared with normal controls. Six months after GHRT withdrawal, both LV mass index and E/A decreased, although remaining within the normal range. Six months after restarting GHRT, cardiac parameters were brought back to the levels measured at study entry, with LV ejection fraction and E/A remaining lower than in normal controls [20]. Two other studies have not identified any echocardiographic abnormalities [19, 23], although concern may be raised at higher doses of GHRT which are associated with significant increases in LV mass index [23].

The clinical relevance of these cardiac changes is not clear. Reassuringly, continuation, discontinuation and recommencement of GHRT have not been shown to have any effect on exercise capacity [17, 19].

Intima-media thickness (IMT) at the common carotid arteries was similar in GHD patients and controls at baseline. In GHD adolescents, despite changes in IGF-1 levels, lipid profile and insulin resistance, 6 months of GHRT withdrawal and 6 months of GHRT reinstitution did not change IMT or systolic and diastolic peak velocities at the common carotid arteries. Thus, the discontinuation of GHRT was not followed by significant alterations within the common carotid arteries [21].

Summary
Despite the experience that GHRT in adults improves the lipid profile, the results in the studies in adolescence are inconsistent. Reassuringly, there were only subtle effects on cardiac morphology and function which improved with recommencement, but no effect was observed on IMT in the common carotid arteries. With more prolonged discontinuation of GHRT, negative effects on the cardiovascular system may occur.

Effect on Quality of Life

GHRT in the transition period has a minimal effect on QoL. One study examined the effect of seamless continuation of GHRT compared with discontinuation and found no effect on QoL at baseline or after 2 years off GHRT [19]. In a study looking at recommencement of GHRT, although QoL was significantly lower than in normal controls (females –0.4 ± 1.2 SDS; males –0.7 ± 1.1 SDS), no change in the overall score was identified with GHRT despite significant improvement in individual parameters that were low at baseline, including sexual arousal and body shape [25]. No such effect on QoL was confirmed by a similar study design [23].

The most marked improvement in QoL in adults with GHRT is seen in subjects with poor QoL. QoL is known to be less affected and to respond less well to GHRT in CO-GHD compared with AO-GHD patients. Therefore, the finding that GHRT does not significantly affect QoL in the transition period is not unexpected. It is possible that with longer duration off GHRT and in subsets of adolescents with poor QoL off GHRT benefit may be seen. The affected dimensions which did improve with GHRT in the study by Attanasio et al. [25] were related to age-specific behavioural and psychological issues which may worsen with age. Thus, some patients may benefit from psychological counselling in the transition period to achieve normal adult behaviour.

Safety

In all GHRT studies, evidence of safety is a priority. In the short term, side effects mostly relate to fluid retention and arthralgia, particularly if high doses of GHRT are employed, whereas in the medium term, there are concerns about alteration in insulin sensitivity and effect on glucose homeostasis, and finally, in the long term, there remain concerns as to whether GHRT increases the risk of malignancy.

Underwood et al. [23] reported similar numbers of most adverse events in the different groups (placebo, GHRT 12.5 μg/kg/day, GHRT 25 μg/kg/day): oedema was reported in 1, 4 and 7 patients and arthralgia in 1, 2 and 2 patients from each of the groups, respectively. Two patients in the placebo and 3 in the higher dose group withdrew because of side effects [23].

Studies have demonstrated an increase in insulin sensitivity [16, 18, 21] with a reduction in fasting glucose [17] on discontinuation of GHRT. Once GHRT is restarted, insulin sensitivity decreases [16, 21], resulting in an increase in fasting glucose levels [17], but glucose tolerance was not impaired [23]. Importantly, there was no major deterioration in insulin sensitivity [16, 18] or fasting glucose with continued GHRT [17].

There appears to be no increase in short- or medium-term safety issues with GHRT in the transition period. Surveillance programs are required to monitor the long-term safety in relation to risk of malignancy and other causes of increased morbidity and mortality in patients with GHD.

Management Strategy in the Transition Period

1 At final height, the adolescent treated with GHRT for GHD should undergo re-evaluation of the underlying diagnosis, adequacy of

other hormone replacements and reassessment of GH status.
2. Some adolescents may not require reassessment of GH status because of the high likelihood of GHD, and in those, GHRT can be continued seamlessly. In adolescents with confirmed severe GHD on reassessment in the transition period, GHRT should be restarted.
3. GHRT should be continued until the mid-twenties, the expected time of adult somatic development, at which point further review of GH status and the need for GHRT in adulthood is required.
4. The dose of GHRT should be altered using IGF-1-based titration using robust gender- and age-matched normative data. The current consensus is to start at a dose of 0.2–0.5 mg/day and aim for an IGF-1 between 0 and +2 SDS, with measurements taken every 6 months.
5. As the attainment of PBM is the most significant clinical goal, bone densitometry should be performed every 2–5 years, with T and Z scores being measured. The aim is to achieve a T score of greater than –1 SDS (height corrected if significant short stature is present).
6. In addition, the current consensus has recommended the following minimum observations to be performed for adolescents on GHRT: yearly – fasting glucose, haemoglobin A_{1c}, height, weight, body mass index, waist/hip ratio, blood pressure, heart rate and QoL; 2–5 yearly – lipids.
7. Adolescents with partial GHD (peak GH ≥5 to <10 µg/l) or with the potential to have evolving GHD should remain under follow-up.

Conclusion

Until recently, GHRT was recommended for the promotion of linear growth in childhood and in adulthood for the normalisztion of QoL and body composition and the reduction in cardiovascular risk factors. It is now recognized that the critical time to achieve full maturational somatic development in those with severe GHD treated with GHRT during childhood is after final height has been achieved. This cannot be attained in the absence of GHRT.

Discontinuation of GHRT at the end of linear growth has been shown to have an adverse impact on somatic development (bone and LBM), and continuation or recommencement has a positive effect. Cardiovascular risk is also maintained at a lower level with continued GHRT. However, there is little evidence of an effect of GHRT on QoL in the transition period.

Therefore, the consensus is that GHRT should be continued after final height to achieve adult somatic development. Recommendations have been made on the biochemical criteria for diagnosis of GHD in the transition period and dosing and duration of GHRT.

However, there remain unresolved issues that require further study.
1. Are the current criteria for diagnosing GHD in adolescence too restrictive?
2. Is there a window of opportunity during which GHRT should be recommenced in the transition period and is this affected by the status of the GH-IGF-1 axis?
3. What surveillance should be provided for those retesting with partial GHD or normal GH status who may evolve to GHD at an older age?
4. What should the management of GHD young adults be once normal somatic development has been achieved?

This change in the therapeutic indication for GHRT has provided an opportunity for paediatric and adult endocrinologists to examine current systems in place for caring for the GHD adolescent. There is a responsibility to organize transitional care in a way that facilitates the physical and psychosocial adjustment of the adolescent with GHD and ensures they can develop autonomy in their own health care decision making.

References

1 Clayton PE, Cuneo RC, Juul A, Monson JP, Shalet SM, Tauber M: Consensus statement on the management of the GH-treated adolescent in the transition to adult care. Eur J Endocrinol 2005; 152:165–170.
2 Matkovic V, Jelic T, Wardlaw GM, Ilich JZ, Goel PK, Wright JK, Andon MB, Smith KT, Heaney RP: Timing of peak bone mass in Caucasian females and its implication for the prevention of osteoporosis. Inference from a cross-sectional model. J Clin Invest 1994;93:799–808.
3 van der Sluis IM, de Ridder MA, Boot AM, Krenning EP, de Muinck Keizer-Schrama SM: Reference data for bone density and body composition measured with dual energy X-ray absorptiometry in white children and young adults. Arch Dis Child 2002;87:341–347; discussion 341–347.
4 Gordon CL, Halton JM, Atkinson SA, Webber CE: The contributions of growth and puberty to peak bone mass. Growth Dev Aging 1991;55:257–262.
5 Drake WM, Carroll PV, Maher KT, Metcalfe KA, Camacho-Hubner C, Shaw NJ, Dunger DB, Cheetham TD, Savage MO, Monson JP: The effect of cessation of growth hormone (GH) therapy on bone mineral accretion in GH-deficient adolescents at the completion of linear growth. J Clin Endocrinol Metab 2003;88:1658–1663.
6 de Boer H, Blok GJ, Van der Veen EA: Clinical aspects of growth hormone deficiency in adults. Endocr Rev 1995; 16:63–86.
7 Boot AM, Engels MA, Boerma GJ, Krenning EP, De Muinck Keizer-Schrama SM: Changes in bone mineral density, body composition, and lipid metabolism during growth hormone (GH) treatment in children with GH deficiency. J Clin Endocrinol Metab 1997;82:2423–2428.
8 Johannsson G, Albertsson-Wikland K, Bengtsson BA: Discontinuation of growth hormone (GH) treatment: metabolic effects in GH-deficient and GH-sufficient adolescent patients compared with control subjects. Swedish Study Group for Growth Hormone Treatment in Children. J Clin Endocrinol Metab 1999;84:4516–4524.
9 Attanasio AF, Howell S, Bates PC, Frewer P, Chipman J, Blum WF, Shalet SM: Body composition, IGF-I and IGFBP-3 concentrations as outcome measures in severely GH-deficient (GHD) patients after childhood GH treatment: a comparison with adult onset GHD patients. J Clin Endocrinol Metab 2002;87:3368–3372.
10 Leger J, Danner S, Simon D, Garel C, Czernichow P: Do all patients with childhood-onset growth hormone deficiency (GHD) and ectopic neurohypophysis have persistent GHD in adulthood? J Clin Endocrinol Metab 2005; 90:650–656.
11 Zadik Z, Chalew SA, McCarter RJ Jr, Meistas M, Kowarski AA: The influence of age on the 24-hour integrated concentration of growth hormone in normal individuals. J Clin Endocrinol Metab 1985;60:513–516.
12 Maghnie M, Aimaretti G, Bellone S, Bona G, Bellone J, Baldelli R, de Sanctis C, Gargantini L, Gastaldi R, Ghizzoni L, Secco A, Tinelli C, Ghigo E: Diagnosis of GH deficiency in the transition period: accuracy of insulin tolerance test and insulin-like growth factor-I measurement. Eur J Endocrinol 2005; 152:589–596.
13 Tauber M, Jouret B, Cartault A, Lounis N, Gayrard M, Marcouyeux C, Pienkowski C, Oliver I, Moulin P, Otal P, Joffre F, Arnaud C, Rochiccioli P: Adolescents with partial growth hormone (GH) deficiency develop alterations of body composition after GH discontinuation and require follow-up. J Clin Endocrinol Metab 2003;88:5101–5106.
14 Fors H, Bjarnason R, Wirent L, Albertsson-Wikland K, Bosaeust L, Bengtsson BA, Johannsson G: Currently used growth-promoting treatment of children results in normal bone mass and density. A prospective trial of discontinuing growth hormone treatment in adolescents. Clin Endocrinol (Oxf) 2001;55:617–624.
15 Hulthen L, Bengtsson BA, Sunnerhagen KS, Hallberg L, Grimby G, Johannsson G: GH is needed for the maturation of muscle mass and strength in adolescents. J Clin Endocrinol Metab 2001;86:4765–4770.
16 Norrelund H, Vahl N, Juul A, Moller N, Alberti KG, Skakkebaek NE, Christiansen JS, Jorgensen JO: Continuation of growth hormone (GH) therapy in GH-deficient patients during transition from childhood to adulthood: impact on insulin sensitivity and substrate metabolism. J Clin Endocrinol Metab 2000;85:1912–1917.
17 Vahl N, Juul A, Jorgensen JO, Orskov H, Skakkebaek NE, Christiansen JS: Continuation of growth hormone (GH) replacement in GH-deficient patients during transition from childhood to adulthood: a two-year placebo-controlled study. J Clin Endocrinol Metab 2000;85:1874–1881.
18 Carroll PV, Drake WM, Maher KT, Metcalfe K, Shaw NJ, Dunger DB, Cheetham TD, Camacho-Hubner C, Savage MO, Monson JP: Comparison of continuation or cessation of growth hormone (GH) therapy on body composition and metabolic status in adolescents with severe GH deficiency at completion of linear growth. J Clin Endocrinol Metab 2004;89:3890–3895.
19 Mauras N, Pescovitz OH, Allada V, Messig M, Wajnrajch MP, Lippe B: Limited efficacy of growth hormone (GH) during transition of GH-deficient patients from adolescence to adulthood: a phase III multicenter, double-blind, randomized two-year trial. J Clin Endocrinol Metab 2005;90:3946–3955.
20 Colao A, Di Somma C, Salerno M, Spinelli L, Orio F, Lombardi G: The cardiovascular risk of GH-deficient adolescents. J Clin Endocrinol Metab 2002; 87:3650–3655.
21 Colao A, Di Somma C, Rota F, Di Maio S, Salerno M, Klain A, Spiezia S, Lombardi G: Common carotid intima-media thickness in growth hormone (GH)-deficient adolescents: a prospective study after GH withdrawal and restarting GH replacement. J Clin Endocrinol Metab 2005;90:2659–2665.
22 Shalet SM, Shavrikova E, Cromer M, Child CJ, Keller E, Zapletalova J, Moshang T, Blum WF, Chipman JJ, Quigley CA, Attanasio AF: Effect of growth hormone (GH) treatment on bone in postpubertal GH-deficient patients: a 2-year randomized, controlled, dose-ranging study. J Clin Endocrinol Metab 2003;88:4124–4129.

23 Underwood LE, Attie KM, Baptista J: Growth hormone (GH) dose-response in young adults with childhood-onset GH deficiency: a two-year, multicenter, multiple-dose, placebo-controlled study. J Clin Endocrinol Metab 2003;88:5273–5280.

24 Attanasio AF, Shavrikova E, Blum WF, Cromer M, Child CJ, Paskova M, Lebl J, Chipman JJ, Shalet SM: Continued growth hormone (GH) treatment after final height is necessary to complete somatic development in childhood-onset GH-deficient patients. J Clin Endocrinol Metab 2004;89:4857–4862.

25 Attanasio AF, Shavrikova EP, Blum WF, Shalet SM: Quality of life in childhood onset growth hormone-deficient patients in the transition phase from childhood to adulthood. J Clin Endocrinol Metab 2005;90:4525–4529.

Effect of Prior Pediatric Growth Hormone Replacement on Serum Lipids and Quality of Life in Young Adults with Reconfirmed Severe Growth Hormone Deficiency: The Combined KIGS and KIMS Experiences

Mitchell E. Geffner[a] Peter Jönsson[b] John P. Monson[c]
Roger Abs[d] Václav Hána[e] Charlotte Höybye[f]
Maria Koltowska-Häggström[b]

[a] The Saban Research Institute, Children's Hospital Los Angeles
4650 Sunset Blvd., Los Angeles, CA 90027 (USA)
[b] Pfizer Endocrine Care
KIGS/KIMS/ACROSTUDY Medical Outcomes
Vetenskapsvägen 10, SE–191 90 Sollentuna (Sweden)
[c] The London Clinic Centre for Endocrinology and Diabetes
145 Harley Street, London W1G 6BJ (UK)
[d] Department of Endocrinology, University Hospital Antwerp
Wilrijkstraat 10, BE–2650 Edegem (Belgium)
[e] 3rd Department of Internal Medicine, Faculty of Medicine 1
Charles University, U nemocnice 1, CZ–128 08 Prague 2
(Czech Republic)
[f] Department of Endocrinology, Metabolism and Diabetes
Karolinska University Hospital, SE–171 76 Stockholm (Sweden)

A predictable grouping of signs and symptoms, known as the adult growth hormone deficiency (AGHD) syndrome, may develop after completion of pediatric GH treatment in young adults previously diagnosed with severe childhood-onset GHD (COGHD) whose GH therapy is interrupted and who have persistent severe GHD [1–4]. To assess the extent to which treatment with GH in childhood affects the clinical presentation of GHD in young adults, we identified a cohort of patients that was followed in KIGS and in KIMS (Pfizer International Metabolic Database) to determine the impact of overall pediatric GH treatment (expressed by average GH dose and duration of pediatric GH replacement) along with the time between termination of pediatric and resumption of adult GH treatment (GH gap) on young adults diagnosed with severe COGHD and treated with GH for typical height indications who were then taken off or stopped GH treatment when maximal linear growth was attained. The factors assessed included serum insulin-like growth factor 1 (IGF-1) and lipid profile, along with quality of life (QoL).

Subjects, Methods and Statistics

The KIMS database was queried for young adults with severe COGHD defined as a peak serum GH concentration during investigator-chosen provocative tests of <3.0 µg/l upon retesting prior to entry into KIMS and who had previously been followed in the KIGS database. An additional inclusion criterion was that pediatric GH replacement was interrupted for a minimum of 3 months before the initiation of adult treatment. GH dose (milligrams/kilogram/week) was calculated as the mean of all GH doses reported from GH start until the end of follow-up in KIGS, including periods without GH treatment. GH duration (years) was computed as the time from KIGS start to the end of follow-up in KIGS, although the possibility exists that some subjects may have received additional GH treatment for short periods beyond this time. GH gap (years) was defined as the time between the final KIGS visit and the date of enrollment into KIMS. These variables were used as proxies for overall GH treatment in childhood and were then correlated with the following assessments obtained at entry into KIMS: (1) serum IGF-1, (2) fasting serum lipids, including total, low-density lipoprotein (LDL) and high-density lipoprotein (HDL) cholesterol and triglycerides (TG), as well as (3) QoL (using the QoL assessment in GHD in adults, or QoL-AGHDA) where a high score denotes poor QoL [5]. The QoL-AGHDA was developed to assess the impact of GHD and GH treatment in adults and has also been used, although not validated, in young adults with GHD [6].

Initially, serum IGF-1 was determined centrally by radioimmunoassay after acid-ethanol extraction of IGF binding proteins (through November 2002) and then by chemiluminescence immunoassay (Nichols Institute Diagnostics, San Juan Capistrano, Calif., USA) [7]. Absolute IGF-1 values were converted into gender- and age-specific standard deviation scores (SDS). Lipid assays were also performed centrally with total cholesterol, HDL cholesterol and TG measured directly, whereas LDL cholesterol concentrations were estimated using Friedewald's formula.

Data are presented as means ± SD. Spearman correlation coefficients were determined separately for comparisons of clinical parameters with GH dose, GH duration and GH gap. In correlations of GH dose and GH gap, correction for the other variable was performed. Correlation of GH duration was also corrected for GH gap. A p value <0.05 defined statistical significance.

Additionally, all correlations were performed separately for subjects with idiopathic or congenital GHD (idiopathic) and for subjects in whom organic disease was the primary cause of GHD (organic) (table 1), as well as for men and women. Furthermore, the correlations in the organic group were analyzed both as a whole and without inclusion of subjects with craniopharyngioma.

Table 1. Etiologies of GHD (n = 240)

Diagnosis	n	%
Idiopathic/congenital	115	45
Organic	125	55
Cranial tumors distant from the hypothalamic-pituitary region	37	15
Craniopharyngioma	32	13
Other causes of acquired GHD	25	13
Tumors in the hypothalamic-pituitary region other than pituitary adenoma	16	7
Treatment for malignancy outside the cranium	12	5
Pituitary adenoma	3	1

Results

There were 240 subjects (62.5% males) with severe GHD found in the KIMS database that had been previously followed in the KIGS database. GHD was idiopathic or congenital in 115 patients and organic in 125, with specific etiologies enumerated in table 1. Twenty-six percent of the total cohort (n = 63) had isolated GHD and 74% (n = 177) had varying patterns of pituitary hormone deficits, including 19% (n = 46) with panhypopituitarism. Of the total cohort, 156 (62.9%) had thyroid-stimulating hormone deficiency, 152 (61.3%) gonadotropin deficiency, 116 (47.0%) adrenocorticotropic hormone deficiency and 58 (23.5%) diabetes insipidus. 131 subjects had medical induction of puberty. In the organic group, 26 underwent neurosurgery, 16 cranial radiation and 29 both treatments.

The mean age was 10.0 ± 4.1 years at entry into KIGS, 17.6 ± 1.9 years at KIGS termination and 21.6 ± 3.3 years at entry into KIMS. The mean pediatric GH dose was 0.18 ± 0.06 mg/kg/week, and the mean duration of GH treatment during childhood was 7.3 ± 3.9 years. The mean duration between pediatric and adult treatment was 3.9 ± 3.0 years. The mean values of the clinical parameters are shown in table 2.

Table 2. Mean (± SD) values of clinical parameters at entry into KIGS, exit from KIGS and start of KIMS

Parameter	KIGS entry	KIGS exit	KIMS start
Age, years	10.0 ± 4.2	17.6 ± 1.9	21.6 ± 3.3
IGF-1 SDS	N/A	N/A	–3.6 ± 2.1
Total cholesterol, mmol/l	N/A	N/A	5.1 ± 1.1
LDL cholesterol, mmol/l	N/A	N/A	3.1 ± 1.0
HDL cholesterol, mmol/l	N/A	N/A	1.3 ± 0.4
TG, mmol/l	N/A	N/A	1.6 ± 1.1
QoL-AGHDA	N/A	N/A	8.7 ± 6.4

N/A = Not available.

Mean GH Dose during Childhood
Correlations of GH dose, controlled for GH gap, yielded a statistically significant negative relationship with LDL at entry into KIMS (fig. 1), but not with other lipid parameters, IGF-1 or with the QoL-AGHDA score. In separate analyses of idiopathic and organic subgroups, correlation coefficients were similar to those of the whole cohort. After exclusion of subjects with craniopharyngioma from the organic group, there were no significant GH dose correlations with any of the study parameters, while analysis solely of data from subjects with craniopharyngioma showed significant negative correlations with QoL-AGHDA, IGF-1 SDS and TG. For the entire group, some gender differences were evident. In men, there was a slight negative correlation with QoL-AGHDA ($r = -0.19$, $p = 0.049$). In women, a negative correlation with TG was noted ($r = -0.29$, $p = 0.03$).

Duration of Pediatric Treatment
GH duration negatively correlated with IGF-1 SDS (fig. 2). For the total cohort, there was no correlation with any other parameter. Subanalyses for subjects with idiopathic and organic disease (with and without patients with craniopharyngioma) produced similar findings, along with a negative correlation with TG in men ($r = -0.21$, $p = 0.04$).

Interruption between Pediatric and Adult Treatment
GH gap correlated positively with total cholesterol (fig. 3a), LDL (fig. 3b), TG (fig. 3c) and QoL-AGHDA scores (fig. 3d). Results from subanalyses of the idiopathic and organic groups showed the same patterns as those found in the total cohort. After excluding subjects with craniopharyngioma from the organic group, there were significant positive correlations with IGF-1 SDS, total cholesterol, LDL and TG, mirroring the findings in the entire cohort. For the craniopharyngioma group alone, GH gap positively correlated with QoL-AGHDA, as was seen for the entire organic group. In men, gender analyses showed a strong positive correlation between GH gap and total cholesterol ($r = 0.41$, $p < 0.0001$), between GH gap and TG ($r = 0.25$, $p = 0.015$), and between GH gap and LDL ($r = 0.40$, $p < 0.0001$). In women, correlations were also positive, but not significant. A strong positive correlation with the QoL-AGHDA score was found in women ($r = 0.45$, $p = 0.0002$) but not in men ($r = 0.11$, $p = $ n.s.).

Discussion

The key features of the AGHD syndrome include abnormal body composition (increased fat and decreased muscle mass), reduced bone mineral

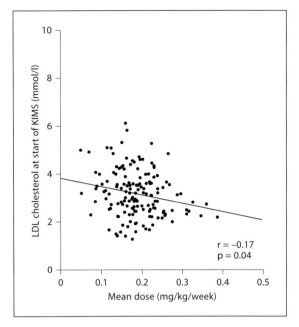

Fig. 1. Correlation between mean pediatric GH dose and LDL cholesterol at entry into KIMS.

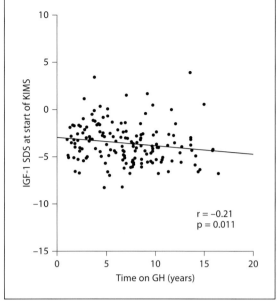

Fig. 2. Correlation between duration of pediatric GH treatment and IGF-1 SDS at entry into KIMS.

density with increased fracture risk, decreased exercise capacity, abnormal serum lipids and impaired QoL (characterized by diminished vitality, life drive and sense of well-being, along with social isolation and depression) [2, 8]. This phenotype manifests in adults who develop GHD in adulthood, or may develop over time in adolescents previously diagnosed with GHD in childhood and treated with GH until completion or near completion of linear growth, who then stop GH treatment. Variations in the phenotype, e.g., failure to accrue normal amounts of bone mass, may even develop with GH treatment to final height [9]. In those patients with COGHD, there is little information as to the rate at which the AGHD syndrome develops after discontinuation of GH therapy.

Thus, using the KIGS and KIMS databases, we set out to determine the clinical effects of pediatric treatment, expressed as GH dose, GH duration and GH gap, in a large cohort of young adults with pediatric GHD treated with GH to adult height who were taken off or stopped GH treatment when height growth was concluded. In our study, GH dose had a moderately beneficial effect on lipids, i.e. the higher the GH dose administered during childhood, the lower the LDL in the total cohort and the lower the TG in women at the time of GH reinitiation, observations that may stem from GH-enhanced clearance of cholesterol by hepatic LDL receptors [10]. Levels of fasting total and HDL cholesterol were uninfluenced by childhood GH dose, but, along with LDL, were higher, particularly in men, as the time off GH between KIGS end and KIMS start increased; these effects are not likely to be explained by age-related physiological rises that occur with advancing age, as the age range in this study is fairly narrow [11] and, overall, the subjects were young. There was no effect of GH dose on subsequent QoL, although a longer treatment gap was associated with a poorer QoL, especially in women.

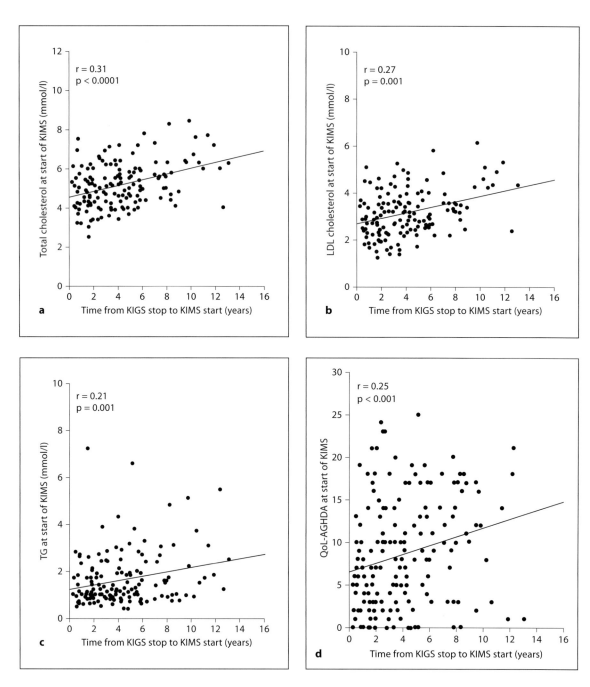

Fig. 3. Correlations between duration of GH interruption between the end of pediatric treatment and the start of adult treatment and total cholesterol (**a**), LDL cholesterol (**b**), TG (**c**) and QoL-AGHDA (**d**).

In previous studies of interruption of GH in adolescents with COGHD after attainment of final height, cardiovascular risk factors worsened within 6 months of treatment cessation (with increases in LDL, TG, HDL-to-total cholesterol ratio and fibrinogen levels, and decreases in left ventricular mass index and early-to-late mitral flow velocity ratio) and were corrected after resumption of GH therapy for 6 months [12]. Similarly, in adolescents and young adults with severe GHD off treatment for an average of 1.3–1.5 years, completion of somatic development (bone, muscle and fat) slows down and is restored with resumption of GH therapy [1, 3, 4, 13]. Finally, 6 months after discontinuation of GH in young adults with COGHD, psychological complaints and depression became apparent with significant improvement in anxiety and QoL 1 year after reinitiation of GH therapy [14]. However, development of the AGHD syndrome (or a beneficial effect of maintenance of GH therapy) during the first 2 years after conclusion of GH for treatment of COGHD to final height is not universally reported [15].

Parenthetically, it should be highlighted that the methodological values associated with these two large observational databases (KIGS and KIMS) run in a similar manner and in common settings that allowed for such subject identification. Bearing in mind the difficulties related to transition from pediatric to adult care in daily practice, having access to data both on pediatric endocrine management and detailed clinical characteristics of the same subjects at restart of GH treatment in adulthood is a truly unique opportunity. In other words, by accessing combined information from these two databases, we could use long-term clinical data derived from two completely different settings (pediatric and adult clinics) that, on average, spanned more than 10 years of the subjects' lives (the mean age at KIGS start was 10 years and at KIMS start 21 years). Additionally, such an approach contributes to viewing a patient's care not in a certain, limited window of 'one practitioner's responsibility', but rather as a continuum that involves multiple practitioners working closely with one another.

In summary, our findings show that the lower the GH dose during pediatric treatment, the shorter its total duration, and the longer the interval before GH is resumed after the end of childhood treatment determine the extent of the severity of GHD in young adults expressed predominantly as an unfavorable lipid profile and poor QoL. Thus, GH treatment of patients with severe COGHD at height completion and beyond should be considered and, when deemed appropriate, requires an individualized approach and an integrated transition strategy between pediatric and internist endocrinologists [16, 17].

Conclusion

The dose of GH used to treat children with severe GHD has effects that extend beyond height achievement in childhood. Furthermore, a long interval after cessation of childhood GH therapy (prior to resumption of adult GH treatment) leads to abnormalities in lipids and QoL. Hence, GH therapy should either be dose transitioned without discontinuation in those with a clear-cut organic basis for GHD or, prior to consideration of resumption of treatment, discontinued for as short a period as possible (for those subjects who require retesting) to avoid adverse health consequences.

References

1 Drake WM, Carroll PV, Maher KT, Metcalfe KA, Camacho-Hubner C, Shaw NJ, Dunger DB, Cheetham TD, Savage MO, Monson JP: The effect of cessation of growth hormone (GH) therapy on bone mineral accretion in GH-deficient adolescents at the completion of linear growth. J Clin Endocrinol Metab 2003;88:1658–1663.

2 Shalet SM: Growth hormone outgrows growth. Clin Endocrinol 2004;61:1–9.

3 Attanasio AF, Shavrikova E, Blum WF, Cromer M, Child CJ, Paskova M, Lebl J, Chipman JJ, Shalet SM, Hypopituitary Developmental Outcome Study Group: Continued growth hormone (GH) treatment after final height is necessary to complete somatic development in childhood-onset GH-deficient patients. J Clin Endocrinol Metab 2004; 89:4857–4862.

4 Carroll PV, Drake WM, Maher KT, Metcalfe K, Shaw NJ, Dunger DB, Cheetham TD, Camacho-Hubner C, Savage MO, Monson JP: Comparison of continuation or cessation of growth hormone (GH) therapy on body composition and metabolic status in adolescents with severe GH deficiency at completion of linear growth. J Clin Endocrinol Metab 2004;89:3890–3895.

5 McKenna SP, Doward LC, Alonso J, Kohlmann T, Niero M, Prieto L, Wiren L: The QoL-AGHDA: an instrument for the assessment of quality of life in adults with growth hormone deficiency. Qual Life Res 1999;8:373–383.

6 Lagrou K, Xhrouet-Heinrichs D, Massa G, Vandeweghe M, Bourguignon JP, De Schepper J, de Zegher F, Ernould C, Heinrichs C, Malvaux P, Craen M: Quality of life and retrospective perception of the effect of growth hormone treatment in adult patients with childhood growth hormone deficiency. J Pediatr Endocrinol Metab 2001;14 (suppl 5):1249–1260.

7 Brabant G, von zur Mühlen A, Ranke MB, Kratzsch J, Kiess W, Ketelslegers JM, Wilhelmsen L, Hulthen L, Saller B, Mattson A, Wilde J, Schemer R, Kann P, German KIMS Board: Serum insulin-like growth factor I reference values for an automated chemiluminescence immunoassay system: results from a multicentre study. Horm Res 2003;60: 53–60.

8 de Boer H, Blok GJ, Van der Veen EA: Clinical aspects of growth hormone deficiency in adults. Endocr Rev 1995; 16:63–86.

9 Papagianni M, Stanhope R: How should we manage growth hormone deficiency in adolescence? Transition from paediatric to adult care. J Pediatr Endocrinol Metab 2003;16:23–25.

10 Lind S, Rudling M, Ericsson S, Olivecrona H, Eriksson M, Borgstrom B, Eggertsen G, Berglund L, Angelin B: Growth hormone induces low-density lipoprotein clearance but not bile acid synthesis in humans. Arterioscler Thromb Vasc Biol 2004;24:349–356.

11 Davis CE, Gordon D, LaRosa J, Wood PD, Halperin M: Correlations of plasma high-density lipoprotein cholesterol levels with other plasma lipid and lipoprotein concentrations. Circulation 1980;62:IV24–IV30.

12 Colao A, Di Somma C, Salerno M, Spinelli L, Orio F, Lombardi G: The cardiovascular risk of GH-deficient adolescents. J Clin Endocrinol Metab 2002; 87:3650–3655.

13 Shalet SM, Shavrikova E, Cromer M, Child CJ, Keller E, Zapletalova J, Moshang T, Blum WF, Chipman JJ, Quigley CA, Attanasio AF: Effect of growth hormone (GH) treatment on bone in postpubertal GH-deficient patients: a 2-year randomized, controlled, dose-ranging study. J Clin Endocrinol Metab 2003;88:4124–4129.

14 Stouthart PJ, Deijen JB, Roffel M, Delemarre-van de Waal HA: Quality of life of growth hormone (GH)-deficient young adults during discontinuation and restart of GH therapy. Psychoneuroendocrinology 2003;28:612–626.

15 Mauras N, Pescovitz OH, Allada V, Messig M, Wajnrajch MP, Lippe B: Limited efficacy of growth hormone (GH) during transition of GH deficient patients from adolescence to adulthood: a phase III multicenter, double-blind, randomized two-year trial. J Clin Endocrinol Metab 2005;90:3946–3955.

16 Clayton PE, Cuneo RC, Juul A, Monson JP, Shalet SM, Tauber M, European Society of Paediatric Endocrinology: Consensus statement on the management of the GH-treated adolescent in the transition to adult care. Eur J Endocrinol 2005;152:165–170.

17 Geffner ME: Transition to the adult endocrine clinic: testing pituitary function – what tests and when? Growth Horm IGF Res 2003;13(suppl A):S117–S121.

13 KIGS

Who Stops Growth Hormone in KIGS – and Why?

Michael B. Ranke

Twenty years after the initiation of KIGS, many patients have terminated their participation within KIGS. The reasons for these terminations are varied. In patients with growth hormone deficiency (GHD), normal adult height may have been reached. In cases with proven permanent GHD [1], treatment may be continued under the supervision of an adult endocrinologist, potentially within the Pfizer International Metabolic Study (KIMS). However, some of these patients may have discontinued treatment, as in adolescent patients in whom severe and permanent GHD could not be confirmed. In all of these instances, normal adult height may or may not have been reached. Similarly, in patients with short stature not caused by GHD (e.g., Turner syndrome), GH therapy may have been terminated when or before a normal adult height was reached. Discontinuation of treatment – within KIGS or generally – may also have occurred for a variety of other reasons, irrespective of whether the treatment goals had been reached or not. In order for KIGS to be a valid evidential tool, it is of utmost importance to document when the patient discontinues treatment, to document the anthropometrical characteristics and to get exact information about the cause for termination. The KIGS case report forms (CRFs), developed and expanded after the first preliminary reports on the subject [2, 3], give the opportunity to investigate who stops within KIGS and why. The analysis was restricted to patients with idiopathic GHD (IGHD) and patients with GHD after tumour treatment.

Methods

Analysis was based on patients with IGHD (KIGS code No. 1.ff) and patients with GHD after tumour treatment (KIGS code Nos. 2.2.1, 2.2.2 and 2.2.3). A subdivision was done according to the nationality of the patients. Information about the patients at the start of GH treatment, after 1 year on GH, at puberty onset and at termination within KIGS was collected. The data analysis related to patient information before and during treatment was done according to the principles and statistical methods outlined before [4]. The reasons for terminating treatment within KIGS were taken from CRF 6:2 of the KIGS documentation. If 'free' information was offered on the CRFs, this was, if possible, grouped (by M.B.R.) into the offered categories of causes for stopping KIGS, as outlined in table 1.

Paediatric Endocrinology Section
University Children's Hospital, University of Tübingen
Hoppe-Seyler-Strasse 1, DE–72076 Tübingen (Germany)

Results

The reasons and frequencies of the 6,258 patients with IGHD who have stopped GH treatment within KIGS are listed in table 1. In more than half of the cases, it can be assumed that the decision to discontinue was part of the normal decision making process. In the majority, GH therapy was stopped because the intended height was reached or the potential for further growth was considered insufficient. The reasons for unplanned termination of GH treatment are more varied and mostly related to parent/patient decisions or non-compliance or loss to follow-up. Adverse events were rare causes for stopping GH treatment prematurely.

The frequencies of causes for stopping GH treatment within KIGS in patients with IGHD – all and according to various countries, i.e. UK, Germany, Japan, France, USA, and the rest of the world – are listed in table 2. Generally, the frequencies in the different categories are quite similar. It is remarkable that in France, bone age is more often used to determine the end of GH treatment than in other countries. In Japan, insufficient funding is the most important cause for terminating participation within KIGS. In Japan and in the US, height velocity is rarely mentioned as a cause for terminating GH treatment.

The reasons for terminating GH therapy according to gender are listed in table 3. The data show a similar pattern, apart from the fact that in females, normal height is mentioned significantly less frequent, and growth plate fusion and height velocity are significantly more frequent than in males.

The frequencies of causes for stopping GH therapy within KIGS in patients with IGHD compared with GHD caused by central nervous system tumours are listed in table 4. In IGHD patients, parent/patient decision, non-compliance and no funds are mentioned more often than in the tumour group. In the tumour group, an insufficient height velocity and adverse events are more frequent causes.

The characteristics of IGHD patients before GH treatment, at treatment start, during the first year on GH and at the end of treatment in relation to the most frequent causes for finishing participation within KIGS are listed in table 5. There is great resemblance between all groups with regard to birth weight, midparental height, degree of GHD, age at GH start, height standard deviation score (SDS) and GH dose. It is noteworthy that in patients who stopped according to normal height reached, the mean documented height was about –1.0 SDS, and the mean height velocity during the recent year was documented to be 3.4 cm/year. In the groups stopping because of growth plate fusion and height velocity, the mean height reached was close to the lower limit or normal. Also in these cases, the mean recent height velocity was recorded to be >2 cm/year.

Table 1. IGHD patient reasons for stopping GH treatment within KIGS (n = 6,258)

	n	%
Causes planned or related to normal treatment process		
Normal height reached	1,418	22.7
Growth plate fusion (bone age)	1,050	16.8
Height velocity diminished	836	13.4
Change: to other doctor, KIMS, adult clinic	116	1.9
All planned	3,420	54.7
Causes not related to normal treatment process		
Patient/parent decision to stop	1,104	17.6
Non-compliance	421	6.7
Lost to follow-up	487	7.8
Moved to unknown place	69	1.1
No more funds for GH	385	6.2
End of treatment trial	71	1.1
Change to other GH brand	99	1.6
Adverse event	93	1.5
Puberty	4	0.1
Other unidentified reasons	105	1.7
All not planned	2,838	45.3

Table 2. IGHD patient reasons for stopping GH treatment within KIGS according to country

	UK		Germany		Japan		France		USA		ROW	
	n	%	n	%	n	%	n	%	n	%	n	%
Causes planned or related to normal treatment process												
Normal height reached	99	18.6	221	27.0	136	17.6	278	22.6	166	15.6	518	28.2
Growth plate fusion (bone age)	27	5.1	137	16.7	71	9.2	353	28.7	146	13.7	316	17.2
Height velocity diminished	125	23.5	111	13.6	43	5.6	176	14.3	42	3.9	339	18.4
Change: to other doctor, KIMS, adult clinic	32	6.0	18	2.2	8	1.0	1	0.1	28	2.6	29	1.6
All planned	283	53.2	487	59.5	258	33.5	808	65.6	382	35.8	1,202	65.4
Causes not related to normal treatment process												
Patient/parent decision to stop	81	15.2	122	14.9	127	16.5	262	21.3	246	23.1	266	14.5
Non-compliance	58	10.9	41	5.0	54	7.0	41	3.3	129	12.1	98	5.3
Lost to follow-up	97	18.2	108	13.2	14	1.8	68	5.5	146	13.7	54	2.9
Moved to unknown place	6	1.1	21	2.6	2	0.3	4	0.3	23	2.2	13	0.7
No more funds for GH	–	–	3	0.4	246	31.9	5	0.4	20	1.9	111	6.0
End of treatment trial	4	0.8	3	0.4	2	0.3	4	0.3	9	0.8	49	2.7
Change to other GH brand	–	–	2	0.2	13	1.7	7	0.6	61	5.7	16	0.9
Adverse event	3	0.6	16	2.0	17	2.2	17	1.4	22	2.1	18	1.0
Puberty	–	–	–	–	2	0.3	2	0.2	–	–	–	–
Other unidentified reasons	–	–	15	1.8	36	4.7	13	1.1	29	2.7	12	0.7
All not planned	249	46.8	331	40.5	513	66.5	423	34.4	685	64.2	637	34.6

ROW = Rest of the world.

Table 3. IGHD patient reasons for stopping GH treatment within KIGS according to gender

	Females		Males	
	n	%	n	%
Causes planned or related to normal treatment process				
Normal height reached	398	19.1	1,020	24.4
Growth plate fusion (bone age)	396	19.0	654	15.7
Height velocity diminished	341	16.4	495	11.9
Change: to other doctor, KIMS, adult clinic	34	1.6	82	2.0
All planned	1,169	56.1	2,251	53.9
Causes not related to normal treatment process				
Patient/parent decision to stop	388	18.6	716	17.2
Non-compliance	109	5.2	312	7.5
Lost to follow-up	123	5.9	364	8.7
Moved to unknown place	19	0.9	50	1.2
No more funds for GH	145	7.0	240	5.6
End of treatment trial	27	1.3	44	1.1
Change to other GH brand	30	1.4	69	1.7
Adverse event	34	1.6	59	1.4
Puberty	1	0.1	3	0.1
Other unidentified reasons	40	1.9	65	1.6
All not planned	916	43.9	1,922	46.1

Table 4. IGHD patient reasons for stopping GH treatment within KIGS according to diagnosis

	IGHD		Tumours		p value
	n	%	n	%	
Causes planned or related to normal treatment process					
Normal height reached	1,418	22.7	314	21.0	n.s.
Growth plate fusion (bone age)	1,050	16.8	245	16.4	n.s.
Height velocity diminished	836	13.4	298	19.9	<0.001
Change: to other doctor, KIMS, adult clinic	116	1.9	128	8.6	<0.001
All planned	3,420	54.7	985	65.9	
Causes not related to normal treatment process					
Patient/parent decision to stop	1,104	17.6	136	9.1	<0.001
Non-compliance	421	6.7	46	3.1	<0.001
Lost to follow-up	487	7.8	99	6.6	n.s.
Moved to unknown place	69	1.1	9	0.6	–
No more funds for GH	385	6.2	38	2.5	<0.001
End of treatment trial	71	1.1	14	0.9	–
Change to other GH brand	99	1.6	10	0.7	–
Adverse event	93	1.5	142	9.5	<0.001
Puberty	4	0.1	5	0.3	–
Other unidentified reasons	105	1.7	11	0.7	–
All not planned	2,838	45.3	510	34.1	

n.s. = Not significant.

In cases terminating participation within KIGS due to causes not related to normal treatment process (patient/parent decision, non-compliance, loss of follow-up) the characteristics at treatment onset and the response to GH during the first year on GH did not differ from the other groups. However, the studentised residual which is indicative of the responsiveness to GH during the first year on GH was significantly lower. This may in part explain some discontent of patients/parents/physicians with the treatment results or reflect relatively poor compliance. These patients also terminated treatment about 2–3 years earlier, were still markedly deficient in height (mean height SDS near –2.0) but showed a (mean) height velocity >5 cm/year.

Discussion

Traditionally, GH treatment in short children is aimed at reaching a height at least within the normal range of the population (more than –2.0 SDS). However, there is no uniform consensus about stopping GH treatment at this margin in case there is still further growth potential. In children with GHD, treatment during adolescence may also be guided by development of puberty and body composition [1]. Usually, in GHD patients, GH treatment is continued as long as there is growth potential and until the adolescent developmental process is completed. Thereafter, GH replacement is interrupted to retest the patients in order to ascertain/exclude permanent and severe GHD [1].

Table 5. Characteristics of IGHD patients stopping GH treatment for various reasons

Variable	Normal height reached	Growth plate fusion	Height velocity	Patient/parent decision	Lost to follow-up	Non-compliance
Background						
Patients	1,418	1,060	836	1,104	487	421
Sex (male), %	71.9	62.3	59.2	64.9	74.7	74.1
Birth weight SDS	–0.6 ± 1.2	–0.7 ± 1.2	–0.7 ± 1.2	–0.7 ± 1.3	–0.7 ± 1.3	–0.8 ± 1.2
MPH SDS	–1.2 ± 1.1	–1.5 ± 1.2	–1.3 ± 1.1	–1.3 ± 1.2	–1.2 ± 1.2	–1.3 ± 1.2
Maximum GH, μg/l	5.8 ± 2.7	6.0 ± 2.7	5.7 ± 2.7	5.9 ± 2.7	5.4 ± 2.9	5.7 ± 2.8
At GH start						
Age, years	11.1 ± 3.4	11.1 ± 3.2	9.8 ± 3.7	10.6 ± 3.6	9.4 ± 4.1	10.2 ± 4.0
Height SDS	–2.8 ± 0.9	–2.9 ± 1.0	–3.2 ± 1.1	–3.1 ± 1.3	–3.2 ± 1.2	–3.3 ± 1.1
Height – MPH SDS	–1.6 ± 1.3	–1.4 ± 1.3	–1.9 ± 1.4	–1.7 ± 1.5	–2.0 ± 1.5	–2.0 ± 1.6
GH dose, mg/kg/week	0.22 ± 0.07	0.21 ± 0.09	0.22 ± 0.08	0.22 ± 0.07	0.24 ± 0.11	0.24 ± 0.10
First year on GH						
Patients	177	129	134	138	76	38
Height velocity, cm/year	9.4 ± 2.5	8.7 ± 2.2	9.0 ± 2.2	8.7 ± 2.2	9.1 ± 2.4	8.7 ± 2.4
Studentised residual	0.2 ± 1.1	0.1 ± 1.0	–0.1 ± 1.0	–0.2 ± 1.0	–0.3 ± 1.1	–0.5 ± 1.0
Latest visit						
Age, years	17.1 ± 1.8	16.7 ± 1.9	16.3 ± 2.7	14.8 ± 3.3	13.4 ± 3.7	14.2 ± 3.8
Bone age, years	15.4 ± 1.4	15.6 ± 1.4	14.3 ± 2.8	13.2 ± 2.9	11.9 ± 3.4	12.5 ± 3.5
Height SDS	–1.0 ± 1.0	–1.6 ± 1.0	–1.8 ± 1.2	–1.8 ± 1.3	–2.0 ± 1.3	–2.3 ± 1.2
Height velocity, cm/year	3.4 ± 2.6	3.2 ± 2.4	2.7 ± 2.3	5.2 ± 2.9	6.2 ± 2.8	5.1 ± 2.7
On GH, years	5.6 ± 3.1	5.2 ± 3.0	6.0 ± 3.5	3.8 ± 2.8	3.9 ± 3.2	3.6 ± 2.9

MPH = Midparental height.

Terminating GH treatment when near adult height is reached is a difficult decision for the physician. Often, the patients and their parents, who are fighting 'for each centimeter', feel deprived of further beneficial height gain when the treatment is stopped or even only interrupted. In accordance with the opinion of Tanner et al. [5], most physicians tend to stop GH therapy when a height velocity <2.0 cm is recorded. However, such a rather crude limit should take the development and the (slowing) growth pattern into consideration. Bone age may be used as a guide. On average, 99% of the adult height is reached when a bone age of 14 years (in girls) and 16 years (in boys) is reached. However, bone age readings may be erroneous and may not accurately reflect the growth potential of the epiphysis. Bone-specific alkaline phosphatase was suggested to be another tool to assist the decision [6]. Given all these uncertainties, efforts need to be undertaken in order to more accurately define when there is such a reduction in growth potential, so that a continuation of the expensive therapy is no longer justified.

These documented data from KIGS confirm our previous analysis [2, 3]: (1) GH therapy is often stopped by the physician despite short stature and despite a preserved growth potential; (2) there is insufficient growth potential, although normal height has not been reached; (3) patients prematurely interrupt GH treatment after many years, although they are still short and have the potential to grow. We assume that more realistic ideas about this therapy, an earlier onset of GH and a more successful treatment during the early years will be strong motives to continue treatment until a normal height has been reached. In disorders with short stature but not GHD (e.g., Turner syndrome), decisions on a long-term therapy should be guided by responsiveness to GH at an early time point in order to avoid psychological burdens, risks and costs.

References

1 Clayton PE, Cuneo RC, Juul A, Monson JP, Shalet SM, Tauber M, European Society of Paediatric Endocrinology: Consensus statement on the management of the GH-treated adolescent in the transition to adult care. Eur J Endocrinol 2005;152:165–170.
2 Ranke MB: Growth hormone therapy in children: when to stop? Horm Res 1995;43:122–125.
3 Ranke MB, Jönson P: Who stops growth hormone in KIGS, the Kabi International Growth Study – and why. KIGS Biannual Report 1995;12:33–39.
4 Preece MA: The assessment of growth; in Ranke MB, Gunnarsson R (eds): Progress in Growth Hormone Therapy – 5 Years of KIGS. Mannheim, J&J Verlag, 1994, pp 10–36.
5 Tanner JM, Whitehouse RH, Hughes PCR, Vince FP: Effect of human growth hormone treatment for 1 to 7 years on growth of 100 children with human growth hormone deficiency, low birth weight, inherited smallness, Turner's syndrome, and other complaints. Arch Dis Child 1991;46:746–782.
6 Tubiume H, Kanzaki S, Hida S, Ono T, Moriwake T, Yamauch S, Tanaka H, Seino Y: Serum bone alkaline phosphatase isoenzyme levels in normal children and children with growth hormone (GH) deficiency: a potential marker for bone formation and response to GH therapy. J Clin Endocrinol Metab 1997;82:2056–2061.

Congenital Growth Hormone Deficiency

Primus E. Mullis

Application of the powerful tool 'molecular biology' has made it possible to ask questions not only about hormone production and action but also to characterize many of the receptor molecules that initiate responses to hormones. We are beginning to understand how cells may regulate the expression of genes and how hormones intervene in regulatory processes to adjust the expression of individual genes. In addition, great strides have been made in understanding how individual cells communicate with each other through locally released factors in order to coordinate growth, differentiation, secretion and other responses within a tissue. Therefore, while focusing on regulatory systems playing a most important role in defining a physiological and/or pathophysiological mechanism, we have to be aware of already having entered the 'post-genomic' area, in which not only a defect at the molecular level but also its functional impact at the cellular level becomes important.

Further, because insulin-like growth factor 1 (IGF-1) plays a pivotal role in growth, where it mediates most, if not all, of the effects of growth hormone (GH), GH deficiency (GHD) could also be somehow considered as IGF-1 deficiency (IGFD) (table 1). Although IGFD can develop at any level of the GH-releasing hormone (GHRH)-GH-IGF axis, we would like to differentiate between GHD (absent to low GH in circulation) and IGFD (normal to high GH in circulation).

Development of the Pituitary Gland and Its Impact on Hormonal Deficiencies

Discovery of transcription factors responsible for pituitary cell differentiation and organogenesis has had an immediate impact on the understanding and diagnosis of pituitary hormone deficiencies. Importantly, combined pituitary hormone deficiencies have been associated with mutations in transcription factor coding genes that control organogenesis or multiple cell lineages, whereas isolated hormone deficiencies are often caused by transcription factors controlling late cell differentiation. However, as there may be a strong phenotypic variability in familial combined pituitary hormone deficiency caused by different transcription factors, e.g., PROP1 (prophet of Pit1), it is of high clinical importance to have some knowledge about these various factors as well as

Department of Paediatric Endocrinology,
Diabetology and Metabolism
University Children's Hospital, Inselspital
CH–3010 Bern (Switzerland)

the steps involved in pituitary gland development (fig. 1) [1–3].

The formation of the pituitary gland involves many factors that control various processes during development, including transcription factors for early patterning (Rathke's pouch: dorsal, Pax6; ventral, Isl-1, Brn-4; early pituitary gland, within the anterior lobe: dorsal, Pax6, Prop1; ventral, Isl-1, Brn-4, Lhx-4, GATA-2; early pituitary gland, within the intermediate lobe: Six-3, Pax-6) and organogenesis, for the control of cell proliferation, and finally, for differentiation of individual lineages [4]. Some of these contribute to more than one process at different times. For example, Pitx-1 and Pitx-2 contribute to very early organogenesis, but they are also involved in late functions such as expansion of the gonadotroph and thyrotroph lineages in Pitx [5] and the control of hormone-coding gene transcription.

Lineage Commitment and Differentiation

All lineages of the anterior and intermediate pituitary gland derive from the epithelial cells of Rathke's pouch, which – in humans – projects as a diverticulum from the roof of the stomadeum at the middle of the fourth week [for a general review, see ref. 4]. Molecular markers indicate that the pouch cells are not equivalent along the dorsoventral axis, and this may be taken as an indication that the commitment to different pituitary lineages may be determined at an early developmental stage. In mice, at stage e9.5–11.5 (embryonic days 9.5–11.5), transcription factors such as Prop1 and Pax6 are preferentially expressed in the dorsal pouch, whereas factors Isl-1, Brn-4, Lhx-4 and GATA-2 are primarily expressed on the ventral side. Only one of these factors, Prop1, may be a commitment factor. It is initially expressed in the dorsal pouch and developing anterior pituitary, where the somatolactotrophs and definitive thyrotrophs will eventually appear. Further, Prop1 is required for the expression of Pit1, which is itself necessary for differentiation of the same lineages. Therefore, if data suggest

Table 1. Alteration in the GHRH-GH axis affecting growth in humans (differential diagnosis of IGFD)

1	Hypothalamus
	a Transcription factors
	b GHRH gene
2	Pituitary gland
	a Transcription factors
	i TPIT
	ii SOX3
	iii HESX1
	iv LHX3
	v LHX4
	vi PROP1
	vii POU1F1
	b GHRH-R
	c GH gene cluster
	i GHD/bioinactivity
3	GH target organs
	a GHR (primary: extracellular, transmembrane, intracellular)
	i GH insensitivity
	ii Signalling (JAK2/STAT5b/ERK)
	b GH insensitivity (secondary)
	i Malnutrition (e.g., anorexia)
	ii Liver disease (e.g., Byler's disease)
	iii Chronic illness
	iv Anti-GH antibodies
4	IGF-1 defects
5	IGF-1 transport/metabolism/clearance
6	IGF-1 resistance
	a IGF-1 receptor defect (type I)
	b IGF-1 signalling (post-receptor defect)

that Prop1 commits the dorsal pituitary to give rise to the somatolactotroph and thyrotroph lineages, there is no evidence of a counterpart of Prop1 that may commit the ventral pituitary to give rise to gonadotroph or corticotroph lineages. IsI-1 and GATA-2 may be candidate factors for this function. Based on the description of gradients of signalling molecules and transcription factors in and around the development of the pituitary gland, a combinatorial model was proposed in which these regulatory molecules define

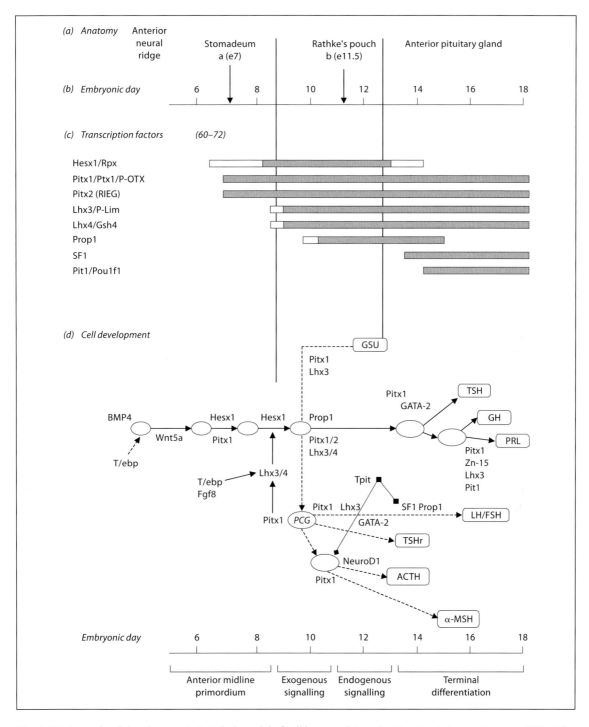

Fig. 1. Pituitary gland development. Detailed model of cell lineage determination in pituitary ontogeny. GSU = Glycoprotein hormone subunit; TSH = thyroid-stimulating hormone; PRL = prolactin; LH = luteinizing hormone; FSH = follicle-stimulating hormone; TSHr = thyroid-stimulating hormone receptor; ACTH = adrenocorticotrophic hormone; MSH = melanocyte-stimulating hormone.

territories within the developing gland. Only a unique combination of signals and/or factors would be responsible for differentiation toward one rather than the other lineages. However, this model reflects that precise relations among all the lineages are not clear at all. As it has been shown that the corticotroph and gonadotroph lineages (both arise ventrally) may have a common precursor, a simple binary model to account for all pituitary differentiation events starting from a common precursor has been proposed (fig. 1d). This model would be consistent with the clear commitment of the dorsal pituitary by Prop1 to form the pre-somato-lacto-thyrotroph precursors, from which thyroid-stimulating hormone, GH and prolactin lineages will later arise through the action of Pit1, GATA-2 and others. Further, pre-cortico-gonadotrophs are committed at a similar time, and later, these will be driven to differentiate into corticotrophs via pre-cortico-melanotrophs under the influence of Tpit or NeuroD1, or even later into gonadotrophs under the influence of SF1 and GATA-2. However, for the time being, it is not clear which factors commit the ventral pituitary to the pre-cortico-gonadotroph fate. Signalling gradients are also likely to be involved and affect differentiation in this model, but these rather act in a stochastic fashion on a cell-by-cell basis than by defining specific territories within the developing gland. The phenotypes caused by the various transcription factors of the pituitary gland are summarized in table 2.

Pituitary Hormones and Maintenance of Normal Cell Function
In addition, it is not only important to have a certain function, but also to maintain it. Therefore, it has to be highlighted that a specific cell function (production of any hormone) might be lost over time because of a lack of cellular cross-talk, as it is suggested in patients suffering from *PROP1* gene defects in terms of adrenocorticotrophic hormone production [6]. Further, not only the different transcription factors but also the distinct and well-tuned hormonal feedback loops, e.g., GHRH, GHRH receptor (GHRH-R), GH, GH receptor (GHR) and IGF-1, may play a major role at the level of maintenance of each hormonal cell activity. For example, GHRH-R-mutant mice (*little* mouse) present with a hypoplastic anterior gland and phenotypically with dwarfism lacking GH secretion.

Different Components of the Growth Hormone Axis

GH is regulated by two hypothalamic peptides, GHRH, which is stimulatory, and GH-inhibiting factor (GHIF), which is inhibitory. There are membrane receptors for both GHRH and GHIF (somatostatin) on anterior pituitary cells. These two peptides are in turn influenced by an array of neurotransmitters. Pituitary GH encoded by the *GH-1* gene is secreted in pulses and binds to GHR in the liver and other target organs. Receptor occupancy increases production and release of IGF-1. This mediator of GH action binds to IGF-1 receptors in target tissues such as growth plates at the end of the long bones. There is a tight feedback control of GH release, involving GH and IGF-1 in the regulation of GHIF and probably GHRH. Further, the classification of genetic defects in the development of the GH axis illustrates that basically, the site of these defects, both reported and hypothetical, may be located at any level from the hypothalamus to the target receptors of skeletal tissues (table 1).

Classification of Isolated GHD

Familial Isolated GHD
Short stature associated with GHD has been estimated to occur in about 1/4,000–1/10,000, as indicated in various studies [7–10]. While most cases are sporadic and believed to result from en-

Table 2. Transcription factors of clinical importance

Gene	Phenotype	Inheritance
Pit1/ POU1F1	hormonal deficiencies: GH, PRL, TSH imaging: anterior pituitary gland, normal to hypo; posterior pituitary gland, normal other manifestations: none	R/D
PROP1	hormonal deficiencies: GH, PRL, TSH, LH, FSH, (ACTH) imaging: anterior pituitary gland, hypo to hyper; posterior pituitary gland, normal other manifestations: none	R
HESX1	hormonal deficiencies: GH, PRL, TSH, LH, FSH, ACTH, IGHD, CPHD imaging: anterior pituitary gland, hypo; posterior pituitary gland, ectopic other manifestations: eyes, brain, septo-optic dysplasia	R/D
LHX3	hormonal deficiencies: GH, PRL, TSH, LH, FSH, (ACTH) imaging: anterior pituitary gland, hypo; posterior pituitary gland, normal other manifestations: neck rotation 75–85° (?) (normal: 160–180°)	R
LHX4	hormonal deficiencies: GH, TSH, ACTH imaging: anterior pituitary gland, hypo; posterior pituitary gland, normal other manifestations: sella turcica/skull defects, cerebellar defects	D
SOX3	hormonal deficiencies: GH imaging: anterior pituitary gland, normal to hypo; posterior pituitary gland, normal, ectopic other manifestations: mental retardation, abnormality of corpus callosum, absent infundibulum	XL

PRL = Prolactin; TSH = thyroid-stimulating hormone; R = autosomal recessively inherited; D = autosomal dominantly inherited; LH = luteinizing hormone; FSH = follicle-stimulating hormone; ACTH = adrenocorticotrophic hormone; CPHD = combined pituitary hormone deficiency; XL = X-linked.

vironmental cerebral insults or developmental anomalies, 3–30% of cases have an affected first-degree relative suggesting a genetic aetiology [8, 9]. Since magnetic resonance examinations detect only about 12–20% of anomalies of either the hypothalamus or pituitary gland in patients suffering from isolated GHD (IGHD), one can assume that many genetic defects are not diagnosed, and a significantly higher proportion of sporadic cases may thus have a genetic cause [11]. Familial IGHD is associated with at least four mendelian disorders (table 3). These include two forms that have autosomal recessive inheritance (IGHD type IA, IB), as well as autosomal dominant (IGHD type II) and X-linked (IGHD type III) forms [4, 12].

IGHD Type IA
IGHD type IA was first described by Illig [13] in 3 Swiss children with unusually severe growth impairment and apparent GHD. Occasionally, affected individuals have short length at birth and hypoglycaemia in infancy but uniformly develop severe growth retardation by the age of 6 months. Their initial good response to exogenous GH is hampered by the development of anti-GH antibodies leading to dramatic slowing of growth [13].

GH-1 Gene Deletions. In 1981, Phillips et al. [14] examined genomic DNA from these Swiss children and, using the Southern blotting technique, discovered that the GH-1 gene was missing. Subsequently, additional cases of GH-1 gene

Table 3. IGHD types

Category	Inheritance	GH radio-immunoassay	Candidate gene	Status
IGHD IA	recessive	absent	hGH-1	deletions/mutations (signal peptide)
IGHD IB	recessive	low	hGH-1	frameshifts
				stop codon
				splice site mutations
			GHRH	unlikely
			GHRH-R	mutations
			trans-acting factors	mutations/deletions
			cis-acting elements	mutations/deletions
IGHD II	dominant	low	hGH-1	splice site mutations
				splice enhancer mutations
				ESE and ISE
				missense mutations
				intervening sequence deletions
IGHD III	X-linked	low	unknown	

deletions have been described responding well to the GH treatment, making the presence of anti-GH antibodies an inconsistent finding in IGHD type IA patients with identical molecular findings (homozygosity for GH-1 gene deletions) [15]. The frequency of GH-1 gene deletions as a cause of GHD varies among different populations and according to the criteria and definition of short stature chosen. Analysing patients with severe IGHD, i.e. less than –4 to –4.5 standard deviation score (SDS), the prevalence reported was 9.4% in Northern European (n = 32), 13.6% in Mediterranean (n = 22), 16.6% in Turkish (n = 24), 38% in Oriental Jewish (n = 13), 12% in Chinese (n = 26) and 0% in Japanese patients (n = 10), respectively [16]. The sizes of the deletions were heterogeneous, with the most frequent (70–80%) being 6.7 kb [16]. The remaining deletions described included 7.6, 7.0 and 45 kb, as well as a double deletion within the GH gene cluster. At the molecular level, these deletions involved unequal recombination and crossing over within the GH gene cluster at meiosis. Interestingly, crossing over is reported to occur in 99% of homologous regions (594 bp) flanking the *GH-1* gene, rather than in *Alu* repeat sequences [17]. Although *Alu* repeats, which are frequent sites of recombination, are adjacent to the *GH-1* gene, they were not involved in any of the recombinational events studied.

IGHD Type IB
Patients with IGHD type IB are characterized by low but detectable levels of GH (<7 mU/l, <2.5 ng/ml), short stature (less than –2 SDS for age and sex), significantly delayed bone age, an autosomal recessive inheritance (e.g., 2 parents of normal height, 2 siblings affected), no demonstrable direct and/or endocrine cause of IGHD, and a positive response and immunological tolerance to treatment with exogenous GH. This subgroup of IGHD patients has been broadened and reclassified on the basis of the nature of their *GH* gene defects and now includes splicing site mutations of the *GH-1* gene; even an apparent lack of GH has been found by radioimmunoassay. There-

fore, the phenotype of IGHD type IB is more variable than that of type IA. In one family, the children may resemble IGHD type IA, whereas in other families, growth during infancy is relatively normal, and growth failure is not noted until mid-childhood. Similarly, GH may be nearly lacking or simply low, following stimulation test. This heterogeneous phenotype suggests that there is more than one candidate gene causing the disorder. Possible candidate genes are noted in table 3.

Splice Site and Nonsense Mutations, as well as Frameshifts within the GH-1 Gene. The *GH-1* gene has often been amplified and screened for small deletions and mutations which have been found and described [4]. However, generally speaking, functional studies are necessary to prove the importance of all these alterations found in any gene. For instance, all the mutations causing a suggested mRNA splicing error need transfection of the mutant gene into a cultured cell system allowing reverse transcription followed by cDNA sequencing. Thereafter, the impact of the changes of the amino acids encoded by the mutant genes is to be studied. Studies with bovine GH mutants have shown that not only the stability and biological activity of the mutants may be altered, but the intracellular targeting of GH protein products to the secretory granules important for secretion may be deranged as well [18, 19].

Candidate Genes in IGHD Type IB

Some of the components of the GH pathway are unique to GH, whereas there are also various components involved in other pathways, therefore unspecific for the GH pathway. However, in patients with IGHD, mutational changes in genes specific to the GHRH-GH axis are of importance, and there is a need to focus on them.

The GHRH Gene. Our and several other laboratories have tried to define *GHRH* gene alterations and have failed so far [20, 21]. Therefore, if *GHRH* mutations do cause IGHD in humans, they must be very rare.

The GHRH-R Gene. In 1992, Kelly Mayo [22] cloned and sequenced the rat and human *GHRH-R* gene, providing the opportunity to examine the role of GHRH-R in growth abnormalities that involve the GH axis. Sequencing of the *GHRH-R* gene in the *little* mouse *(lit/lit)* showed a single nucleotide substitution in codon 60 that changed aspartic acid to glycine (D60G), eliminating the binding of GHRH to its own receptor [23]. As the phenotype of IGHD type IB in humans has much in common with the phenotype of homozygous *lit/lit* mice, including autosomal recessive inheritance, time of onset of growth retardation, diminished secretion of GH and IGF-1, proportional reduction in weight and skeletal size, and delay in sexual maturation, the *GHRH-R* gene was searched for alterations in patients suffering from IGHD type IB [24]. The GHRH-R is a member of a large family of heptahelical transmembrane receptors that couple to G proteins upon receptor activation. Binding of GHRH to GHRH-R expressed on the surface of somatotroph cells activate G_s and lead to a consequent increase in cAMP synthesis that induces cellular proliferation and GH secretion. Wajnrajch et al. [24] reported a nonsense mutation similar to the *little* mouse in an Indian Moslem kindred. Furthermore, in two villages in the Sindh area of Pakistan, Baumann and Maheshwari [25] reported another form of severe short stature caused by a point mutation in the *GHRH-R* gene, resulting in a truncation of the extracellular domain of this receptor. Individuals who are homozygous for this mutation are very short (–7.4 SDS) but normally proportioned. They appear of normal intelligence, and at least some are fertile. Biochemical testing revealed that they have normal levels of GHRH and GH binding protein (GHBP), but undetectable levels of GH and extremely low levels of IGF-1. Mutations in the *GHRH-R* gene have been described as the basis of a syndrome characterized by autosomal recessive IGHD and anterior pituitary hypoplasia, defined as a pituitary height >2 SD below the age-adjusted normal, which is likely due to the depletion of the somatotroph cells (OMIM: 139190); however, certain variability in anterior pituitary size, even in siblings with the same mutation, has been described [26].

Specific trans-*Acting Factor to GH Gene.* Any alteration to the specific transcriptional regulation of the *GH-1* gene may produce IGHD type IB. Mullis et al. [27] have reported a heterozygous 211-bp deletion within the retinoic acid receptor α gene causing the phenotype of IGHD type IB.

IGHD Type II

Focusing on the autosomal dominant form of IGHD, IGHD type II (IGHD II) is mainly caused by mutations within the first 6 bp of intervening sequences 3 (5′IVS-3), which result in a mis-splicing at the mRNA level and the subsequent loss of exon 3, producing a 17.5-kDa human GH (hGH) isoform [4]. This GH product lacks amino acids 32–71 (del32–71 GH), which is the entire loop that connects helix 1 and helix 2 in the tertiary structure of hGH [28, 29]. Skipping of exon 3 caused by *GH-1* gene alterations other than those at the donor splice site in 5′IVS-3 has also been reported in other patients with IGHD II. These include mutations in exon splice enhancer [ESE1 and ESE2 in exon 3 (E3); E3 + 1 G→T: ESE1m1; E3 + 2 A→C: ESE1m2; E3 + 5 A→G: ESE1m3; ESE2: Δ721–735] and within suggested intron splice enhancer (ISE; IVS-3 + 28 G→A: ISEm1; IVS-3 del + 28–45: ISEm2) sequences [4, 30, 31].

Such mutations lie within purine-rich sequences and cause increased levels of exon 3 skipped transcripts [4, 30, 31], suggesting that the usage of the normal splicing elements (ESE1 at the 5′ end of exon 3 as well as ISE in intron 3) may be disrupted [30, 31]. The first 7 nucleotides in exon 3 (ESE1) are crucial for the splicing of GH mRNA [32], such that some nonsense mutations might cause skipping of one or even more exons during mRNA splicing in the nucleus. This phenomenon is called 'nonsense-mediated altered splicing', and its underlying mechanisms are still unknown [33]. Furthermore, intron 3 of the *GH-1* gene is 92 nt in length, well above the approximately 50-nt minimum intron length required for spliceosome assembly. Nevertheless, deletion analysis within intron 3 allowed to suggest that exon skipping observed within deletions of at least 12 nt is due to the decreasing size of the intron, rather than the actual sequence deleted [32]. A recent report of a novel deletion including IVS-3 (5′IVS-3 del + 56–77) confirmed this former hypothesis in a child and her mother [34]. In addition to the above described splice site mutations and deletions that result in the production of del32–71 GH, three other mutations within the *GH-1* gene (missense mutations) are reported to be responsible for IGHD II, namely, the substitution of leucine for proline, histidine for arginine and phenylalanine for valine at amino acid positions 89 (P89V), 183 (R183H) and 110 (V110F), respectively [4].

At the functional level, the 17.5-kDa isoform exhibits a dominant-negative effect on the secretion of the 22-kDa isoforms in both tissue cultures as well as in transgenic animals [35–37]. The 17.5-kDa isoform is initially retained in the endoplasmic reticulum, disrupts the Golgi apparatus, impairs both GH and other hormonal trafficking [38], and partially reduces the stability of the 22-kDa isoform [35]. Furthermore, transgenic mice over-expressing the 17.5-kDa isoform exhibit a defect in the maturation of GH secretory vesicles and anterior pituitary gland hypoplasia due to a loss of the majority of somatotrophs [30, 35, 36]. However, trace amounts of the 17.5-kDa isoforms are normally present in children and adults of normal growth and stature [39], and heterozygosity for A731G mutation (K41R) within the newly defined ESE2 (which is important for exon 3 inclusion) led to approximately 20% exon 3 skipping, resulting in both normal as well as short stature [30, 32]. From the clinical point of view, severe short stature (less than –4.5 SDS) is not present in all affected individuals, indicating that in some forms, growth failure in IGHD II is less severe than one might expect [40]. It has been hypothesized that children with splice site mutations are younger and shorter at diagnosis than their counterparts with missense mutations [40]. Furthermore, more recent in vitro and animal data suggest that both a quantitative and qualitative difference in phenotype may result from variable splice site mutations causing differing degrees of exon 3 skipping [4, 36]. To summarize, the data of these actual studies highlight that the variable phenotype of autosomal dominant GHD may reflect a threshold and a dose dependency effect of the amount of 17.5 kDa relative to 22-kDa hGH [36, 37, 41]. Specifically, this has a variable impact on pituitary size, onset and severity of GHD, and, unexpectedly, the most severe, rapid onset forms of GHD might be subsequently associated with the evolution of other pituitary hormone deficiencies [42, 43].

General Aspects of the Dominant-Negative Nature of IGHD II. IGHD II is a rare autosomal dominant form of GHD, usually caused by hGH splicing mutations that generate internally truncated GH forms that block the secretion of wild-type GH produced from the normal allele [12]. From the clinical point of view, there is evidence of great variability in the IGHD II phenotype in terms of onset, severity and rate of progression according to the mutation (splice site vs. missense) within the *GH-1* gene [4, 40–43]. Severe short stature was only present in one third of the affected individuals at diagnosis in the study by Binder et al. [40]. Furthermore, it has to be stressed that in a recent study, we described 5 families, clinically clearly autosomal dominant GH deficient, where we could not find any *GH-1* gene alterations [44]. In these subjects, not only the whole *GH-1* gene but also *HESX-1* was sequenced, as in mice and humans, monoallelic *hesx-1/HESX-1* alterations may cause mild forms of GHD.

Variable Clinical Course Depending on the GH-1 Gene Alteration. We studied a total of 89 subjects on a clinical basis and sequenced the whole *GH-1,* introns and exons included, in the index cases of 32 families with IGHD II [42, 43]. Sixty-nine subjects belonging to 27 families suffered from different splice site as well as missense mutations within the *GH-1* gene. The subjects presenting with a 5′IVS-3 +1/+2 bp splice site mutation leading to a skipping of exon 3 were found to be more likely to present with other pituitary hormone deficiencies during follow-up [42]. In addition, although patients with missense mutations have previously been reported to be less affected, a number of patients presenting with the P89L missense GH form showed some pituitary hormone impairment [42, 43]. The development of multiple hormonal deficiencies is not age dependent and there is a clear variability in onset, severity and progression, even within the same families presenting with identical *GH-1* gene alterations. The most important message gained from these studies was that other hormone deficits can develop in IGHD II patients, underscoring the clinical importance of maintaining vigilance for the development of other hormonal deficiencies over the years [42, 43].

IGHD Type III

This reported type is X-linked recessively inherited. In these families, the affected males were immunoglobulin as well as GH deficient [45, 46]. Recent studies have shown that the long arm of chromosome X may be involved and that the disorder may be caused by mutations and/or deletions of a portion of the X chromosome containing two loci, one necessary for normal immunoglobulin production and the other for GH expression [47]. In addition, Duriez et al. [48] reported an exon skipping mutation in the *btk* gene of a patient with X-linked agammaglobulinemia and IGHD.

GH Insensitivity

A variety of studies have indicated that approximately 25% of children evaluated for idiopathic short stature have primary IGFD presenting with abnormally low IGF-1 in the face of normal to high GH in circulation [49, 50]. In its purest and most dramatic forms, primary IGFD has been identified with three classes of molecular defects: (1) GH insensitivity resulting from mutations within the *GHR* gene primarily called 'Laron's syndrome' [51, 52], (2) genetic defects affecting the GH signalling pathway, mainly the Janus kinase 2 (JAK2) signal transducer and activator of transcription 5b (STAT5b) [53–55], and (3) deletions or mutations of the *IGF-1* gene itself [56, 57]. Furthermore, the concept of dysfunctional GH variants and/or bioactive GH molecules has been proposed for years [58] and opens an interesting platform to study the elements between GHD and IGFD, as some of these patients excellently respond to the exogenous GH treatment. In addition, there are reports on abnormal GHR signalling in children with idiopathic short stature in the absence of any *GHR* or *GH-1* gene alteration [59, 60].

Syndrome of Bioinactive GH

The diagnosis 'syndrome of bioactive GH' has often been discussed and suggested in short children with a phenotype resembling IGHD but who had normal or even slightly elevated basal GH levels in combination with low IGF-1 concentrations that increased after treatment with exogenous GH excluding the diagnosis of Laron's syndrome. Takahashi et al. [61–63] described 2 cases heterozygous for point mutations in the *GH-1* gene (R77C and D112G). The R77C GH mutant bound with unusually high affinity to the GHBP and abnormally to the GHR. Further, it was able to inhibit tyrosine phosphorylation in the GH signalling pathway, presumably acting in a dominant-negative fashion as a GH antagonist, as IGF-1 levels were not measurable following exogenous recombinant hGH treatment. However, as the patient's father, who was also heterozygous for the same mutations, was phenotypically normal and of normal stature [61], many questions remain unanswered. The D112G mutant involved a single A→G substitution in exon 4 in a girl with short stature [63]. The locus of the mutation was found within site 2 of the GH molecule in binding to the GHR/GHBP that purportedly prevented dimerization of the GHR [63]. The patient presented with high levels of GH and low levels of IGF-1, but responded well to the recombinant hGH: not only IGF-1 but also height velocity increased, leading to an improved somatic growth (11 cm/year compared with 4.5 cm/year before therapy). Therefore, the authors claimed to report the first patient affected with a 'real' bioactive GH. In addition, in a most recent report, Millar et al. [41] described several dysfunctional GH variants associated with a significantly reduced ability to activate GHR-mediated JAK/STAT signal transduction. However, we described a homozygous missense mutation, C53S, in the GH molecule of 1 Serbian patient with growth retardation showing all the clinical characteristics of a bioactive GH. The bioactivity of this mutant has been confirmed on a molecular and cellular basis and is due to lower affinity of the C53S variant for the GHR, presumably caused by the disruption of the disulfide bond between Cys-53 and Cys-165. Therefore, this research contributes new evidence, highlighting the importance of these conserved cysteines in mediating the biological effects of this hormone [64].

Cell Biology/Post-Genomic Defects

As we have already entered the 'post-genomic' area, it is most important to broaden our views and, having defined the possible disorders at the DNA/RNA level, to focus on function and re-analyse the specific defects at the cellular level.

The autosomal dominant IGHD II is stated as an example. Heterozygous *GH-1* gene mutations yielding an un- or misfolded GH protein do not necessarily cause ultimate GHD. Some are dominant, others are recessive. This fact is of importance and suggests possible mechanisms in the secretory pathway. All these mechanisms are far from being confirmed and are still a major challenge to the whole scientific community focusing on the pathway of secretory proteins. Of particular interest is the fact that identical phenotypes might be caused by different genotypes causing completely different defects at the cellular and therefore functional level [42, 43].

Acknowledgements

This work was supported by the Swiss National Science Foundation 3200B0-105853/1 (to P.E.M.).

References

1 Mullis PE: Transcription factors in pituitary development. Mol Cell Endocrinol 2001;185:1–16.
2 Pulichino AM, Vallette-Kasic S, Drouin J: Transcriptional regulation of pituitary gland development: binary choices for cell differentiation. Curr Opin Endocrinol Diabet 2004;11:13–17.
3 Dattani MT: Growth hormone deficiency and combined pituitary hormone deficiency: does the genotype matter? Clin Endocrinol (Oxf) 2005;63:121–130.
4 Mullis PE: Genetic control of growth. Eur J Endocrinol 2005;152:11–31.
5 Szeto DP, Rodriguez-Esteban C, Ryan AK, O'Connell SM, Liu F, Kioussi C, Gleiberman AS, Izpisua-Belmonte JC, Rosenfeld MG: Role of the bicoid-related homeodomain factor Pitx1 in specifying hindlimb morphogenesis and pituitary development. Genes Dev 1999;13:484–494.
6 Vallette-Kasic S, Barlier A, Teinturier C, Diaz A, Manavela M, Berthezene F, Bouchard P, Chaussain JL, Brauner R, Pellegrini-Bouiller I, Jaquet P, Enjalbert A, Brue T: PROP1 gene screening in patients with multiple pituitary hormone deficiency reveals two sites of hypermutability and a high incidence of corticotroph deficiency. J Clin Endocrinol Metab 2001;86:4529–4535.
7 Vimpani GV, Vimpani AF, Lidgard GP, Cameron EH, Farquhar JW: Prevalence of severe growth hormone deficiency. Br Med J 1977;2:427–430.
8 Rona RJ, Tanner JM: Aetiology of idiopathic growth hormone deficiency in England and Wales. Arch Dis Child 1977;52:197–208.
9 Lacey KA, Parkin JM: Causes of short stature: a community study of children in Newcastle upon Tyne. Lancet 1974;i:42–45.
10 Lindsay R, Feldkamp M, Harris D, Robertson J, Rallison M: Utah growth study: growth standards and the prevalence of growth hormone deficiency. J Pediatr 1994;125:29–35.
11 Cacciari E, Zucchini S, Carla G, Pirazzoli P, Cicognani A, Mandini M, Busacca M, Trevisan C: Endocrine function and morphological findings in patients with disorders of the hypothalamo-pituitary area: a study with magnetic resonance. Arch Dis Child 1990;65:1199–1202.
12 Phillips JA 3rd: Inherited defects in growth hormone synthesis and action; in Scriver C, Beaudet AL, Sly WS, Valle D (eds): The Metabolic Basis of Inherited Disease, ed 7. New York, McGraw-Hill, 1995, pp 3023–3044.
13 Illig R: Growth hormone antibodies in patients treated with different preparations of human growth hormone (hGH). J Clin Endocrinol Metab 1970;31:679–688.
14 Phillips III JA, Hjelle B, Seeburg PH, Zachmann M: Molecular basis for familial isolated growth hormone deficiency. Proc Natl Acad Sci USA 1981;78:6372–6375.
15 Laron Z, Kelijman M, Pertzelan A, Keret R, Shoffner JM, Parks JS: Human growth hormone deletion without antibody formation or growth arrest during treatment: a new disease entity? Isr J Med Sci 1985;250:999–1006.
16 Mullis PE, Akinci A, Kanaka C, Eble A, Brook CG: Prevalence of human growth hormone-1 gene deletions among patients with isolated growth hormone deficiency from different populations. Pediatr Res 1992;31:532–534.
17 Vnencak-Jones CL, Phillips JA 3rd: Hot spots for growth hormone gene deletions in homologous regions outside Alu repeats. Science 1990;250:1745–1748.
18 Chen WY, Wight DC, Chen NY, Coleman TA, Wagner TE, Kopchick JJ: Mutations in the third α-helix of bovine growth hormone dramatically affect its intracellular distribution in vitro and growth enhancement in transgenic mice. J Biol Chem 1991;266:2252–2258.
19 McAndrew SJ, Chen NY, Wiehl P, DiCaprio L, Yun J, Wagner TE, Okada S, Kopchick JJ: Expression of truncated forms of the bovine growth hormone gene in cultured mouse cells. J Biol Chem 1991;266:20965–20969.
20 Mullis PE, Patel M, Brickell PM, Brook CG: Isolated growth hormone deficiency: analysis of the growth hormone (GH) releasing hormone gene and the GH gene cluster. J Clin Endocrinol Metab 1990;70:187–191.
21 Perez-Jurado LA, Phillips JA 3rd, Francke U: Exclusion of growth hormone (GH)-releasing hormone gene mutations in familial isolated GH deficiency by linkage and single strand conformation analysis. J Clin Endocrinol Metab 1994;78:622–628.

22 Mayo K: Molecular cloning and expression of a pituitary-specific receptor for growth hormone-releasing hormone. Mol Endocrinol 1992;6:1734–1744.

23 Lin SC, Lin CR, Gukovsky I: Molecular basis of the *little* mouse phenotype and implications for cell type-specific growth. Nature 1993;364:208–213.

24 Wajnrajch MP, Gertner JM, Harbison MD, Chua SC Jr, Leibel RL: Nonsense mutation in the human growth hormone receptor causes growth failure analogous to the little *(lit)* mouse. Nat Genet 1996;12:88–90.

25 Baumann G, Maheshwari H: The Dwarfs of Sindh: severe growth hormone (GH) deficiency caused by a mutation in the GH-releasing hormone receptor gene. Acta Paediatr Suppl 1997;423:33–38.

26 Alba M, Hall CM, Whatmore AJ, Clayton PE, Price DA, Salvatori R: Variability in anterior pituitary size within members of a family with GH deficiency due to a new splice mutation in the GHRH receptor gene. Clin Endocrinol (Oxf) 2004;60:470–475.

27 Mullis PE, Eblé A, Wagner JK: Isolated growth hormone deficiency is associated with a 211 bp deletion within RAR α gene (abstract). Horm Res 1994;41:61.

28 de Vos AM, Ultsch M, Kossiakoff AA: Human growth hormone and extracellular domain of its receptor: crystal structure of the complex. Science 1992;255:306–312.

29 Cunningham BC, Ultsch M, De Vos AM, Mulkerrin MG, Clauser KR, Wells JA: Dimerization of the extracellular domain of the human growth hormone receptor by a single hormone molecule. Science 1991;25:821–825.

30 Ryther RC, McGuinness LM, Phillips JA 3rd, Moseley CT, Magoulas CB, Robinson IC, Patton JG: Disruption of exon definition produces a dominant-negative growth hormone isoform that causes somatotroph death and IGHD II. Hum Genet 2003;113:140–148.

31 McCarthy EMS, Phillips JA 3rd: Characterization of an intron splice enhancer that regulates alternative splicing of human GH pre-mRNA. Hum Mol Genet 1998;7:1491–1496.

32 Ryther RC, Flynt AS, Harris BD, Phillips JA 3rd, Patton JG: GH1 splicing is regulated by multiple enhancers whose mutation produces a dominant-negative GH isoform that can be degraded by allele-specific siRNA. Endocrinology 2004;145:2988–2996.

33 Vivenza D, Guazzarotti L, Godi M, Frasca D, di Natale B, Momigliano-Richiardi P, Bona G, Giordano M: A novel deletion in the GH1 gene including the IVS3 branch site responsible for autosomal dominant isolated growth hormone deficiency (IGHD II). J Clin Endocrinol Metab 2006;91:980–986.

34 Dietz HC: Nonsense mutations and altered splice-site selections. Am J Hum Genet 1997;60:729–730.

35 Lee MS, Wajnrajch MP, Kim SS, Plotnick LP, Wang J, Gertner JM, Leibel RL, Dannies PS: Autosomal dominant growth hormone (GH) deficiency type II: the Del32–71-GH deletion mutant suppresses secretion of wild-type GH. Endocrinology 2000;141:883–890.

36 McGuinness L, Magoulas C, Sesay AK, Mathers K, Carmignac D, Manneville JB, Christian H, Phillips JA 3rd, Robinson IC: Autosomal dominant growth hormone deficiency disrupts secretory vesicles in vitro and in vivo in transgenic mice. Endocrinology 2003;144:720–731.

37 Hayashi Y, Yamamoto M, Ohmori S, Kamijo T, Ogawa M, Seo H: Inhibition of growth hormone (GH) secretion by a mutant GH-I gene product in neuroendocrine cells containing secretory granules: an implication for isolated GH deficiency inherited in an autosomal dominant manner. J Clin Endocrinol Metab 1999;84:2134–2139.

38 Graves TK, Patel S, Dannies PS, Hinkle PM: Misfolded growth hormone causes fragmentation of the Golgi apparatus and disrupts endoplasmic reticulum-to-Golgi traffic. J Cell Sci 2001;114:3685–3694.

39 Lewis UJ, Sinha YN, Haro LS: Variant forms and fragments of human growth hormone in serum. Acta Paediatr Suppl 1994;399:29–31.

40 Binder G, Keller E, Mix M, Massa GG, Stokvis-Brantsma WH, Wit JM, Ranke MB: Isolated GH deficiency with dominant inheritance: new mutations, new insights. J Clin Endocrinol Metab 2001;86:3877–3881.

41 Millar DS, Lewis MD, Horan M, Newsway V, Easter TE, Gregory JW, Fryklund L, Norin M, Crowne EC, Davies SJ, Edwards P, Kirk J, Waldron K, Smith PJ, Phillips JA 3rd, Scanlon MF, Krawczak M, Cooper DN, Procter AM: Novel mutations of the growth hormone 1 (GH1) gene disclosed by modulation of the clinical selection criteria for individuals with short stature. Hum Mutat 2003;21:424–440.

42 Mullis PE, Robinson IC, Salemi S, Eblé A, Besson A, Vuissoz JM, Deladoey J, Simon D, Czernichow P, Binder G: Isolated autosomal dominant growth hormone deficiency: an evolving pituitary deficit? A multicenter follow-up study. J Clin Endocrinol Metab 2005;90:2089–2096.

43 Salemi S, Yousefi S, Baltensberger K, Robinson IC, Eblé A, Simon D, Czernichow P, Binder G, Sonnet E, Mullis PE: Variability of isolated autosomal dominant GH deficiency (IGHD II): impact of the P89L GH mutation on clinical follow-up and GH secretion. Eur J Endocrinol 2005;153:791–802.

44 Fintini D, Salvatori R, Salemi S, Otten B, Ubertini GN, Cambiaso P, Mullis PE: Autosomal dominant growth hormone deficiency (IGHD II) with normal GH-1 gene. Horm Res 2006;65:76–82.

45 Fleisher TA, White RM, Broder S, Nissley SP, Blaese RM, Mulvihill JJ, Olive G, Waldmann TA: X-linked hypogammaglobulinemia and isolated growth hormone deficiency. N Engl J Med 1980;302:1429–1439.

46 Sitz KV, Burks AW, Williams LW, Kemp SF, Steele RW: Confirmation of X-linked hyogammaglobulinemia with isolated growth hormone deficiency as a disease entity. J Pediatr 1990;116:292–294.

47 Conley ME, Burks AW, Herrod, HG, Puck JM: Molecular analysis of X-linked agammaglobulinemia and isolated growth hormone deficiency. J Pediatr 1991;119:392–397.

48 Duriez B, Duquesnoy P, Dastot F, Bougnères P, Amselem S, Goossens M: An exon-skipping mutation in the btk gene of a patient with X-linked agammaglobulinemia and isolated growth hormone deficiency. FEBS Lett 1994;346:165–170.

49 Attie KM, Carlsson LM, Rundle AC, Sherman BM: Evidence for partial growth hormone insensitivity among patients with idiopathic short stature. The National Cooperative Growth Study. J Pediatr 1995;127:244–250.
50 Buckway CK, Guevara-Aguirre J, Pratt KL, Burren CP, Rosenfeld RG: The IGF-I generation test revisited: a marker of GH sensitivity. J Clin Endocrinol Metab 2001;86:5176–5183.
51 Laron Z, Pertzelan A, Mannheimer S: Genetic pituitary dwarfism with high serum concentration of growth hormone: a new inborn error of metabolism? Isr J Med Sci 1966;2:152–155.
52 Woods KA, Dastot F, Preece MA, Clark AJ, Postel-Vinay MC, Chatelain PG, Ranke MB, Rosenfeld RG, Amselem S, Savage MO: Phenotype: genotype relationships in growth hormone insensitivity syndrome. J Clin Endocrinol Metab 1997;82:3529–3535.
53 Hwa V, Little B, Kofoed EM, Rosenfeld RG: Transcriptional regulation of insulin-like growth factor-I by interferon-γ requires STAT-5b. J Biol Chem 2004; 279:2728–2736.
54 Kofoed EM, Hwa V, Little B, Woods KA, Buckway CK, Tsubaki J, Pratt KL, Bezrodnik L, Jasper H, Tepper A, Heinrich JJ, Rosenfeld RG: Growth hormone insensitivity associated with a STAT5b mutation. N Engl J Med 2003;349: 1139–1147.
55 Hwa V, Little B, Adiyaman P, Kofoed EM, Pratt KL, Ocal G, Berberoglu M, Rosenfeld RG: Severe growth hormone insensitivity resulting from total absence of signal transducer and activator of transcription 5b. J Clin Endocrinol Metab 2005;90:4260–4266.
56 Woods KA, Camacho-Hubner C, Savage MO, Clark AJ: Intrauterine growth retardation and postnatal growth failure associated with deletion of the insulin-like growth factor I gene. N Engl J Med 1996;335:1363–1367.
57 Walenkamp MJ, Karperien M, Pereira AM, Hilhorst-Hofstee Y, van Doorn J, Chen JW, Mohan S, Denley A, Forbes B, van Duyvenvoorde HA, van Thiel SW, Sluimers CA, Bax JJ, de Laat JA, Breuning MB, Romijn JA, Wit JM: Homozygous and heterozygous expression of a novel insulin-like growth factor-I mutation. J Clin Endocrinol Metab 2005; 90:2855–2864.
58 Kowarski AA, Schneider J, Ben-Galim E, Weldon VV, Daughaday WH: Growth failure with normal serum RIA-GH and low somatomedin activity: somatomedin restoration and growth acceleration after exogenous GH. J Clin Endocrinol Metab 1978;47: 461–464.
59 Salerno M, Balestrieri B, Matrecano E, Officioso A, Rosenfeld RG, Di Maio S, Fimiani G, Ursini MV, Pignata C: Abnormal GH receptor signaling in children with idiopathic short stature. J Clin Endocrinol Metab 2001;86:3882–3888.
60 Binder G, Benz MR, Elmlinger M, Pflaum CD, Strasburger CJ, Ranke MB: Reduced human growth hormone (hGH) bioactivity without a defect of the *GH-1* gene in three patients with rhGH responsive growth failure. Clin Endocrinol (Oxf) 1999;51:89–95.
61 Takahashi Y, Kaji H, Okimura Y, Goji K, Abe H, Chihara K: Brief report: short stature caused by a mutant growth hormone. N Engl J Med 1996;334:432–436.
62 Takahashi Y, Chihara K: Clinical significance and molecular mechanisms of bioinactive growth hormone. Int J Mol Med 1998;2:287–291.
63 Takahashi Y, Shirono H, Arisaka O, Takahashi K, Yagi T, Koga J, Kaji H, Okimura Y, Abe H, Tanaka T, Chihara K: Biologically inactive growth hormone caused by an amino acid substitution. J Clin Invest 1997;100:1159–1165.
64 Besson A, Salemi S, Deladoey J, Vuissoz JM, Eble A, Bidlingmaier M, Burgi S, Honegger U, Fluck C, Mullis PE: Short stature caused by a biologically inactive mutant growth hormone (GH-C53S). J Clin Endocrinol Metab 2005;90:2493–2499.

Growth Hormone Deficiency of Known Origin within KIGS (Code No. 2.1.1–2.1.6)

Michael B. Ranke[a] Hanna Karlsson[b]

The group of patients with growth hormone deficiency (GHD) of known origin (code No. 2 ff.) consists of two major categories: (1) patients with congenital forms of GHD (code No. 2.1 ff.) and (2) patients with acquired forms of GHD (code No. 2.2 ff.). Patients with acquired forms are discussed by Jostel [this vol., pp. 240–249]. The various causes of congenital forms of GHD are discussed in the chapters by Mullis [this vol., pp. 189–201] and Darendeliler [this vol., pp. 213–239]. Table 1 lists the frequency of reported diagnoses with code No. 2.1 ff. according to the KIGS Aetiology Classification List. There were a total of 2,272 cases reported within this diagnostic category.

Commentary

The exact classification into the various diagnostic groups is difficult since it requires a detailed phenotypical description and analysis, modern imaging techniques and sophisticated biochemical and molecular genetic techniques. During the 20-year course of KIGS, many of the necessary techniques have just emerged recently and are not available to all investigators. In addition, the reporting to KIGS was/is not structured to collect the information which is required to make a fair appraisal of the plausibility of the diagnoses given by the investigators. Thus, the data were analysed according to the diagnoses provided by the investigators. The data show a multitude of patients within KIGS with diagnoses which are very rare and usually not seen by single investigators during their professional life. Thus, in a second step, a follow-up of these patients is needed in order to make a more thorough analysis. For example, it appears to be of interest to find out why 187 patients were classified under 'other' genetic causes of GHD (code No. 2.1.1.9), or which prenatal infections were considered the basis of GHD in the 19 patients coded under 2.1.4.9. The 173 patients with 'bioactive GH syndrome' and the 65 patients with 'functional GHD' also need a de-

[a] Paediatric Endocrinology Section
University Children's Hospital, University of Tübingen
Hoppe-Seyler-Strasse 1, DE–72076 Tübingen (Germany)
[b] Pfizer Endocrine Care
KIGS/KIMS/ACROSTUDY Medical Outcomes
Vetenskapsvägen 10, SE–191 90 Sollentuna (Sweden)

tailed analysis, since during the past years, only little information/evidence has emerged in the literature on these entities.

Amongst the patients within this diagnostic group, about half suffer from septo-optic dysplasia (SOD; n = 466) and empty sella syndrome (ESS) including pituitary aplasia (n = 578). There are sufficient data at the start of GH treatment, during prepubertal growth on GH and at near adult height (NAH) to analyse data in more detail. In order to allow for a comparison with idiopathic GHD (IGHD), two subcohorts were formed: (1) a very early onset GHD group (e.g., GH replacement at <2 years of age, multiple pituitary hormone deficiency) and (2) a group with GH onset between 7 and 8 years of age. The latter represents a typical prepubertal cohort of children with IGHD.

The cohorts with IGHD at the start of GH treatment (all), during the first prepubertal year on GH and at NAH are listed in table 2. At the start of GH therapy, the two groups showed a distinct quantitative difference. In comparison with prepubertal children (total n = 1,379), children with very early onset GHD (n = 227) had a higher birth length, whereas the midparental height (MPH) was less reduced and the maximum GH levels during testing and the basal insulin-like growth factor 1 (IGF-1) levels were lower. Height reduction was more severe in the early onset group, but the body mass index was lower. The GH dose at treatment start was higher. In both groups, the relative frequency of male patients was similar.

One hundred and eighty children with early onset GH and 1,064 prepubertal children were observed during at least 1 full prepubertal year on GH. The characteristics of these cohorts at the start of GH therapy did not differ significantly from the total cohorts of the two groups documented within KIGS. However, there were differences in the observed height response: height velocity (measured in centimetres/year) was higher in the early onset group, but height velocity ex-

Table 1. Frequency of cases according to diagnostic categories of the KIGS Aetiology Classification List (code No. 2.1 ff.)

KIGS code	Diagnosis	Cases (total n = 2,272)
2.1.1	Genetic cause of GHD	228
2.1.1.1	GH gene defect (type IA)	21
2.1.1.2	GH gene defect	16
2.1.1.3	GH-releasing hormone gene defect	4
2.1.1.9	Others	187
2.1.2	Central malformations	1,696
2.1.2.1	SOD	466
2.1.2.2	ESS (including pituitary aplasia)	578
2.1.2.3	Solitary central maxillary incisor syndrome	18
2.1.2.4	Midline palate cleft	91
2.1.2.5	Arachnoid cyst	55
2.1.2.6	Congenital hydrocephalus	76
2.1.2.7	Hypoplastic pituitary, missing stalk, ectopic posterior pituitary (hemimegalencephaly)	19
2.1.2.9	Others	377
2.1.3	Complex syndromes with congenital GHD	88
2.1.3.1	Fanconi pancytopenia	27
2.1.3.2	Rieger syndrome	1
2.1.3.3	Ectrodactyly-ectodermal dysplasia-clefting syndrome	3
2.1.3.9	Others	57
2.1.4	Prenatal infections	20
2.1.4.1	Rubella	1
2.1.4.9	Others	19
2.1.5	Bioinactive GH syndrome	173
2.1.5.1	Kowarski type	116
2.1.5.9	Others	57
2.1.6	Functional GHD	83
2.1.6.1	GH receptor defect (Laron type)	6
2.1.6.2	GH receptor/postreceptor defect	8
2.1.6.3	IGF resistance	4
2.1.6.9	Others	65

Table 2. IGHD patients <2 years (MPHD) and 7–8 years old at GH start

	<2 years			7–8 years			p
	median	10th centile	90th centile	median	10th centile	90th centile	
Background							
Patients	227 (65.6)			1,379 (65.9)			
Birth weight SDS	–0.2	–2.0	1.2	–0.8	–2.3	0.7	
Birth length SDS	–0.4	–2.6	1.5	–0.5	–2.3	1.2	
MPH SDS (Prader)	–0.4	–2.3	1.1	–1.5	–3.0	0.1	<0.01
Maximum GH, μg/l	1.9	0.2	7.0	6.1	1.5	9.3	<0.01
IGF-1 SDS	–2.6	–3.6	–0.7	–1.9	–3.4	–0.5	<0.01
MPHD, %	all			19.4			
At GH start							
Age, years	1.2	0.2	1.8	7.5	7.1	7.9	<0.01
Height SDS (Prader)	–3.7	–7.1	–1.0	–3.3	–4.8	–2.4	<0.01
BMI SDS	–0.7	–2.6	1.2	–0.3	–1.7	1.1	<0.01
GH dose, mg/kg/week	0.25	0.16	0.47	0.20	0.15	0.30	<0.01
First year on GH							
Patients	180 (66.1)			1,064 (65.8)			
Height velocity, cm/year	14.6	9.8	21.2	8.1	6.0	11.1	<0.01
Height velocity SDS (Prader)	0.8	–0.7	3.5	3.2	0.4	7.1	<0.01
Δ height SDS (Prader)	1.5	0.0	3.5	0.6	0.2	1.2	<0.01
Studentised residual (without maximum GH)	n.a.			–0.3	–1.4	1.0	
NAH							
Patients	38 (68.4)			185 (55.1)			
Age, years	17.7	16.4	21.1	17.2	14.9	20.0	
Height SDS (Prader)	–0.6	–2.7	1.0	–1.4	–3.1	0.0	<0.01
Height – MPH SDS (Prader)	–0.3	–2.0	1.2	–0.2	–2.0	1.1	
Total Δ height SDS (Prader)	4.1	0.8	6.4	2.2	0.9	3.6	<0.01

Figures in parentheses are percentages of male patients. MPHD = Multiple pituitary hormone deficiency; BMI = body mass index; n.a. = not available.

pressed in terms of the standard deviation score (SDS) was lower (due to the higher distribution of height velocity references during this age), and the change in the height SDS was higher.

Of the prepubertal group, 185 children had reached NAH. The height SDS was lower than in the normal population (median SDS –1.4) but almost the same if corrected for MPH (median SDS –0.2). The total (median) SDS gain was 2.2.

In the early onset group, only 38 had reached NAH. The median height SDS reached –0.6 SDS and was greater than in the prepubertal group; however, the height SDS corrected for MPH was similar (–0.3 SDS). The overall gain in height SDS was 4.1 SDS, being almost twice that observed in the prepubertal group.

The cohorts with SOD and ESS at the start of GH treatment (all), during the first prepubertal year on GH and at NAH are listed in table 3. At the start of GH treatment, the two groups showed a distinct quantitative difference. The frequency of boys was lower in the SOD (56%) compared

Table 3. SOD and ESS patients

	SOD			ESS			p
	median	10th centile	90th centile	median	10th centile	90th centile	
Background							
Patients	466 (55.6)			578 (69)			<0.01
Birth weight SDS	–0.3	–1.6	1.2	–0.5	–2.2	1.1	
Birth length SDS	0.3	–1.3	2.0	–0.3	–2.0	1.5	<0.01
MPH SDS (Prader)	0.3	–1.7	1.2	–0.9	–2.5	0.6	<0.01
Maximum GH, μg/l	2.5	0.7	7.1	2.4	0.4	9.2	
IGF-1 SDS	–2.8	–4.4	–1.7	–2.8	–4.3	–0.9	
MPHD, %	59.7			50.0			
At GH start							
Age, years	4.3	1.0	11.3	7.7	1.3	14.6	<0.01
Height SDS (Prader)	–3.0	–4.8	–0.7	–3.5	–5.8	–1.9	<0.01
BMI SDS	0.3	–1.7	2.2	–0.2	–2.0	1.8	<0.01
GH dose, mg/kg/week	0.24	0.15	0.33	0.20	0.14	0.31	
First year on GH							
Patients	331 (55.6)			382 (70.7)			
Height velocity, cm/year	10.8	6.8	15.1	10.7	6.9	16.8	
Height velocity SDS (Prader)	3.0	–0.9	8.7	4.3	0.2	9.8	<0.01
Δ height SDS (Prader)	1.0	0.1	2.0	1.1	0.4	2.3	
Studentised residual (without maximum GH)	–0.1	–2.4	2.0	0.5	–1.2	2.4	<0.01
NAH							
Patients	44 (43.2)			52 (65.4)			
Age, years	17.3	15.1	19.7	17.6	15.6	19.9	
Height SDS (Prader)	–1.1	–3.0	0.4	–1.3	–2.2	0.3	
Height – MPH SDS (Prader)	–0.8	–2.3	0.8	–0.3	–1.1	1.4	
Total Δ height SDS (Prader)	2.5	0.5	4.2	2.4	1.4	4.7	

Figures in parentheses are percentages of male patients. MPHD = Multiple pituitary hormone deficiency; BMI = body mass index.

with the ESS (69%) group. In comparison with SOD children (n = 466), those with ESS (n = 578) had a lower birth length, and MPH was more reduced. These parameters were higher than in the prepubertal group with IGHD. The maximum GH levels during testing and the basal IGF-1 levels were almost identical in SOD and ESS children and lower than in the GHD groups. The relative frequency of multiple pituitary hormone deficiency was 59.7% in SOD and 50.0% in ESS children. The age at GH treatment averaged 4.3 years in SOD patients. In ESS patients, the age was 7.7 years and resembled the prepubertal IGHD group. Height reduction was more severe in children with ESS, but the body mass index was lower. The GH dose at treatment start was similar. Overall, the ESS group resembled the prepubertal IGHD cohort.

Three hundred and thirty-one children with SOD and 382 with ESS were observed during at least 1 full prepubertal year on GH. The characteristics of these cohorts at the start of GH thera-

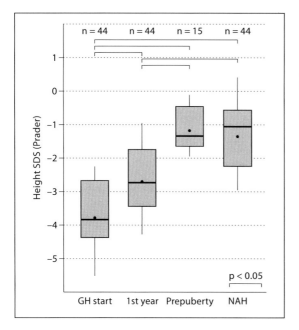

Fig. 1. Height SDS of the SOD cohort followed to NAH. Data at the start of treatment, after 1 year on GH, at puberty onset and at NAH are illustrated.

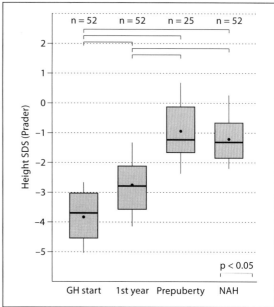

Fig. 2. Height SDS of the ESS cohort followed to NAH. Data at the start of treatment, after 1 year on GH, at puberty onset and at NAH are illustrated.

py did not differ significantly from the total cohorts of the two groups documented within KIGS. However, there were differences in the observed height response: height velocity (measured in centimetres/year) and the change in the height SDS were similar in both groups, whereas height velocity expressed in terms of the SDS was higher, and the studentised residual (score of observed – predicted height velocity) was higher in the ESS cohort. The first-year response to GH was equal (SOD) or better (ESS) in the two groups compared with prepubertal IGHD and early onset GHD.

Forty-four children of the SOD group and 52 of the ESS group had reached NAH. In contrast to the ESS group, the male to female ratio was near unity in the SOD group. The height SDS was lower than in the reference population (median SOD SDS –1.1; median ESS SDS –1.3), and if corrected for MPH, near normal in ESS (median SDS –0.3) but not much lower in SOD patients (median SDS –0.8). The total gain was a median SOD SDS of 2.5 and a median ESS SDS of 2.4. The course of height development in these groups is illustrated in figures 1 and 2.

Conclusion

Patient groups with early onset GHD, prepubertal IGHD, SOD and ESS differ in terms of their background, their presentation, their first prepubertal year of response to GH and their overall height outcomes. Differences in NAH occur despite the similarity of GH doses applied. This suggests that the various causes of GHD need to be treated according to the underlying cause and the individual response to GH. Identifying the causes of congenital GHD is thus an important task for treating physicians. In the future, detailed information about the aetiology of congenital forms of GH needs to be collected.

Growth Hormone Treatment of Children with Previous Craniopharyngioma: The KIGS Experience

David A. Price

The occurrence of craniopharyngioma (CP) is so rare that it has been difficult to define the optimal manner of tumour management, and after 5 decades, there is still controversy. The incidence of CP was recently reported as 1.4 per million children per year [1] confirming a much earlier report of 1.2 per million in the age range of 0–14 years [2]. The usual dilemma for tumour management is whether there should be an attempt at radical tumour surgery ('total' excision) with its potential for damage to surrounding central nervous system structures or whether there should be a deliberately more conservative surgical approach with postoperative radiotherapy to prevent recurrence of the tumour. However rarely a child with CP may present to the neurosurgeon, there is a larger population of survivors who have a very high incidence of pituitary insufficiency. These children fall under the aegis of paediatric endocrinologists and then adult endocrinologists. Presently, the number of survivors entered into international studies such as the Pfizer International Growth Study (KIGS) and the Pfizer International Metabolic Study is relatively large, being well over 1,000 in KIGS. There have been previous reports when the database was smaller [3–6].

This analysis studies three aspects of growth hormone (GH) treatment of children who had previously suffered a CP, namely the short-term response to GH over 1 year, prepubertal growth on GH treatment, and the final height outcome.

Methods

Two cohorts were selected and their case report forms examined.

Group 1
All children with CP entered into KIGS who had completed 1 year of GH treatment. The first year of treatment was defined by the minimal availability of height measurements at the start of treatment and also at 9–15 months after onset.

Group 2
Group 2 included those who had reached near adult height, defined as the height observed when GH therapy

Royal Manchester Children's Hospital, Hospital Road Pendlebury, Swinton, Manchester M27 4HA (UK)

Table 1. Characteristics of children with prior CP who completed 1 year of GH treatment before and at the start of GH treatment

Variable	n	Median	10th centile	90th centile
Birth weight SDS	922	−0.3	−1.6	1.1
Birth length SDS	611	0.2	−1.2	1.7
MPH SDS (Prader)	965	−0.4	−2.0	0.9
Maximum peak GH, μg/l	936	1.2	0.2	4.4
IGF-1 SDS	213	−3.1	−4.8	−1.2
At the start of GH treatment				
Age, years	1,141	10.5	5.2	15.6
Bone age, years	453	9.0	3.2	13.0
Height SDS (Prader)	1,141	−2.3	−4.2	−0.5
Height − MPH SDS	965	−1.8	−3.6	−0.9
Height velocity, cm/year	586	3.1	0.9	6.2
BMI SDS	1,140	1.2	−1.0	2.9

MPH = Midparental height; IGF-1 = insulin-like growth factor 1.

was discontinued, provided that treatment had lasted at least 1 year and was not terminated before the ages of 16 years in boys and 14 years in girls. Longitudinal growth on GH treatment was then divided into a prepubertal component and the remaining component. The onset of puberty was defined as the documentation of breast development B2 in girls and 4-ml testicular size in boys. Group 2 was compared with a group of children with idiopathic GH deficiency (IGHD) who had multiple pituitary hormone deficiencies (MPHD) and who had reached near adult height. Comparisons were also made between subgroups who had received different modes of tumour treatment (data not shown).

Results

First-Year Response

One thousand one hundred and forty-one children (649 boys and 492 girls) had completed a year's treatment with GH, and their characteristics at the start of GH treatment are documented in table 1. Parental heights were relatively low compared with the normal population, as was the child's birth weight. The affected children had severe GH deficiency and their insulin-like growth factor 1 levels were low before treatment. Heights before GH therapy were not necessarily below the normal centiles, but growth velocity was low. The median body mass index standard deviation score (BMI SDS) was raised, but not greatly so. There were minor differences between males and females, namely that the boys were slightly older at the start of GH treatment and had a slightly greater BMI. Only 14.5% of either sex were in puberty.

Limiting the first-year growth in response to GH to those who remained prepubertal (table 2), height velocity increased from 3.0 to 9.0 cm/year. This was greater than predicted from a model developed for prepubertal children with IGHD (which did not contain the predictor of the peak GH level during testing). Thus, the CP children were very sensitive to GH. Median BMI SDS fell from 1.2 to 0.9 over the year.

Prepubertal Growth on GH Treatment

Table 3 tabulates the longitudinal growth of 79 males and 89 females to near adult height and describes the prepubertal and pubertal components. There was no statistically significant difference between the sexes, but normally, there would have been an earlier onset of puberty in the girls. This may indicate a reluctance to induce puberty in females whilst on treatment with GH. Although both males and females started

Table 2. First-year growth response to GH in prepubertal children with prior CP

Variable	n	Median	10th centile	90th centile
At the start of GH treatment				
Age, years	657	9.0	4.6	14.0
Bone age, years	260	6.8	2.9	11.6
Height SDS (Prader)	657	−2.2	−4.0	−0.1
Height − MPH SDS	562	−1.7	−3.5	0.1
Height velocity, cm/year	355	3.0	1.0	6.1
BMI SDS	657	1.2	−0.9	3.0
Dose of GH, mg/kg/week	657	0.17	0.11	0.26
Frequency of injections	657	6	3	7
After 1 year of GH treatment				
Height SDS (Prader)	657	−1.4	−3.1	0.3
Height velocity, cm/year	657	9.0	5.6	12.9
BMI SDS	652	0.9	−1.1	2.8
Studentised residual of actual − predicted height velocity	272	0.4	−1.6	2.4

MPH = Midparental height.

Table 3. Longitudinal growth on GH treatment until onset of puberty and to near adult height in boys and girls

Variable	Males				Females			
	n	median	10th centile	90th centile	n	median	10th centile	90th centile
At the start of GH treatment								
Age, years	79	9.7	4.9	13.6	89	9.0	5.2	11.8
Height SDS (Prader)	79	−2.3	−3.8	−0.5	89	−2.2	−4.4	−0.6
Height − MPH SDS	70	−1.7	−3.4	0.1	74	−1.8	−4.0	−0.2
BMI SDS	79	1.2	−1.1	2.5	89	0.9	−0.8	2.6
At the start of puberty								
Age, years	42	13.7	12.2	16.9	49	13.5	11.6	16.0
Height SDS (Prader)	42	−0.2	−1.8	1.1	49	−0.5	−1.7	1.4
Height − MPH SDS	37	−0.3	−1.6	1.8	40	0.1	−2.0	1.3
Δ height SDS from GH start	42	1.6	0.9	2.8	49	1.6	0.5	3.8
BMI SDS	42	1.0	−1.1	2.6	49	0.5	−1.3	2.9
Mean prepubertal GH dose, mg/kg/week	42	0.16	0.09	0.24	49	0.16	0.09	0.27
At near adult height								
Age, years	79	18.6	16.9	20.7	89	17.5	15.5	20.7
Height SDS (Prader)	79	−0.5	−2.2	1.3	89	−0.5	−2.5	1.5
Height − MPH SDS	70	−0.2	−1.6	1.6	74	0.0	−1.6	1.4
Δ height SDS from GH start	79	1.6	0.3	3.0	89	1.7	−0.6	4.1
Δ height SDS from puberty start	42	−0.2	−0.9	1.5	49	0.1	−1.7	1.4
BMI SDS	77	1.0	−1.2	3.0	89	1.1	−0.6	2.8
Mean pubertal GH dose, mg/kg/week	42	0.17	0.09	0.24	49	0.15	0.08	0.26
Years on GH	79	8.1	4.6	12.7	89	7.3	4.7	12.0

MPH = Midparental height.

Table 4. Comparison of height and BMI at the start and end of GH treatment between children with prior CP and children with MPHD associated with IGHD

Variable	CP median	n	MPHD median	n	p value
Height SDS at the start of GH	–0.1	168	–1.0	686	0.0001
BMI SDS at the start of GH	1.0	166	0.1	670	0.0001
Near adult height SDS	–0.1	168	–1.0	686	0.0001
BMI SDS at the end of GH	1.0	166	0.1	670	0.0001

GH treatment at a median height SDS of –2.3 and –2.2, respectively, by the onset of puberty, both median values for the height SDS fell within the normal centiles, the Δ increments being 1.6 SDS. There was no useful increment in the SDS during puberty as reflected by the median values, although there were individuals who gained a great deal during puberty. Median values for the near adult height SDS show that normal heights were achieved. The BMI SDS at the start of GH therapy had positive values and showed a decrease by onset of puberty as in the first-year growth above, but by the end of treatment, there was a tendency to increase again. The doses of GH used tended to be modest.

Effects of the Mode of Tumour Treatment
Tumour treatment was done by surgery alone in 599 children, by surgery and irradiation in 310, and by irradiation alone in 36. There were no consistent statistical differences in auxological outcome according to tumour treatment modalities.

Comparison of Near Adult Height and BMI of Children with Prior CP and IGHD Children with MPHD
The height SDS and BMI SDS at the start and end of GH treatment are compared in table 4. Children with CP were taller at the start of GH treatment and had a greater BMI SDS than children with MPHD. These differences continued at the completion of GH treatment.

Discussion

Children with prior CP have been consistently reported in KIGS [3–7]. Now, one can report on over 600 children who have completed 1 year of treatment with GH. The caveats made previously [7] about the selection of patients in a safety and efficacy study need to be repeated. Presumably, patients who are recognised early in the disease process to have a bad prognosis, perhaps with very early recurrence or with severe hypothalamic damage, are less likely to be considered for GH treatment and would be excluded from such a study, and thus, a more optimistic picture of the condition is given. An earlier report indicated that recurrence during GH treatment did not have a significant effect on growth response [6]. This might be misleading in that KIGS does not necessarily record the exact reasons for withdrawal from the study, although we believe there would be good documentation from clinics committed to the study.

There is evidence that the mode of tumour treatment does affect tumour recurrence in that surgery alone without postoperative irradiation carries a greater risk of recurrence than surgery combined with radiotherapy [8, 9], although there is one dissenting view that radiotherapy does not lower the risk [10]. Furthermore, there is concern that more radical or aggressive surgery may cause greater surrounding neural damage, especially to the hypothalamus [9], and this can result in severe morbidity. Therefore, it is of value to know that the growth response is not worsened in the group which received more conservative surgery followed by irradiation. It is also reassuring that GH treatment itself does not increase the recurrence rate [8, 11, 12].

It is puzzling to note that the birth weight SDS and midparental height are slightly lower than expected in the normal population. Could they represent unknown genetic or environmental aetiologies? Other characteristics at the start of GH treatment are representative of acquired GH deficiency, the children being relatively tall and having severe GH deficiency. Obesity is often a characteristic of children and adults who had prior CP, and it is noteworthy that the median BMI SDS at the start of GH therapy is positive. Geffner et al. [13] showed evidence from KIGS that children with CP were more prone to weight gain than children with other forms of acquired GH deficiency and that GH treatment had only a slight benefit on gain in BMI. This is consistent with the present findings that although there was a decrease in BMI in the short term, this was not sustained after longer GH treatment.

There is great interest in long-term quality of life, morbidity and mortality in patients with prior CP. Tomlinson et al. [14] found that mortality in those with CP was nearly 10 times greater than for other causes of hypopituitarism. Decreased quality of life in adults with prior CP has been recorded and analysed in the Pfizer International Metabolic Database [15, 16] and by other groups [17, 18]. Müller et al. [18] found that hypothalamic involvement, tumour progression and relapse had long-term negative effects on the quality of life of survivors and emphasised the effect of severe obesity. GH treatment can have no effect on factors involved with tumour management but may have a beneficial effect on lipid metabolism, if unable to prevent an increase in BMI over the long term.

During the first year of GH treatment, there was a good response, in fact superior to that of patients with IGHD, as evidenced by the studentised residual of observed minus predicted response. Given this good sensitivity to GH, better results may have been achieved by less modest doses of GH. The BMI SDS fell during the first year and up to the onset of puberty.

The gain in the height SDS was good up until the onset of puberty. Thereafter, there was no biologically significant increase in the median height SDS at near adult height. However, there was a wide range of pubertal growth, and some individuals made good continuing gains. The end result was better than that previously reported [7, 19, 20]. The Δ height SDS gain was +1.6 in males and +1.7 in females, with resulting adult heights within the normal range in most and within the midparental target range in all. Interestingly, there was a rise in the BMI SDS by the end of GH treatment. There is a marked contrast between the auxology of children with CP and those with idiopathic hypopituitarism as shown in table 4. The latter do not do so well in terms of adult height but remain slim with a normal BMI.

Conclusions

As reported previously from KIGS, there was a good response to GH in the short and long term with correction of the height deficit caused by severe GH deficiency. This sensitivity to GH is unaffected by the mode of tumour treatment. GH replacement is now a standard, safe and integral part of management of children with CP. In the future, more attention will need to be paid to the prevention and amelioration of long-term morbidity of survivors.

References

1 Haupt R, Magnani C, Pavaello M, Caruso S, Dama E, Garre ML: Epidemiological aspects of craniopharyngioma. J Pediatr Endocrinol Metab 2006; 19(suppl 1):289–293.
2 Blair V, Birch LM: Patterns and temporal trends in the incidence of malignant disease in children. 2. Solid tumours of childhood. Eur J Cancer 1994;30A: 1498–1511.
3 Price DA: Growth response in the first year of growth hormone treatment in prepubertal children with organic growth hormone deficiency. Acta Paediatr Scand Suppl 1990;130:131–137.
4 Price DA: Characteristics and first year response to growth hormone of children with craniopharyngioma. Kabi International Growth Study Report 1990;5:25–28.
5 Price DA, Jonsson P: Effect of growth hormone treatment in children with craniopharyngioma with reference to the KIGS database. Acta Paediatr Suppl 1996;417:83–85.
6 Price DA, Wilton P, Jonsson P, Albertsson-Wikland K, Chatelain P, Cutfield W, Rank MB: Efficacy and safety of growth hormone treatment in children with prior craniopharyngioma: an analysis of the Pharmacia and Upjohn International Growth Database (KIGS) from 1988 to 1996. Horm Res 1998;49: 91–97.
7 Price DA: Growth hormone treatment in children with craniopharygioma in KIGS; in Ranke MB, Wilton P (eds): Growth Hormone Therapy in KIGS – 10 Years' Experience. Leipzig, Heidelberg, 1999, pp 189–198.
8 Clayton PE, Price DA, Shalet SM, Gattamanemi HR: Craniopharyngioma recurrence and growth hormone therapy (letter). Lancet 1988;i:642.
9 Merchant TE, Kiehna EN, Sanford RA, Mulhern RK, Thompson SJ, Wison MW, Lustig RH, Kun LE: Craniopharyngioma: the St Jude Children's Research Hospital experience 1984–2001. Int J Radiat Oncol Biol Phys 2002;53: 533–542.
10 Bulow B, Attewell R, Hagmar L, Malmstrom P, Nordstrom C-H, Erfurth EM: Postoperative prognosis in craniopharyngioma with respect to cardiovascular mortality, survival and tumor recurrence. J Clin Endocrinol Metab 1998;83:3897–3904.
11 Wilton P: Rate of relapse of craniopharyngioma in children treated with growth hormone. KIGS Biannual Report 1992;8:42–47.
12 Karavitaki N, Warner JT, Marland A, Shine B, Ryan F, Arnold J, Turner HE, Wass JA: GH replacement does not increase the risk of recurrence in patients with craniopharyngioma. Clin Endocrinol (Oxf) 2006;64:556–560.
13 Geffner M, Lundberg ML, Kotowska-Haggstrom, Abs R, Verhelst J, Erfurth E, Kendall-Taylor P, Price DA, Jonsson P, Bakker B: Changes in height, weight, and BMI in children with craniopharyngioma after three years of growth hormone therapy: analysis of KIGS (Pfizer International Growth Database). J Clin Endocrinol Metab 2004; 89:5435–5440.
14 Tomlinson JW, Holden N, Hills RK, Wheatley K, Bates AS, Sheppard MC, Stewart PM, the West Midlands Prospective Hypopituitary Study Group: Association between premature mortality and hypopituitarism. Lancet 2001;357:425–431.
15 Kendall-Taylor P, Jonsson P, Abs R, Erfurth E, Koltowska-Haggstrom M, Price DA, Verhelst J: The clinical, metabolic, endocrine features and quality of life in adults with childhood-onset craniopharyngioma compared with adult-onset craniopharyngioma. Eur J Endocrinol 2005;152:557–567.
16 Verhelst J, Kendall-Taylor P, Erfurth EM, Price DA, Geffner M, Koltowska-Haggstrom M, Jonsson P, Wilton P, Abs R: Baseline characteristics and response to 2 years of growth hormone (GH) replacement of hypopituitary patients with GH deficiency due to adult-onset craniopharyngioma in comparison with non-functioning pituitary adenoma: data from KIMS (Pfizer International Metabolic Database). J Clin Endocrinol Metab 2005;90:4636–4643.
17 Müller HL, Bueb K, Bartels U, Roth C, Harz K, Graf N, Korinthenberg R, Bettendorf M, Kuhl J, Gutjahr P, Sorensen N, Calaminus G: Obesity after childhood craniopharyngioma – German multicenter study on pre-operative risk factors and quality of life. Klin Pädiatr 2001;213:244–249.
18 Müller HL, Bruhnken G, Emser A, Faldum A, Etavard-Gorris N, Gebhardt U, Kolb R, Sörensen N: Longitudinal study on quality of life in 102 survivors of childhood craniopharyngioma. Childs Nerv Syst 2005;21:975–980.
19 Burns EC, Tanner JM, Preece MA, Cameron N: Growth hormone treatment in children with craniopharyngioma: final height status. Clin Endocrinol 1981;14:587–595.
20 De Vile CJ, Grant DB, Hayward RD, Stanhope R: Growth and sequelae of craniopharyngioma. Arch Dis Child 1996;75:108–114.

Growth Hormone Treatment in Rare Disorders: The KIGS Experience

Feyza Darendeliler

Short stature is a common feature of many types of genetic syndromes. Poor growth in these conditions reflects either some unknown abnormality in growth hormone (GH) action or an intrinsic defect of growth at the cellular level. GH deficiency (GHD) may also be encountered in some of these syndromes [1]. Since the advent of recombinant GH, several researchers have investigated the effect of GH treatment on genetic syndromes with short stature, whether associated with GHD or not. This chapter will discuss clinical findings and growth characteristics in some of these syndromes, as well as results of GH treatment reported in the literature, if any. The literature review of each syndrome will be followed by the auxological characteristics and treatment results obtained from the KIGS database regarding the respective syndrome.

The disorders will be presented in two parts. Part 1 consists of rare syndromes and part 2 mainly of rare disorders associated with the central nervous system or pituitary malformations. The diagnosis of the patients is based on the data submitted by the reporting physicians. It should be kept in mind that the diagnosis in most of the syndromes in part 1, except for Down syndrome (DS) and Fanconi anemia (FA), depends on the clinical findings. The diagnoses in some of the rare disorders in part 2 mainly depend on cranial imaging, for example, the diagnosis of empty sella. The imaging techniques that the investigators have used may have varied in the course of time and may not have been reported in full detail to the KIGS database. The sensitivity of the imaging method may vary among reporting centers. Genetic analyses might have contributed to the diagnosis of some of these disorders, like in hypoplastic anterior pituitary, had it been possible. Therefore, it should be kept in mind that the diagnoses mainly depend on the findings reported by the physicians, and these drawbacks may be taken as the weak point in this presentation. However, the large number of patients in each disorder should be considered as the strong part of the presentation.

Department of Pediatrics, Istanbul Faculty of Medicine
Istanbul University, TR–34390 Capa – Istanbul (Turkey)

Table 1. Results of GH treatment in rare syndromes with longitudinal data in the KIGS database

	AS				CdLS				DS			
	n	median	10th centile	90th centile	n	median	10th centile	90th centile	n	median	10th centile	90th centile
Start of GH treatment												
Age, years	17	7.8	5.1	11.2	12	8.0	1.8	11.0	46	4.8	1.2	11.6
Height SDS (Prader)	17	–3.4	–4.4	–2.3	12	–3.8	–7.3	–2.7	46	–4.0	–6.3	–2.8
Height – MPH SDS (Prader)	17	–2.3	–2.8	–0.2	11	–3.5	–5.3	–1.4	38	–3.2	–4.8	–1.1
Height velocity SDS	5	–1.8	–2.3	–0.6	6	–1.0	–3.0	–0.4	22	–2.2	–4.5	–0.8
BMI SDS	17	0.1	–2.3	1.2	12	–0.4	–3.5	0.4	46	0.2	–1.8	1.7
GH dose, mg/kg/week	17	0.22	0.15	0.31	12	0.23	0.15	0.42	46	0.21	0.17	0.31
Injection/week	17	6	4	7	12	6	4	7	46	7	4	7
1 year of GH therapy												
Age, years	17	8.7	6.1	12.2	12	9.0	2.7	12.2	46	6.0	2.2	12.5
Height SDS (Prader)	17	–2.9	–4.3	–1.9	12	–3.2	–6.2	–2.4	46	–3.5*	–5.6	–1.5
Height – MPH SDS (Prader)	17	–1.8	–2.5	–0.3	11	–3.0	–5.1	–0.8	38	–2.3*	–4.2	–0.7
Height velocity SDS	17	2.5*	–1.1	4.6	12	0.9*	–1.9	2.7	46	1.5*	–0.7	7.0
Δ height SDS	17	0.6	0.1	0.7	12	0.5	0.2	0.9	46	0.7	0.1	1.3
BMI SDS	17	–0.2	–0.8	1.3	12	–0.7	–3.0	0.9	46	0.4	–1.8	2.0
SR	10	–0.9	–2.4	0.3	4	–1.5	–3.2	–1.0	23	–1.2	–2.4	0.0

BMI = Body mass index. * $p < 0.05$, comparison of values between the start and 1 year of GH therapy.

Methods

The methodology for analyzing the growth data of the patients described in this chapter corresponds to that used for other growth disorders in this book, using Prader standards for the calculation of standard deviation scores (SDS) for growth parameters. Growth data of the longitudinally followed prepubertal children for each disorder are given if the numbers are adequate (n ≥ 10). These are summarized in tables 1 and 2. Otherwise, results of cross-sectional data are given, summarized in table 3. Studentized residuals (SR), the difference between the actual height velocity and predicted height velocity based on the KIGS model for idiopathic GHD (IGHD), is used for comparison of the child's growth response with what would have been observed in IGHD [2]. Median values are given with the 10th and 90th percentile values. Nonparametric tests were used in comparison with the medians only in the longitudinally followed prepubertal children. If the number of subjects in each group was <10, even if there is a significant difference between the groups, it was not taken for granted. Significance is denoted for $p < 0.05$.

Rare Syndromes

Aarskog Syndrome

Aarskog syndrome (AS), first described by Aarskog in 1970 [3], is characterized by a typical facies, shawl scrotum and short stature. Since the inclusion of new features in the definition of AS, the term 'faciogenital dysplasia' is now commonly used to designate the syndrome [4].

Clinical Criteria for Diagnosis. Phenotypic variability exists between family members and variability of expression between the sexes, males typically being more severely affected than females [5]. The primary diagnostic criteria of AS [5] include short stature, hypertelorism, a broad nasal bridge, a short nose with anteverted nares, a long philtrum, maxillary hypoplasia with or without malocclusion, a crease below the lower lip, abnormal auricles with fleshy lobules, short and broad hands, short fifth fingers with clinodactyly and a shawl scrotum. The secondary criteria include 'widow's peak' hair pattern, ptosis,

	KS				WBS				FA				DBA			
	n	median	10th centile	90th centile	n	median	10th centile	90th centile	n	median	10th centile	90th centile	n	median	10th centile	90th centile
	10	7.6	4.5	13.5	13	5.2	2.8	8.1	22	10.1	1.2	13.3	11	10.6	7.9	13.0
	10	−3.4	−4.8	−2.4	13	−4.3	−6.6	−2.9	22	−4.9	−6.4	−1.7	11	−2.4	−4.7	−2.0
	6	−2.0	−2.7	−0.8	13	−2.9	−5.4	−1.8	21	−3.5	−5.8	−0.5	10	−2.6	−4.3	−1.3
	4	−1.8	−6.8	−0.7	9	−1.8	−4.1	−1.0	8	−1.9	−9.8	4.0	8	−2.0	−3.8	1.1
	10	0.3	−1.5	1.9	13	−0.8	−2.3	0.2	22	−0.7	−2.4	1.4	11	0.4	−2.3	0.8
	10	0.17	0.14	0.33	13	0.22	0.16	0.34	22	0.19	0.14	0.33	11	0.20	0.17	0.32
	10	5.5	2.5	7	13	6	3	7	22	7	3	7	11	7	6	7
	10	8.5	5.5	14.5	13	6.3	3.8	9.2	22	11.1	2.3	14.3	11	11.6	8.9	13.9
	10	−2.8	−4.3	−1.7	13	−3.7	−5.2	−2.6	22	−3.5	−5.7	−1.0	11	−2.1	−4.1	−1.8
	6	−1.3	−1.7	−0.6	13	−2.5	−4.9	−0.7	21	−2.4	−5.3	0.3	10	−2.1	−3.7	−1.1
	10	1.8*	−0.9	3.8	13	0.8*	−0.7	4.0	22	1.5	−0.6	3.7	11	1.3*	−1.6	4.1
	10	0.7	0.2	1.0	13	0.4	0.2	1.1	22	0.7	0.3	1.9	11	0.4	0.2	0.8
	10	0.1	−2.0	1.9	13	−1.3	−2.0	0.6	22	−1.5	−2.6	0.9	11	0.2	−2.3	0.4
	2	−0.9	−0.9	−0.9	9	−1.7	−2.3	−1.1	7	−1.4	−2.2	1.7	3	−2.3	−2.4	−1.1

downward slanting palpebral fissures, joint hyperextensibility, broad feet with bulbous toes, cryptorchidism, inguinal hernia and mild interdigital webbing. Short stature, present in up to 90% of children with AS, is usually disproportionate, with an increased upper to lower segment ratio [5, 6]. Head circumference is usually normal, but macrocephaly may be encountered [5]. Ophthalmological findings, including strabismus, ophthalmoplegia, large cornea, esotropia, nystagmus and amblyopia, have been reported [7]. Dental findings include delayed eruption of permanent teeth, hypodontia, dental malocclusion and enamel hypoplasia [8]. There is partial expression of the syndrome in girls, which mainly consists of short stature, short and broad hands and feet, and mild facial features [5]. Intelligence is reported as normal or in the mildly retarded range [3, 5, 9]. Hyperactive behavior and symptoms of attention deficit disorder are frequently present. Behavioral problems regress after adolescence, and social integration of adults is satisfactory. The lifespan is normal, as is fertility, except in cases which had undergone orchiopexy for cryptorchidism at older ages [3].

Molecular Genetics. The inheritance is X-linked recessive in most cases [10]. Male-to-male transmission has been reported, which suggests autosomal dominant inheritance with a strong sex influence [11]. The faciogenital dysplasia gene (FGD1) has been mapped to chromosome Xp11.21 [12]. Mutations in the FGD1 gene have been reported in some families; however, the low frequency of mutations suggests that other genes may be involved [12, 13].

Growth. Disproportionate short stature is one of the main features of AS. Birth weight and length are usually in the lower half of the normal range [6, 14]. In about a third of children, growth becomes impaired during the first year of life due to feeding difficulties or recurrent respiratory tract infections [14]. In the remaining children, growth becomes impaired between 1 and 3 years of age. Nearly all children drop below the third

Table 2. Results of GH treatment in other rare disorders with longitudinal data in the KIGS database

	Arachnoid cyst				Empty sella			
	n	median	10th centile	90th centile	n	median	10th centile	90th centile
Start of GH treatment								
Age, years	30	7.0	3.5	12.4	382	6.2	1.1	13.1
Height SDS (Prader)	30	−2.6	−4.9	−1.0	382	−3.6	−5.7	−1.8
Height − MPH SDS (Prader)	28	−1.7	−3.1	−0.1	347	−2.7	−5.0	−0.7
Height velocity SDS	15	−2.6	−3.7	−0.1	144	−2.1	−4.6	0.6
BMI SDS	30	0.4	−1.5	2.9	382	−0.3	−1.9	1.6
GH dose, mg/kg/week	30	0.22	0.13	0.33	382	0.20	0.15	0.31
Injection/week	30	7	3	7	382	7	5	7
1 year of GH therapy								
Age, years	30	7.8	4.5	13.4	382	7.1	2.2	14.0
Height SDS (Prader)	30	−1.8*	−3.8	−0.1	382	−2.4*	−4.5	−0.5
Height − MPH SDS (Prader)	28	−0.7*	−2.7	−0.5	347	−1.6*	−3.5	0.4
Height velocity SDS	30	4.2*	0.0	9.5	379	4.3*	0.2	9.8
Δ height SDS	30	0.9	0.3	1.8	378	1.1	0.4	2.3
BMI SDS	30	0.2	−1.8	2.7	382	−0.5	−1.9	1.1
SR	17	0.4	−0.2	2.0	197	0.5	−1.2	2.4

BMI = Body mass index. * $p < 0.05$, comparison of values between the start and 1 year of GH therapy.

Table 3. Results of GH treatment in rare syndromes with cross-sectional data in the KIGS database

	Floating-Harbor syndrome				RTS			
	n	median	10th centile	90th centile	n	median	10th centile	90th centile
Start of GH treatment								
Age, years	12	7.7	5.5	12.0	13	10.4	2.3	14.4
Height SDS (Prader)	12	−4.6	−5.5	−3.3	13	−4.0	−6.0	−2.9
Height − MPH SDS (Prader)	12	−4.4	−4.8	−2.2	10	−3.1	−8.2	−2.0
Height velocity SDS	5	−1.2	−4.1	0.5	4	−0.9	−2.7	1.5
BMI SDS	12	0.4	−1.9	0.8	13	0.0	−2.9	1.5
GH dose, mg/kg/week	12	0.24	0.14	0.46	13	0.23	0.15	0.33
Injection/week	12	7	6	7	13	7	6	7
1 year of GH therapy								
Age, years	9	8.7	6.0	13.0	9	11.4	3.4	13.6
Height SDS (Prader)	9	−4.2	−6.1	−1.5	9	−3.5	−8.6	−2.2
Height − MPH SDS (Prader)	9	−3.9	−4.9	−1.0	7	−2.9	−7.4	−1.3
Height velocity SDS	9	1.5	−4.4	5.6	9	1.6	−1.5	4.8
Δ height SDS	9	0.6	0.6	1.0	9	0.7	0.3	1.9
BMI SDS	9	−0.7	−3.5	2.4	9	−0.3	−2.9	2.4

BMI = Body mass index.

Midline palate cleft				SMMCI syndrome				Congenital hydrocephalus			
n	median	10th centile	90th centile	n	median	10th centile	90th centile	n	median	10th centile	90th centile
66	4.7	0.4	10.8	11	6.6	1.2	11.4	52	6.0	3.8	10.6
66	−4.1	−6.5	−2.2	11	−4.8	−5.0	−3.3	52	−3.7	−5.7	−2.5
61	−3.0	−5.5	−1.1	10	−3.8	−5.1	−2.3	43	−2.9	−5.3	−1.3
27	−1.7	−3.0	0.8	5	−2.0	−3.2	0.2	27	−1.5	−4.5	1.7
66	−0.4	−2.7	1.4	11	0.3	−1.7	0.8	52	0.1	−1.6	1.7
66	0.20	0.12	0.32	11	0.22	0.16	0.33	52	0.18	0.14	0.30
66	6.5	3	7	11	6	4	7	52	7	3	7
66	5.6	1.5	11.8	11	7.5	2.4	12.2	52	7.0	4.9	11.8
66	−3.0*	−5.1	−0.9	11	−2.7*	−4.1	−1.7	52	−3.1*	−4.7	−1.4
61	−2.0*	−4.4	0.0	10	−1.7*	−3.5	−1.1	43	−2.4*	−4.1	−0.3
66	2.5*	−0.6	7.3	11	3.7*	−2.2	6.9	52	2.7*	−1.0	9.2
66	1.1	0.2	2.6	11	0.8	0.7	2.6	52	0.7	0.2	1.7
66	−0.4	−2.9	1.2	11	0.0	−2.5	0.4	52	−0.4	−1.9	1.5
25	0.2	−1.2	2.1	7	0.2	−0.4	3.0	27	−0.5	−2.5	2.1

CHH				KFS				Hypoplastic anterior pituitary			
n	median	10th centile	90th centile	n	median	10th centile	90th centile	n	median	10th centile	90th centile
14	9.1	3.1	11.2	12	7.8	2.3	12.6	19	9.7	1.0	14.5
14	−5.2	−6.7	−3.5	12	−3.8	−6.1	−2.5	19	−3.2	−6.8	−1.7
12	−4.4	−7.2	−2.4	10	−2.6	−5.1	−0.2	18	−2.8	−4.2	−0.7
3	−1.7	−2.8	−1.6	5	−1.4	−2.7	−0.7	3	−3.8	−4.4	−0.6
14	0.8	−0.3	2.0	12	0.6	−1.7	1.4	19	−0.5	−2.5	1.4
14	0.26	0.14	0.33	12	0.24	0.19	0.38	19	0.23	0.17	0.38
14	7	6	7	12	7	6	7	19	7	6	7
7	5.8	2.2	12.1	6	8.8	4.0	12.8	8	9.3	2.0	15.4
7	−5.2	−6.8	−2.7	6	−2.9	−4.7	−1.4	8	−2.6	−5.6	−2.2
6	−4.3	−7.0	0.4	5	−1.5	−3.7	−1.3	7	−1.3	−2.9	0.0
7	0.1	−4.6	3.8	6	2.7	−2.2	5.2	8	6.4	0.7	14.9
7	0.5	−0.5	1.6	6	0.6	−0.2	1.1	8	1.3	0.1	2.3
7	0.4	−2.6	2.8	6	−0.1	−2.3	0.8	8	−0.8	−1.6	1.2

centile line around 3 years of age. Growth is slow during childhood. Puberty is usually delayed with a delayed bone age, and pubertal height gain is suppressed. Final height is reported to be between 150 and 160 cm in males and 140 and 150 cm in females, corresponding to a height SDS of approximately –2.5 [10, 14]. With the exception of 1 reported case [15], AS patients are not GH deficient.

There is one report of a large series of 19 (16 male) AS patients treated with GH [16]. The height SDS increased by 1.0 ± 0.8 over a mean of 4 years of therapy at a dose of 0.3 ± 0.1 mg/kg/week. In those patients (n = 6) who have completed GH treatment, the median final height was 167.8 cm, ranging from 160 to 170.2 cm. There were no side effects, except for gynecomastia and hepatomegaly in 1 case. The second paper is on the analysis of patients with AS registered in the KIGS database [17], in which the height SDS improved from a median value of –2.8 to –2.3 (n = 13) over 1 year and to –1.8 (n = 7) over 3 years in longitudinally followed prepubertal children.

KIGS Data. Twenty-six (25 male) patients with AS were enrolled in the KIGS database, with a birth weight and length SDS of –1.0 (–2.4 to 0.1) and –1.3 (–2.7 to 0.2). The results of the longitudinally followed prepubertal children (n = 17, 16 males), as seen in table 1, showed that the patients increased their height SDS from a median value of –3.4 to –2.9. However, this increase was not significant. Height velocity increased from a pretreatment value of 4.8 cm/year (3.2–5.7) to 7.7 cm/year (4.8–8.5) over the first year of therapy. The maximum GH peak (n = 14) was 11.3 μg/l (9.0–21.0) in stimulation tests, excluding GHD. However, there were low insulin-like growth factor 1 (IGF-1) levels, with the IGF-1 SDS (n = 5) ranging from –5.1 to 0.8 (median –1.4). The SR was –0.9 (–2.4 to 0.3) indicating a growth response within the expected ranges, but less in magnitude compared with that of IGHD children. It should be noted that the median dose of GH used in this series is at the lower end of the doses used in GHD. In conclusion, GH treatment did not cause a significant increase in overall height SDS in this group of children with AS; however, as is evident from the wide ranges, there was a great individual variability, with some patients showing a satisfactory increase in height velocity up to 8.5 cm/year on GH treatment. As in other non-GHD conditions where GH treatment is used, it would be desirable to be able to identify those children that would respond to therapy. More data are needed for long-term results on the efficacy of GH treatment in this disorder. There were no major or minor adverse events that may be related to GH treatment, except for facial edema in 1 patient.

Cornelia de Lange Syndrome

Described in 1933 by Cornelia de Lange [18], this syndrome (CdLS) is characterized by a distinct facial appearance, limb abnormalities and retardation of growth and neuromotor development. Its incidence is reported to 1/10,000 [19].

Clinical Criteria for Diagnosis. The typical facial appearance includes a long philtrum, thin lips, downturned angles of the mouth (crescent-shaped mouth), depressed and/or broad nasal bridge, anteverted nostrils and micrognathia [20, 21]. Orbital ridges and zygomatic arches are underdeveloped. Generalized hirsutism or hypertrichosis, together with a low posterior hairline, long eyelashes and especially neat, well-defined and arched (penciled) and confluent eyebrows (synophrys) constitute the most frequently encountered findings. Microbrachycephaly is present.

Upper limb abnormalities including oligodactyly or phocomelia may be seen in a quarter of the patients [20]. However, in many of the patients, the limb abnormalities are limited to subtle changes in the phalanges and metacarpal bones, including single palmar flexion creases, clinodactyly and limitation of elbow extension. Hands and/or feet are almost always small. Ophthalmological abnormalities, which occur quite frequently, include myopia, ptosis and nystagmus. Mild to severe hearing loss has been reported in 50–100% of these children [20, 21].

Gastroesophageal reflux and various forms of obstruction such as malrotation with volvulus and congenital diaphragmatic hernia are the main abnormalities involving the gastrointestinal tract. Gastroesophageal reflux is exceedingly common and may explain the frequent respiratory tract infections, episodes of aspiration, feeding difficulties and failure to thrive encountered in the infancy period [22]. Cardiac defects include ventricular (VSD) and atrial septal defects (ASD), pulmonary stenosis, tetralogy of Fallot and several others [20, 23].

Mental retardation is usually moderate to severe. However, intelligence can also be normal or slightly below normal [24]. Behavior has been described as autistic like, showing a stereotype behavior pattern [20, 25]. Hyperactivity is also a frequent finding. Other findings include cryptorchidism, genital hypoplasia, hypospadias, and frequently, renal findings [20, 21].

The clinical variability within CdLS has led to the recognition of classical (severe, full) and mild forms of the syndrome [19, 20, 26], which account for 20–30% of the cases and may remain unrecognized until older ages.

Molecular Genetics. CdLS patients are mostly sporadic. Familial occurrences have been reported and point to an autosomal dominant inheritance in most of the cases [27]. Mutations in the NIPBL gene (5p13.1), the human homolog of the *Drosophila melanogaster* Nipped-B gene, have recently been reported to cause CdLS [28] and found to occur in approximately 50% of patients [29]. This gene encodes a component of the cohesin complex. Phenotype-genotype correlation has been shown. An X-linked form of CdLS with SMC1L1 mutations (Xp11.22-p11.21) also encoding this complex has been reported [30].

Growth. Growth retardation, more prominent in the classical phenotype, is one of the main features of CdLS. In a study by Kline et al. [31] in which serial measurements were taken in 180 patients with CdLS from birth to adult ages, birth weight and length were found to be lower than 3,000 g in 89% of the patients. The frequency of premature birth was 31%. The growth parameters obtained from this study showed that mean adult height is 155.8 cm in males and 131.1 cm in females. Height, weight and head circumference curves in both sexes up to 19 years of age are available in this paper. Mean height and weight values fall below the normal 5th centile line by 6 months and remain so until puberty, which occurs at normal ages. Pubertal height gain is suppressed. Obesity is seen especially in males after puberty. The head circumference, below the 2nd centile at birth, continues to be so until adulthood.

GHD has been implicated in some studies [32] as the etiology of short stature. Abnormalities in GH secretion and/or defects at end organ level have been shown [33]. Neonatal-onset panhypopituitarism was reported in 1 patient [34]. A spectrum of endocrinopathies was reported in another study [35], including GHD, increased gonadotropin response suggestive of primary gonadal failure, increased prolactin response, abnormalities in osmoregulation and empty sella.

KIGS Data. Twenty-one (9 male) patients with CdLS were enrolled in the KIGS database with a birth weight and length SDS of –2.3 (–3.8 to –0.5) and –2.4 (–3.5 to –0.2). The results of the longitudinally followed prepubertal children (n = 12, 3 males), as seen in table 1, showed that the patients increased their height SDS over 1 year of therapy, but not significantly. Pretreatment height velocity was 5.2 cm/year (3.1–12.2) and 6.3 cm/year (5.1–8.4) after 1 year of therapy. The maximum GH peak (n = 12) was 13.9 µg/l (3.9–34.8) and the IGF-1 SDS (n = 4) –0.3 (–1.7 to 0.4). Although the numbers are limited, it may be concluded that there was no adequate response to GH therapy in CdLS at short term. The response was quite lower than that in IGHD, with a median SR of –1.5. There were no major or minor adverse events that may be related to GH treatment.

Down Syndrome

DS was first described in 1866 by Down [36]. The syndrome, shown to be due to trisomy of chromosome 21, is characterized by distinctive dysmorphic features and mental retardation. DS is the most frequent cause of mental retardation.

Clinical Criteria for Diagnosis. The well-known distinctive physical phenotype of DS includes upslanting palpebral fissures, a flat nasal bridge, epicanthal folds, macroglossia, brachycephaly, folded and small ears, a short neck, short and incurved fifth fingers, a transverse palmar crease, hyperflexibility and short and broad hands [37]. Other clinical findings include excessive skinfolds on the neck, increased distance between the first and second toes and Brushfield spots on the iris. These features, together with a series of dermatoglyphic features, permit a reasonably accurate diagnosis of DS. Although there may be individual differences, developmental milestones and intelligence quotient (IQ) show a progressive delay throughout childhood [38]. DS is frequently accompanied by major congenital malformations pertaining mainly to the cardiac and gastrointestinal systems. Congenital heart defects may be present in up to 62% of children [39]. These consist mainly of atrioventricular canal defects, which are found in nearly 50% of cases. Gastrointestinal tract defects, which are less frequent, encompass duodenal stenosis or atresia, imperforate anus, Hirschsprung's disease and tracheoesophageal fistula or atresia [37]. The risk of leukemia is 10–20 times higher in DS patients than in normal children [40], with peaks in the newborn period and between 3 and 6 years of age. Ninety percent of all DS patients have conductive-type hearing loss and external pinna malformations [41]. Otitis media is seen in 50–70% of DS patients. Several endocrine abnormalities, such as type 1 diabetes mellitus and thyroid abnormalities, including congenital and autoimmune hypothyroidism and celiac disease, are also known to occur more frequently in DS children compared with normal children [42].

Molecular Genetics. DS results from trisomy of chromosome 21. About 95% of patients have three free copies of chromosome 21 (47, +21). In about 5% of patients, one copy is translocated to another acrocentric chromosome, often chromosome 14 or 21 [42]. The trisomy encompasses all or a critical portion of chromosome 21, also called the 'DS critical region', which is the region responsible for the DS phenotype.

Growth. Growth retardation is one of the main features of DS. This retardation starts prenatally and is apparent in ultrasound images as early as 15–16 weeks of gestation.

Birth size is compromised by 0.5–1.5 SD [43]. Height deficit increases with age, becoming more than 3 SD by 3–5 years of age [43, 44]. Short stature is disproportionate, with an increased upper to lower segment ratio. A long-term study of growth in DS indicated poor growth, especially between 6 and 18 months of age, with a height velocity compromised by 20%, and also during adolescence, when height velocity decreased by 27% in girls and 50% in boys. Growth velocity was diminished by 5–10% during mid-childhood [45]. The mean final heights for girls and boys were 145 and 153 cm, respectively, in the longitudinal study by Cronk et al. [45]. Recently published Swedish DS growth charts yielded a final height of 161.5 cm in males and 147.5 cm in females [46]. Although puberty is somewhat earlier, pubertal spurt is suppressed. This has also been shown in a Japanese DS growth chart [47]. Congenital heart defects contribute 1–2 cm to the height deficit. DS patients tend to be overweight from late infancy, which may be due to environmental and/or genetic factors. Bone age has been reported to be retarded. Head circumference, reduced by 1 SD at birth, falls below 2 SD after 5–6 months of age [46, 48].

GHD does not account for the poor growth in DS [49]. However, abnormalities in GH secretion have been reported [50]. Serum levels of IGF-1 were found to be normal during infancy, but did not show the expected increase in puberty [51].

Serum IGF-2 [52], insulin and IGF receptors in the brains of fetuses were reported to be normal [53]. Treatment with GH causes a short-term increase in growth velocity, which doubles over 6–12 months of therapy [49, 50], with concomitant increases in IGF-1 and IGF-2 levels. In fact, it has been speculated that GH, by increasing IGF-1, can positively affect central nervous system functions. In the study by Torrado et al. [50], there was a significant increase in the head circumference of patients on GH therapy.

In a long-term study by Anneren et al. [54], 15 DS patients, started on GH therapy (0.2 mg/kg/week) at a mean age of 7.4 months, increased their height SDS from –1.8 to –0.8 over 3 years of therapy, while the control DS patients had a decrease in height SDS from –1.7 to –2.2. Although some improvement in fine motor development was noted in the GH-treated group, there was no effect on head growth and no difference in mental or gross motor development. Growth velocity declined after stopping treatment. No side effects of short-term GH therapy were reported in these studies. However, there is some concern regarding the long-term use of GH in DS. One of these is the possible development of leukemia, which may be associated with GH therapy. Although recent evaluations have not proven an association between GH and leukemia, it is recommended that these children be followed closely. Another concern is whether GH therapy results in an improved quality of life.

KIGS Data. Seventy-two (44 male) patients with DS were enrolled in the KIGS database with a birth weight and length SDS of –0.6 (–2.8 to 0.6) and –1.0 (–2.4 to 0.6). Longitudinal analysis, as seen in table 1, revealed that the prepubertal patients (n = 46, 30 males) were severely short at onset of treatment and significantly increased their height SDS, height velocity SDS and height – midparental height (MPH) SDS on GH treatment ($p < 0.05$). The maximum GH peak (n = 40) was 8.0 μg/l (1.2–21.4). The IGF-1 SDS (n = 9) was –1.7 (–4.1 to –0.1), showing that patients have low GH and/or IGF-1 levels. Height velocity increased from 4.7 cm/year (2.4–7.1) to 8.3 cm/year (5.6–12.5; $p < 0.05$). The body mass index did not show a significant change during therapy. The median SR was –1.2 (–2.4 to 0.0), indicating a relatively lower response compared with that of IGHD children; however, the number of children for the prediction model decreased to 23 in the analysis, and again, there is a wide individual variability. With similar baseline data, the Δ height SDS over 1 year was similar in girls (0.6) and in boys (0.7). It may be concluded that GH given at early prepubertal ages causes a significant increase in height SDS over 1 year of therapy in short children with DS. GHD may explain short statute at least in some patients. This is the series with the highest number of patients with DS on GH treatment at short term. However, data on long-term efficacy of GH treatment are needed. There were no major adverse events that may be related to GH treatment. Among minor events, edema was reported in 1 patient.

Floating-Harbor Syndrome
Floating-Harbor syndrome was named after the descriptions of similar patients from Boston Floating Hospital and Harbor General Hospital, California, USA, by Pelletier et al. [55] and Leisti et al. [56]. The three central features are short stature with delayed bone maturation, expressive language delay and normal motor development, and typical facies.

Clinical Criteria for Diagnosis. Typical triangular-shaped facies with a prominent nose with an overhanging bulbous tip, a long mouth with thin lips, and seemingly deep-set eyes are seen. Long eyelashes, a short philtrum and wide columella, posteriorly rotated ears and low posterior hairline are usually present. Head size is usually normal, giving the appearance of a large head compared with body size [57]. Other features include digital findings [58] like broad fingers and toes, clinodactyly, hypoplastic thumb, clubbing, distal broadening of the phalanges, small nails on the 4th and 5th toes and associated loss of ossification centers under the 4th and 5th toes. Several children have been reported to develop celiac disease [57]. Cardiac anomalies have been reported. High-pitched voice and supernumerary upper incisors are additional findings [59]. There is delay in expressive language development with normal intelligence or mild mental retardation.

Molecular Genetics. The genetic basis is unknown, but nearly all recognized cases have been sporadic. There is one report of a mother and daughter who both had major features of the syndrome [60, 61], suggesting dominant inheritance. No laboratory tests are available for diagnosis.

Growth. Birth length is often compromised [57]. Height is lost rapidly in the first 2 years of life and then tends to increase parallel with the lowest centile line. There is extreme short stature with a height in childhood between –4 and –6 SDS [57]. Eventual adult height is very low with reports of heights between 131 and 142 cm. Bone maturation is very delayed, but puberty is usually normally timed, and bone maturation and epiphyseal fusion occur normally and result in extreme short adult stature. Immaturity of bone development is seen especially in the capital femoral epiphysis. GHD has been reported [62] with a dramatic increase in growth on GH therapy over 18 months. Two other patients have increased their height during GH therapy [63]. A patient who had been on GH therapy [64] was suggested to have unmasked tethered cord due to increased growth velocity. Of particular relevance if GH treatment is being considered is the report of Perthes' disease in 1 child [57].

KIGS Data. Twelve (5 male) patients with Floating-Harbor syndrome were enrolled in the KIGS database with a birth weight and length SDS of –1.7 (–2.9 to 0.0) and –2.0 (–3.1 to 1.2). As seen in table 3, cross-sectional analysis revealed that patients (2 pubertal) showed a small increment in height SDS after 1 year of GH treatment. Pretreatment height velocity increased from 5.6 cm/year (3.2–6.4) to 6.3 cm/year (3.1–10.0). The maximum GH peak (n = 9) was 14.3 µg/l (3.4–53.5) at onset of treatment, indicating GH resistance in some patients. In favor of this, the IGF-1 SDS (n = 4) was –2.0 (–3.7 to –1.0). There are no adequate data on longitudinal follow-up of prepubertal children to conclude on the results of GH treatment in this disorder. There were no major adverse events that may be related to GH treatment. Among minor events, headache was reported in 1 patient.

Kabuki Syndrome

Kabuki syndrome (KS), first described by Niikawa et al. [65] and Kuroki et al. [66] in 1981, is a mental retardation-malformation syndrome affecting multiple organ systems. It is characterized by five main features: developmental delay, distinct facial anomalies, limb and skeletal anomalies, dermatoglyphic abnormalities and postnatal growth retardation [67–69]. Males and females are similarly affected. It is more common in Japanese people with a prevalence of 1/32,000 [67]. However, in recent years, a growing number of patients have been recognized outside of Japan [68].

Clinical Criteria for Diagnosis. The facial appearance is characterized by eversion of the lower lateral eyelid, arched eyebrows with sparse or dispersed lateral one third, long palpebral fissures, long eyelashes, epicanthus, short nasal septum, micrognathia, a depressed nasal tip, large and prominent ears with preauricular pits, and cleft lip and/or palate. Microcephaly is seen in half of the patients [70]. Limb and skeletal anomalies include a deformed spinal column with or without vertebral clefts, congenital dislocation of the hips and brachydactyly. Dermatoglyphic abnormalities include frequent finger ulnar loop patterns, hypothenar loop patterns and persistence of finger tip pads [71].

Congenital heart defects are reported in 30–55% and mostly include coarctation of the aorta, single ventricle with a common atrium, VSD,

ASD, tetralogy of Fallot, patent ductus arteriosus, as well as some other types [72]. In general, mental development is mild to moderately retarded; however, children with average intelligence have been reported. There may be behavioral problems such as inattention and/or hyperactivity [70, 73]. Hypotonia and feeding difficulties are common in infancy [70]. Seizures are seen in less than half of the patients [70]. Dysplasia of the inner ear may result in hearing loss. Recurrent otitis media and ophthalmologic problems are frequent.

Immune deficiency and autoimmune disorders like Hashimito's thyroiditis, autoimmune hemolytic anemia and vitiligo may be encountered quite frequently [74].

Molecular Genetics. Most cases are sporadic. Familial cases suggest autosomal dominant inheritance with different expressivity [75]. No common abnormalities or breakpoints of the putative KS genes have been demonstrated until today.

Growth. Size at birth is usually normal [70], but postnatal progressive growth deficiency is one of the hallmarks of the syndrome [65, 66, 70]. However, normal height has also been reported in approximately 20% of the patients [67, 76], although the heights of these patients do not exceed the 50th percentile. GHD or neurosecretory dysfunction has been noted in some reports [69, 70, 77–80]. Very few patients have been treated with GH, either with no change in growth velocity [71], a good catch-up growth at short term [77, 78] or a moderate response at long term [79, 80]. Early breast development is seen in 23% [67], either as isolated premature thelarche or as full-blown early puberty. Excess weight gain over 5 years and in puberty may be a serious long-term complication [81]. Type 1 diabetes mellitus [82] and central diabetes insipidus [77] may also be associated findings.

KIGS Data. Seventeen (14 male) patients with KS were enrolled in the KIGS database with a birth weight and length SDS of –1.3 (–2.3 to –0.2) and –0.9 (–2.0 to 0.7). Longitudinal analysis (table 1) revealed that 10 (8 male) patients showed an insignificant increment in height SDS on GH treatment. Pretreatment height velocity was 4.1 cm/year (1.1–5.8) and increased to 7.9 cm/year (5.8–9.5) on therapy. The maximum GH peak (n = 9) was 8.7 µg/l (6.1–25.8). The numbers to evaluate the SR were too few. The dose of GH used was much lower than the dose used in GHD. Although the number of children is limited, GH therapy does not seem to be effective in this syndrome; however, there is much individual variability in the growth response in compliance with the literature [71, 77–80]. There were no major or minor adverse events that may be related to GH treatment.

Williams-Beuren Syndrome

Williams-Beuren syndrome (WBS) is a disorder characterized by a distinctive facial appearance, psychomotor retardation and cardiovascular malformations, mostly supravalvular aortic stenosis [83, 84]. The incidence of WBS is reported as 1/10,000.

Clinical Criteria for Diagnosis. The features are variable among patients and also within family members [85]. The facial appearance described as elfin face and mental deficiency are the most consistent findings, as well as growth retardation [86, 87]. Facial characteristics include flat nasal bridge, medial eyebrow flare, periorbital fullness, epicanthal folds, long philtrum, wide mouth with thick lips, anteverted nares with full nasal tip and flat malar region with full cheeks. The 'lacey' or 'stellate' iris pattern constitutes the main ocular finding and is seen in 50–74% of the patients [88]. Other than the frequently noted dental malocclusion [84], microdontia and enamel hypoplasia may be seen in half of the patients. Cardiac defects which are reported in 80–100% of the patients mainly include supravalvular aortic stenosis [89]. Hypertension, which may be of diverse etiology, has been encountered in up to 40–60% of the patients [90]. Renal anomalies, which may also be frequently present, consist of nephrocalcinosis, asymmetrical or small kidneys and renal artery stenosis [91], which may all be associated with functional abnormalities. Mental retardation is one of the main features of WBS, with average IQs ranging between 40 and 79 [92]. The patients have a friendly behavior with no reserve to strangers. Musculoskeletal findings including joint limitation, kyphosis, scoliosis, lordosis, pectus excavatum and awkward gait may be present in half of the children. Hypercalcemia, which resolves after infancy, is reported in a number of the infants [93]. A scoring system has been developed by Preus [94].

Molecular Genetics. WBS is usually sporadic; however, familial occurrence with autosomal dominant inheritance has also been reported [95]. WBS is caused by a hemizygote microdeletion mapped to the long arm of chromosome 7 at 7q11.23, which contains the elastin gene [96]. The deletion is detected in over 90% of the patients [97]. Besides the elastin gene, several other genes have been identified within the deleted region [98].

Growth. Intrauterine growth retardation is a frequent finding in WBS [86, 93, 94]. Birth length and weight are low or of low normal values. In early infancy, there is a loss of weight and height due to feeding difficulties. In a large series of patients with WBS followed longitudinally [99], evaluation of growth showed that in boys, birth length is decreased and accounts for one fourth of the overall height deficit. The height deficit increased over the first 6 months of life, and this trend continued up to 10 years of age. Pubertal height gain was suppressed, resulting in a further height deficit of about 20%. Final height of the males was 165.2 ± 10.9 cm, which was 10.1 ± 5.8 cm lower than their target height. Peak height velocity (8.7 ± 2.3 cm/year) occurred at ages 11–12 years, 2 years earlier than the reference population. In girls, growth followed a similar pattern up to the age of 8 years. A group of girls had early puberty with peak height velocity (7.8 ± 2.1 cm/year) at age 9 and another group at age 11 (7.5 ± 1.1 cm/year). The girls showed a relative catch-up in height growth during puberty. Increased height velocity compensated for the shorter duration of puberty. Final height of the girls was 152.4 ± 5.7 cm when the target height was 163.1 ± 5.1 cm. Bone age was delayed in both sexes during childhood and accelerated markedly during puberty. Cardiac defects have not been found to make a difference in growth prognosis [86]. There are a few case reports [100, 101] on GH therapy in WBS. GHD is not a likely cause of short stature in WBS. Thyroid abnormalities are frequent [102].

KIGS Data. Twenty (9 male) patients with WBS were enrolled in the KIGS database with a birth weight and length SDS of –1.1 (–3.0 to –0.1) and –1.4 (–2.9 to –0.5). Longitudinal analysis revealed (table 1) an insignificant increase in height SDS in 13 (6 male) patients. Pretreatment height velocity was 4.9 cm/year (3.3–8.4) and increased to 6.9 cm/year (5.6–10.0) on therapy. The maximum GH peak (n = 9) was 9.1 µg/l (1.8–33.2). The IGF-1 SDS (n = 3) was –0.9 (–2.8 to 1.1). GHD does not seem to be present in most of the children. The growth response on GH treatment is quite low, at least in this series of patients with WBS. Among the major adverse events, malignant lymphoma was reported in 1 patient at age 14.2 years. This patient had received kidney transplantation for renal insufficiency due to congenital malformation and was on immunosuppressive therapy, which may be a risk factor for malignancy, and had been on GH for 0.4 years at the diagnosis, thus making the association of GH and lymphoma unlikely. Although very rare, this has been reported in literature without GH treatment [103]. Chromosome 7 is the most frequent chromosome involved in the cytogenetic aberrations observed in human malignancies [104], and thus, patients with WBS should be followed in this respect. Among minor events, abnormality in liver function tests was reported in 1 and albuminuria and hematuria in 2 patients each, which may be encountered in WBS.

Fanconi Anemia

FA, first described by Fanconi [105], is an autosomal recessive disorder that is characterized by a variety of congenital malformations, dermal pigmentary changes and a predisposition to bone marrow failure and malignancy [106, 107]. FA has a carrier frequency of 1/300 [106].

Clinical Criteria for Diagnosis. There is a wide clinical variability, both intra- and interfamilial [108], and there is an overlap with a variety of genetic and nongenetic diseases; thus, diagnosis of FA on clinical grounds is difficult.

According to the International Fanconi Anemia Registry (IFAR) [106, 107, 109–111], analysis of more than 700 subjects showed that major congenital malformations in FA included radial ray (49.1%), skeletal (21.6%), renal (33.8%), male genital (19.7%), gastrointestinal (14.3%), heart (13.2%) and central nervous system (7.7%) malformations and hearing loss (11.3%). Radial ray abnormalities can be bi- or unilateral and consist of absent or hypoplastic radii and/or thumbs. Gastrointestinal malformations include anorectal malformation in 5.1% and duodenal atresia in 4.6% as the two most frequent malformations. Hydrocephalus or ventriculomegaly was the most frequent central nervous system malformation (4.6%). Congenital hip and vertebral abnormalities were also noted in addition to several other skeletal malformations [106]. The analysis of patients in the IFAR showed that patients with congenital malformations are usually diagnosed after the onset of hematological abnormalities. Café-au-lait spots, hyper- or hypopigmentation are frequent. Many FA patients have distinct facial characteristics, including microphthalmia, small facial size, flattened nasal bridge, low-set protruding ears, thin upper lip and prominent forehead. Thenar hypoplasia, clinodactyly and syndactyly of fingers, as well as hyperextensible thumbs are noted.

About one third of patients do not have congenital malformations. Of these, 85% have at least one of the following: skin pigmentation, microphthalmos or height, weight or head circumference at or below the 5th centile line [109].

Among 754 subjects with FA [111], 80% had bone marrow failure and 23% had neoplasms. Of these neoplasms, 60% were hematologic, mainly acute myeloid leukemia, and 40% nonhematologic, most commonly gastrointestinal and gynecologic tumors. The risk of bone marrow failure and neoplasm increases with age. All bone marrow elements are affected, resulting in anemia, leukopenia and thrombocytopenia. Leukemia is a fatal complication and may occur in family members who lack major stigma.

Molecular Genetics. The clinical variability reflects genetic heterogeneity. Diagnosis is based on the unique hypersensitivity of FA cells to DNA crosslinking agents such as diepoxybutane [112, 113]. FA can be caused by a mutation in any of at least 7 genes: FANCA (16q24.3), FANCC (9q22.3), FANCD (3p22-26), FANCG (9p13), FANCE (6p21.2–21.3) and FANCF (11p15) [106, 114]. FA-A is the most prevalent group. Soulier et al. [115] reported that the proteins encoded are part of a nuclear multiprotein core complex that have a role in the repair of DNA damage.

Growth. FA is associated with growth failure which starts prenatally. Short stature may be the initial presenting symptom in patients without congenital malformation [109]. The mean height SDS of FA patients registered in the IFAR (n = 54) was slightly below –2 SD. Weight and head circumference were also at or less than –2 SD. Nearly all children had GHD on pharmacological tests and/or physiological evaluation, and a third had primary hypothyroidism [116]. GHD worsens the height prognosis. Bone age is delayed and pubertal growth is suppressed. A significant number of patients had insulin resistance, impaired glucose tolerance or overt diabetes mellitus [106, 116]. Hypogonadism may be seen and is hypergonadotropic [107, 117, 118]. Older females have irregular menses but pregnancy can occur in FA patients. Genital malformations and hypoplasia of gonads are common in males, and there is abnormality in spermatogenesis [106]. Data on GH treatment are scarce [116] and not conclusive.

KIGS Data. Twenty-nine (24 male) patients with FA were enrolled in the KIGS database with a birth weight and length SDS of –2.5 (–3.5 to –0.1) and –1.8 (–4.7 to 0.7). The results of the longitudinally followed prepubertal children (n = 22, 20 males) (table 1) showed that the severely short patients had an insignificant increase in height SDS during treatment. The maximum GH peak (n = 20) was 4.4 µg/l (0.4–11.8) in stimulation tests indicating a subnormal GH response. Height velocity increased from 4.5 cm/year (1.3–7.7) to 7.3 cm/year (4.5–14.1). The SR was –1.4 (–2.2 to 1.7; n = 7) indicating a growth response at the lower end compared with that of IGHD children; however, this interpretation needs caution because of the low numbers in the analysis. It may be concluded that short-term growth response was not satisfactory in FA in this database; however, there was a great individual variability, and the median dose of GH used was low in face of the low GH levels. There were no major adverse events that may be related to GH treatment except for diabetes mellitus (n = 2), pancytopenia, acute leukemia, biliary cirrhosis and renal disease, each in 1 patient, which may be expected findings in FA. Among minor events, edema was reported in 1 patient. There was one reported death among the patients at age 10.6 years, whereas the cause was not identified.

Rubinstein-Taybi Syndrome

Rubinstein-Taybi syndrome (RTS), with an estimated birth prevalence of 1/100,000–1/125,000 [119], is characterized by a characteristic face, broad thumbs, broad big toes and mental retardation.

Clinical Criteria for Diagnosis. Facial appearance includes microcephaly, prominent forehead, downslanting palpebral fissures, epicanthal folds, strabismus, broad nasal bridge, beaked nose and highly arched palate [120, 121]. Unusual smile is frequent. Findings related to the eye (ptosis, glaucoma, refractive errors, cataracts) and to the ears, including hearing loss and frequent otitis media, may be seen [120, 122]. Talon cusps (markedly enlarged cingulum on maxillary incisor teeth) have been observed in 90% of children [123]. Broad thumbs and big toes are present in all cases. Clinodactyly of the 5th finger and overlapping of toes are present in half of the patients.

Skeletal findings include pectus excavatum, rib defects, scoliosis, kyphosis and several others [120]. Laxity of the ligaments, hyperextensibility of the joints and increased fracture frequency have been noted [124]. The anterior fontanelle is large, and there is a delay in its closure. Cryptorchidism is very frequent. Urinary tract abnormalities and urinary infections may be seen [120, 125]. A number of other physical findings have been reported, the most common being cardiac defects, including patent ductus arteriosus and ASD or VSD [120, 124–126].

Mental deficiency is a consistent finding in RTS [125], with a mean IQ of 36. These patients are usually friendly. They have a short attention span, poor coordination and sudden mood changes [127]. Electroencephalogram abnormalities and seizures are quite frequent [120, 124, 125]. There is an increased rate of malignancy [128] including rhabdomyosarcoma, pheochromocytoma, meningioma and other brain tumors and leukemia. Keloid formation is common [120, 125, 129].

Molecular Genetics. RTS is a de novo occurring autosomal dominant trait. It has been mapped to 16p13.3 [130]. CREB binding protein (CBP) gene mutations on 16p13.3 are found in 15–20% of cases [131]. CBP is a large nuclear protein involved in transcription. It is expressed in all tissue types. Evidence suggests that RTS is caused by haploinsufficiency of CBP during fetal development [119]. Mutations in EP300 (E1A binding protein, 300 kDa; 22q13) have also been shown in some patients with RTS [132].

Growth. Birth weight and length and head circumference are in the normal ranges, between the 25th and 50th centile line [124, 133]. Gestational age is normal. Weight gain is poor in infancy, with a history of respiratory and feeding problems. Growth retardation becomes evident in infancy. Pubertal spurt is suppressed, and bone age is delayed. Final height is reported as 153.1 cm for males and 146.7 cm for females [133]. Overweight is a frequent problem. Thyroid functions and growth hormone secretion are normal [134]. Hyperinsulinemia has been reported, and premature thelarche may be seen.

KIGS Data. Thirteen (8 male) patients with RTS were enrolled in the KIGS database with a birth weight and length SDS of –1.1 (–2.1 to –0.1) and –0.9 (–6.5 to 0.9). As seen in table 3, cross-sectional analysis revealed that patients (2 pubertal) increased their height SDS from –4.0 to –3.5 SD. Pretreatment height velocity increased from 5.1 cm/year (3.8–6.3) to 7.2 cm/year (5.5–13.8) after 1 year of therapy. The maximum GH peak (n = 12) was 7.9 μg/l (4.1–19.3). The IGF-1 SDS (n = 5) was –2.2 (–2.2 to –1.7). There are no adequate data on longitudinal follow-up of prepubertal children to conclude on the results of GH treatment in this disorder. There were no major and minor adverse events that may be related to GH treatment.

Cartilage-Hair Hypoplasia
Cartilage-hair hypoplasia (CHH), also known as McKusick type metaphyseal chondrodysplasia, is characterized by short-limbed short stature, hypoplastic hair, defective immunity and diminished erythrocyte generation. It is a rare disease, but its prevalence is higher in the Old Order Amish in the USA, as first described by McKusick et al. [135], and in the Finnish population [136].

Clinical Criteria for Diagnosis. There is a remarkable degree of phenotypic variability. In most patients, but not all, the hair is sparse, fine and light colored. Skeletal features besides short-limbed growth failure include ligament laxity, increased lumbar lordosis, bowing of the lower limbs, chest deformity, limited extension at the elbows and mild scoliosis. The fibula is relatively longer than the tibia [135, 136]. Individuals with CHH have defective cellular immunity, but humoral immunity may also be impaired. The defective immunity may be more evident during childhood, and varicella infections may even be fatal. Patients are unusually prone to infections [137, 138].

Increased incidence of malignancies (lymphoma, skin neoplasms, leukemia) has been shown both in the Amish and the Finnish patients [139]. A failure of erythrocyte production may be mild or severe, even fatal [140, 141]. Anemia is seen in approximately 80%, accompanied by macrocytosis. Hirschsprung's disease is a significantly associated finding [136]. The diagnosis is mainly based on typical radiographic findings. In childhood, the tubular bones are short with flared and scalloped metaphyseal ends and show irregular and sclerotic areas. After epiphyseal closure, the bone ends remain flared and angulated [142, 143]. Bone age is delayed.

Molecular Genetics. The disease shows an autosomal recessive trait. The defect was mapped to 9p21-p12. It was shown that CHH is caused by several mutations in the RNA component of the endoribonuclease RNase MRP gene which is involved in several cellular and mitochondrial functions [144, 145].

Growth. The growth failure is already evident at birth, and the short limbs may be noticed in the neonatal period. The growth failure is progressive and leads to a median adult height of 131.1 cm in males and 122.5 cm in females [146]. Growth curves for Finnish individuals with CHH can be found in this paper. There is no correlation between final height and parental height. The short limbs are evident in almost all individuals. Pubertal growth is suppressed. The weight for height is slightly above normal. The adult head circumference SDS is –0.9 SD. Spermatogenesis has been found impaired [147]. The number of patients treated with GH is small. One patient increased height from –4.2 to –2.1 SD on GH therapy plus limb lengthening [148], whereas 4 other children did benefit fairly from the therapy [149]. The tendency for multiple malignancies in CHH may be seen as a handicap for GH treatment; however, there are no reports of malignancies after GH in CHH, and the overall adverse events are only mild infections and skin rash.

KIGS Data. Fourteen (6 male) patients with CHH were enrolled in the KIGS database with a birth weight and length SDS of –0.9 (–2.5 to 1.9) and –2.6 (–4.3 to 0.1). Cross-sectional analysis (table 3) revealed that patients (all prepubertal) did not show an increase in height SDS on GH treatment. Pretreatment height velocity was 5.1 cm/year (3.5–11.1) and 6.6 cm/year (3.1–7.7) after 1 year of therapy. The maximum GH peak (n = 12) was 10.5 µg/l (5.4–21.0), and the IGF-1 SDS (n = 3) was –1.3 (–3.5 to –0.5). There are no adequate data on longitudinal follow-up of prepubertal children to conclude on the results of GH treatment in this disorder. There were no major and minor adverse events that may be related to GH treatment.

Klippel-Feil Syndrome
Klippel-Feil syndrome (KFS) consists of a short neck, low posterior hairline and limited neck movement, first described in 1912. The incidence is 1/40,000.

Clinical Criteria for Diagnosis. Less than 50% of patients show all of these three features [150]. The main finding is the presence of a congenital defect in the formation or segmentation of the cervical spine, resulting in a fused appearance. Scoliosis may also be seen. Deafness is a well-known feature [151], mostly sensorineural. According to the morphologic types of cervical vertebral fusion, type 1 is associated with the most rostral fusion of C1 and severe anomalies like cardiac defects and craniofacial anomalies with autosomal recessive inheritance. Type 2 is associated with dominant C2–3 fusion which becomes apparent postnatally, and type 3 shows an isolated fusion, most rostral at C3. Type 4 shows vertebral fusion and ocular anomalies with possible X-linked inheritance [152]. Autosomal recessive KFS is associated with absent ulna and ulnar ray.

Moleculer Genetics. Most cases are sporadic. Besides recessive inheritance, autosomal dominant inheritance has been reported as well [153]. Cytogenetic analyses have not yielded conclusive evidence.

Growth. Growth data on KFS are scarce. GHD has been reported in a child with KFS and other associated findings [154].

KIGS Data. Twelve (8 male) patients with KFS were enrolled in the KIGS database with a birth weight and length SDS of –1.4 (–3.1 to 0.2) and –2.0 (–3.1 to –0.5). Cross-sectional analysis (table 3) revealed that patients (3 pubertal) were severely short at onset of GH treatment and showed a reasonable increase in height SDS. Pretreatment height velocity increased from 4.4 cm/year (3.0–8.2) to 7.6 cm/year (5.0–11.3) after 1 year. The maximum GH peak (n = 9) was 9.7 µg/l (0.5–20.3). The IGF-1 SDS (n = 3) was –2.4 (–2.7 to –1.9). Although the response is satisfactory in this analysis, there are no adequate data on longitudinal follow-up of prepubertal children to conclude on the results of GH treatment in this disorder. There were no major adverse events that may be related to GH treatment except for arthralgia in 1 patient which may be associated with the disease itself.

Diamond-Blackfan Anemia
Diamond-Blackfan anemia (DBA) is an entity that is associated with congenital erythroid aplasia and other congenital anomalies, especially of the upper limbs and craniofacial region, first described in 1938 [155].

Clinical Criteria for Diagnosis. In the retrospective analysis of 80 cases registered in the UK DBA registry [156], anemia presented at birth or by the age of 3 months in nearly all patients. Macrocytosis was seen in two thirds of the patients. Craniofacial anomalies were seen in 37%, and 18% had thumb anomalies. Height was below the 3rd centile in 28%, whereas 31% had normal stature and no physical anomalies. In another series that analyzed 229 patients registered in the European Society for Pediatric Hematology and Immunology DBA working group, 40% of children had associated physical findings, including thumb anomalies, short stature, VSD, kidney hypoplasia, low hairline and congenital glaucoma [157, 158].

Molecular Genetics. Approximately 10–25% of DBA cases are familial [156] with autosomal dominant inheritance [157], although most are sporadic. Twenty-five percent of cases of DBA are caused by mutation in the gene encoding ribosomal protein SI9 (RPS19; 19q13.2) [159]. Another locus has been mapped to 8p23-p22 (DBA2) [160]. The genotype-phenotype correlation is not clear.

Growth. Short stature is seen in approximately 10–30% of the patients as either an isolated finding or associated with other malformations [156, 158, 160]. One possible cause of short stature may be chronic steroid use; however, GHD has been reported in some cases [161, 162]. A satisfactory increase in height velocity in some cases over short term on GH therapy has been observed [161, 163], but patients should be followed carefully for malignancies.

KIGS Data. Twenty-two (10 male) patients with DBA were enrolled in the KIGS database with a birth weight and length SDS of −0.7 (−4.1 to 0.8) and −0.4 (−2.7 to 1.4). Longitudinal analysis (table 1) revealed that 11 (5 male) patients showed an insignificant increase in height SDS. Pretreatment height velocity was 4.3 cm/year (2.5–6.7) and 6.3 cm/year (4.9–8.3) after 1 year of therapy. The maximum GH peak (n = 7) was 9.3 μg/l (0.4–28.0). The median SR was −2.3 (−2.4 to −1.0), indicating a much lower response than that seen in IGHD. However, the numbers are too low for evaluation. There were no major adverse events that may be related to GH treatment. Among minor events, hyperglycemia and hypoparathyroidism were reported in 1 patient each, which may be due to hemochromatosis seen in the course of the disease.

Some Other Rare Disorders Associated with Short Stature

Arachnoid cysts are frequently associated with other malformations of the brain like holoprosencephaly, absence of the corpus callosum [164] and are accompanied by a wide spectrum of endocrine disorders including isolated or multiple pituitary hormone deficiency (MPHD) [165, 166]. Precocious puberty may be seen frequently.

Another finding on magnetic resonance imaging that may be associated with GHD is empty sella. The term 'empty sella' describes that the sella turcica does not contain normal pituitary structures. Although this does not give a definite clue to pituitary function, in many cases with isolated GHD and MPHD, empty sella is a reported finding [167]. Cacciari et al. [167] examined 339 children and adolescents with hypothalamo-pituitary disorders and found empty sella in 10.9% of the patients. It was mainly associated with MPHD. Empty sella and pituitary aplasia may be in the spectrum of pituitary stalk interruption syndrome [168]. Pituitary stalk interruption syndrome probably constitutes a continuum ranging from total stalk interruption with severe hormonal deficits to milder forms with partial pituitary activity, with images including ectopic posterior pituitary, pituitary hypoplasia or aplasia and interrupted pituitary stalk on magnetic resonance imaging.

Midline palatal cleft and lip defects as well as solitary median maxillary central incisor (SMMCI) syndrome are midline defects that may be associated with GHD. SMMCI syndrome consists of multiple, mainly midline defects of development and may be associated with other anomalies like holoprosencephaly. Varying degrees of hypothalamo-pituitary function are seen in this disorder, with 50% of the children having short stature. GHD accounts for 33% of short stature. In 50%, there is intellectual disability of varying degree. The etiology is uncertain. Missense mutations in the SHH gene (7q36) may be associated with SMMCI syndrome [for a review, see ref. 169]. Midline palatal and lip defects have been associated with hypothalamo-pituitary dysfunction [170, 171] and GHD. GHD is seen 40 times more often in children with cleft lip and palate than in those without [170]. Diabetes insipidus may also be observed.

Congenital hydrocephalus associated with or without meningomyelocele is frequently accompanied by GHD or neurosecretory dysfunction. GHD may be isolated or part of MPHD. Early puberty is also frequently encountered [172, 173].

KIGS Data

Arachnoid Cyst. Fifty-five (38 male) patients with this diagnosis were enrolled in the KIGS database. They had a birth weight and length SDS of –0.2 (–1.6 to 1.0) and 0.3 (–1.6 to 1.6). The longitudinal analysis of 30 (21 male) prepubertal patients, as seen in table 2, shows that the height SDS and the height velocity SDS increased significantly on GH therapy over the first year, with an increment in the height velocity from 4.0 cm/year (3.4–6.2) to 10.2 cm/year (6.0–13.8; p<0.05). The height – MPH SDS also showed a significant increase. The SR showed that the growth response obtained was even above the median response for IGHD. The maximum GH peak (n = 22) was 4.1 µg/l (0.7–10.8), showing GHD in nearly all children. The IGF-1 SDS (n = 8) was low as well, –2.1 (–2.3 to –1.3). When analyzed by gender, the Δ height SDS of females (n = 9), 1.5 (0.2–2.4) was higher than that observed in males (n = 21), 0.8 (0.3–1.5), over the first year of therapy. The median dose of GH used in females (0.17 mg/kg/week) was lower than that used in males (0.23 mg/kg/week), but girls were slightly younger at onset of treatment which may account for this difference. When analyzed by the presence of other hormone deficiencies, isolated GHD was present in 19 (63.3%) and multiple GHD in 11 (36.7%) of the patients. The Δ height SDS was 1.1 (0.2–2.0) in isolated and 0.7 (0.5–1.5) in multiple GHD and did not show a significant difference. In conclusion, children with GHD with an associated arachnoid cyst responded well to GH therapy at short term, as expected. There were no major adverse events that may be related to GH treatment. Intracranial hemorrhage, autism and bacterial infection were three reported serious events. Among minor events, headache was reported in 5 patients in addition to less specific frequently observed childhood infections.

Empty Sella. A total of 578 (399 male) patients with this diagnosis were enrolled in the KIGS database. They had a birth weight and length SDS of –0.5 (–2.2 to 1.1) and –0.3 (–2.0 to 1.5). The longitudinal analysis of 382 (270 male) prepubertal patients, as seen in table 2, shows that the height and height velocity SDS increased significantly on GH therapy over the first year, with an increment in the height velocity from 4.9 cm/year (2.3–8.5) to 10.7 cm/year (6.9–16.8; p<0.05). The height – MPH SDS also showed a significant increase. The maximum GH peak (n = 348) was 2.1 µg/l (0.4–8.8), indicating that all children had GHD. The IGF-1 SDS (n = 78) was low in all children, with a median value of –2.8 (–4.3 to –0.9). The SR showed that the growth response was parallel to the response for IGHD. When analyzed by gender, over the first year of therapy, the Δ height SDS of females (n = 112), 1.4 (0.6–2.4), was higher than that observed in males (n = 270), 1.0 (0.4–2.1). When analyzed by the presence of other hormone deficiencies, among the available data, isolated GHD was present in 172 (45%) and multiple GHD in 205 (53.7%) of the patients. The Δ height SDS over 1 year of therapy was 1.0 (0.4–2.0) in isolated and 1.2 (0.3–2.3) in multiple GHD (p < 0.01). Multiple GHD patients were younger than isolated GHD patients at onset of therapy

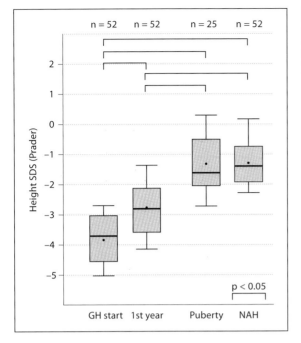
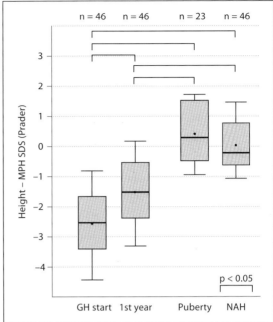

Fig. 1. Height SDS at onset, during GH treatment and at near adult height in longitudinally followed children with empty sella.

Fig. 2. Height – MPH SDS at onset, during GH treatment and at near adult height in longitudinally followed children with empty sella.

(6.0 vs. 8.2 years; p < 0.001), which may explain their higher response. Near adult height (NAH) in 52 (34 male) patients longitudinally followed from the onset of GH treatment and through puberty showed that there was a significant increase in height SDS and height – MPH SDS on GH treatment (fig. 1, 2). As seen in table 4, children reached their MPH even at relatively low GH doses, and some even exceeded it. The largest gain in height SDS was during prepubertal ages. NAH was –1.3 (–2.2 to 0.2) in males and –1.2 (–3.7 to 0.5) in females and did not differ from each other. Height – MPH SDS at NAH was –0.4 (–1.1 to 1.4) in females and –0.1 (–1.6 to 1.4) in males. There was no difference between the NAH of the isolated (n = 25) and multiple (n = 27) GHD patients with empty sella, although the Δ height SDS was slightly higher in the multiple GHD patients. The number of patients in each group may be too small to detect a difference. In conclusion, children with GHD and associated empty sella respond well to GH therapy. However, the drawbacks in the diagnosis of empty sella on cranial imaging should be taken into account. There were no major adverse events that may be related to GH treatment. Somnolence in 1, gastrointestinal disturbances like diarrhea and vomiting in 6, dehydration in 1, hypoglycemia in 5, adrenal insufficiency in 3, arrhythmia in 1, pneumonia in 3, cerebral thrombosis in 1, convulsions in 3, and infections in 4 patients were reported as serious events, probably mostly associated with adrenal insufficiency. There was pain at injection in 2 patients. Spine malformation (n = 2), aseptic bone necrosis (n = 2) and intracranial hypertension (n = 1, with recovery) were other reported serious events. Among minor events, abnormal glucose tolerance in 1, gynecomastia in 2, nevus in 1, ede-

Table 4. NAH in empty sella

	Empty sella			
	n	median	10th centile	90th centile
Start of GH treatment				
Age, years	52	7.8	3.4	11.6
Height SDS (Prader)	52	–3.7	–5.0	–2.7
Height – MPH SDS (Prader)	46	–2.6	–4.5	–0.9
Height velocity SDS	24	–2.2	–4.2	0.6
BMI SDS	52	–0.3	–1.7	1.5
GH dose, mg/kg/week	52	0.20	0.14	0.28
Injections/week	52	6	3	7
NAH				
Age, years	52	17.6	15.6	19.9
Height SDS (Prader)	52	–1.3*	–2.2	0.3
Height – MPH SDS (Prader)	46	–0.3*	–1.1	1.4
Δ height (latest to puberty) SDS (Prader)	25	0.0	–1.0	0.7
Δ height (latest to start) SDS (Prader)	52	2.4	1.4	4.7
BMI SDS	51	–0.1	–1.7	1.8
Years on GH	52	9.3	5.5	13.6
Pubertal years on GH	25	3.8	1.6	5.5
Mean prepubertal GH dose, mg/kg/week	52	0.18	0.14	0.24
Mean pubertal GH dose, mg/kg/week	25	0.18	0.13	0.26

BMI = Body mass index. * $p < 0.05$, comparison of values between the start and at NAH.

ma in 1 and headache in 8 patients were reported, in addition to less specific frequently observed childhood disorders.

Midline Palatal Cleft. A total of 91 (50 male) patients with this diagnosis were enrolled in the KIGS database. They had a birth weight and length SDS of –0.9 (–2.2 to 0.6) and –1.1 (–2.9 to 0.6). The longitudinal analysis of 66 (39 male) prepubertal patients, as seen in table 2, shows that the height and height velocity SDS increased significantly on GH therapy over the first year, with an increment in the pretreatment height velocity from 5.7 cm/year (3.6–14.1) to 10.3 cm/year (5.4–19.3; $p < 0.05$). The height – MPH SDS also showed a significant increase. The maximum GH peak (n = 60) was 3.2 μg/l (0.2–9.0), indicating that all children had GHD. The IGF-1 SDS was also low, with a median value of –2.6 (–4.9 to –1.9). The SR showed that the growth response was parallel to the response for IGHD. When analyzed by gender, the Δ height SDS of females (n = 27), 1.3 (0.4–3.0), was higher than that observed in males (n = 39), 0.8 (0.1–2.4), over 1 year of therapy. When analyzed by the presence of other hormone deficiencies, among the available data, isolated GHD was present in 30 (45.5%) and multiple GHD in 31 (47%) of the patients. The Δ height SDS over 1 year of therapy was 0.8 (0.3–1.6) in isolated and 1.8 (0.2–3.0) in multiple GHD patients ($p < 0.01$). Age at onset of therapy was younger in multiple (2.2 years) compared with isolated (7.3 years; $p < 0.001$) GHD patients and the dose of GH higher (0.23 vs. 0.17 mg/kg/week; $p < 0.01$), accounting for the higher response in this group. In conclusion, GHD which may be associated with midline defects responds well to

GH therapy. There were no major adverse events that may be related to GH treatment except for spine malformation in 3 patients and convulsions in 2 patients, as a result of hypoglycemia and epilepsy in each. Death was reported in 1 patient at age 2.7 years. The patient had a medical history of hypoglycemia and anophthalmia and was on hydrocortisone and thyroxine therapy. Among minor events, headache was reported in 2 patients in addition to less specific frequently observed childhood disorders.

SMMCI Syndrome. A total of 18 (7 male) patients with this diagnosis were enrolled in the KIGS database. They had a birth weight and length SDS of –0.6 (–2.5 to 1.4) and –0.6 (–1.7 to 1.8). The longitudinal analysis of 11 (4 male) prepubertal patients, as seen in table 2, shows that the height SDS increased significantly on GH therapy over the first year, with an increment in the pretreatment height velocity from 4.5 cm/year (2.9–5.2) to 9.0 cm/year (8.6–16.7). The height – MPH SDS also showed a significant increase. The maximum GH peak (n = 9) was 4.2 µg/l (0.8–22.0), indicating that most of the children had GHD. When analyzed by the presence of other hormone deficiencies, isolated GHD was present in 7 (63.6%) and multiple GHD in 4 (36.4%) of the patients. The SR showed that the growth response was parallel to the response for IGHD, although the numbers are low in the analysis. There were no major or minor adverse events that may be related to GH treatment.

Congenital Hydrocephalus. A total of 72 patients (39 males, excluding 4 meningomyelocele patients) with this diagnosis were enrolled in the KIGS database. They had a birth weight and length SDS of –0.8 (–2.3 to 0.9) and –0.4 (–2.5 to 0.8). The longitudinal analysis of 52 (29 male) prepubertal patients, as seen in table 2, shows that the height and height velocity SDS increased significantly on GH therapy over the first year, with an increment in the pretreatment height velocity from 4.6 cm/year (2.6–7.5) to 8.1 cm/year (5.4–13.4; $p < 0.05$). The height – MPH SDS also showed a significant increase. The maximum GH peak (n = 45) was 7.1 µg/l (1.7–13.4). The IGF-1 SDS was low in 11 children, with a median value of –2.4 (–4.0 to –0.5). The SR showed that the growth response was within the ranges observed for IGHD. The Δ height SDS in females (0.8) was similar to that of males (0.6) over the first year of therapy. When analyzed by the presence of other hormone deficiencies, among the available data, isolated GHD was present in 39 (75%) and multiple GHD in 6 (11.5%) of the patients. In conclusion, congenital hydrocephalus, not related to meningomyelocele in this series, and mostly associated with GHD, responds well to GH therapy. There were no major adverse events that may be related to GH treatment except for headache in 3 and edema in 1 patient. Among minor events, nevus was reported in 1 patient in addition to less specific frequently observed childhood disorders. Early puberty was noted in 2 patients.

Hypoplastic Anterior Pituitary. Nineteen (9 male) patients with hypoplastic anterior pituitary were enrolled in the KIGS database with a birth weight and length SDS of –0.7 (–2.7 to 0.9) and –0.9 (–2.3 to 0.9). Cross-sectional analysis (table 3) revealed that patients (2 pubertal) showed a remarkable increase in height SDS, increasing their pretreatment height velocity from 3.0 cm/year (2.3–4.5) to 11.3 cm/year (7.9–16.5). The maximum GH peak (n = 18) was 9.7 µg/l (0.5–20.3), and the IGF-1 SDS (n = 14) was –2.1 (–3.7 to –1.6), pointing to GH and/or IGF-1 deficiency. The growth response is satisfactory at least in this cross-sectional analysis. There were no major or minor adverse events that may be related to GH treatment.

There was no significant difference in the body mass index between onset and 1 year of therapy in any of the disorders.

References

1 Rimoin DL, Borochowitz Z, Horton WA: Short stature: physiology and pathology. West J Med 1986;144:710–721.
2 Ranke MB, Guilbaud O: Growth response in prepubertal children with idiopathic growth hormone deficiency during the first two years of treatment of human growth hormone: analysis of the Kabi Pharmacia International Growth Study. Acta Paediatr Scand Suppl 1991;379:109–115.
3 Aarskog D: A familial syndrome of short stature associated with facial dysplasia and genital anomalies. J Pediatr 1970;77:856–861.
4 Glover TW, Verga V, Rafael J, Barcroft C, Gorski JL, Bawle EV, Higgins JV: Translocation breakpoint in Aarskog syndrome maps to Xp11.21. Hum Mol Genet 1993;2:1717–1718.
5 Teebi AS, Rucquoi JK, Meyn MS: Aarskog syndrome: report of a family with review and discussion of nosology. Am J Med Genet 1993;46:501–509.
6 Duncan PA, Klein RM, Wilmat PL, Shapiro LR: Additional features of the Aarskog syndrome. J Pediatr 1977;91:769–770.
7 Brodsky MC, Keppen LD, Rice CD, Ranells JD: Ocular and systemic findings in the Aarskog (facial-digital-genital) syndrome. Am J Ophthalmol 1990;109:450–456.
8 Halse A, Bjorvatn K, Aarskog D: Dental findings in patients with Aarskog syndrome. Scand J Dent Res 1979;87:253–259.
9 Logie LJ, Porteous ME: Intelligence and development in Aarskog syndrome. Arch Dis Child 1998;79:359–360.
10 Furukawa CT, Hall BD, Smith DW: The Aarskog syndrome. J Pediatr 1972;81:1117–1122.
11 Grier RE, Farrington FH, Kendig R, Mamunes P: Autosomal dominant inheritance of the Aarskog syndrome. Am J Med Genet 1983;15:39–46.
12 Pasteris NG, Cadle A, Logie LJ, Porteous ME, Schwartz CE, Stevenson RE, Glover TW, Wilray RS, Gorski JL: Isolation and characterization of the faciogenital dysplasia (Aarskog-Scott syndrome) gene: a putative Rho/Rac guanine nucleotide exchange factor. Cell 1994;79:669–678.
13 Orrico A, Galli L, Cavaliere ML, Garavelli L, Fryns JP, Crushell E, Rinaldi MM, Medeira A, Sorrentino V: Phenotypic and molecular characterisation of the Aarskog-Scott syndrome: a survey of the clinical variability in light of FGD1 mutation analysis in 46 patients. Eur J Hum Genet 2004;12:16–23.
14 Fryns JP: Aarskog syndrome: the changing phenotype with age. Am J Med Genet 1992;43:420–427.
15 Kodama M, Fujimoto S, Namikazoa T, Matsuda I: Aarskog syndrome with isolated growth hormone deficiency. Eur J Pediatr 1981;135:273–276.
16 Petryk A, Richton S, Sy JP, Blethen SL: The effect of growth hormone treatment on stature in Aarskog syndrome. J Pediatr Endocrinol Metab 1999;12:161–165.
17 Darendeliler F, Larsson P, Neyzi O, Price AD, Hagenas L, Sipila I, Lindgren AC, Otten B, Bakker B, KIGS International Board: Growth hormone treatment in Aarskog syndrome: analysis of the KIGS (Pharmacia International Growth Database) data. J Pediatr Endocrinol Metab 2003;16:1137–1142.
18 de Lange C: Sur un type nouveau de dégénération (typus amstelodamensis). Arch Med Enf 1933;36:713–718.
19 Opitz JM: Editorial comment: The Brachmann-de Lange syndrome. Am J Med Genet 1985;22:89–102.
20 Jackson L, Kline AD, Barr MA, Koch S: De Lange syndrome: a clinical review of 310 individuals. Am J Med Genet 1993;47:940–946.
21 Hawley PP, Jackson LG, Kurnit DM: Sixty-four patients with Brachmann-de Lange syndrome: a survey. Am J Med Genet 1985;20:453–459.
22 Bull MJ, Fitzgerald JF, Heifetz SA, Brei TJ: Gastrointestinal abnormalities: a significant cause of feeding difficulties and failure to thrive in Brachmann-de Lange syndrome. Am J Med Genet 1993;47:1029–1034.
23 Tsukahara M, Okamoto N, Ohashi H, Kuwajima K, Kondo I, Sugie H, Nagai T, Naritomi K, Hasegawa T, Fukushima Y, Masuno M, Kuroki Y: Brachmann-de Lange syndrome and congenital heart disease. Am J Med Genet 1998;75:441–442.
24 Lacassie Y, Bobadilla O, Cambias RD: A boy with a mild case of Cornelia de Lange syndrome with above average intelligence. J Intellect Dev Disabil 1997;22:293–299.
25 Berney TP, Ireland M, Burn J: Behavioural phenotype of Cornelia de Lange syndrome. Arch Dis Child 1999;81:333–336.
26 Allanson JE, Hennekam RCM, Ireland M: De Lange syndrome: subjective and objective comparison of the classical and mild phenotypes. J Med Genet 1997;34:645–650.
27 Russell KL, Ming JE, Patel K, Jukofsky L, Magnusson M, Krantz ID: Dominant paternal transmission of Cornelia de Lange syndrome: a new case and review of 25 previously reported familial recurrences. Am J Med Genet 2001;104:267–276.
28 Krantz ID, McCallum J, DeScipio C, Kaur M, Gillis LA, Yaeger D, Jukofsly L, Wasserman N, Bottani A, Morris CA, Nowaczyk MJ, Toriello H, Bamshad MJ, Carey JC, Rappaport E, Kawauchi S, Lander AD, Calof AL, Li HH, Devoto M, Jackson LG: Cornelia de Lange syndrome is caused by mutations in NIPBL, the human homolog of *Drosophila melanogaster* Nipped-B. Nat Genet 2004;36:631–635.
29 Bhuiyan ZA, Klein M, Hammond P, van Haeringen A, Mannens MM, Van Berckelaer-Onnes I, Hennekam RC: Genotype-phenotype correlations of 39 patients with Cornelia de Lange syndrome: the Dutch experience. Med Genet 2006;43:568–575.
30 Musio A, Selicorni A, Focarelli ML, Gervasini C, Milani D, Russo S, Vezzoni P, Larizza L: X-linked Cornelia de Lange syndrome owing to SMC1L1 mutations. Nat Genet 2006;38:528–530.
31 Kline AD, Barr M, Jackson LG: Growth manifestations in the Brachmann-de Lange syndrome. Am J Med Genet 1993;47:1042–1049.
32 Hillman JC, Hammond J, Neo O, Reiss M: Endocrine investigations in de Lange's and Seckel's syndromes. J Ment Defic 1968;3:30–33.
33 Kousseff BG, Thomson-Meares J, Newkirk P, Root AW: Physical growth in Brachmann-de Lange syndrome. Am J Med Genet 1993;47:1050–1052.

34 Tonini G, Marinoni S: Neonatal-onset panhypopituitarism in a girl with Brachmann-de Lange syndrome. Am J Med Genet 1990;36:102–103.
35 Schwartz DI, Schwartz KJ, Kousseff BG, Bercu BB, Root AW: Endocrinopathies in Cornelia de Lange syndrome. J Pediatr 1990;117:920–923.
36 Down JLH: Observation on an ethnic classification of idiots. London Hosp Clin Lect Rep 1866;3:259–262.
37 Pueschel SM: Clinical aspects of Down syndrome from infancy to adulthood. Am J Med Genet Suppl 1990;7:52–56.
38 Carr J: Six weeks to twenty-one years old: longitudinal study of children with Down's syndrome and their families. J Child Psychol Psychiatry 1988;29:407–431.
39 Källén B, Mastroiacovo P, Robert E: Major congenital malformations in Down syndrome. Am J Med Genet 1996;65:160–166.
40 Dixon N, Kishnani PS, Zimmerman S: Clinical manifestations of hematologic and oncologic disorders in patients with Down syndrome. Am J Med Genet C Semin Med Genet 2006;142:149–157.
41 Mazzoni DS, Ackley RS, Nash DJ: Abnormal pinna type and hearing loss correlations in Down's syndrome. J Intellect Disabil Res 1994;38:549–560.
42 Epstein CJ: Down syndrome (trisomy 21); in Scriver CR, Beaudet AL, Sly WS, Valle D (eds): The Metabolic and Molecular Bases of Inherited Disease, ed 8. New York, McGraw-Hill, 2001, vol 1, pp 1223–1256.
43 Cronk CE: Growth of children with Down's syndrome: birth to age 3 years. Pediatrics 1978;61:564–568.
44 Rarick GL, Seefeldt V: Observations from longitudinal data on growth in stature and sitting height of children with Down's syndrome. J Ment Defic Res 1974;18:63–78.
45 Cronk C, Crocker AC, Pueschel SM, Shea AM, Zackai E, Pickens G, Reed RB: Growth charts for children with Down syndrome: 1 month to 18 years of age. Pediatrics 1988;81:102–110.
46 Myrelid A, Gustafsson J, Ollars B, Anneren G: Growth charts for Down's syndrome from birth to 18 years of age. Arch Dis Child 2002;87:97–103.
47 Kimura J, Tachibana K, Imaizumi K, Kurosawa K, Kuroki Y: Longitudinal growth and height velocity of Japanese children with Down's syndrome. Acta Paediatr 2003;92:1039–1042.
48 Palmer CGS, Cronk C, Pueschel SM, Wisniewski KE, Laxova R, Crocker AC, Pauli RM: Head circumference of children with Down syndrome (0–36 months). Am J Med Genet 1992;42:61–67.
49 Anneren G, Sara VR, Hall K, Tuvemo T: Growth and somatomedin response to growth hormone in Down's syndrome. Arch Dis Child 1986;61:48–52.
50 Torrado C, Bastian W, Wisniewski EK, Castelis S: Treatment of children with Down syndrome and growth retardation with recombinant human growth hormone. J Pediatr 1991;119:478–483.
51 Sara VR, Gustavson KH, Anneren G, Hall K, Wetterberg L: Somatomedins in Down's syndrome. Biol Psychiatry 1983;18:803–811.
52 Anneren G, Enberg G, Sara VR: The presence of normal levels of serum immunoreactive insulin-like growth factor 2 (IGF-2) in patients with Down's syndrome. Ups J Med Sci 1984;89:274–278.
53 Sara VR, Sjögren B, Anneren G, Gustavson KH, Forsman A, Hall K, Vahlström J, Wetterberg L: The presence of normal receptors for somatomedin and insulin in fetuses with Down's syndrome. Biol Psychiatry 1984;19:591–598.
54 Anneren G, Tuvemo T, Carlssom-Skwirut C, Lonnerholm T, Bang P, Sara VR, Gustafsson J: Growth hormone treatment in young children with Down's syndrome: effects on growth and psychomotor development. Arch Dis Child 1999;80:334–338.
55 Pelletier G, Feingold M: Case report 1; in Bergsma D (ed): Syndrome Identification. White Plains, National Foundation – March of Dimes, 1973, vol 1, pp 8–9.
56 Leisti J, Hollister DW, Rimoin DL: The Floating-Harbor syndrome. Birth Defects Orig Artic Ser 1975;11:305.
57 Robinson PL, Shohat M, Winter RM, Conte WJ, Gordon-Nesbitt D, Feingold M, Paron Z, Rimoin DL: A unique association of short stature, dysmorphic features, and speech impairment (Floating-Harbor syndrome). J Pediatr 1988;113:703–706.
58 Majewski F, Lenard HG: The Floating-Harbor syndrome. Eur J Pediatr 1991;150:250–252.
59 Ala-Mello S, Peippo M: Two more diagnostic signs in the Floating-Harbor syndrome. Clin Dysmorphol 1996;5:85–88.
60 Lacombe D, Patton MA, Elleau C, Battin J: Floating-Harbor syndrome: description of a further patient, review of the literature, and suggestion of autosomal dominance inheritance. Eur J Pediatr 1995;154:658–661.
61 Rosen AC, Newby RF, Sauer CM, Lacey T, Hammeke TA, Lubinsky MS: A further report on a case of Floating-Harbor syndrome in a mother and daughter. J Clin Exp Neuropsychol 1998;20:483–495.
62 Cannavo S, Bartolone L, Lapa D, Venturino M, Almoto B, Violi A, Trimarchi F: Abnormalities of GH secretion in a young girl with Floating-Harbor syndrome. J Endocrinol Invest 2002;25:58–64.
63 Wieczorek D, Wusthof A, Harms E, Meinecke P: Floating-Harbor syndrome in two unrelated girls: mild short stature in one patient and effective growth hormone therapy in the other. Am J Med Genet 2001;104:47–52.
64 Wiltshire E, Wickremesekera A, Dixon J: Floating-Harbor syndrome complicated by tethered cord: a new association and potential contribution from growth hormone therapy. Am J Med Genet A 2005;136:81–83.
65 Niikawa N, Matsuura N, Fukushima Y, Ohsawa T, Kajii T: Kabuki make-up syndrome: a syndrome of mental retardation, unusual facies, large and protruding ears, and postnatal growth deficiency. J Pediatr 1981;99:565–569.
66 Kuroki Y, Suzuki Y, Chiyo H, Hata A, Matsui I: A new malformation syndrome of long palpebral fissures, large ears, depressed nasal tip and skeletal anomalies associated with postnatal dwarfism and mental retardation. J Pediatr 1981;99:570–573.
67 Niikawa N, Kuroki Y, Kajii T, Matsuura N, Ishikiriyama S, Tonoki H, Ishikawa N, Yamada Y, Fujita M, Umemoto H, Iwama Y, Kondoh I, et al: Kabuki make-up (Niikawa-Kuroki) syndrome: a study of 62 patients. Am J Med Genet 1988;31:565–589.
68 Wilson GN: Thirteen cases of Niikawa-Kuroki syndrome: report and review with emphasis on medical complications and preventive management. Am J Med Genet 1998;79:112–120.

69 Wessels MW, Brooks AS, Hoogeboom J, Niermeijer MF, Willems PJ: Kabuki syndrome: a review study of three hundred patients. Clin Dysmorphol 2002; 11:95–102.
70 Kawame, H, Hannibal MC, Hudgins L, Pagon RA: Phenotypic spectrum and management issues in Kabuki syndrome. J Pediatr 1999;134:480–485.
71 Niikawa N, Kuroki Y, Kajii T: The dermatoglyphic pattern of the Kabuki make-up syndrome. Clin Genet 1982; 21:315–320.
72 Digilio MC, Marino B, Toscano A, Giannotti A, Dallapiccola B: Congenital heart defects in Kabuki syndrome. Am J Med Genet 2001;100:269–274.
73 Mervis CB, Becerra AM, Rowe ML, Hersh JH, Morris CA: Intellectual abilities and adaptive behavior of children and adolescents with Kabuki syndrome: a preliminary study. Am J Med Genet A 2005;132:248–255.
74 Ming JE, Russell KL, McDonald McGinn DM, Zackai EH: Autoimmune disorders in Kabuki syndrome. Am J Med Genet A 2005;132:260–262.
75 Armstrong L, Abd El Moneim A, Aleck K, Aughton DJ, Baumann C, Braddock SR, Gillessen-Kaesbach G, Graham JM Jr, Grebe TA, Gripp KW, Hall BD, Hennekam R, Hunter A, Keppler-Noreuil K, Lacombe D, Lin AE, Ming JE, Kokitsu-Nakata NM, Nikkel SM, Philip N, Raas-Rothschild A, Sommer A, Verloes A, Walter C, Wieczorek D, Williams MS, Zackai E, Allanson JE: Further delineation of Kabuki syndrome in 48 well-defined new individuals. Am J Med Genet A 2005;132:265–272.
76 White SM, Thompson EM, Kidd A, Savarirayan R, Turner A, Amor D, Delatycki MB, Fahey M, Baxendale A, White S, Haan E, Gibson K, Halliday JL, Bankier A: Growth, behavior and clinical findings in 27 patients with Kabuki (Niikawa-Kuroki) syndrome. Am J Med Genet A 2004;127:118–127.
77 Tawa R, Kaino Y, Ito T, Goto Y, Kida K, Matsuda H: A case of Kabuki make-up syndrome with central diabetes insipidus and growth hormone neurosecretory dysfunction. Acta Paediatr Jpn 1994;36:412–415.
78 Devriendt K, Lemli L, Craen M, de Zegher F: Growth hormone deficiency and premature thelarche in a female infant with Kabuki makeup syndrome. Horm Res 1995;43:303–306.
79 Gabrielli O, Carloni I, Coppa GV, Bedeschi MF, Petroncini MM, Selicorni A: Long-term hormone replacement therapy in two patients with Kabuki syndrome and growth hormone deficiency. Minerva Pediatr 2000;52:47–53.
80 Gabrielli O, Bruni S, Bruschi B, Carloni I, Coppa GV: Kabuki syndrome and growth hormone deficiency: description of a case treated by long-term hormone replacement. Clin Dysmorphol 2002;11:71–72.
81 Schrander-Stumpel CT, Spruyt L, Curfs LM, Defloor T, Schrander JJ: Kabuki syndrome: clinical data in 20 patients, literature review, and further guidelines for preventive management. Am J Med Genet A 2005;132:234–243.
82 Fujishiro M, Ogihara T, Tsukuda K, Shojima N, Fukushima Y, Kimura S, Oka Y, Asano T: A case showing an association between type 1 diabetes mellitus and Kabuki syndrome. Diabetes Res Clin Pract 2003;60:25–31.
83 Williams JCP, Barrat-Boyes BG, Lowe JB: Supravalvular aortic stenosis. Circulation 1961;24:1311–1318.
84 Beuren AJ, Schulze C, Eberle P, Harmjanz D, Apitz J: The syndrome of supravalvular aortic stenosis, peripheral pulmonary stenosis, mental retardation and similar facial appearance. Am J Cardiol 1964;13:471–483.
85 Pankau R, Siebert R, Kautza M, Schneppenheim R, Gosch A, Wessel A, Partsch CJ: Familial Williams-Beuren syndrome showing varying clinical expression. Am J Med Genet 2001;98:324–329.
86 Pankau R, Partsch CJ, Gosch A, Opperman IC, Wessel A: Statural growth in Williams-Beuren syndrome. Eur J Pediatr 1992;151:751–755.
87 Franceschini P, Guala A, Vardeu MP, Signorile F, Franceschini D, Mastroiacovo P, Gianotti A, Livini E, Lalatta F, Selicorni A, Andria G, Scaranao G, Della Monica M, Rizzo R, Zelante L, Stabile M, Gabrielli O, Neri G: The Williams syndrome: an Italian collaborative study. Minerva Pediatr 1996;48:421–428.
88 Winter M, Pankau R, Amm M, Gosch A, Wessel A: The spectrum of ocular features in the Williams-Beuren syndrome. Clin Genet 1996;49:28–31.
89 Hallidie-Smith KA, Karas S: Cardiac anomalies in Williams-Beuren syndrome. Arch Dis Child 1988;63:809–813.
90 Broder K, Reinhardt E, Ahern J, Lifton R, Tamborlane W, Pober B: Elevated ambulatory blood pressure in 20 subjects with Williams syndrome. Am J Med Genet 1999;83:356–360.
91 Pankau R, Partsch CJ, Winter M, Gosch A: Incidence and spectrum of renal abnormalities in Williams-Beuren syndrome. Am J Med Genet 1996;63:301–304.
92 Gosch A, Stading G, Pankau R: Linguistic abilities in children with Williams-Beuren syndrome. Am J Med Genet 1994;52:291–296.
93 Morris CA, Demsey SA, Leonoral CO, Dilts C, Blackburn BL: Natural history of Williams syndrome: physical characteristics. J Pediatr 1988;113:318–326.
94 Preus M: The Williams syndrome: objective definition and diagnosis. Clin Genet 1984;25:422–428.
95 Ounap K, Laidre P, Partsch O, Rein R, Lipping-Sitska M: Familial Williams-Beuren syndrome. Am J Med Genet 1998;80:491–493.
96 Ewart AK, Morris CA, Atkinson D, Jin W, Sternes K, Spallone P, Stock AD, Leppert M, Keating MT: Hemizygosity at the elastin locus in a developmental disorder, Williams syndrome. Nature Genet 1993;5:11–16.
97 Nickerson E, Greenberg F, Keating MT, McCaskill C, Shaffer LG: Deletions of the elastin gene at 7q11.23 occur in approximately 90% of patients with Williams syndrome. Am J Hum Genet 1995;56:1156–1161.
98 De Silva U, Massa H, Trask BJ, Green ED: Comparative mapping of the region of human chromosome 7 deleted in Williams syndrome. Genome Res 1999;9:428–436.
99 Partsch CJ, Dreyer G, Gosch A, Winter M, Scheppenheim R, Wessel A, Pankau R: Longitudinal evaluation of growth, puberty and bone maturation in children with Williams syndrome. J Pediatr 1999;134:82–89.
100 Kuijpers GM, De Vroede M, Knol HE, Jansen M: Growth hormone treatment in a child with Williams-Beuren syndrome: a case report. Eur J Pediatr 1999;158:451–454.

101 Xekouki P, Fryssira H, Maniati-Christidi M, Amenta S, Karavitakis EM, Kanaka-Gantenbein C, Dacou Voutetakis C: Growth hormone deficiency in a child with Williams-Beuren syndrome. The response to growth hormone therapy. J Pediatr Endocrinol Metab 2005;18:205–207.

102 Selicorni A, Fratoni A, Pavesi MA, Bottigelli M, Arnaboldi E, Milani D: Thyroid anomalies in Williams syndrome: investigation of 95 patients. Am J Med Genet A 2006;140:1098–1101.

103 Amenta S, Moschovi M, Sofocleous C, Kostaridou S, Mavrou A, Fryssira H: Non-Hodgkin lymphoma in a child with Williams syndrome. Cancer Genet Cytogenet 2004;154:86–88.

104 Hasle H, Olsen JH, Hansen J, Friedrich U, Tommerup N: Occurrence of cancer in a cohort of 183 persons with constitutional chromosome 7 abnormalities. Cancer Genet Cytogenet 1998;105:39–42.

105 Fanconi G: Familäre infantile perniziosaartige Anämie (perniziöses Blutbild und Konstitution). Jahre Kinderh 1927;117:257.

106 Auerbach AD, Buchwald M, Joenje H: Fanconi anemia; in Scriver CR, Beaudet AI, Sly WS, Valle D (eds): The Metabolic and Moleculer Bases of Inherited Disease, ed 8. New York, McGraw-Hill, 2001, vol 1, pp 753–768.

107 Giampietro PF, Adler-Brecher B, Verlander PC, Pavlakis SG, Davis JG, Auerbach AD: The need for more accurate and timely diagnosis in Fanconi anemia: a report from the International Fanconi Anemia Registry. Pediatrics 1993;91:1116–1120.

108 Giampietro PF, Verlander PC, Maschan A, Davis JG, Auerbach AD: Fanconi anemia: a model for somatic gene mutation during development. Am J Genet 1994;52:36.

109 Giampietro PF, Verlander PC, Davis JG, Auerbach AD: Diagnosis of Fanconi anemia in patients without congenital malformations: an international Fanconi Anemia Registry Study. Am J Med Genet 1997;68:58–61.

110 Kutler DI, Singh B, Satagopan J, Batish SD, Berwick M, Giampietro PF, Hanenberg H, Auerbach AD: A 20-year perspective on the International Fanconi Anemia Registry (IFAR). Blood 2003;101:1249–1256.

111 Butturini A, Gale RP, Verlander PC, Adler-Brecher B, Gillio AP, Auerbach AD: Hematologic abnormalities in Fanconi anemia: an International Fanconi Anemia Registry study. Blood 1994;84:1650.

112 Auerbach AD, Adler B, Chaganti RSK: Prenatal and postnatal diagnosis and carrier detection of Fanconi anemia by a cytogenetic method. Pediatrics 1981;67:128–135.

113 Auerbach AD, Rogatko A, Schroeder-Kurth TM: International Fanconi Anemia Registry: relation of clinical symptoms to diepoxybutane sensitivity. Blood 1989;73:391–396.

114 Strathdee CA, Gavish H, Shannon W, Buchwald M: Cloning of cDNAs for Fanconi anaemia by functional complementation. Nature 1992;356:763–767.

115 Soulier J, Leblanc T, Larghero J, Dastot H, Shimamura A, Guardiola P, Esperou H, Ferry C, Jubert C, Feugeas JP, Henri A, Toubert A, Socie G, Baruchel A, Sigaux F, D'Andrea AD, Gluckman E: Detection of somatic mosaicism and classification of Fanconi anemia patients by analysis of the FA/BRCA pathway. Blood 2005; 105:1329–1336.

116 Wajnrajch MP, Gertner JM, Huma Z, Popovic J, Lin K, Verlander PC, Batish SD, Giampietro PF, Davis JG, New MI, Auerbach AD: Evaluation of growth and hormonal status in patients referred to the International Fanconi Anemia Registry. Pediatrics 2001;107: 744–754.

117 Berkovitz GD, Zinkham WH, Migeon CJ: Gonadal function in two siblings with Fanconi's anemia. Horm Res 1984;19:137–141.

118 Massa GG, Heinrichs C, Vamos E, Van Vliet G: Hypergonadotropic hypogonadism in a boy with Fanconi anemia with growth hormone deficiency and pituitary stalk interruption. J Pediatr 2002;140:277.

119 Petrij F, Giles RH, Breuning MH, Hennekam RCM: Rubinstein-Taybi syndrome; in Scriver CR, Beaudet AI, Sly WS, Valle D (eds): The Metabolic and Molecular Bases of Inherited Disease, ed 8. New York, McGraw-Hill, 2001, vol 4, pp 6167–6182.

120 Hennekam RCM, Van den Boogaard MJ, Sibbles BJ, Van Spijker HG: Rubinstein-Taybi syndrome in the Netherlands. Am J Med Genet 1990;6(suppl):17–29.

121 Allanson JE: Rubinstein-Taybi syndrome: the changing face. Am J Med Genet 1990;6(suppl):38–41.

122 Filippi G: The Rubinstein-Taybi syndrome: report of 7 cases. Clin Genet 1972;3:303–318.

123 Hennekam RCM, Van Doome JM: Oral aspects of Rubinstein-Taybi syndrome. Am J Med Genet 1990;6(suppl):42–47.

124 Rubinstein JH: Broad thumb-hallux (Rubinstein-Taybi) syndrome 1957–1988. Am J Med Genet 1990;6(suppl):3–16.

125 Stevens CA, Carey JC, Blackburn BL: Rubinstein-Taybi syndrome: a natural history study. Am J Med Genet 1990; 6(suppl):30–37.

126 Stevens CA, Bhakta MG: Cardiac abnormalities in the Rubinstein-Taybi syndrome. Am J Med Genet 1995;59: 346–348.

127 Hennekam RC, Baselier AC, Beyaert E, Bos A, Blok JB, Jansma HB, Thorbecke-NiIsen VV, Veerman H: Psychological and speech studies in Rubinstein-Taybi syndrome. Am J Ment Retard 1992;96:645–660.

128 Miller RW, Rubinstein JH: Tumors in Rubinstein-Taybi syndrome. Am J Med Genet 1995;56:112–115.

129 Goodfellow A, Emmerson RW, Calvert HT: Rubinstein-Taybi syndrome and spontaneous keloids. Clin Exp Dermatol 1980;5:369–370.

130 Lacombe D, Saura R, Taine L, Battin J: Confirmation of assignment of a locus for Rubinstein-Taybi syndrome gene to 16pI3.3. Am J Med Genet 1992;44: 126–128.

131 Hou JW: Rubinstein-Taybi syndrome: clinical and molecular cytogenetic studies. Acta Paediatr Taiwan 2005; 46:143–148.

132 Roelfsema JH, White SJ, Ariyürek Y, Bartholdi D, Niedrist D, Papadia F, Bacino CA, den Dunnen JT, van Ommen GJ, Breuning MH, Hennekam RC, Peters DJ: Genetic heterogeneity in Rubinstein-Taybi syndrome: mutations in both the CBP and EP300 genes cause disease. Am J Hum Genet 2005;76:572–580.

133 Stevens CA, Hennekam RCM, Blackburn BL: Growth in the Rubinstein-Taybi syndrome. Am J Med Genet 1990;6(suppl):51–55.
134 Olson DP, Koenig RJ: Thyroid function in Rubinstein-Taybi syndrome. J Clin Endocrinol Metab 1997;82:3264–3266.
135 McCusick VA, Eldridge R, Hostetler JA, Egeland JA, Ruangwit U: Dwarfism in the Amish. 2. Cartilage-hair hypoplasia. Bull Johns Hopkins Hosp 1965;116:285–326.
136 Mäkitie O, Sulisalo T, de la Chapelle A, Kaitila I: Cartilage-hair hypoplasia. J Med Genet 1995;32:39–43.
137 Mäkitie O, Kaitila I, Savilahti E: Deficiency of humoral immunity in cartilage-hair hypoplasia. J Pediatr 2000;137:487–492.
138 Mäkitie O, Pukkala E, Kaitila I: Increased mortality in cartilage-hair dysplasia. Arch Dis Child 2001;84:65–67.
139 Mäkitie O, Pukkala E, Teppo L, Kaitila I: Increased incidence of cancer in patients with cartilage-hair dysplasia. J Pediatr 1999;134:315–318.
140 Mäkitie O, Kaitilia I: Cartilage-hair hypoplasia – clinical manifestations in 108 Finnish patients. Eur J Pediatr 1993;152:211–217.
141 Williams MS, Ettinger RS, Hermanns P, Lee B, Carlson G, Taskinen M, Mäkitie O: The natural history of severe anemia in cartilage – hair hypoplasia. Am J Med Genet A 2005;138:35–40.
142 Mäkitie O, Marttinen E, Kaitila I: Skeletal growth in cartilage-hair dysplasia. A radiological study in 82 patients. Pediatr Radiol 1992;22:434–439.
143 Glass RB, Tift CJ: Radiologic changes in infancy in McKusick cartilage hair hypoplasia. Am J Med Genet 1990;86:312–315.
144 Ridanpää M, van Eenennaam H, Pelin K, Chadwick R, Johnson C, Yuan B, vanVenrooij W, Pruijn G, Salmela R, Rockas R, Makitie O, Kaitila I, de la Chapella A: Mutations in the RNA component of RNase MRP cause a pleotropic human disease, cartilage-hair dysplasia. Cell 2001;104:195–203.
145 Hermanns P, Tran A, Munivez A, Carter S, Zabel B, Lee B, Leroy JG: RMRP mutations in cartilage-hair hypoplasia. Am J Med Genet A 2006;140:2121–2130.

146 Mäkitie O, Perheentupa J, Kaitila I: Growth in cartilage-hair hypoplasia. Pediatr Res 1992;31:176–180.
147 Mäkitie OM, Tapanainen PJ, Dunkel L, Siimes MA: Impaired spermatogenesis: an unrecognized feature of cartilage-hair hypoplasia. Am Med 2001;33:201–205.
148 Harada D, Yamanaka Y, Ueda K, Shimizu J, Inoue M, SeinoY, Tanaka H: An effective case of growth hormone treatment on cartilage-hair hypoplasia. Bone 2005;36:317–322.
149 Bocca G, Weemaes CM, van der Burgt I, Otten BJ: Growth hormone treatment in cartilage-hair hypoplasia: effect on growth and the immune system. J Pediatr Endocrinol Metab 2004;17:47–54.
150 Tracy MR, Dormans JP, Kusumi K: Klippel-Feil syndrome: clinical features and current understanding of etiology. Clin Orthop Relat Res 2004;424:183–190.
151 McGaughran JM, Kuna P, Das V: Audiological abnormalities in the Klippel-Feil syndrome. Arch Dis Child 1998;79:352–355.
152 Clarke RA, Catalan G, Diwan AD, Kearsley JH: Heterogeneity in Klippel-Feil syndrome: a new classification. Pediatr Radiol 1998;28:967–974.
153 Thompson E, Haan E, Sheffield L: Autosomal dominant Klippel-Feil anomaly with cleft palate. Clin Dysmorphol 1998;7:11–15.
154 Tubbs RS, Oakes WJ, Blount JP: Isolated atlantal stenosis in a patient with idiopathic growth hormone deficiency, and Klippel-Feil and Duane's syndromes. Childs Nerv Syst 2005;21:421–424.
155 Diamond LK, Allen DM, Magill FB: Congenital (erythroid) hypoplastic anemia. A 25-year study. Am J Dis Child 1961;102:403–415.
156 Ball SE, McGuckin CP, Jenkins G, Gordon-Smith EC: Diamond-Blackfan anaemia in the UK: analysis of 80 cases from a 20-year birth cohort. Br J Haematol 1996;94:645–653.

157 Willig TN, Draptchinskaia N, Dianzami I, Ball S, Niemeyer C, Ramenghi U, Orfali K, Gustavsson P, Garelli E, Brusco A, Tiemann C, Perignon JL, Bouchier C, Cicchiello L, Dahl N, Mohandas N, Tchernia G: Mutations in ribosomal protein S19 gene and Diamond-Blackfan anemia: wide variations in phenotypic expression. Blood 1999;94:4294–4306.
158 Willig TN, Niemeyer CM, Leblanc T, Tiemann C, Robert A, Budde J, Lambiliotte A, Kohne E, Souillet G, Eber S, Stephan JL, Girot R, Bordigoni P, Cornu G, Blanche S, Guillard JM, Mohandas N, Tchernia G: Identification of new prognosis factors from the clinical and epidemiologic analysis of a registry of 229 Diamond-Blackfan anemia patients. DBA group of Société d'Hématologie et d'Immunologie Pédiatrique (SHIP), Gesellschaft für Pädiatrische Onkologie und Hämatologie (GPOH), and the European Society for Pediatric Hematology and Immunology (ESPHI). Pediatr Res 1999;46:553–561.
159 Draptchinskaia N, Gustavsson P, Andersson B, Pettersson M, Willig TN, Dianzani I, Ball S, Tchernia G, Klar J, Matsson H, Tentler D, Mohandas N, Carlsson B, Dahl N: The gene encoding ribosomal protein S19 is mutated in Diamond-Blackfan anaemia. Nat Genet 1999;21:169–175.
160 Gazda H, Lipton JM, Willig TN, Ball S, Niemeyer CM, Tchernia G, Mohandas N, Daly MJ, Ploszynska A, Orfali KA, Vlachos A, Glader BE, Rokicka-Milewska R, Ohara A, Baker D, Pospisilova D, Webber A, Viskochil DH, Nathan DG, Beggs AH, Sieff CA: Evidence for linkage of familial Diamond-Blackfan anemia to chromosome 8p23.3–p22 and for non-19q non-8p disease. Blood 2001;97:2145–2150.
161 Lanes R, Muller A, Palacios A: Multiple endocrine abnormalities in a child with Blackfan-Diamond anemia and hemochromatosis. Significant improvement of growth velocity and predicted adult height following growth hormone treatment despite liver damage. J Pediatr Endocrinol Metab 2000;13:325–328.

162 Leblanc T, Gluckman E, Brauner R: Growth hormone deficiency caused by pituitary stalk interruption in Diamond-Blackfan anemia. J Pediatr 2003;142:358.

163 Scott EG, Haider A, Hord J: Growth hormone therapy for short stature in Diamond-Blackfan anemia. Pediatr Blood Cancer 2004;43:542–544.

164 Hoffman HJ, Hendrick EB, Humphreys RP, Armstrong EA: Investigation and management of suprasellar arachnoid cysts. J Neurosurg 1982;57: 597–601.

165 Adan L, Bussieres L, Dinand V, Zerah M, Pierre-Kahn A, Brauner R: Growth, puberty and hypothalamic-pituitary function in children with suprasellar arachnoid cyst. Eur J Pediatr 2000;159:348–355.

166 Mohn A, Schoof E, Fahlbusch R, Wenzel D, Dorr HG: The endocrine spectrum of arachnoid cysts in childhood. Pediatr Neurosurg 1999;31:316–321.

167 Cacciari E, Zucchini S, Ambrosetto P, Tani G, Carla G, Cicognani A, Pirazzoli P, Sganga T, Balsamo A, Cassio A: Empty sella in children and adolescents with possible hypothalamic-pituitary disorders. J Clin Enodcrinol Metab 1994;78:767–771.

168 DiNatale B, Scotti G, Pellini C, del Maschino A, Triulzi F, Petecca C, Uboldi F, Chiumello G: Empty sella in children with pituitary dwarfism: does it exist? Pediatrician 1987;14: 246–252.

169 Hall RK: Solitary median maxillary central incisor (SMMCI) syndrome. Orphanet J Rare Dis 2006;1:1–9.

170 Rudman D, Davis T, Priest JH, Patterson JH, Kutner MH, Heymsfield SB, Bethel RA: Prevalence of growth hormone deficiency in children with cleft lip or palate. J Pediatr 1978;93:378–382.

171 Traggiai C, Stanhope R: Endocrinopathies associated with midline cerebral and cranial malformations. J Pediatr 2002;140:252–255.

172 Hochhaus F, Butenandt O, Schwarz HP, Ring-Mrozik E: Auxological and endocrinological evaluation of children with hydrocephalus and/or meningomyelocele. Eur J Pediatr 1997; 156:597–601.

173 Cholley F, Trivin C, Sainte-Rose C, Souberbielle JC, Cinalli G, Brauner A: Disorders of growth and puberty in children with non-tumoral hydrocephalus. J Pediatr Endocrinol Metab 2001;14:319–327.

Childhood Brain Tumours and Growth Hormone Treatment

Andreas Jostel   Stephen M. Shalet

Childhood brain tumours (CBTs) cause more deaths than any other paediatric cancer. They are the most common solid tumours in childhood accounting for one sixth of all malignancies. Advances in diagnosis and treatment have increased long-term survival in these children, but most of them remain at high risk of developing complications later in life as a result of their disease or its treatment. Endocrinopathies are the most commonly encountered late effects in these cancer survivors, with growth hormone (GH) deficiency being the most frequent abnormality of the hypothalamic-pituitary axis after cranial irradiation. Many late effects are of delayed onset or may progress with time, and life-long monitoring is mandatory.

Clinical Presentation and Classification

The clinical presentation is primarily determined by the age of the child and the location of the tumour. The most common location is infratentorial (45–60% of all CBTs), followed by supratentorial hemispheric (25–40%) and supratentorial midline (15–20%) location [1]. Infants may present with failure to thrive, increased head circumference or vomiting due to hydrocephalus caused by infratentorial or midline tumours. Children may lose previously attained milestones, may have seizures unrelated to fever or develop headaches and focal neurological deficits with supratentorial tumours. Tumours of the brainstem often cause ataxia, cranial nerve deficits or pyramidal signs, whereas those arising in the suprasellar region may cause visual loss or endocrine dysfunction, e.g., growth abnormalities or precocious puberty [2].

The revised World Health Organization classification [3] of brain tumours is the internationally most widely adopted histological classification system. It is based primarily on histological features and describes the tumours based on the cell of origin (table 1).

Department of Endocrinology, Christie Hospital
Wilmslow Road
Manchester M20 4BX (UK)

Astrocytomas account for 46% of all tumours, followed by medulloblastomas/primitive neuroectodermal tumours with 22%, other gliomas with 17% and ependymomas with 11% [4].

The improved histological classification criteria have been a step forward in standardizing histological reporting, but they do not eliminate diagnostic inaccuracy from subjective interpretation of the histological features, which are not always reliably and reproducibly identified by different observers. Additionally, the histological appearance of a brain tumour is often heterogeneous, which adds to the potential diagnostic confusion.

Epidemiology

Over recent decades, a wealth of epidemiological data on CBTs has been gathered. However, the analysis of these data with regard to epidemiological trends is not straightforward. Very few populations have been studied with inclusive tumour registries, i.e. most national statistics are extrapolations of figures derived from smaller areas. This approach may misrepresent geographical heterogeneity in tumour incidence or the effects of variations in ethnicity, urbanization and affluence. Furthermore, trend analysis is hampered by changes in diagnostic classifications (e.g., non-malignant CBT have only been included in major US cancer registries since 2004) and improvements in diagnostic methods, e.g., imaging technology.

The Surveillance, Epidemiology and End Results (SEER) Program in the United States has been a main source of population-based CBT incidence and survival data since 1973. It collects data from several cancer registries, including five US states and four metropolitan areas across the US, representing 9% of the whole population. The combined data from the SEER Program and the National Program of Cancer Registries in 2002 estimated the annual incidence and mortal-

Table 1. World Health Organization brain tumour classification and examples

Tumours of neuroepithelial tissue
Astrocytic tumours
    Diffuse astrocytoma, anaplastic astrocytoma, glioblastoma
Oligodendroglial tumours
    Oligodendroglioma, ependymoma
Mixed tumours
    Oligoastrocytoma
Choroid plexus tumours
    Choroid plexus papilloma
Neuronal and mixed neuronal-glial tumours
    Gangliocytoma, cerebellar liponeurocytoma
Pineal tumours
    Pineoblastoma
Embryonal tumours
    Medulloblastoma, supratentorial primitive neuroectodermal tumours
Neuroblastic tumours
    Olfactory neuroepithelioma
Glial tumours of uncertain aetiology
    Gliomatosis cerebri

Tumours of peripheral nerves
Schwannoma, neurofibroma

Tumours of the meninges
Meningioma, rhabdomyosarcoma

Lymphomas and haemopoietic neoplasms, germ cell tumours
Germinoma, yolk sac tumour, choriocarcinoma, teratoma

Tumours of the sellar region
Craniopharyngioma

Metastatic tumours

ity rates as 3.2 [5] and 0.8 per 100,000 US population (in children <15 years of age, and non-malignant brain tumours excluded) [4], which is similar to European statistics [5]. Joinpoint regression analysis of the SEER data identified two distinct trends of annual incidence rates: (1) a brain cancer increase in all age groups until 1987 and (2) stabilization of the incidence rate in children [6], whereas rates declined for non-elderly adults. Studies from Europe and other parts of the world have shown similar incidence rates, and trends of increasing CBT in the early 1980s were also documented.

Various investigators employed different statistical models to best describe the change in incidence rates before the late 1980s, including a 'jump model' of a single upward shift occurring in the early 1980s, coinciding in time with the general introduction of superior imaging techniques in the form of magnetic resonance (MR) scanning [7], although the assumption by some authors of a causal relationship between the two is regarded as controversial by others.

Only a few risk factors for the development of CBT are well established: heritable tumour syndromes (e.g., neurofibromatosis I and II, von Hippel-Lindau syndrome, Gorlin syndrome), immunosuppression in central nervous system lymphomas (e.g., HIV, post-transplant) and cranial ionizing irradiation. It was originally thought that only high-dose ionizing radiation was etiologically linked to brain tumour development. Yet a large-scale epidemiological Israeli study in 1988 demonstrated that previous exposure even to very small radiation doses (e.g., as low as 2.5 Gy, used historically in that cohort of 10,834 children for treatment of tinea capitis) was associated with a nearly 20-fold relative brain tumour risk compared with non-irradiated siblings [8].

A German population-based study [9] found links between increased brain tumour risk and low birth weight, maternal smoking during pregnancy and exposure to wood preservatives. The most recent SEER data suggested Caucasian race, male sex and residence in a metropolitan county as age-independent risk associations with brain tumours [6]. Public concerns about possible links between non-ionizing electromagnetic fields or wireless mobile phones and brain tumour incidence were not supported by several epidemiological studies examining these issues. Other potential environmental factors have been postulated, including exposure to nitrosamines, viral infections, certain medications and vitamins, parental occupation, as well as seasonality of birth, but consistent evidence is lacking.

Diagnosis and Treatment

Nowadays, the main imaging tool for the diagnosis of CBT is MR imaging, although for certain CBT subtypes, e.g., craniopharyngiomas, computed tomography may add information about typical calcification within the tumour. Most CBT diagnoses require histological confirmation in order to select the most appropriate treatment strategy, which, at present, consists of surgery for most of the children (95%), often with radiotherapy (RT, 70%) and additional chemotherapy (30%) [10].

Treatment options vary considerably according to the histological diagnosis.

Low-grade gliomas – the most common CBT – are likely to be cured, if gross total resection is possible. If resection is incomplete, RT can be employed for progressive or recurrent disease or chemotherapy in children under the age of 10 years.

Medulloblastomas – the most common malignant CBT – may present with disseminated disease in 20% of cases. Gross or near-total tumour resection is prognostically beneficial, but RT (craniospinal irradiation and posterior fossa boost) and chemotherapy are the standard treatment for children older than 3 years [2] and required to minimize the risk of recurrence. Disease in very young children has been shown to respond to more intense chemotherapy and autologous stem cell rescue, allowing RT to be postponed or avoided altogether in some cases.

Patients with high-grade gliomas have the best chance of survival, if tumour resection of more than 90% can be achieved, although the overall survival rate even with additional RT and chemotherapy remains <50% at 5 years.

Standard treatment for ependymomas includes resection and focal RT, resulting in overall survival rates of 50–60%. Craniopharyngiomas may be treated with surgery or RT; however, it is still debated, which of the two is the best choice. Intracranial germinomas are extremely radiosensitive, and excellent survival rates are achieved. Brain stem tumours are not amenable to surgery due to their location, and prognosis is dismal despite intensified RT and computed tomography regimes.

Novel Diagnostic Strategies

The evolution of diagnostic classification schemes for CBTs is driven by advances in scientific knowledge and available technology, as well as by the ambition to improve the accuracy of prognosis and optimize therapy of CBTs. Some histological features of CBTs correlate with clinical outcome, e.g., the histopathological degree of anaplasia in medulloblastomas is strongly linked to the degree of aggressive clinical behaviour of such tumours [11], and the histological grade of localized ependymomas influences the survival rate in ependymomas [12]. However, for other tumour types, the histological grade is less useful, e.g., neither the original nor the revised World Health Organization sub-classification of supratentorial astrocytomas is able to separate these tumours prognostically [13], and histological sub-classification of low-grade cerebellar astrocytomas is generally of no prognostic value [14].

The ever-increasing understanding of molecular pathology will undoubtedly shape future diagnostic cancer classifications, including those of CBTs, and some novel molecular markers have already been shown not only to reliably differentiate tumour subtypes, but also to provide unequivocal additional prognostic information.

Pomeroy et al. [15] studied gene expression in 99 tissue samples of embryonal brain tumours using DNA microarrays. Their data showed that medulloblastoma is a distinct entity which clearly differs on a molecular level from other brain tumours, including primitive neuroectodermal tumours. The authors also demonstrated that clinical outcome was strongly correlated with gene expression profiles of the individual tumours. Similar gene profiling allowed risk stratification independent of all clinical variables in medulloblastomas [16].

With increased knowledge about molecular pathways involved in tumorigenesis, individual molecular risk markers have been identified and studied in the clinical context. Over-expression versus low expression of p53 in malignant gliomas in childhood is strongly associated with an improved 5-year progression-free survival (17 vs. 44%; $p < 0.001$) [17]. Laminin-8 – a vascular basement membrane component – has been found over-expressed in highly invasive glioblastoma multiforme tumours, and its expression level correlated with the duration until tumour relapse [18]. Expression of tumour ERBB2 protein in cells of clinically average-risk medulloblastomas was associated with a 54% 5-year overall survival rate compared with 100% in ERBB2-negative tumours [19]. Mutations of genes encoding components of the Wnt/Wg signalling pathway (which have been implicated in the pathogenesis of some medulloblastomas), e.g., *CTNNB1*, can lead to abnormal activation of the pathway and subsequent accumulation of β-catenin protein (encoded by *CTNNB1*) within the cell nucleus. Such mutations occur in approximately 15% of sporadic medulloblastomas and were found to be associated with a statistically highly significant survival benefit [20]. Epidermal growth factor receptor (EGFR) is another marker for biological behaviour of supratentorial glioblastoma multiforme, possibly corresponding to alterations in radiosensitivity; EGFR immunonegativity was associated with a significantly longer survival [21, 22].

Apart from being a valid prognostic marker for the biological behaviour of supratentorial glioblastoma multiforme, EGFR is also an example target of molecular targeted therapy of EGFR immunopositive tumours with EGFR tyrosine kinase inhibitors (e.g., erlotinib), which are currently being studied.

New imaging technologies are being applied in the clinical context of adult brain tumours as well as CBTs. Some of these techniques add functional and metabolic information to corresponding anatomical images. Development of advanced MR imaging technology has led to various new modalities: proton MR spectroscopy may help distinguish tumour tissue from normal tissue by detecting differences in concentrations of certain neurochemicals, e.g., N-acetylaspartate; MR perfusion imaging differentiates therapy-related brain injury from residual or recurrent tumour; magnetic source imaging is the superimposition of magnetoencephalography data on co-localized MR images and may help in cortical mapping before neurosurgery. Modern nuclear medicine technologies (single photon emission computed tomography, positron emission tomography) may be used for grading of neoplasm, detection of tumour recurrence [23] or the preoperative localization and therefore avoidance of eloquent cortices at surgery [24].

Novel Therapeutic Strategies

Advances in neurosurgical techniques include neuronavigation based on high-resolution MR imaging, which allows 3-dimensional guidance and simulation of surgical tumour access routes before or during the operation. Functional imaging and cortical mapping before or during the operation allow increased tumour resection while minimizing injury to the surrounding brain [2, 24].

Advances in radiation therapy include precision-guided dose delivery with 3-dimensional conformal RT and intensity-modulated RT, which allow optimization of radiation beam shapes and modulation of the radiation dose, as well as stereotactic radiosurgery. These techniques provide a more precise target volume, allowing higher dose delivery to the tumour while sparing surrounding structures (e.g., healthy brain, cochlea and pituitary gland). Proton beam therapy is useful for deeper located tumours and is characterized by a rapid dose fall-off beyond the tumour margins.

Chemotherapy has been increasingly employed in order to reduce relapse rates. It has also been used as an alternative to RT, or as a means of allowing RT to be postponed or applied at lower doses, in particular in very young children, in the hope of reducing late sequelae of RT, which are most severe in that age group. Stem cell rescue procedures have facilitated the use of newer, more aggressive, potentially myeloablative chemotherapy regimens for treatment of CBTs. Novel chemotherapeutic agents have been used for their radiosensitizing properties (e.g., temozolomide). Other studies have been directed at improving delivery of chemotherapeutic agents to tumour tissue: implantation of biodegradable carmustine wafers and convection-enhanced delivery are aimed at achieving much higher than systemically tolerated doses within the tumour tissue. Procedures to overcome the natural blood-brain barrier (e.g., intracarotid hypotonic mannitol infusion) have been used with some success, and co-administration of P-glycoprotein inhibitors is being studied as a potential facilitator of drug entry into tumour cells.

A better understanding of molecular pathology, immune mechanisms and genetic aberrations that contribute to brain tumorigenesis will encourage the development of specifically targeted molecular, immuno- and gene therapy for CBTs.

Growth Hormone Deficiency in Childhood Brain Tumour Survivors

With increasing numbers of long-term survivors of CBT, clinicians focus more and more on the long-term sequelae of the disease and its treatment. Numerous physical and mental handicaps may occur and are often summarized under the term 'late effects'. Common late effects in CBT survivors include neuropsychological problems and impaired cognitive function, endocrinopathies, short stature, second malignancies, increased overall mortality, strokes, epilepsy, osteopenia and impaired quality of life.

In contrast to most other late effects, treatment of endocrinopathies and hormone deficiencies is relatively straightforward with currently available hormone replacement therapies. The most commonly encountered hypothalamic-pituitary abnormality in CBT survivors is GH deficiency, which may manifest itself as short stature, although the aetiology of short stature in cancer survivors is often multifactorial.

In 1973, Probert et al. [25] published evidence of growth retardation as a result of spinal irradiation in 22 children. It had been known since the 1920s that high-dose radiation to the brain can cause damage to cerebral and pituitary tissue, but it was not until 1976 that publications from our unit described impaired GH responses to stimulation tests in short-statured children who had previously been irradiated for either CBT or prophylactically for acute lymphoblastic leukaemia [26–28].

The risk of having a subnormal GH response correlated with the radiation dose [29]. Subsequent investigations [30] revealed the presence of other hypothalamic-pituitary hormone deficiencies as a result of previous radiotherapy. The rate at which stimulated peak GH responses decline over the first 5 years following cranial irradiation is dose dependent, although ultimately, most patients receiving high-dose cranial irradiation will develop subnormal GH responses, if monitored long enough [31].

In 1981, Shalet et al. [32] reported the first results of the experience of our unit with GH treatment in 6 children who had survived a brain tumour. All responded to GH therapy, and growth rates increased to 6.0–10.1 cm during the first year. Final height outcomes in CBT survivors treated with GH were subsequently reported by various centres, with a significant proportion of children reaching final heights above the third centile [33]. The response to GH treatment in prepubertal children occurred regardless of spinal irradiation [34], supporting the theory that impaired spinal growth during the pubertal growth spurt was the main factor contributing to lack of 'catch-up' growth in these spinally irradiated children, compared with the better auxological outcome after GH treatment in cranially-only irradiated children or children with idiopathic GH deficiency.

A study of the effects of spinal irradiation on final height in 79 CBT patients (not treated with GH) in our unit estimated the radiation-related spinal height loss to be at least 9 versus 7 versus 5.5 cm when irradiation was given at the age of 1 versus 5 versus 10 years, highlighting the vulnerability of very young children to suffer the most severe spinal growth retardation [35]. Early reports pointed out the poor response of spinal growth to GH treatment in those spinally irradiated children, although treatment was able to prevent further reduction in height standard deviation scores. Other studies [36, 37] also reported a pronounced effect of spinal irradiation on height outcome, particularly in boys, which is in keeping with the greater contribution of pubertal growth to final height in males.

Another factor, often encountered in CBT survivors, contributes to the relatively poor spinal growth response: early (although less frequent true precocious) puberty, which tends to be of normal duration. The predicted age of onset of puberty is positively correlated with the age at cranial irradiation, i.e. the younger the patient at irradiation, the earlier the predicted age of onset of puberty [38]. Mean ages of pubertal onset were 8.5 years in girls and 9.2 in boys in our patient cohort (fig. 1). The associated earlier completion of puberty also meant that there was only limited time available for augmentation of spinal growth during the pubertal growth spurt by GH treat-

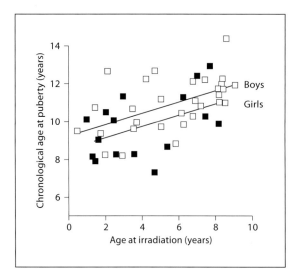
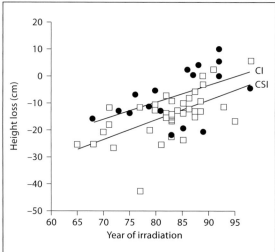

Fig. 1. Estimated and fitted chronological ages at the onset of puberty for age at irradiation. ■ = Girls; □ = boys. With permission from Ogilvy-Stuart et al. [38].

Fig. 2. Improvements in height loss from 1975 to 2000. ● = Cranial irradiation; □ = craniospinal irradiation. With permission from Gleeson et al. [41].

ment, especially in comparison with idiopathic GH deficiency, where the duration of puberty tends to be prolonged. Both the radiation osteitis of the spine and abnormal pubertal tempo in the context of early onset contribute to the poor response of sitting height to GH treatment, causing segmental disproportion in most GH-treated children who had received previous spinal irradiation.

Over recent decades, auxological outcome improved significantly with GH treatment. After our initial studies, subsequent reports in larger cohorts recorded even better responses in height gain, if higher doses of GH were used, e.g., increases in height velocity of 5 cm per year in the first year of treatment, but the spinal growth deficit remained [39, 40].

Strategies to circumvent the dilemma of final height loss secondary to spinal growth limitation include the earlier initiation of GH treatment, the use of gonadotropin-releasing hormone (GnRH) analogues to delay early puberty, and the search for improved CBT treatment strategies that allow the elimination or postponement of spinal irradiation or dose reduction, since the deleterious long-term effects are most severe after high-dose spinal irradiation in very young children.

Analysis of auxological data of the last 25 years of GH treatment in CBT survivors in our unit revealed a gradual improvement in final height outcome for both cranial irradiation ($r = 0.5$, $p = 0.03$) and craniospinal irradiation patients ($r = 0.6$, $p < 0.001$) [41] (fig. 2). The main factors contributing to that success were the improved and higher GH dosing regimes, the earlier introduction of GH treatment after completion of radiotherapy and the additional use of GnRH analogue therapy for early puberty in selected patients. Before 1985, children received 5 mg pituitary-derived GH 3 times a week by intramuscular injection, whereas afterwards, synthetic GH was used, and weight-based regimes of GH dosing (e.g., 0.5 IU/kg/week) were the standard therapy from 1988 onwards. Lag times between completion of RT and initiation of GH therapy were reduced from a mean 5.8 years to 3.3 years for patients treated before versus after 1988. GnRH analogue therapy conferred additional height benefits in selected patients, although final height gains were often achieved at the expense of increased segmental disproportion between sitting height and leg length.

Second Malignant Neoplasms and Growth Hormone

The mitogenic properties of GH in vitro, the excess risk of malignancy in acromegaly, and epidemiological links between insulin-like growth factor 1 and cancer are some of the reasons why the use of GH in cancer survivors may be regarded as potentially hazardous in terms of triggering tumour recurrence. On the other hand, many children are at high risk of developing severe short stature and reduced bone mass if the highly prevalent GH deficiency among cranially irradiated children remains untreated.

One inherent problem of secondary malignant neoplasm (SMN) in CBT survivors is that they are already at a very high risk of developing SMN even before starting GH treatment. This may be related to the disease itself: many children may harbour a genetic predisposition from known or not yet elucidated tumour syndromes that led to the primary CBT in the first place. An early study by Farwell and Flannery [42] of 670 CBT survivors, 9 of whom developed an SMN, not only found that there was a 9 times higher risk of developing a second cancer, but also that siblings of the patients were significantly more affected by cancer than expected, suggesting a familial clustering of cancer risk in these patients.

Secondly, radiation therapy is a major risk factor for the development of further cancers, and a variety of cases with second CBT after previous different CBTs have been published. Common tumour types include meningiomas within the radiation field and malignant gliomas. They can occur after long latency periods and tend to be biologically more aggressive than the equivalent primary CBTs.

Ever since GH treatment was introduced for GH-deficient CBT survivors, surveillance and long-term monitoring for tumour recurrence has been an integral part of GH treatment in these children. The gold standard of assessing whether GH can be implicated in tumorigenesis would be a long-term, randomized placebo-controlled trial of GH treatment in CBT survivors. However, such a trial is neither ethical nor realistically feasible on a large scale over a long period of time.

Therefore, current evidence has to rely on epidemiological data, typically from large cancer study groups, e.g., the International Late Effects Study Group and the Childhood Cancer Survivor Study (CCSS) in the US, and from pharmacosurveillance programs. The data from the CCSS have the benefit of a control population, whereas pharmacosurveillance programs excel in the availability of a large total number of enrolled patients exposed to exogenous GH.

Early published data from the UK on CBT recurrence came from single centres [43], followed by combining data from smaller cancer registries [44] and a dedicated national study in 2000 that included 180 GH-treated CBT survivors from three large cancer treatment centres [45]. None of these studies found an increase in tumour recurrence rate. A safety report from the largest North American pharmacosurveillance program (the National Cooperative Growth Study) in 1996 found no increased incidence of CBT recurrence in those 1,262 CBT survivors treated with GH [46].

A safety analysis by the Growth Hormone Research Society in 2001 found no convincing evidence that there was an increased risk of tumour recurrence in those 20% of GH-treated children with a history of malignancy [47].

A first report [48] of the CCSS on the risk of tumour recurrence and SMN concluded that there did not appear to be an increased risk of disease recurrence in survivors of childhood cancer, although repeated findings of slightly but significantly increased rates of SMNs in GH-treated

CBT survivors highlight the importance of continued vigilance.

The significant but very small increase in SMNs does not constitute a good enough reason to withhold GH treatment in CBT survivors, but ultimately, the decision to treat or not to treat has to be made on an individual basis for each patient.

For most CBT survivors, GHD remains an important issue beyond final height: the benefits of adult GH treatment, e.g., in terms of body composition and quality of life, have been shown to extend to GH-deficient CBT survivors [49, 50], but neuroimaging surveillance must remain an essential part of monitoring therapy in those patients in order to detect asymptomatic SMNs, in particular meningiomas [51].

References

1 Pollack IF: Brain tumors in children. N Engl J Med 1994;331:1500–1507.
2 Levy AS: Brain tumors in children: evaluation and management. Curr Probl Pediatr Adolesc Health Care 2005;35:230–245.
3 Kleihues P, Cavenee WK: Pathology and Genetics of Tumours of the Nervous System. Lyon, IARC Press, 2000.
4 US Cancer Statistics Working Group: United States Cancer Statistics: 2002 Incidence and Mortality. Atlanta, US Department of Health and Human Services, Centers for Disease Control and Prevention and National Cancer Institute, 2005. http://www.cdc.gov/cancer/npcr/uscs/pdf/2002_USCS.pdf (accessed June 12, 2006).
5 McNally RJ, Kelsey AM, Cairns DP, Taylor GM, Eden OB, Birch JM: Temporal increases in the incidence of childhood solid tumors seen in Northwest England (1954–1998) are likely to be real. Cancer 2001;92:1967–1976.
6 Deorah S, Lynch CF, Sibenaller ZA, Ryken TC: Trends in brain cancer incidence and survival in the United States: Surveillance, Epidemiology, and End Results Program, 1973 to 2001. Neurosurg Focus 2006;20:E1.
7 Smith MA, Freidlin B, Ries LA, Simon R: Trends in reported incidence of primary malignant brain tumors in children in the United States. J Natl Cancer Inst 1998;90:1269–1277.
8 Ron E, Modan B, Boice JD Jr, Alfandary E, Stovall M, Chetrit A, Katz L, et al: Tumors of the brain and nervous system after radiotherapy in childhood. N Engl J Med 1988;319:1033–1039.
9 Schuz J, Kaletsch U, Kaatsch P, Meinert R, Michaelis J: Risk factors for pediatric tumors of the central nervous system: results from a German population-based case-control study. Med Pediatr Oncol 2001;36:274–282.
10 Sklar CA: Childhood brain tumors. J Pediatr Endocrinol Metab 2002;15 (suppl 2):669–673.
11 Eberhart CG, Kepner JL, Goldthwaite PT, Kun LE, Duffner PK, Friedman HS, Strother DR, et al: Histopathologic grading of medulloblastomas: a Pediatric Oncology Group study. Cancer 2002;94:552–560.
12 Merchant TE, Jenkins JJ, Burger PC, Sanford RA, Sherwood SH, Jones-Wallace D, Heideman RL, et al: Influence of tumor grade on time to progression after irradiation for localized ependymoma in children. Int J Radiat Oncol Biol Phys 2002;53.52–57.
13 Gilles FH, Brown WD, Leviton A, Tavare CJ, Adelman L, Rorke LB, Davis RL, et al: Limitations of the World Health Organization classification of childhood supratentorial astrocytic tumors. Children Brain Tumor Consortium. Cancer 2000;88:1477–1483.
14 Bernhardtsen T, Laursen H, Bojsen-Moller M, Gjerris F: Sub-classification of low-grade cerebellar astrocytoma: is it clinically meaningful? Childs Nerv Syst 2003;19:729–735.
15 Pomeroy SL, Tamayo P, Gaasenbeek M, Sturla LM, Angelo M, McLaughlin ME, Kim JY, et al: Prediction of central nervous system embryonal tumour outcome based on gene expression. Nature 2002;415:436–442.
16 Fernandez-Teijeiro A, Betensky RA, Sturla LM, Kim JY, Tamayo P, Pomeroy SL: Combining gene expression profiles and clinical parameters for risk stratification in medulloblastomas. J Clin Oncol 2004;22:994–998.
17 Pollack IF, Finkelstein SD, Woods J, Burnham J, Holmes EJ, Hamilton RL, Yates AJ, et al: Expression of p53 and prognosis in children with malignant gliomas. N Engl J Med 2002;346:420–427.
18 Ljubimova JY, Fugita M, Khazenzon NM, Das A, Pikul BB, Newman D, Sekiguchi K, et al: Association between laminin-8 and glial tumor grade, recurrence, and patient survival. Cancer 2004;101:604–612.
19 Gajjar A, Hernan R, Kocak M, Fuller C, Lee Y, McKinnon PJ, Wallace D, et al: Clinical, histopathologic, and molecular markers of prognosis: toward a new disease risk stratification system for medulloblastoma. J Clin Oncol 2004; 22:984–993.
20 Ellison DW, Onilude OE, Lindsey JC, Lusher ME, Weston CL, Taylor RE, Pearson AD, et al: β-Catenin status predicts a favorable outcome in childhood medulloblastoma: the United Kingdom Children's Cancer Study Group Brain Tumour Committee. J Clin Oncol 2005;23:7951–7957.
21 Saito T, Hama S, Kajiwara Y, Sugiyama K, Yamasaki F, Arifin MT, Arita K, et al: Prognosis of cerebellar glioblastomas: correlation between prognosis and immunoreactivity for epidermal growth factor receptor compared with supratentorial glioblastomas. Anticancer Res 2006;26:1351–1357.

22 Halatsch ME, Schmidt U, Behnke-Mursch J, Unterberg A, Wirtz CR: Epidermal growth factor receptor inhibition for the treatment of glioblastoma multiforme and other malignant brain tumours. Cancer Treat Rev 2006;32:74–89.
23 Henze M, Mohammed A, Schlemmer HP, Herfarth KK, Hoffner S, Haufe S, Mier W, et al: PET and SPECT for detection of tumor progression in irradiated low-grade astrocytoma: a receiver-operating-characteristic analysis. J Nucl Med 2004;45:579–586.
24 Gupta N, Banerjee A, Haas-Kogan D: Pediatric CNS Tumors. Berlin, Springer, 2004.
25 Probert JC, Parker BR, Kaplan HS: Growth retardation in children after megavoltage irradiation of the spine. Cancer 1973;32:634–639.
26 Shalet SM, Beardwell CG, Morris-Jones P, Bamford FN, Ribeiro GG, Pearson D: Growth hormone deficiency in children with brain tumors. Cancer 1976;37(suppl 2):1144–1148.
27 Shalet SM, Beardwell CG, Jones PH, Pearson D: Growth hormone deficiency after treatment of acute leukaemia in children. Arch Dis Child 1976;51:489–493.
28 Shalet SM, Beardwell CG, Twomey JA, Jones PH, Pearson D: Endocrine function following the treatment of acute leukemia in childhood. J Pediatr 1977;90:920–923.
29 Shalet SM, Beardwell CG, Pearson D, Jones PH: The effect of varying doses of cerebral irradiation on growth hormone production in childhood. Clin Endocrinol (Oxf) 1976;5:287–290.
30 Shalet SM, Beardwell CG, MacFarlane IA, Jones PH, Pearson D: Endocrine morbidity in adults treated with cerebral irradiation for brain tumours during childhood. Acta Endocrinol (Copenh) 1977;84:673–680.
31 Clayton PE, Shalet SM: Dose dependency of time of onset of radiation-induced growth hormone deficiency. J Pediatr 1991;118:226–228.
32 Shalet SM, Whitehead E, Chapman AJ, Beardwell CG: The effects of growth hormone therapy in children with radiation-induced growth hormone deficiency. Acta Paediatr Scand 1981;70:81–86.
33 Herber SM, Dunsmore IR, Milner RD: Final stature in brain tumours other than craniopharyngioma: effect of growth hormone. Horm Res 1985;22:63–67.
34 Clayton PE, Shalet SM: The evolution of spinal growth after irradiation. Clin Oncol (R Coll Radiol) 1991;3:220–222.
35 Shalet SM, Gibson B, Swindell R, Pearson D: Effect of spinal irradiation on growth. Arch Dis Child 1987;62:461–464.
36 Brownstein CM, Mertens AC, Mitby PA, Stovall M, Qin J, Heller G, Robison LL, et al: Factors that affect final height and change in height standard deviation scores in survivors of childhood cancer treated with growth hormone: a report from the childhood cancer survivor study. J Clin Endocrinol Metab 2004;89:4422–4427.
37 Lerner SE, Huang GJ, McMahon D, Sklar CA, Oberfield SE: Growth hormone therapy in children after cranial/craniospinal radiation therapy: sexually dimorphic outcomes. J Clin Endocrinol Metab 2004;89:6100–6104.
38 Ogilvy-Stuart AL, Clayton PE, Shalet SM: Cranial irradiation and early puberty. J Clin Endocrinol Metab 1994;78:1282–1286.
39 Lannering B, Albertsson-Wikland K: Improved growth response to GH treatment in irradiated children. Acta Paediatr Scand 1989;78:562–567.
40 Xu W, Janss A, Moshang T: Adult height and adult sitting height in childhood medulloblastoma survivors. J Clin Endocrinol Metab 2003;88:4677–4681.
41 Gleeson HK, Stoeter R, Ogilvy-Stuart AL, Gattamaneni HR, Brennan BM, Shalet SM: Improvements in final height over 25 years in growth hormone (GH)-deficient childhood survivors of brain tumors receiving GH replacement. J Clin Endocrinol Metab 2003;88:3682–3689.
42 Farwell J, Flannery JT: Second primaries in children with central nervous system tumors. J Neurooncol 1984;2:371–375.
43 Clayton PE, Shalet SM, Gattamaneni HR, Price DA: Does growth hormone cause relapse of brain tumours? Lancet 1987;i:711–713.
44 Ogilvy-Stuart AL, Ryder WD, Gattamaneni HR, Clayton PE, Shalet SM: Growth hormone and tumour recurrence. BMJ 1992;304:1601–1605.
45 Swerdlow AJ, Reddingius RE, Higgins CD, Spoudeas HA, Phipps K, Qiao Z, Ryder WD, et al: Growth hormone treatment of children with brain tumors and risk of tumor recurrence. J Clin Endocrinol Metab 2000;85:4444–4449.
46 Moshang T Jr, Rundle AC, Graves DA, Nickas J, Johanson A, Meadows A: Brain tumor recurrence in children treated with growth hormone: the National Cooperative Growth Study experience. J Pediatr 1996;128:S4–S7.
47 Growth Hormone Research Society: Critical evaluation of the safety of recombinant human growth hormone administration: statement from the Growth Hormone Research Society. J Clin Endocrinol Metab 2001;86:1868–1870.
48 Sklar CA, Mertens AC, Mitby P, Occhiogrosso G, Qin J, Heller G, Yasui Y, et al: Risk of disease recurrence and second neoplasms in survivors of childhood cancer treated with growth hormone: a report from the Childhood Cancer Survivor Study. J Clin Endocrinol Metab 2002;87:3136–3141.
49 Murray RD, Darzy KH, Gleeson HK, Shalet SM: GH-deficient survivors of childhood cancer: GH replacement during adult life. J Clin Endocrinol Metab 2002;87:129–135.
50 Mukherjee A, Tolhurst-Cleaver S, Ryder WD, Smethurst L, Shalet SM: The characteristics of quality of life impairment in adult growth hormone (GH)-deficient survivors of cancer and their response to GH replacement therapy. J Clin Endocrinol Metab 2005;90:1542–1549.
51 Jostel A, Mukherjee A, Hulse PA, Shalet SM: Adult growth hormone replacement therapy and neuroimaging surveillance in brain tumour survivors. Clin Endocrinol (Oxf) 2005;62:698–705.

KIGS Patients with Acquired Growth Hormone Deficiency (Code No. 2.2 ff.)

Michael B. Ranke

Context

Patients with acquired growth hormone deficiency (GHD) are a large group within KIGS (n = 5,134; 9%). The causes of GHD are varied: tumours of the pituitary area (code No. 2.2.1 ff.), cranial tumours distant from the pituitary (code No. 2.2.2 ff.), malignancies outside the cranium (code No. 2.2.3 ff.) and other causes (code No. 2.2.4 ff.). The primary disorders themselves or their treatments (surgery, X-ray therapy, chemotherapy) often lead to combined pituitary hormonal deficits and potentially to an impaired responsiveness to GH. Aside from the issue of efficacy of GH treatment there are safety aspects.

Various aspects related to these patients are discussed in detail within the chapters of Jostel and Shalet [this vol., pp. 240–249] and Polak [this vol., pp. 269–276] and have been dealt with in previous analyses from KIGS.

Paediatric Endocrinology Section
University Children's Hospital, University of Tübingen
Hoppe-Seyler-Strasse 1, DE–72076 Tübingen (Germany)

Methods

The analysis of the data was restricted to: (1) characteristics of patients at the start of GH treatment; (2) characteristics and response to GH during the first prepubertal year; (3) characteristics at GH start, puberty onset and near adult height (NAH). The data are purely descriptive. More details on patients with craniopharyngioma are given in the chapter by Price [this vol., pp. 207–212].

The response to GH during the first prepubertal year was also analysed and compared with idiopathic GHD (IGHD) using the first-year prediction model without GH maximum. The results are expressed in terms of studentised residuals (negative values indicate a response worse than IGHD). For further reading see chapter by Ranke and Lindberg [this vol., pp. 422–431].

Results

Characteristics of Patients at the Start of GH Treatment

The characteristics of patients at the start of GH treatment are listed in tables 1–4. Confidence ranges are usually in the order of magnitude as described in detail in the chapter by Price [this vol., pp. 207–212].

- Craniopharyngioma and germinoma are the most frequent causes of tumours within the

Table 1. Tumour of the pituitary/hypothalamic area: patients documented at the start of GH therapy

	Craniopharyngioma (code No. 2.2.1.1)	Germinoma (code No. 2.2.1.2)	Others (code No. 2.2.1.9)
Background			
Patients	1,140	336	313
Males, %	57	48	63
Birth weight SDS	−0.3	−0.3	−0.2
Birth length SDS	0.2	0.2	0.1
MPH SDS	−0.4	−0.7	−0.5
Maximum GH, μg/l	1.2	1.5	2.0
MPHD, %	93	89	66
IGF-1 SDS	−3.1	−2.8	−3.0
At GH start			
Age, years	10.5	12.6	11.9
Bone age, years	9.0	11.0	11.0
Height SDS	−2.3	−2.1	−2.1
BMI SDS	1.2	0.6	1.0
GH dose, mg/kg/week	0.17	0.17	0.18

Data are medians. MPHD = Multiple pituitary hormone deficiency; IGF-1 = insulin-like growth factor 1.

Table 2. Cranial tumour distant from the pituitary/hypothalamic area: patients documented at the start of GH therapy

	Astrocytoma (code No. 2.2.2.1)	Ependymoma (code No. 2.2.2.2)	Glioma (code No. 2.2.2.3)	Medulloblastoma (code No. 2.2.2.4)	Nasopharyngeal tumour (code No. 2.2.2.5)	Others (code No. 2.2.2.9)
Background						
Patients	227	141	145	754	68	206
Males, %	57	60	55	66	63	55
Birth weight SDS	−0.3	−0.2	−0.2	−0.1	0.2	−0.3
Birth length SDS	0.2	0.2	−0.2	0.1	0.6	0.1
MPH SDS	−0.3	−0.4	−0.5	−0.3	0.0	−0.7
Maximum GH, μg/l	2.6	4.9	2.5	4.8	3.2	3.4
MPHD, %	52	40	54	53	46	50
IGF-1 SDS	−2.2	−1.7	−2.9	−2.2	−2.6	−2.7
At GH start						
Age, years	10.3	9.7	10.1	10.4	10.1	10.2
Bone age, years	9.1	8.7	9.1	9.4	8.8	9.1
Height SDS	−1.3	−1.9	−1.6	−1.9	−1.9	−2.2
BMI SDS	1.1	0.7	1.1	0.2	−0.1	0.5
GH dose, mg/kg/week	0.18	0.19	0.18	0.20	0.21	0.18

Data are medians. MPHD = Multiple pituitary hormone deficiency; IGF-1 = insulin-like growth factor 1.

Table 3. Treatment for malignancy outside the cranium: patients documented at the start of GH therapy

	Lymphatic leukaemia (code No. 2.2.3.1.1)	Myeloid leukaemia (code No. 2.2.3.1.2)	Others (code No. 2.2.3.1.9)	Solid tumours (code No. 2.2.3.2)	Others (code No. 2.2.3.2.9)
Background					
Patients	470	85	139	101	60
Males, %	62	54	58	62	72
Birth weight SDS	−0.2	0.0	0.1	−0.3	−0.4
Birth length SDS	0.2	0.1	0.3	0.1	−0.2
MPH SDS	−0.5	−0.3	−0.4	−0.2	−0.7
Maximum GH, µg/l	6.0	6.4	6.5	4.9	6.5
MPHD, %	46	60	29	48	58
IGF-1 SDS	−1.9	−2.2	−2.2	−2.2	−2.0
At GH start					
Age, years	11.8	11.8	11.6	10.9	12.1
Bone age, years	11.1	10.5	11.0	10.5	10.7
Height SDS	−1.8	−1.9	−1.9	−2.1	−2.3
BMI SDS	0.4	−0.1	0.2	−0.2	0.3
GH dose, mg/kg/week	0.20	0.22	0.18	0.21	0.18

Data are medians. MPHD = Multiple pituitary hormone deficiency; IGF-1 = insulin-like growth factor 1.

Table 4. Other causes of acquired GHD: patients documented at the start of GH therapy

	Head trauma (code No. 2.2.4.1)	CNS infection (code No. 2.2.4.2)	Hydrocephalus (code No. 2.2.4.3)
Background			
Patients	121	45	61
Males, %	63	56	69
Birth weight SDS	−0.7	−0.4	−0.3
Birth length SDS	−0.4	0.1	0.0
MPH SDS	−0.9	−1.0	−0.9
Maximum GH, µg/l	3.0	3.4	6.6
MPHD, %	58	49	18
IGF-1 SDS	−2.9	−1.1	−2.5
At GH start			
Age, years	10.7	9.9	8.2
Bone age, years	7.8	9.8	6.5
Height SDS	−3.1	−3.5	−3.6
BMI SDS	0.2	0.3	−0.4
GH dose, mg/kg/week	0.19	0.19	0.19

Data are medians. CNS = Central nervous system; MPHD = multiple pituitary hormone deficiency; IGF-1 = insulin-like growth factor 1.

Table 5. Tumour of the pituitary/hypothalamic area: patients treated for 1 prepubertal year

	Cranio-pharyngioma (code No. 2.2.1.1)	Germinoma (code No. 2.2.1.2)	Others (code No. 2.2.1.9)
At GH start			
Patients	656	163	122
Males, %	59	41	70
Age, years	9.0	11.9	9.4
Height SDS	−2.2	−1.8	−2.2
Height velocity, cm/year	3.0	2.8	3.7
Height velocity SDS	−3.3	−4.3	−2.7
BMI SDS	1.2	0.7	0.9
GH dose, mg/kg/week	0.17	0.17	0.17
After 1 year			
Age, years	10.0	12.9	10.5
Height SDS	−1.4	−1.2	−1.5
Height velocity, cm/year	9.0	7.1	8.4
Height velocity SDS	4.4	2.6	3.6
Δ height SDS	0.8	0.5	0.7
Studentised residual	0.4	0.0	0.2
BMI SDS	0.9	0.6	0.6

Data are medians.

pituitary area (code No. 2.2.1 ff.). The patients are severely GH deficient. Height is moderately decreased and the BMI is increased. The patients tend to receive GH in doses common for the replacement of IGHD.

– Astrocytoma, ependymoma, glioma, medulloblastoma and nasopharyngeal tumour are the most frequent causes of tumours distant from the pituitary area (code No. 2.2.2 ff.). The patients are severely to moderately GH deficient. Height is moderately decreased and the body mass index (BMI) varies (normal in medulloblastoma, nasopharyngeal tumour). The patients tend to receive GH in doses common for the replacement of IGHD.

– Lymphatic and myeloid leukaemia and lymphoma are the most frequent causes of malignancies outside the cranium (code No. 2.2.3 ff.). The patients are moderately GH deficient. Height is moderately decreased and the BMI is normal. The patients tend to receive GH in doses common for the replacement of IGHD.

– Head trauma, central nervous system infections and hydrocephalus are the most frequent 'other' causes of acquired GHD (code No. 2.2.4 ff.). The patients are moderately to severely GH deficient. Height is moderately decreased and the BMI is normal. The patients tend to receive GH in doses common for the replacement of IGHD.

Characteristics and Response to GH during the First Prepubertal Year

The characteristics at the start of GH and after the first prepubertal year of treatment are listed in tables 5–8. Confidence ranges are usually in the order of magnitude as described in detail in the chapter by Price [this vol., pp. 207–212].

– In children with GHD, as a result of a pituitary/hypothalamic tumour (code No. 2.2.1

Table 6. Tumour distant from the pituitary/hypothalamic area: patients treated for 1 prepubertal year

	Astrocytoma (code No. 2.2.2.1)	Ependymoma (code No. 2.2.2.2)	Glioma (code No. 2.2.2.3)	Medullo-blastoma (code No. 2.2.2.4)	Others (code No. 2.2.2.9)
At GH start					
Patients	64	65	61	328	96
Males, %	64	69	64	74	57
Age, years	8.9	8.3	8.5	8.7	9.1
Height SDS	−2.0	−2.2	−1.8	−2.0	−2.3
Height velocity, cm/year	3.4	3.6	4.5	3.6	3.4
Height velocity SDS	−2.8	−3.3	−2.3	−2.7	−3.1
BMI SDS	0.7	0.7	1.3	0.3	0.3
GH dose, mg/kg/week	0.18	0.19	0.17	0.19	0.18
After 1 year					
Age, years	9.9	9.3	9.3	9.6	10.1
Height SDS	−1.1	−1.4	−1.3	−1.5	−1.7
Height velocity, cm/year	8.6	8.0	8.2	7.6	8.3
Height velocity SDS	4.5	3.3	3.1	2.8	3.8
Δ height SDS	0.7	0.6	0.6	0.5	0.7
Studentised residual	0.1	−0.5	−0.3	−0.8	−0.3
BMI SDS	0.8	0.4	1.1	0.1	0.0

Data are medians.

Table 7. Treatment for malignancy outside the cranium: patients treated for 1 prepubertal year

	Lymphatic leukaemia (code No. 2.2.3.1.1)	Myeloid leukaemia (code No. 2.2.3.1.2)	Others (code No. 2.2.3.1.9)	Lymphoma (code No. 2.2.3.2)	Others (code No. 2.2.3.2.9)
At GH start					
Patients	185	30	50	49	24
Males, %	72	50	79	69	75
Age, years	10.7	9.7	10.6	9.5	11.3
Height SDS	−1.9	−2.0	−2.1	−2.7	−2.2
Height velocity, cm/year	3.7	3.5	3.5	4.1	3.8
Height velocity SDS	−2.7	−2.7	−2.4	−1.6	−2.2
BMI SDS	0.3	−0.3	0.2	−0.2	0.1
GH dose, mg/kg/week	0.20	0.21	0.17	0.2	0.18
After 1 year					
Age, years	11.7	10.6	11.6	10.5	12.1
Height SDS	−1.5	−1.7	−1.7	−2.2	−1.7
Height velocity, cm/year	7.0	6.5	6.9	8.2	7.7
Height velocity SDS	2.1	1.8	2.4	3.0	3.4
Δ height SDS	0.5	0.4	0.4	0.5	0.5
Studentised residual	−1.1	−1.3	−1.0	−0.6	−0.1
BMI SDS	−0.1	−0.4	0.1	−0.6	−0.4

Data are medians.

Table 8. Other causes of acquired GHD: patients treated for 1 prepubertal year

	Head trauma (code No. 2.2.4.1)	CNS infection (code No. 2.2.4.2)	Hydrocephalus (code No. 2.2.4.3)
At GH start			
Patients	66	25	40
Males, %	70	64	75
Age, years	8.6	8.2	6.7
Height SDS	–3.2	–4.0	–3.7
Height velocity, cm/year	3.9	4.8	3.7
Height velocity SDS	–2.7	–1.4	–2.8
BMI SDS	0.1	0.2	–0.4
GH dose, mg/kg/week	0.19	0.19	0.22
After 1 year			
Age, years	9.6	9.2	7.6
Height SDS	–2.3	–2.8	–3.0
Height velocity, cm/year	9.1	9.3	8.5
Height velocity SDS	4.7	5.5	3.5
Δ height SDS	0.9	1.3	0.7
Studentised residual	0.3	0.7	–0.8
BMI SDS	–0.2	–0.4	–0.3

Data are medians. CNS = Central nervous system.

ff.), the responsiveness to GH tended to be greater than in IGHD.
- In children with GHD, as a result of a cranial tumour distant to the pituitary (code No. 2.2.2 ff.), the responsiveness to GH tended to be lower than in IGHD, particularly in medulloblastoma.
- In children with GHD, as a result of malignancies outside the cranium (code No. 2.2.3 ff.), the responsiveness to GH tended to be much lower than in IGHD.
- In children with GHD, as a result of head trauma and central nervous system infections, the responsiveness to GH tended to be higher and, in cases with hydrocephalus, lower than in IGHD.

Height standard deviation scores (SDS) at GH start and after the first year in patients with craniopharyngioma, germinoma, medulloblastoma, lymphatic leukaemia and head trauma are illustrated in figure 1.

Characteristics at GH Start, Puberty Onset and NAH

The characteristics at the start of GH treatment, at puberty onset and at NAH are listed in table 9. Confidence ranges are usually in the order of magnitude as described in detail in the chapter by Price [this vol., pp. 207–212].

Height SDS at treatment start, after 1 year, at puberty onset and at NAH in patients with craniopharyngioma, germinoma, medulloblastoma and lymphatic leukaemia are illustrated in figure 2.

Height SDS – midparental height (MPH) at GH start, after 1 year, at puberty onset and at NAH in patients with craniopharyngioma, germinoma, medulloblastoma and lymphatic leukaemia are illustrated in figure 3.

In patients with craniopharyngioma, NAH was close to normal (fig. 4). In medulloblastoma and lymphatic leukaemia, more than half of the patients did not reach normal height. All groups

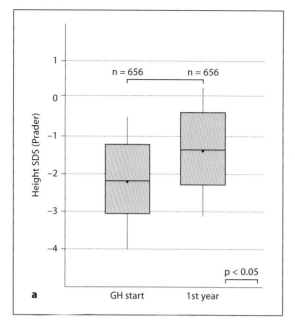
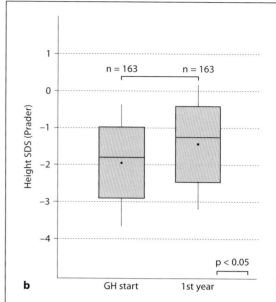
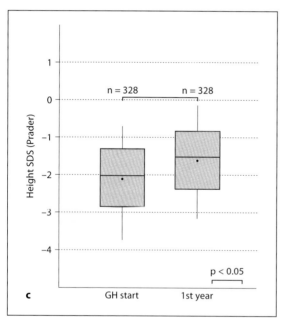

Fig. 1. a Height SDS at GH start and after 1 year of treatment in prepubertal patients with craniopharyngioma (**a**), germinoma (**b**), medulloblastoma (**c**), lymphatic leukaemia (**d**) and head trauma (**e**).

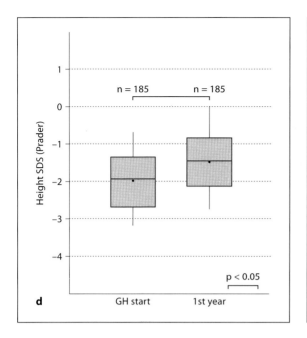
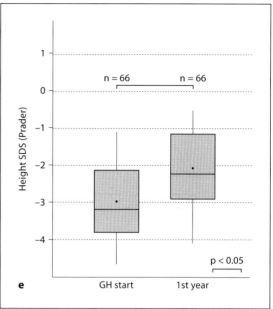

Table 9. Acquired GHD – patients treated to NAH

	Craniopharyngioma (code No. 2.2.1.1)	Germinoma (code No. 2.2.2.2)	Medulloblastoma (code No. 2.2.2.4)	Lymphatic leukaemia (code No. 2.2.3.1.1)
At GH start				
Patients, n	168	45	111	59
Males, %	47	31	63	71
Age, years	9.3	11.2	8.7	10.3
Bone age, years	7.0	9.6	6.2	9.3
Height SDS	−2.3	−1.7	−2.2	−2.1
BMI SDS	1.1	0.9	0.3	0.4
GH dose, mg/kg/week	0.17	0.16	0.19	0.20
At puberty				
Age, years	13.6	14.5	11.6	12.3
Height SDS	−0.5	−0.7	−1.0	−0.4
Δ height SDS (start – puberty)	1.6	0.9	1.1	0.8
BMI SDS	0.7	0.8	0.2	−0.2
At adult height				
Age, years	18.0	18.3	17.3	17.6
Height SDS (Prader)	−0.5	−1.2	−2.3	−2.1
Δ height SDS (puberty – end)	0.0	−0.1	−1.1	−0.9
Δ height SDS (start – end)	1.7	0.9	−0.1	0.2
BMI SDS	1.0	1.3	0.3	0.1
Puberty on GH, years	3.4	3.4	4.0	3.9
Total years on GH	7.7	6.6	7.2	6.3

Data are medians.

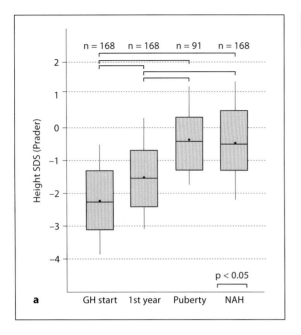
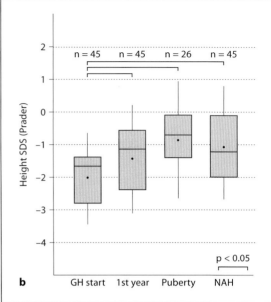
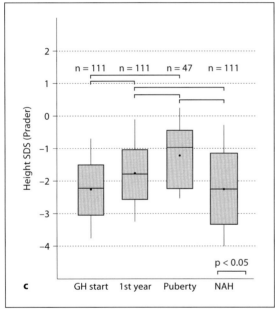
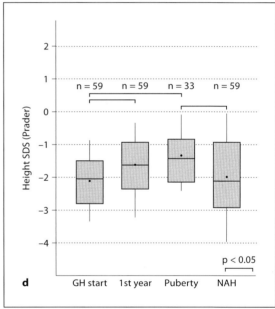

Fig. 2. Height SDS at GH start, after the 1st year of treatment, at puberty and at NAH in patients with craniopharyngioma (**a**), germinoma (**b**), medulloblastoma (**c**) and lymphatic leukaemia (**d**).

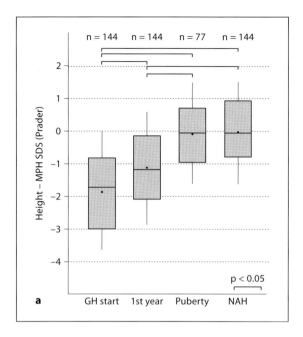
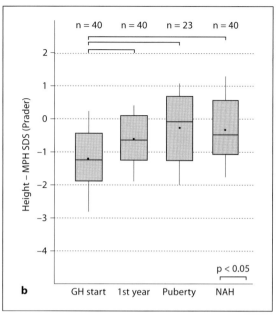
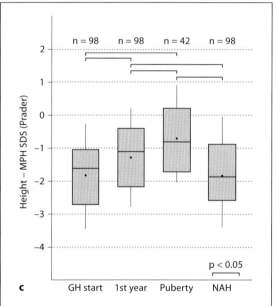
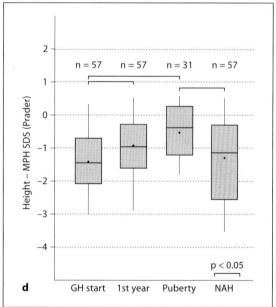

Fig. 3. Height – MPH SDS at GH start, after the 1st year of treatment, at puberty and at NAH in patients with craniopharyngioma (**a**), germinoma (**b**), medulloblastoma (**c**) and lymphatic leukaemia (**d**).

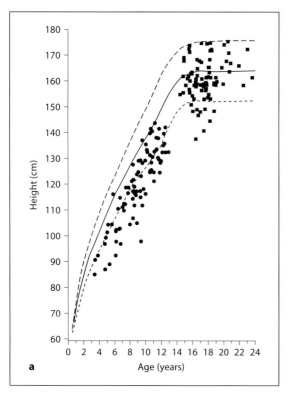
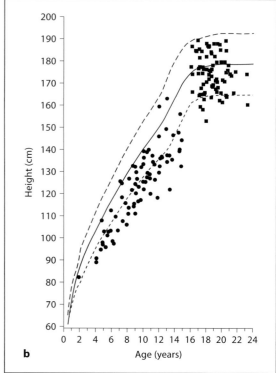

Fig. 4. Height at GH start (●) and NAH (■) in girls (**a**) and boys (**b**) with craniopharyngioma. Dashed lines = ± 2 SD; solid line = 0 SD.

gained some height before puberty. In medulloblastoma and lymphatic leukaemia patients, there were substantial losses in height during puberty, which started at a normal age.

Commentary

Responses to GH in children with acquired GHD vary greatly according to the underlying disorder. In most cases with a malignancy as the primary disorder, both the response and the responsiveness to GH are low. This is probably the cause of too low doses of GH (response) and too high an age and tissues altered by modes of treatment (responsiveness). Growth in response to GH treatment in puberty is particularly unsatisfactory. Treatment in these disorders needs to be optimised in the future.

Growth Hormone Treatment of Children with Previous Leukaemia and Lymphoma: The KIGS Experience

David A. Price[a]   Hanna Karlsson[b]

In recent years, there have been remarkable improvements in outcome for children with acute leukaemia and lymphoma. European children affected by cancer have increasingly survived their disease, and this improvement in prognosis has been most marked in leukaemias and lymphomas [1]. Five-year survival from acute lymphoid leukaemia increased from less than 80% in 1983–1985 to over 80% 10 years later. Over the same period, survival improved comparably in non-Hodgkin's lymphoma (NHL), and although prognosis was generally poorer in leukaemias other than lymphoid leukaemia, there were considerably more survivors during this time period. Survivors from these diseases have been well represented in KIGS since its inception. Numbers of children treated with growth hormone (GH) who had previously had acute lymphoblastic leukaemia (ALL), acute myeloid leukaemia (AML) and non-Hodgkin's lymphoma (NHL) reported within KIGS have increased since 1994 from 103, 14 and 13 [2] to 470, 85 and 30, respectively. During the development of KIGS, there have been many changes in the treatment of childhood malignancies, but this chapter will not attempt to unravel their effects on response to GH, with the exception of some data on the influence of types of prophylactic irradiation.

Patients

The case report forms of all children with a previous history of ALL, AML and NHL were analysed. There were 470 children with ALL, 85 with AML and 30 with NHL. Cross-sectional data were examined in these 3 cohorts. Those who had completed 1 year of GH treatment and remained prepubertal were analysed, namely 185 with ALL, 30 with AML and 12 with NHL. Lastly, 59 patients who had reached near adult height and who had previous ALL were analysed. The onset of puberty was defined as a testicular volume of >3 ml in boys and as breast budding (Tanner stage 2) in girls. Swiss data were used for auxological reference [3, 4].

[a] Royal Manchester Children's Hospital, Hospital Road Pendlebury, Swinton, Manchester M27 4HA (UK)
[b] Pfizer Endocrine Care
KIGS/KIMS/ACROSTUDY Medical Outcomes
Vetenskapsvägen 10, SE–191 90 Sollentuna (Sweden)

Table 1. Cross-sectional data at the start of GH treatment for children with prior ALL, AML and NHL

	ALL				AML				NHL			
	n	median	10th percentile	90th percentile	n	median	10th percentile	90th percentile	n	median	10th percentile	90th percentile
Background												
Age at diagnosis, years	447	3.7	1.8	7.5	83	5.4	1.9	11.5	28	5.3	2.7	11.0
Maximum GH, μg/l	379	6.0	2.1	12.0	66	6.4	3.2	15.8	26	6.6	2.3	19.4
IGF-1 SDS	55	−1.9	−3.8	0.2	17	−2.2	−4.9	−1.4	3	−1.3	−3.6	0.7
Start of GH treatment												
Age, years	470	11.8	8.3	14.7	85	11.8	8.0	15.7	30	12.6	8.0	15.9
Bone age, years	181	11.1	7.8	14.0	29	10.5	6.5	15.3	13	12.5	8.0	14.0
In puberty	403	(36.2)			68	(38.2)			25	(36.0)		
Height SDS (Prader)	470	−1.8	−3.1	−0.5	85	−1.9	−3.8	−0.6	30	−2.4	−3.4	−0.9
Height − MPH SDS (Prader)	416	−1.3	−3.0	0.2	76	−1.5	−3.7	−0.1	29	−1.5	−3.0	−0.2
Height velocity, cm/year	265	4.0	2.1	6.2	44	3.6	1.9	5.2	15	4.5	1.0	5.8
BMI SDS	470	0.4	−1.2	1.9	85	−0.1	−1.4	1.5	30	0.4	−1.6	2.5
Sitting height ratio SDS	170	0.2	−1.1	1.4	37	−0.1	−1.1	0.6	9	0.3	−4.3	1.7
GH dose, mg/kg/week	470	0.20	0.13	0.29	85	0.22	0.15	0.29	30	0.19	0.13	0.28
Injection frequency	470	7	6	7	85	7	6	7	30	7	6	7

Male/female ratios were 1.6 for ALL, 1.2 for AML and 2.0 for NHL. Figures in parentheses are percentages. IGF-1 = Insulin-like growth factor 1.

Results

Cross-Sectional Data at the Onset of GH Treatment

It is noteworthy that despite evidence of GH deficiency (GHD), height in relation to midparental height was not exceptionally low before GH treatment, and bone age was close to chronological age. This is probably related to evidence of relatively early pubertal maturation as seen by the proportion (over a third) in puberty. The body mass index (BMI) standard deviation score (SDS) and the ratio of sitting height to leg length were positive in the diagnostic groups of ALL and NHL (table 1).

Comparison of Males and Females with ALL at Onset of GH Treatment

It is seen that boys presented with ALL at a significantly older age (p = 0.003), and thus, started GH treatment later (p = 0.0001), despite being of similar short stature to girls. A higher percentage of girls was established in puberty despite their younger age, and there was no delay in bone maturation. GH dose was lower in boys (p = 0.002) (table 2).

First-Year Response to GH Treatment

The auxological response to the first year of GH treatment is summarised in table 3 and figures 1 and 2. Although height velocity clearly rose, the achieved velocity was less than that predicted from the first-year response of prepubertal children with idiopathic GHD (IGHD) (fig. 2). Those with NHL responded slightly better than the other two groups despite being shorter at onset. There was improvement in leg length as a proportion of total height for ALL and AML groups, and the BMI SDS fell in all 3 diagnostic groups.

Near Adult Height

Near adult height or height at the end of GH treatment has been recorded in 59 individuals treated for ALL. Their results are summarised in table 4.

This smaller cohort with previous ALL (59 in total) started GH treatment at 10.3 years with a total duration of 6.3 years. The height SDS rose

Table 2. Comparison of cross-sectional data at onset of GH treatment for males and females with prior ALL

	Males				Females			
	n	median	10th percentile	90th percentile	n	median	10th percentile	90th percentile
Background								
Age at diagnosis, years	276	4.0	1.9	7.9	171	3.3	1.2	6.7
Maximum GH, μg/l	236	6.2	2.2	12.4	143	5.7	1.8	11.9
IGF-1 SDS	28	−2.3	−4.3	0.3	27	−1.5	−3.0	0.2
Start of GH treatment								
Age, years	291	12.4	8.9	15.0	179	10.8	8.0	13.4
Bone age, years	111	11.5	8.0	14.0	70	10.8	6.8	13.6
In puberty	248	(25.4)			155	(53.5)		
Height SDS (Prader)	291	−1.8	−3.0	−0.5	179	−1.9	−3.4	−0.3
Height − MPH SDS (Prader)	264	−1.3	−2.8	0.2	152	−1.3	−3.1	0.2
Height velocity, cm/year	169	3.9	2.3	6.1	96	4.2	2.0	6.2
BMI SDS	291	0.4	−1.3	1.9	179	0.5	−1.2	1.9
Sitting height ratio SDS	102	0.1	−1.1	1.4	68	0.3	−1.0	1.3
GH dose, mg/kg/week	291	0.19	0.13	0.29	179	0.22	0.14	0.29
Injection frequency	291	7	5	7	179	7	6	7

Figures in parentheses are percentages. IGF-1 = Insulin-like growth factor 1.

Table 3. Response to GH treatment during the first year in the 3 diagnostic groups

	ALL				AML				NHL			
	n	median	10th percentile	90th percentile	n	median	10th percentile	90th percentile	n	median	10th percentile	90th percentile
Start of GH treatment												
Age, years	185	10.7	7.3	14.0	30	9.7	6.2	11.9	12	11.5	6.0	14.7
Height SDS (Prader)	185	−1.9	−3.2	−0.7	30	−2.0	−3.9	−1.2	12	−2.6	−3.4	−0.7
Height velocity, cm/year	106	3.7	2.3	5.5	16	3.5	1.7	4.4	8	4.2	−0.5	5.8
BMI SDS	185	0.3	−1.4	1.8	30	−0.3	−1.4	1.0	12	0.3	−1.4	2.6
Sitting height ratio SDS	50	0.3	−0.7	1.6	11	0.0	−1.0	0.3	3	0.3	−1.2	1.7
GH dose, mg/kg/week	185	0.20	0.13	0.30	30	0.21	0.15	0.27	12	0.19	0.12	0.26
Injection frequency	185	7	3	7	30	7	6	7	12	7	6	7
After 1 year												
Height SDS (Prader)	185	−1.5	−2.8	0.0	30	−1.7	−3.7	−0.7	12	−2.0	−2.9	−0.5
Height velocity, cm/year	185	7.0	4.9	9.8	30	6.5	4.7	9.1	12	8.2	5.3	10.2
BMI SDS	184	−0.1	−1.9	1.5	30	−0.4	−1.9	0.5	12	−0.2	−1.5	2.3
Sitting height ratio SDS	64	0.2	−0.8	1.4	11	−0.1	−1.4	0.6	5	0.4	−1.6	0.9
Studentised residual of height velocity	84	−1.1	−2.6	0.6	17	−1.3	−3.3	0.1	4	−0.4	−2.0	0.8

The studentised residual of the first-year velocity was calculated by comparison with the response of prepubertal children with IGHD and therefore related to leukaemia subgroups that had not entered puberty.

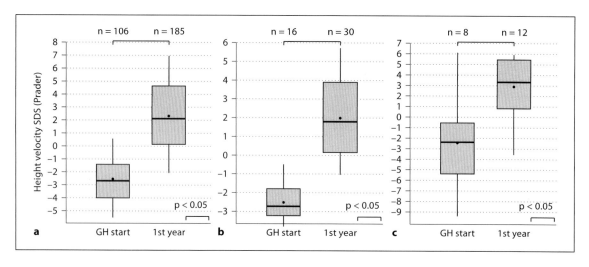

Fig. 1. Height velocity of ALL (**a**), AML (**b**) and NHL cohorts (**c**) before and during the first year of GH treatment (25th–75th percentiles represented by boxes, and 10th–90th percentiles represented by whiskers).

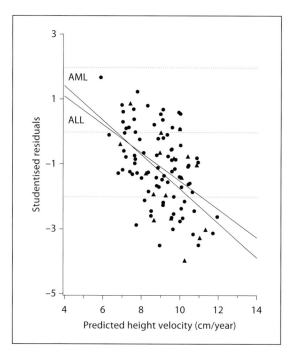

Fig. 2. Studentised residuals of observed first-year height velocities compared with predicted height velocities (predicted from prepubertal IGHD children) in prepubertal ALL (●) and AML (▲) children (insufficient numbers of NHL children) with lines of regression for both groups.

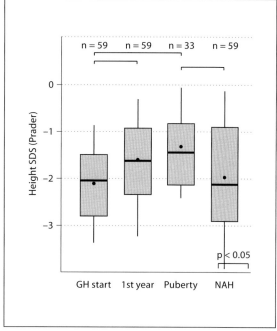

Fig. 3. Height SDS of patients with ALL who had reached near adult height at GH start, at 1 year of GH treatment, at onset of puberty and at near adult height (25th–75th percentiles represented by boxes, and 10th–90th percentiles represented by whiskers).

Table 4. Characteristics of children with ALL who had completed GH treatment

	n	Median	10th percentile	90th percentile
Start of GH treatment				
Age, years	59	10.3	8.1	13.1
Height SDS (Prader)	59	–2.1	–3.4	–0.9
BMI SDS	59	0.4	–1.3	1.8
Sitting height ratio SDS	18	0.4	–0.7	1.7
After 1 year				
Age, years	59	11.3	9.0	14.0
Height SDS (Prader)	59	–1.6	–3.2	–0.3
BMI SDS	58	–0.1	–1.9	1.4
Sitting height ratio SDS	27	0.2	–0.9	1.5
At puberty onset				
Age, years	33	12.3	11.4	15.5
Height SDS (Prader)	33	–1.5	–2.4	–0.1
BMI SDS	33	–0.2	–1.7	1.5
Sitting height ratio SDS	18	0.0	–1.1	2.3
At completion of GH treatment				
Age, years	59	17.6	15.6	19.5
Height SDS (Prader)	59	–2.1	–3.9	–0.2
BMI SDS	56	0.1	–1.7	1.8
Sitting height ratio SDS	27	–0.1	–3.2	1.8

Data at the start of GH treatment, after 1 year of GH, at puberty onset and at the end of GH treatment in a cohort of 59 patients who had completed GH treatment with a median treatment duration of 6.3 years.

Table 5. ALL cohort subdivided according to irradiation schedule, CR, CS and any schedule including TBI, and further subdivided according to the length of time treated with GH

Irradiation schedule	CR	CS	TBI
Start of GH treatment			
Patients	164	59	187
Age, years	12.2[a]	11.6	11.5
Bone age, years	11.3	11.0	11.5
Height SDS (Prader)	–1.8	–1.8	–1.9
Sitting height ratio SDS	0.2	–0.2	0.2
BMI SDS	0.4	0.7[b]	0.38
After 1 year			
Patients	54	17	85
Height velocity at 1 year, cm/year	7.2[a]	6.9	6.5
Predicted height velocity, cm/year	9.1	9.0	9.1
Studentised residual	–0.6	–0.2	–1.3
Having reached near adult height			
Patients	21		27
Δ height SDS at puberty onset	0.7		0.9
Δ height SDS at adult height from puberty onset	0.2[c]		–1.3
Δ height SDS at adult height from start of GH	0.6[c]		–0.4
Sitting height ratio SDS	0.4		–0.3
BMI SDS	0.3		0

It should be noted that there are differing numbers of patients at the entry into KIGS, after completion of 1 year of treatment and after reaching near adult height.
[a] p = 0.01, CR versus TBI.
[b] p = 0.01, CS versus TBI.
[c] p = 0.0001, CR versus TBI.

appreciably in the first year, but had fallen to the starting value by the end of treatment (fig. 3). The BMI SDS fell during the first year, and a reduced level continued until completion. Disproportion of sitting height and leg length changed from a longer trunk length to leg length at treatment start to the opposite at the end of treatment, i.e. trunk length gradually diminished with time compared with leg length. There were differences in behaviour between males and females during this time period. Males started and finished GH treatment later, with a median duration of 6.4 years compared with 6.0 years in females. From the start of GH therapy to completion of treatment, the height SDS changed from –2.0 to –1.8 in males and from –2.4 to –2.5 in females. The BMI SDS fell in both sexes by the end of treatment, and there was a greater disproportion at the end of treatment in females. Both sexes had negative studentised residuals of observed to predicted height velocities in the first year (–0.7 in males and –1.3 in females).

Influence of Radiation Schedules
Table 5 shows some comparisons between those children with ALL who had received cranial irradiation (CR), craniospinal irradiation (CS) and

Table 6. Age correlations

	ALL			AML			NHL		
	n	correlation	p value	n	correlation	p value	n	correlation	p value
Age at diagnosis									
Age at GH start	447	0.43	<0.001	83	0.74	<0.001	28	0.64	<0.001
Age at puberty start	114	0.41	<0.001	26	0.50	0.01	5	0.50	NS
Age at GH start									
Age at puberty start	124	0.81	<0.001	27	0.58	0.001	5	0.90	0.037

NS = Not significant.

any schedule that included total body irradiation (TBI). There were insufficient numbers to show data for CS patients who had reached near adult height.

At the start of GH treatment, those that had received TBI were younger than those who had had CR alone. First-year height velocities on GH treatment were higher in the CR group than in the TBI group, and Δ increments in the height SDS from the start of GH therapy and from the onset of puberty to near adult height were greater in the CR group than in the TBI group.

Correlations between Ages at Diagnosis of Malignancy and at Start of GH Treatment
Correlations of ages at diagnosis of malignancy with ages at GH start and puberty, as well as correlations of ages at GH start with ages at puberty onset are shown in table 6.

Discussion

Despite extensive experience of the use of GH replacement treatment of acquired GHD in long-term survivors of acute leukaemias and lymphomas, studies of effects of GH treatment on quality of life have only just begun [5]. Predominantly, attention has been placed on improvement in height deficit, but possible effects of GHD on body metabolism may need to be factored into our assessment of the value of GH treatment [6–8].

The case for correction of height deficit has been well made. Muller et al. [9] showed that CR and CS led to a decrease in adult height in long-term survivors of ALL who had not received GH treatment, and Bongers et al. [10] used a more sensitive measure of adult height impairment, namely distance from target height, to show that the majority of long-term survivors of ALL were adversely affected, attributable to irradiation-induced GHD. The possibility that chemotherapy alone in newer treatment schedules may affect hypothalamo-pituitary function in the long term is not ruled out [11], but it is likely to be less common.

At entry into KIGS, there is a height deficit (modest compared with IGHD) in the face of biochemically confirmed GHD. Assuming that the start of GH treatment in KIGS approximates to the timing of GHD, the age at malignancy diagnosis and the appearance of GHD appear to be strongly correlated, confirming the concept that the pathogenesis of hypothalamic impairment after irradiation (at prophylactic doses) takes several years to appear. Already a third of individuals are in puberty at a relatively early age, probably another effect of hypothalamic impairment by irradiation. The conjunction of these two epiphenomena constrains the time available for effective GH treatment for height deficit.

Despite evidence of poorer responsiveness in these diagnostic groups, the GH doses are similar to those in IGHD. During the first year of GH treatment, there were significant increases in height velocity and in the height SDS for ALL patients. However, when compared with the responses seen in prepubertal IGHD patients, the studentised residuals were negative, especially in the ALL and AML groups. The studentised residuals are controlled for GH dose, and it is likely that greater growth responses would have been seen with higher doses in these more GH-resistant groups.

The analysis of near adult height was restricted to ALL patients, because there were too few in the other subgroups reaching the end of GH treatment for height. The failure to increase the height SDS over the whole duration of treatment is misleading in that it is very likely that patients would have lost more height without replacement GH. The pattern of gain in the first year or until onset of puberty and then loss during puberty is clinically significant. It seems to indicate that every effort should be made to maximise catch-up growth by the onset of puberty. Could GH replacement have been started earlier in the evolution of GHD and should greater doses of GH have been used throughout treatment for height deficit? Evidence for those strategies is not yet available, but it seems clinically likely. The alternative strategy of delaying unduly early pubertal onset might also be considered. However, all these manipulations have to be considered in the light of a patient population which has been through a prolonged therapeutic ordeal in managing the original malignancy. The very limited data [5] on attitude to GH injections suggest that this group perceives injections as painful, and at the same time, parents may be disappointed in the growth response achieved. These two observations make strategies such as parental monitoring of injections and insulin-like growth factor 1 measurements in order to ensure good compliance very important.

At the end of GH treatment for height deficit of ALL patients, the BMI SDS had lessened and the trunk to leg length disproportion had been mitigated. The links between metabolic syndrome and cardiovascular risk factors on the one hand and CR and GHD on the other [6–8] indicate that after near adult height is achieved, the patient should be retested for ongoing GHD with a view to continuing GH replacement when necessary for metabolic objectives. Again, the attitudes towards GH treatment in this special group of malignancy survivors would be critical to success in long-term replacement.

The influence of TBI within any treatment protocol is seen in table 5. Growth response to GH is particularly poor as evidenced by the negative studentised residual of achieved over predicted height velocity, as well as the loss of the height SDS within puberty and over the whole duration of treatment. Those patients with ALL who did not receive TBI gained 0.6 SDS by adult height and those who did receive TBI lost 0.4 SDS. This negative influence of TBI on epiphyseal behaviour will no doubt be considered when therapeutic protocols are devised.

In summary, the data in KIGS relating to this group of patients with secondary GHD indicate that there is an important role for replacement GH treatment in addressing height deficit and adverse metabolic changes, but practices have not yet been modified to accommodate the special circumstances that surround this group of long-term survivors of childhood malignancy, which include GH resistance, a shorter window of opportunity for GH due to early puberty, and possibly different psychological perspectives of the families.

References

1 Gatta G, Capocacia R, Stiller C, Kaatsch P, Berrino F, Terenziana M, the EUROCARE Working Group: Childhood cancer survival trends in Europe: a EUROCARE Working Group study. J Clin Oncol 2005;23:3742–3751.
2 Price DA, Clayton PE: Growth hormone treatment in children in remission from leukaemia and lymphoma; in Ranke MB, Gunnarsson R (eds): Progress in Growth Hormone Therapy – 5 Years of KIGS. Mannheim, J & J Verlag, 1996, pp 157–172.
3 Largo AD, Prader A: Pubertal development in Swiss boys. Helv Paediatr Acta 1983;38:211–228.
4 Largo AD, Prader A: Pubertal development in Swiss girls. Helv Paediatr Acta 1983;38:229–243.
5 Eiser C, Vance YH, Glaser A, Galvin H, Horne B, Picton S, Stoner A, Butler G: Growth hormone treatment and quality of life among survivors of childhood cancer. Horm Res 2005;63:300–304.
6 Link K, Moell C, Garwicz S, Cavallin-Stahl E, Bjork J, Thilen U, Ahren B, Erfurth EM: Growth hormone deficiency predicts cardiovascular risk in young adults treated for acute lymphoblastic leukaemia in childhood. J Clin Endocrinol Metab 2004;89:5003–5012.
7 Jarfelt N, Lannering B, Bosaeus I, Johannsson G, Bjarnason R: Body composition in young adult survivors of childhood acute lymphoblastic leukaemia. Eur J Endocrinol 2005;153:81–89.
8 Gurney JG, Ness KK, Sibley SD, O'Leary M, Dengel DR, Lee JM, Youngren NM, Glasser SP, Baker KS: Metabolic syndrome and growth hormone deficiency in adult survivors of childhood acute lymphoblastic leukaemia. Cancer 2006; 107:1303–1312.
9 Muller HL, Klinkhammer-Schalke M, Kuhl J: Final height and weight of long-term survivors of childhood malignancies. Exp Clin Endocrinol Diabetes 1998;106:135–139.
10 Bongers ME, Francken AB, Rouwe C, Kamps WA, Postma A: Reduction of adult height in childhood acute lymphoblastic leukaemia survivors after prophylactic cranial irradiation. Pediatr Blood Cancer 2005;34:139–143.
11 Haddy TB, Mosher RB, Nunez SB, Reaman GH: Growth hormone deficiency after chemotherapy for acute lymphoblastic leukaemia in children who have not received cranial irradiation. Pediatr Blood Cancer 2006;46:258–261.

Growth Hormone, Langerhans Cell Histiocytosis and Neurofibromatosis

Michel Polak

Langerhans Cell Histiocytosis

Introduction

Langerhans cell histiocytosis (LCH) is characterized by excessive proliferation and accumulation of Langerhans cells [1]. The clinical manifestations and outcome are highly variable, ranging from an isolated, spontaneously remitting bone lesion to multisystem involvement with life-threatening organ dysfunction [2]. The pathophysiology of LCH is largely unknown [3]. The pituitary is a well-known target of LCH.

Growth Hormone Deficiency

Growth hormone deficiency (GHD) is the most frequent anterior pituitary hormone deficiency among patients with LCH and pituitary dysfunction (table 1). GHD is usually diagnosed years after posterior pituitary deficiency and is responsible for growth retardation. Described initially as a rare complication [4–7], GHD is now estimated to affect up to 42% of LCH patients with diabetes insipidus (DI) [8].

The 10-year cumulative incidence of GHD in the French nationwide LCH survey (n = 589) was 53.7% among patients with DI (fig. 1) [9, 10]. GHD was the second most common endocrine deficiency, confirming the results of a single-center survey [8]. Two early findings were associated with subsequent GHD in patients who apparently had isolated posterior pituitary involvement, namely early loss of growth velocity and a magnetic resonance imaging (MRI)-documented decrease in anterior pituitary height. In the year after DI onset, a growth deficiency of 0.5 standard deviation (SD) appeared among patients without GHD (probably resulting from the disease itself and/or from its treatment), compared with 1.5 SD among patients who subsequently developed GHD. A further loss was noted between GHD diagnosis and the outset of GH treatment, which was implemented at a median height SD score (SDS) of –2. This delay in treatment may have been due to reluctance to use GH in this immunological disorder and to a focus on controlling disease activity. This point will be discussed below. The value of MRI for early detection of pa-

Service d'Endocrinologie Pédiatrique
INSERM EMI 363, Hôpital Necker-Enfants Malades
149 Rue de Sèvres
FR–75015 Paris (France)

Table 1. Endocrine dysfunctions and their combinations in the French LCH Study (n = 593 LCH patients)

	n	Characteristics
DI	141	77 alone 35 DI + GHD only 29 DI + 1 or more endocrinopathies
GHD	61	4 without DI: 3 isolated GHD 1 GHD + TSH deficiency
Central hypothyroidism	23	all in association
Primary hypothyroidism	2	
Primary hyperthyroidism	1	Graves' disease
Gonadotrophin deficiency	17	all in association
Corticotroph deficiency	10	all in association
Panhypopituitarism	9	

TSH = Thyroid-stimulating hormone.

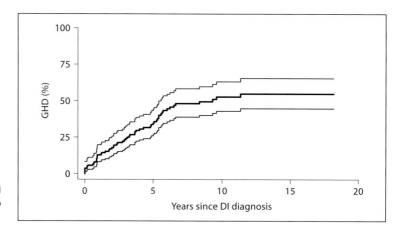

Fig. 1. Cumulative risk of GHD among the 141 patients with DI, with 95% confidence intervals.

tients at high risk of GHD must be confirmed in a prospective study, as it has not been reported previously [8].

Radiotherapy, despite the use of low doses (10–15 Gy), was associated with an increased risk of GHD, as previously reported with higher doses [7, 11]. As the benefit of radiotherapy is probably limited in LCH, this increased risk of GHD is a further reason to avoid it [12].

To identify further risk factors for GHD, clinical features and the main therapeutic parameters of the 61 patients with GHD were compared with those of our 528 patients without GHD. Only ear, nose and throat involvement (sinus, mastoid, external auditory tract and gums) and neurological LCH involvement were significantly associated with the risk of GHD [9, 10].

Efficacy and Safety of GH Treatment in the French LCH Study
GH Treatment. Forty-seven patients were treated with GH for GHD, at a median dose of 0.18 mg/kg/week (range 0.03–0.26), representing 0.54 units/kg/week. Among these 47 patients, the 5 pa-

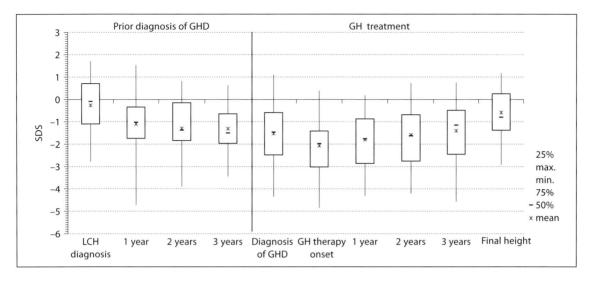

Fig. 2. Growth in patients with GHD according to GH therapy. The results are expressed as SDS, with 95% confidence intervals.

tients treated before 1985 received low-dose extractive GH. All the other patients received biosynthetic human GH. Fourteen GH-deficient patients were not treated for various reasons [9, 10].

Growth Response to GH Treatment. Median growth velocity increased from –1.7 to 1.8 SDS after 1 year of GH treatment. Mean height increased gradually with the year of treatment (fig. 2). The final median height SDS, based on data for 28 GH-treated patients, was –0.8, a value significantly higher than at the diagnosis of GHD (–1.6 SD), and at GH treatment outset (–2 SD). The difference in final height – target height between the non-GH-deficient group and the GH-deficient GH-treated group (0.3 SD) was not significant. Final height SD among GH-deficient GH-untreated patients was –2.8 SD (n = 6), a value far below the target height (final stature – midparental height = –3 SD).

The long-term response to GH therapy in children with GHD due to causes other than LCH is dependent on early treatment, before the onset of significant growth failure [13–16]. In our study, GH therapy was started when most patients already had severe growth failure. It is noteworthy that the final height of the 6 children with GHD who were not treated with GH was almost –3 SD, compared with only –0.8 SD in treated children.

The median final height among non-GH-deficient LCH patients was normal, suggesting that the disease and its treatment are not growth-limiting factors in the long run. The final height of treated GHD patients remained moderately below the midparental (target) height [9, 10]. The less satisfactory final heights obtained in this study, compared with other settings, may have been due to the use of relatively low doses in a subgroup of 5 patients treated with extractive hormone, as the dose of GH is known to influence final stature [13].

Safety of GH Therapy. No adverse effects clearly related to GH therapy were observed in the 47 treated patients. A total of 19 new LCH events occurred among 12 of the 47 patients, with first relapses after a median of 1.4 years on GH therapy (range 0.3–6.9). Three patients receiving recombinant GH developed a LCH neurodegenerative

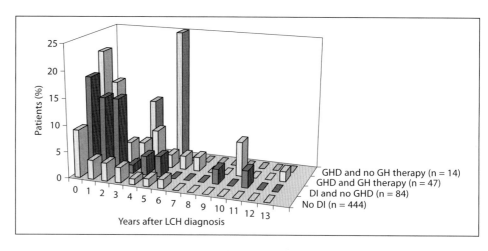

Fig. 3. Proportion of patients with new LCH disease events according to the year after LCH diagnosis, pituitary status and GH therapy. Patients with pituitary involvement had significantly more events than patients without pituitary involvement (p < 0.001) during the first 3 years after LCH diagnosis, but no significant difference was observed according to GH therapy among patients with pituitary involvement.

syndrome. In 2 patients, osseous involvement was the first nonpituitary site of LCH. Lung involvement was diagnosed 6 years after LCH onset (and after 1.4 years on GH) in a teenager who had started to smoke. In the 6 remaining patients, the events consisted solely of bone lesions. Before GH treatment, relapses were significantly more frequent in patients with pituitary involvement than in patients without. Interestingly, among patients with pituitary involvement, the relapse rate was not significantly influenced by GHD or GH therapy, arguing against a deleterious effect of GH therapy on LCH disease activity. Finally, 36 of the events observed in GHD patients occurred during periods without GH therapy, compared with 19 during GH therapy (fig. 3).

Our results appear reassuring as regards the potential adverse effects of GH treatment in LCH. In particular, the frequency of new LCH events was low during GH therapy relative to periods without GH therapy, but this observation was based on a limited number of patients (n = 47) and has to be confirmed by reports of distinct teams.

Conclusion

In pediatric-onset LCH, GHD is the most frequent anterior pituitary hormone deficiency and is commonly associated with DI. Its frequency increases with time, underlining the need for long-term follow-up. GHD can be detected by monitoring growth velocity and maybe by measuring anterior pituitary size by MRI. Radiotherapy to fields including the pituitary appeared to favor the onset of GHD and should therefore be avoided. GH therapy was efficacious and did not appear to increase the frequency of LCH disease events. These findings remain to be confirmed in a prospective study.

Neurofibromatosis

Introduction

Neurofibromatosis type 1 (NF1), also known as von Recklinghausen disease, is an autosomal dominant disease, generally inherited, affecting 1 in 3,000 individuals [17]. Seven key components of the disease (table 2) have been identified

[18]; 2 at least must be present in order to establish the diagnosis.

A feature of NF1, known for some time now, is short stature (height ≥2 SDS below the population mean); it affects approximately 13–24% of prepubertal patients and more than 40% of adults [19, 20].

Short Stature and GHD

Short stature associated with NF1 usually affects the skeleton symmetrically [21]. The etiology of short stature in patients with NF1 does not correlate with disease severity; it is multifactorial and due to the disease itself or its complications. These complications may include problems that interfere with normal skeletal development, such as scoliosis [22, 23] or deep plexiform neurofibromas, or the use of psychostimulant medications [24] for the treatment of attention deficit disorder [25], a frequent behavioral problem in children with NF1. Risk factors for suboptimal growth are listed in table 3. In a cross-section study of the National Neurofibromatosis Foundation International Database, the distribution of heights in 569 Caucasian North American children with NF1 was analyzed [26]; the mean height SDS among their patients was found to be lower than that of the reference population. Thirteen percent of the NF1 patients fell more than 2 SD below the reference population mean, compared with only 2% of controls. Authors concluded that the distributions of stature are shifted among NF1 patients. The parameters of growth, puberty and final height of 89 children with NF1 were evaluated in a prospective study [19]. Short stature was observed in 25.5% of the patients during the prepubertal period, with a significant gradual reduction in relative height for age during puberty. Forty-three percent of patients had a short adult height; of these, 58% had short stature attributable to familial NF1. Short adult height was more often attributed to central nervous system pathology when the father was the affected parent, less when both parents were affected, and rarely when neither parent was affected. There was also a 4-fold higher frequency of central precocious puberty (CPP) among the patients compared with that observed in the general population, but the frequency of short stature remained the same even when patients with CPP were excluded. GHD as the cause of short stature was found only after neurosurgery and irradiation in a minority of short patients.

GHD is an important complication in children with NF1, and the etiology in some patients

Table 2. Diagnostic criteria

1.	Six or more café-au-lait macules, the greatest diameter being >5 mm in prepubertal patients and >15 mm in postpubertal patients
2.	Freckling in the axillary or inguinal region
3.	Two or more neurofibromas of any type or one plexiform neurofibroma
4.	Two or more Lisch nodules in the iris
5.	Optic glioma
6.	A distinctive osseous lesion such as sphenoid dysplasia or pseudoarthritis
7.	A first-degree relative with NF1 diagnosed according to the preceding criteria

Table 3. Risk factors associated with short stature in children with NF1

Suprasellar lesions
Surgery or radiotheraypy for intracranial lesions
GHD
Thyroid-stimulating hormone deficiency
Central precocious puberty
Delayed puberty
Scoliosis
Plexiform neurofibromas
Familial NF1
Familial short stature
Methylphenidate use for attention deficit disorder

remains unclear. In the majority of children with NF1, GHD occurs primarily in those with an intracranial tumor who undergo intracranial surgery and cranial irradiation therapy. In a study of 24 patients with optic pathway gliomas (OPGs) [27], half had NF1; GHD was found in 15 out of the 18 patients who were evaluated following treatment with radiotherapy. Huguenin et al. [28] evaluated the relationship of adult height after cranial radiation for OPG with NF1, CPP and GHD caused by the tumor itself or its management. Cranial irradiation resulted in GHD in 100% of cases. Reduced adult height resulted when there was GHD and CPP in the presence of NF1. A 2.5% prevalence of GHD was reported in children with NF1 without an intracranial mass and before surgical or radiation therapy for OPG, a frequency significantly higher than the 0.03% observed in the general pediatric population [29]. An OPG was detected in 1 of 3 children with GHD, suggesting that GHD may appear independently of the presence of OPG. The causal mechanism of increased frequency of GHD in patients with NF1 requires further explanation.

Efficacy and Safety of GH
In a cohort including children with NF1 and GHD without suprasellar lesions, recombinant human GH (rhGH) replacement therapy increased the patients' annual growth rate (from a pretreatment average) of 5–9 cm/year during the first year, 8.3 cm/year during the second year and 6 cm/year during years 3–5 of rhGH therapy [30]. Further data obtained from the KIGS database will be detailed elsewhere. The response to treatment was modest and less than that observed in patients with idiopathic GHD.

While therapy with rhGH has been shown to be safe, theoretical concerns remain that rhGH treatment may potentially increase an individual's risk of developing cancer de novo or increase the risk of recurrence of primary tumors and/or the incidence of second tumors in cancer survivors. The natural history of OPG in children with NF1, as reported in previous studies [31], suggests an incidence of tumor recurrence of 11–14%. A 30% recurrence rate of OPG after 10 years in NF1 patients under the age of 20 treated with surgery has also been reported [32]. The occurrence of second intracranial tumors has also been frequently reported in children with NF1 and OPG. Second tumors were reported in 21% [33] and 52% [34] during a 9-year follow-up. There does not appear to be an increased risk of primary tumor recurrence nor development of a second malignancy in children with NF1 treated with rhGH [35]. However, all such patients should undergo continuous surveillance [36].

Progression of NF1 Features
It is well documented that café-au-lait macule size increases during puberty [37]. It is also known that neurofibromas increase both in size and in number in pubertal patients. Superficial growth of neurofibromas can lead to underlying segmental hypertrophy, whereas deeper structure invasion of the spine and paraspinal areas can create anatomical problems, the most dangerous of which is spinal cord compression. Whether rhGH treatment can accelerate or increase the growth of these lesions with harmful sequelae remains of concern. Indeed, 13% of the NF1 patients in the KIGS database [38], many of whom were pubertal, had changes in café-au-lait macules and neurofibromas.

There are no reports that the increase in disease progression was accelerated secondary to rhGH, although 1 patient had an increase in the size of a prelumbar mass thought to be a neurofibroma. Cnossen et al. [29] reported no growth of neurofibromas that could be attributed to rhGH replacement in their patient population. Although these results are reassuring, close monitoring of the growth of neurocutaneous lesions is still warranted in rhGH-treated NF1 patients until larger-scale observations are made available.

Conclusion

Current knowledge suggests that increased prevalence of GHD exists in NF1 and that GH treatment does not influence the progression of any of the features of NF1, including the incidence of recurrence of primary or the development of secondary intracranial tumors. Hence, it appears that the use of GH is efficacious and safe in children with NF1 and GHD, although continuous surveillance is necessary.

Acknowledgments

We thank Jean Donadieu, MD, PhD and the French study group for LCH (GEH) who made the studies on the endocrine aspects of LCH possible.

References

1. Egeler RM, D'Angio GJ: Langerhans cell histiocytosis. J Pediatr 1995;127:1–11.
2. French Langerhans' Cell Histiocytosis Study Group: A multicentre retrospective survey of Langerhans' cell histiocytosis: 348 cases observed between 1983 and 1993. Arch Dis Child 1996;75:17–24.
3. Geissmann F, Lepelletier Y, Fraitag S, Valladeau J, Bodemer C, Debré M, et al: Differentiation of Langerhans cells in Langerhans cell histiocytosis. Blood 2001;97:1241–1248.
4. Braunstein GD, Kohler PO: Pituitary function in Hand-Schuller-Christian disease. N Engl J Med 1972;286:1225–1229.
5. Braunstein GD, Raiti S, Hansen JW, Kohler PO: Response of growth-retarded patients with Hand-Schuller-Christian disease to growth hormone therapy. N Engl J Med 1975;292:332–333.
6. Braunstein GD, Kolher PO: Endocrine manifestations of histiocytosis. Am J Pediatr Hematol Oncol 1981;3:67–75.
7. Dean HJ, Bishop A, Winter JS: Growth hormone deficiency in patients with histiocytosis X. J Pediatr 1986;109:615–618.
8. Nanduri VR, Bareille P, Pritchard J, Stanhope R: Growth and endocrine disorders in multisystem Langerhans' cell histiocytosis. Clin Endocrinol (Oxf) 2000;53:509–515.
9. Donadieu J, Rolon MA, Pion I, Thomas C, Doz F, Barkaoui M, Robert A, Deville A, Mazingue F, David M, Brauner R, Cabrol S, Garel C, Polak M, French LCH Study Group: Incidence of growth hormone deficiency in pediatric-onset Langerhans cell histiocytosis: efficacy and safety of growth hormone treatment. J Clin Endocrinol Metab 2004;89:604–609.
10. Donadieu J, Rolon MA, Thomas C, Brugieres L, Plantaz D, Emile JF, Frappaz D, David M, Brauner R, Genereau T, Debray D, Cabrol S, Barthez MA, Hoang-Xuan K, Polak M, French LCH Study Group: Endocrine involvement in pediatric-onset Langerhans' cell histiocytosis: a population-based study. J Pediatr 2004;144:344–350.
11. Rozenzweig KE, Arceci RJ, Tarbell NJ: Diabetes insipidus secondary to Langerhans cell histiocytosis: is radiation therapy indicated? Med Pediatr Oncol 1997;29:36–40.
12. El-Sayed S, Brewin TB: Histiocytosis X: does radiotherapy still have a role? Clin Oncol (R Coll Radiol) 1992;4:27–31.
13. Blethen SL, Compton P, Lippe BM, Rosenfeld RG, August GP, Johanson A: Factors predicting the response to growth hormone (GH) therapy in prepubertal children with GH deficiency. J Clin Endocrinol Metab 1993;76:574–579.
14. Blethen SL, Baptista J, Kuntze J, Foley T, LaFranchi S, Johanson A: Adult height in growth hormone (GH)-deficient children treated with biosynthetic GH. The Genentech Growth Study Group. J Clin Endocrinol Metab 1997;82:418–420.
15. Ranke MB, Price DA, Albertsson-Wikland K, Maes M, Lindberg A: Factors determining pubertal growth and final height in growth hormone treatment of idiopathic growth hormone deficiency. Analysis of 195 Patients of the Kabi Pharmacia International Growth Study. Horm Res 1997;48:62–71.
16. Rappaport R, Mugnier E, Limoni C, Crosnier H, Czernichow P, Leger J, Limal JM, Rochiccioli P, Soskin S: A 5-year prospective study of growth hormone (GH)-deficient children treated with GH before the age of 3 years. French Serono Study Group. J Clin Endocrinol Metab 1997;82:452–456.
17. Riccardi VM, Eichner JE: Neurofibromatosis: Phenotype, Natural History and Pathogenesis. Baltimore, Johns Hopkins University Press, 1986, pp 29–36.
18. National Institutes of Health Consensus Development Conference: Neurofibromatosis. Conference statement. Arch Neurol 1988;45:575–578.
19. Carmi D, Shohat M, Metzker A, Dickerman Z: Growth, puberty, and endocrine functions in patients with sporadic or familial neurofibromatosis type 1: a longitudinal study. Pediatrics 1999;103:1257–1262.
20. Vassilopoulou-Sellin R, Woods D, Quintos MT, Needle M, Klein MJ: Short stature in children and adults with neurofibromatosis. Pediatr Nurs 1995;21:149–153.
21. Riccardi VM: Neurofibromatosis: Phenotype, Natural History and Pathogenesis, ed 2. Baltimore, Johns Hopkins University Press, 1992.

22 Chaglassian JH, Riseborough EJ, Hall JE: Neurofibromatous scoliosis. Natural history and results of treatment in thirty-seven cases. J Bone Joint Surg Am 1976;58:695–702.
23 DiSimone RE, Berman AT, Schwentker EP: The orthopaedic manifestation of neurofibromatosis. A clinical experience and review of the literature. Clin Orthop Relat Res 1988;(230):277–283.
24 Pizzi WJ, Rode EC, Barnhart JE: Methylphenidate and growth: demonstration of a growth impairment and a growth-rebound phenomenon. Dev Pharmacol Ther 1986;9:361–368.
25 North K: Neurofibromatosis type 1. Am J Med Genet 2000;97:119–127.
26 Szudek J, Birch P, Friedman JM: Growth in North American white children with neurofibromatosis 1 (NF1). J Med Genet 2000;37:933–938.
27 Pierce SM, Barnes PD, Loeffler JS, McGinn C, Tarbell NJ: Definitive radiation therapy in the management of symptomatic patients with optic glioma. Survival and long-term effects. Cancer 1990;65:45–52.
28 Huguenin M, Trivin C, Zerah M, Doz F, Brugieres L, Brauner R: Adult height after cranial irradiation for optic pathway tumors: relationship with neurofibromatosis. J Pediatr 2003;142:699–703.
29 Cnossen MH, Stam EN, Cooiman LC, Simonsz HJ, Stroink H, Oranje AP, Halley DJ, de Goede-Bolder A, Niermeijer MF, de Muinck Keizer-Schrama SM: Endocrinologic disorders and optic pathway gliomas in children with neurofibromatosis type 1. Pediatrics 1997;100:667–670.
30 Vassilopoulou-Sellin R, Klein MJ, Slopis JK: Growth hormone deficiency in children with neurofibromatosis type 1 without suprasellar lesions. Pediatr Neurol 2000;22:355–358.
31 Janss AJ, Grundy R, Cnaan A, Savino PJ, Packer RJ, Zackai EH, Goldwein JW, Sutton LN, Radcliffe J, Molloy PT, et al: Optic pathway and hypothalamic/chiasmatic gliomas in children younger than age 5 years with a 6-year follow-up. Cancer 1995;75:1051–1059.
32 Alvord EC Jr, Lofton S: Gliomas of the optic nerve or chiasm. Outcome by patients' age, tumor site, and treatment. J Neurosurg 1988;68:85–98.
33 Hochstrasser H, Boltshauser E, Valavanis A: Brain tumors in children with von Recklinghausen neurofibromatosis. Neurofibromatosis 1988;1:233–239.
34 Kuenzle C, Weissert M, Roulet E, Bode H, Schefer S, Huisman T, Landau K, Boltshauser E: Follow-up of optic pathway gliomas in children with neurofibromatosis type 1. Neuropediatrics 1994;25:295–300.
35 Sklar CA: Growth hormone treatment: cancer risk. Horm Res 2004;62(suppl 3):30–34.
36 Saenger P: Growth hormone in von Recklinghausen's disease: reckless or recommended? J Pediatr 1998;133:172–174.
37 Listernick R, Charrow J: Neurofibromatosis type 1 in childhood. J Pediatr 1990;116:845–853.
38 Howell SJ, Wilton P, Lindberg A, Shalet SM: Growth hormone and neurofibromatosis. Horm Res 2000;53(suppl 1):70–76.

Growth Hormone Treatment in Neurofibrosis Type 1 Involving Central Nervous System Tumours and Pituitary Langerhans Cell Histiocytosis within KIGS

Michael B. Ranke[a]   Wayne S. Cutfield[b]

Background

Many details related to the topic have been discussed and reviewed in the article by Polak [this vol., pp. 269–276].

Neurofibromatosis type 1 (NF1, also known as von Recklinghausen disease) is a frequent autosomal dominant disease with an incidence of about 1 in 3,000 [1]. It is caused by a mutation of the NF1 gene located on chromosome 17q11.2, which encodes the protein neurofibromin [2]. This protein is considered to be a tumour suppressor gene. Its inactivation leads to a variety of tumours, such as neurofibromas, peripheral nerve sheath tumours, optic gliomas and pheochromocytomas, among others [3]. Since the molecular genetics of the disorder is complex, the diagnosis is usually still based on clinical criteria, such as café-au-lait spots, cutaneous neurofibromas, opticus glioma, freckles in the axillae, first-degree NF1 relative, or changes in bone structure [4]. Central nervous system tumours occur either along the optic pathway (approximately 70%) or outside it, with varying histological dignity, such as pilocytic, anaplastic or low-grade astrocytoma, and glioblastoma [5, 6]. The location of the tumour and the extent of its growth or infiltration in the pituitary region determines the endocrine-related symptoms, such as growth hormone deficiency (GHD) and precocious puberty [1, 7, 8]. Treatment varies due to the great individual variability of the tumours and includes surgery, X-ray therapy and chemotherapy. These methods may affect pituitary function and thus influence the overall prognosis [5]. Howell et al. [9] reported on the short-term effect of GH treatment on growth in such patients, including those followed in KIGS. Since central nervous system tumours related to NF1 cannot be completely eradicated, the application of GH treatment must be discussed in terms of tumour growth and the risk of malignancies [10, 11].

[a]Paediatric Endocrinology Section
University Children's Hospital, University of Tübingen
Hoppe-Seyler-Strasse 1, DE–72076 Tübingen (Germany)
[b]Liggins Institute, University of Auckland
2–6 Park Avenue, Grafton, Auckland (New Zealand)

Table 1. Characteristics of patients with NF1 at GH therapy start

	All				Females		Males	
	n	median	10th centile	90th centile	n	median	n	median
Background								
Birth weight SDS	193	−0.3	−1.9	1.0	87	−0.3	106	−0.2
Birth length SDS	132	−0.4	−1.8	1.0	62	−0.2	70	−0.4
MPH SDS	209	−1.4	−2.9	0.2	89	−1.4	120	−1.3
Maximum GH, μg/l	208	7.1	1.5	16.0	92	6.4	116	7.3
IGF-1 SDS	36	−2.2	−3.4	−1.2	8	−2.2	28	−2.1
Start of GH therapy								
Chronological age, years	235	10.1	5.8	13.8	103	9.9	132	10.3
Bone age, years	106	9.0	3.8	12.8	48	9.5	58	8.0
In puberty, n	201	62 (31)			89	31 (35)	112	31 (28)
Height SDS	235	−3.0	−4.3	−0.5	103	−3.2	132	−2.7
Height − MPH SDS	209	−1.3	−3.2	0.3	89	−1.6	120	−1.1
BMI SDS	235	0.2	−1.6	1.9	103	0.3	132	0.2
GH dose, mg/kg/week	235	0.19	0.14	0.29	103	0.19	132	0.19

Figures in parentheses are percentages. MPH = Midparental height; IGF-1 = insulin-like growth factor 1; BMI = body mass index.

Langerhans cell histiocytosis (LCH, also known as eosinophilic granuloma, histiocytosis X, Hand-Schüller-Christian disease, and Abt-Lettere-Siwe disease) is a disease whose aetiology is yet unknown. It manifests itself as a clonal proliferation of dendritic histiocytes, either through isolated lesions in bones or as a systemic affection [12]. Infiltrations of the pituitary-hypothalamic region are associated with a varied picture when imaging is done [13, 14]. It is common practice to apply chemotherapy (e.g., glucocorticoids and/or vincristine) or X-ray treatment for this semi-malignant disorder. Histiocytic infiltration in the posterior pituitary region is associated with diabetes insipidus, which is the most frequent endocrine abnormality [15, 16]. However, dysfunction of the anterior pituitary is mainly associated with GHD and is less common [15–17]. Several articles have dealt with the short-term growth response to GH [for a review, see chapter by Polak, this vol., pp. 269–276] and include previous data from KIGS [17].

Methods

This article is based on data taken from the KIGS database: NF1 has the KIGS code No. 3.3.3 and LCH the KIGS code No. 2.2.4.5. The analysis of data was done as outlined in this volume. The Swiss references (Prader) were used to illustrate and calculate height data. The analysis of the data was restricted to (1) characteristics of patients at the start of GH treatment, (2) characteristics and response to GH during the first prepubertal year and (3) characteristics at GH start and near adult height (NAH). The data are purely descriptive.

Results

Patients with NF1

The characteristics of the 235 patients with NF1 at the start of GH treatment are listed in table 1. The height in comparison with normal references at GH start, for girls and boys, is illustrated in figure 1. The majority (56%) of patients were boys. In 3%, diabetes insipidus was observed. In 31%, pituitary deficiencies other than GHD were

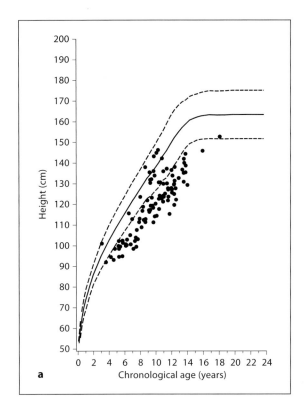 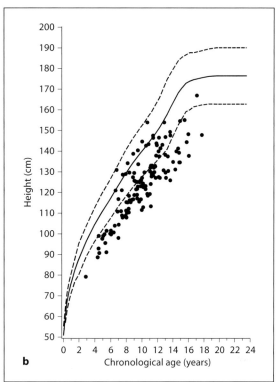

Fig. 1. Height at the start of GH therapy of girls (**a**) and boys (**b**) with NF1 within KIGS. The lines represent normal ranges and the 50th centile of the Prader references.

documented. The size at birth was only marginally below average. On average, the patients were moderately GH deficient, i.e. maximum GH to tests (median) 7.1 μg/l. Midparental height (−1.4 standard deviation score, SDS) was markedly reduced in comparison with normal parents. Chronological age averaged 10.1 years, and the height was severely reduced (−3.0 SDS). The GH dose given (0.19 mg/kg week) was in the same order of magnitude as in other patient groups with central nervous tumours (and idiopathic GHD, IGHD).

The characteristics of the 115 patients who received GH treatment for a full prepubertal year are listed in table 2. The background data relating to birth characteristics, parental height and the degree of GHD were very similar to the total cohort. Age at GH therapy start averaged 9.1 years at a height of −3.0 SDS. The height velocity SDS during the first year was 2.4 and the Δ height SDS 0.4. In comparison with children with IGHD (using the model without maximum GH to tests), the studentized residual was significantly diminished (−0.7; p < 0.001), thus indicating an impaired responsiveness to GH treatment.

In 23 patients (14 boys), treatment with GH was followed to NAH. The data at GH start, during the first year on GH and at NAH are listed in table 3. The height of these patients at GH start and at NAH is also illustrated in figure 2. At a median age of 17.6 years and after a median of 6.1 years on GH, the cohort reached a height of −1.6 SDS. Corrected for parental height, the NAH reached was −0.1 SDS.

Table 2. Characteristics of patients with NF1: first-year prepubertal growth on GH

	Prepubertal longitudinal growth				females		males	
	all							
	n	median	10th centile	90th centile	n	median	n	median
Start of GH therapy								
Chronological age, years	115	9.1	5.3	12.7	42	8.8	73	9.2
Bone age, years	53	7.0	3.4	12.0	20	6.0	33	7.1
Height SDS	115	−3.0	−4.2	−1.4	42	−3.1	73	−2.9
Height − MPH SDS	104	−1.3	−2.7	−0.1	37	−1.5	67	−1.3
BMI SDS	115	0.1	−1.7	1.5	42	0.1	73	0.1
GH dose, mg/kg/week	115	0.19	0.15	0.27	42	0.19	73	0.19
After 1 year on GH								
Chronological age, years	115	10.1	6.3	13.8	42	9.7	73	10.3
Height SDS	115	−2.4	−3.7	−0.8	42	−2.5	73	−2.4
Height − MPH SDS	104	−0.7	−2.2	0.4	37	−0.9	67	−0.6
Height velocity, cm/year	115	7.1	5.3	9.3	42	7.0	73	7.2
Height velocity SDS	115	2.4	−0.6	5.6	42	2.2	73	2.5
Δ height SDS	115	0.4	−0.5	0.8	42	0.3	73	0.4
BMI SDS	114	−0.1	−1.6	1.1	41	0.0	73	−0.1
Studentized residual[1]	56	−0.7	−2.2	0.4	17	−0.8	39	−0.7

BMI = Body mass index. [1] IGHD model without maximum GH.

Table 3. Characteristics of NF1 patients treated to NAH

	n	All		
		median	10th centile	90th centile
Start of GH treatment				
Chronological age, years	23	10.3	6.2	13.0
Height SDS	23	−2.8	−4.6	−2.2
Height − MPH SDS	21	−1.2	−2.7	−0.5
BMI SDS	23	0.1	−1.7	1.4
GH dose, mg/kg/week	23	0.19	0.15	0.31
After 1 year of GH therapy				
Chronological age, years	23	11.3	7.2	14.0
Height SDS	23	−2.4	−3.9	−1.3
Height − MPH SDS	21	−0.7	−2.1	0.2
Height velocity, cm/year	23	7.2	5.8	9.6
Height velocity SDS	23	1.9	−0.4	5.0
Δ height SDS	23	0.4	0.1	0.8
At NAH				
Chronological age, years	23	17.6	16.7	20.0
Height SDS	23	−1.6	−3.0	−0.4
Height − MPH SDS	21	−0.1	−1.2	1.1
Δ height SDS (latest − start, Prader)	23	1.3	−0.1	2.7
BMI SDS	22	0.2	−0.9	1.4

MPH = Midparental height; BMI = body mass index.

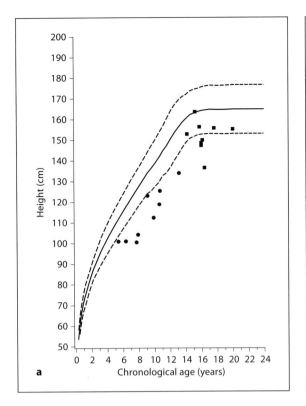 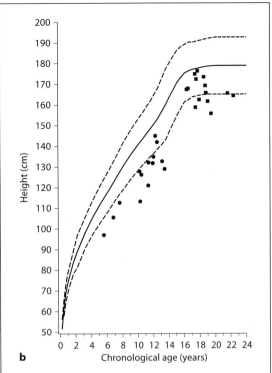

Fig. 2. Height at the start of GH therapy (●) and at NAH (■) of girls (**a**) and boys (**b**) with NF1 within KIGS. The lines represent normal ranges and the 50th centile of the Prader references.

Patients with LCH

The characteristics of the 158 patients with LCH at the start of GH treatment are listed in table 4. The height in comparison with the normal references at GH start for girls and boys is illustrated in figure 3. The majority (61%) of patients were boys. In 67%, diabetes insipidus was observed. In 85%, pituitary deficiencies other than GHD were documented. The size at birth was only marginally below average. Midparental height (–0.8 SDS) was moderately reduced in comparison with normal parents. On average, the patients were severely GH deficient, i.e. maximum GH to tests (median) 3.9 μg/l. Chronological age averaged 8.8 years, and the height was severely reduced (–2.5 SDS). The GH dose given (0.18 mg/kg/week) was in the same order of magnitude as in other groups of patients with central nervous tumours (and IGHD).

The characteristics of the 92 patients who received GH treatment for a full prepubertal year are listed in table 5. The background data relating to birth characteristics, parental height and the degree of GHD were very similar to the total cohort. Age at GH start averaged 7.6 years at a height of –2.7 SDS. The height velocity SDS during the first year was 4.1 and the Δ height SDS 0.8. In comparison with children with IGHD (using the model without maximum GH to tests), the studentized residual was slightly diminished (–0.3; p < 0.01), thus indicating an impaired responsiveness to GH treatment.

Table 4. Characteristics of patients with LCH at GH therapy start

	All				Females		Males	
	n	median	10th centile	90th centile	n	median	n	median
Background								
Birth weight SDS	131	−0.2	−1.3	1.2	52	−0.1	79	−0.2
Birth length SDS	80	0.2	−1.4	1.8	29	0.5	51	−0.0
MPH SDS	134	−0.8	−2.1	0.7	52	−0.5	82	−0.9
Maximum GH, μg/l	138	3.9	1.0	9.6	54	3.3	84	4.5
IGF-1 SDS	33	−3.0	−4.2	−1.6	18	−3.1	15	−2.7
Start of GH therapy								
Chronological age, years	158	8.8	5.3	14.6	62	8.2	96	9.3
Bone age, years	60	6.8	3.3	13.2	22	7.4	38	5.5
In puberty, n	136	23 (17)			58	14 (24)	78	9 (12)
Height SDS	158	−2.5	−3.9	−1.1	62	−2.4	96	−2.6
Height − MPH SDS	134	−1.8	−3.4	−0.1	52	−2.1	82	−1.6
BMI SDS	158	17.6	14.7	23.0	62	17.7	96	17.2
GH dose, mg/kg/week	158	0.18	0.13	0.28	62	0.18	96	0.17

Figures in parentheses are percentages. MPH = Midparental height; IGF-1 = insulin-like growth factor 1; BMI = body mass index.

Table 5. Characteristics of patients with LCH: first-year prepubertal growth on GH

	Prepubertal longitudinal growth							
	all				females		males	
	n	median	10th centile	90th centile	n	median	n	median
Start of GH therapy								
Chronological age, years	92	7.6	5.2	11.3	32	7.0	60	7.9
Bone age, years	37	5.9	3.5	9.5	8	6.0	29	5.5
Height SDS	92	−2.7	−4.1	−1.5	32	−2.5	60	−2.8
Height − MPH SDS	76	−2.1	−4.0	−0.4	25	−2.3	51	−1.9
BMI SDS	92	0.6	−1.2	2.1	32	0.8	60	0.4
GH dose, mg/kg/week	92	0.18	0.14	0.26	32	0.19	60	0.18
After 1 year on GH								
Chronological age, years	92	8.6	6.2	12.4	32	8.0	60	9.0
Height SDS	92	−1.8	−3.7	−0.6	32	−1.5	60	−2.0
Height − MPH SDS	76	−1.3	−2.8	0.1	25	−1.4	51	−1.3
Height velocity, cm/year	92	9.0	5.6	11.9	32	9.0	60	9.0
Height velocity SDS	92	4.1	−0.7	8.7	32	3.8	60	4.1
Δ height SDS	92	0.8	−0.1	1.4	32	0.8	60	0.7
BMI SDS	90	0.3	−1.3	1.6	32	0.6	58	0.1
Studentized residual[1]	48	−0.3	−1.6	1.1	19	−0.4	29	−0.2

MPH = Midparental height; BMI = body mass index. [1] IGHD model without maximum GH.

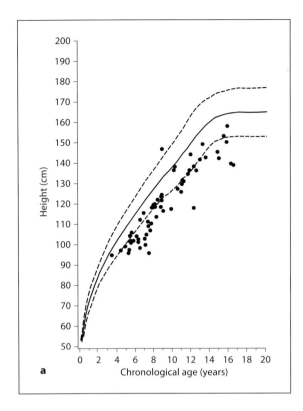 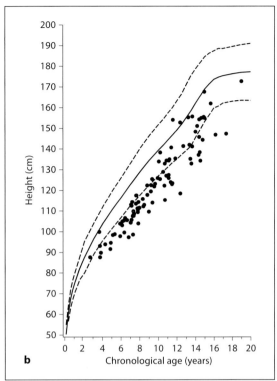

Fig. 3. Height of girls (**a**) and boys (**b**) with LCH within KIGS at the start of GH therapy. The lines represent normal ranges and the 50th centile of the Prader references.

Comparison of NF1 and LCH with Craniopharyngioma

The characteristics (medians) of the patients with NF1 and LCH at GH start, during the first prepubertal year on GH and at NAH (not for LCH) are listed in table 6, in comparison with those observed in patients with craniopharyngioma [see also chapter on acquired GHD, Ranke, this vol., pp. 250–260].

Patients with NF1 have smaller parents than those with LCH or craniopharyngioma, mainly because NF1 is a disorder with autosomal dominant inheritance, and also due to the fact that NF1 is associated with short stature, irrespective of a pituitary affection. In both NF1 and LCH, the body mass index is not as high as in craniopharyngioma, since in the latter, the hypothalamus is more frequently affected. The extent of GHD is more severe in craniopharyngioma, followed by LCH. Patients with LCH are somewhat younger at the start of GH therapy; however, in relation, patients with NF1 are the shortest, which again may be attributable to the additional underlying growth disorder in NF1.

The response to GH during the first prepubertal year on GH is similar in craniopharyngioma and LCH, but lower in NF1. The responsiveness to GH as determined through a comparison of the predicted and the observed growth velocity (studentized residual = 'index of responsiveness') is lower in LCH and lowest in NF1. NAH differs between NF1 and craniopharyngioma patients, but both groups have reached their respective target height; Ht-MPH SDS is −0.1 and 0.0, respectively.

Table 6. Characteristics of patients with NF1 and LCH treated to NAH

	Craniopharyngioma (code No. 2.2.1.1)	NF1 (code No. 3.3.3)	NF1 versus craniopharyngioma	LCH (code No. 2.2.4.5)	LCH versus craniopharyngioma	LCH versus NF1
Background						
Total patients, n	1,140	235		158		
Males, %	57	56	n.s.	61	n.s.	n.s.
Birth weight SDS	−0.3	−0.3	n.s.	−0.2	n.s.	n.s.
Birth length SDS	0.2	−0.4	<0.001	0.2	n.s.	<0.001
MPH SDS (Prader)	−0.4	−1.4	<0.001	−0.8	<0.01	<0.001
Maximum GH, μg/l	1.2	7.1	<0.001	3.9	<0.001	<0.001
MPHD, %	93	31	<0.001	85	<0.01	<0.001
IGF-1 SDS	−3.1	−2.2	<0.001	−3.0	n.s.	<0.01
At GH start						
Age, years	10.5	10.1	n.s.	8.8	<0.001	<0.05
Bone age, years	9.0	9.1	n.s.	6.8	<0.05	<0.05
Height SDS (Prader)	−2.3	−3.0	<0.001	−2.5	n.s.	<0.05
BMI SDS	1.2	0.2	<0.001	0.5	<0.001	<0.05
GH dose, mg/kg/week	0.17	0.19	<0.001	0.18	<0.05	<0.05
First year on GH						
Patients, n	656	115		92		
Males, %	59	64	n.s.	65	n.s.	n.s.
Age, years	10.0	10.1	n.s.	8.6	<0.01	<0.01
Height SDS (Prader)	−1.4	−2.4	<0.001	−1.8	<0.001	<0.001
Height velocity, cm/year	9.0	7.1	<0.001	9.0	n.s.	<0.001
Height velocity SDS (Prader)	4.4	2.4	<0.001	4.1	n.s.	<0.001
Δ height SDS (Prader)	0.8	0.4	<0.001	0.8	n.s.	<0.001
Studentized residual SDS[1]	0.4	−0.7	<0.001	−0.3	<0.001	n.s.
BMI SDS	0.9	−0.1	<0.001	0.3	<0.001	<0.01
At NAH						
Patients, n	168	23				
Males, %	47	61	n.s.			
Age, years	18.0	17.6	n.s.			
Height SDS (Prader)	−0.5	−1.6	<0.001			
Δ height SDS (start – end, Prader)	1.7	1.3	n.s.			
BMI SDS	1.0	0.2	<0.01			
Total years on GH	7.7	6.1	n.s.			

Data are medians. n.s. = Not significant; MPH = midparental height; MPHD = multiple pituitary hormone deficiency; IGF-1 = insulin-like growth factor 1; BMI = body mass index.
[1] IGHD model without maximum GH.

Conclusions

Responses to exogenous GH in children with NF1 and LCH – as in other disorders with acquired GHD – vary greatly according to the underlying disorder. In most cases with a (semi)malignancy as the primary disorder, both the response and the responsiveness to GH are low in comparison with IGHD and craniopharyngioma. This is probably caused by very low doses of GH (response), GH therapy start when the child is much older, and also by tissue which is altered due to the genetic background and/or modes of treatment (responsiveness). In the future, treatment in these disorders needs to be further optimized. The individual risks of GH treatment in children with these disorders need to be considered.

References

1 Cnossen MH, Stam EN, Cooiman LC, Simonsz HJ, Stroink H, Oranje AP, Halley DJ, de Goede-Bolder A, Niermeijer MF, de Muinck Keizer-Schrama SM: Endocrinologic disorders and optic pathway gliomas in children with neurofibromatosis type 1. Pediatrics 1997; 100:667–670.

2 Barker D, Wright E, Nguyen K, Cannon L, Fain P, Goldgar D, Bishop DT, Carey J, Baty B, Kivlin J, et al: Gene for von Recklinghausen neurofibromatosis is in the pericentromeric region of chromosome 17. Science 1987;236:1100–1102.

3 Dasgupta B, Gutmann DH: Neurofibromin regulates neural stem cell proliferation, survival, and astroglial differentiation in vitro and in vivo. J Neurosci 2005;25:5584–5594.

4 National Institute of Health Consensus Development Conference: Neurofibromatosis conference statement. Arch Neurol 1988;45:575–578.

5 Guillamo JS, Creange A, Kalifa C, Grill J, et al: Prognostic factors of CNS tumours in neurofibromatosis 1 (NF1) – a retrospective study of 104 patients. Brain 2003;126:152–160.

6 Kleihues P, Cavenee WK (eds): Pathology and Genetics of Tumours of the Nervous System. Lyon, IARC Press, 2000.

7 Hochstrasser H, Boltshauser E, Valavanis A: Brain tumours in children with von Recklinghausen neurofibromatosis. Neurofibromatosis 1988;1:233–239.

8 Vassilopoulou-Sellin R, Klein MJ, Slopis JK: Growth hormone deficiency in children with neurofibromatosis type 1 without suprasellar lesions. Pediatr Neurol 2000;22:355–358.

9 Howell SJ, Wilton P, Lindberg A, Shalet SM: Growth hormone and neurofibromatosis. Horm Res 2000;53(suppl 1):70–76.

10 Sklar CA: Growth hormone treatment: cancer risk. Horm Res 2004;62(suppl 3):30–34.

11 Cunha KS, Barboza EP, Da Fonseca EC: Identification of growth hormone receptor in localised neurofibromas of patients with neurofibromatosis type 1. J Clin Pathol 2003;56:758–763.

12 Willman CL, Busque L, Griffith BB, Favara BE, McClain KL, Duncan MH, Gilliland DG: Langerhans' cell histiocytosis (histiocytosis X) – a clonal proliferative disease. N Engl J Med 1994; 331:154–160.

13 Manghie M, Arico M, Villa A, Genovese E, Beluffi G, Severi F: MR of the hypothalamic-pituitary axis in Langerhans cell histiocytosis. AJNR Am J Neuroradiol 1992;13:1365–1371.

14 Manghie M, Bossi G, Klersy C, Cosi G, Genovese E, Arico M: Dynamic endocrine testing and magnetic resonance imaging in the long-term follow-up of children with Langerhans cell histiocytosis. J Clin Endocrinol Metab 1998;83: 3089–3094.

15 Donadieu J, Rolon MA, Pion I, Thomas C, Doz F, et al: Incidence of growth hormone deficiency in pediatric-onset Langerhans cell histiocytosis: efficacy and safety of growth hormone treatment. J Clin Endocrinol Metab 2004; 89:604–609.

16 Nanduri VR, Bareille P, Pritchard J, Stanhope R: Growth and endocrine disorders in multisystem Langerhans' cell histiocytosis. Clin Endocrinol 2000;53:509–515.

17 Howell SJ, Wilton P, Shalet SM: Growth hormone replacement in patients with Langerhans cell histiocytosis. Arch Dis Child 1998;78:469–473.

Growth and GH Treatment in Patients with Juvenile Idiopathic Arthritis

Paul Czernichow

Growth failure is one of the major features of children with chronic disease. In most situations, abnormal growth velocity occurs during the most active part of the course of the disease. Decreased growth velocity induces a loss of height and a delayed bone maturation that are usually correlated with the severity and the duration of the disease. Some catch-up may occur when the disease is less active and the treatment less aggressive. Unfortunately, in most instances, the catch-up is incomplete.

This chapter will describe the anomaly of growth observed in juvenile idiopathic arthritis (JIA).

Juvenile Idiopathic Arthritis and Growth

Growth retardation is a prominent feature of children with idiopathic arthritis. It is present in patients given glucocorticoids (GCs), but short stature was described long before the era of modern treatment. In 1887, Sir George Still wrote about JIA: 'A remarkable feature in these cases is the general arrest of development that occurs when the disease begins before the second dentition. A child of 12 and a half years would easily have been mistaken for 6 or 7 years, which another of 4 years looked more like 2 and a half or 3 years' [1].

Although growth retardation has been described a long time ago, few precise studies are available on cohorts of patients treated with corticoids. A group of patients whose disease onset started at the age of 3.4 years was followed until they reached final height [2]. As shown in figure 1, a significant loss of height of -2.7 ± 1.5 standard deviation score (SDS) occurred during the first years of the disease and was correlated with prednisone therapy duration. Consequently, the mean height for chronological age (about 12 years) at prednisone discontinuation was significantly lower than the mean target height (-2.6 ± 1.4 vs. -0.3 ± 0.9 SDS). After prednisone discontinuation, 17 patients (70%) had catch-up growth, but 7 patients (30%) had a persistent loss of height. Consequently, the mean final height was significantly different between these two groups, i.e. -3.6 ± 1.2 SDS in the group without

Department of Endocrinology and Growth Diseases
Hôpital Necker
149 rue de Sèvres
FR–75015 Paris (France)

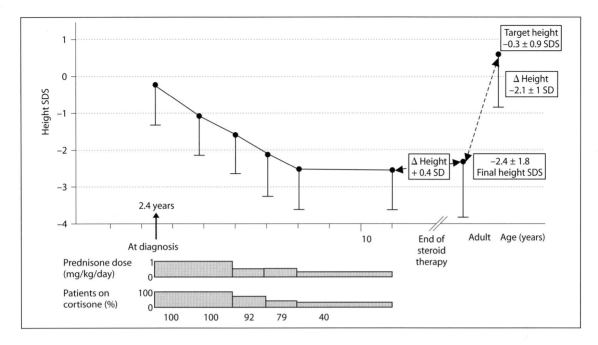

Fig. 1. Changes in height SDS throughout follow-up in a group of 24 patients suffering from JIA. Note the marked loss of height during GC therapy and the partial catch-up growth after prednisone discontinuation [2].

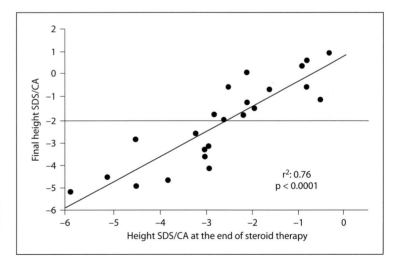

Fig. 2. Correlation between final height SDS/chronological age (CA) and height SDS at the discontinuation of GCs [2].

catch-up growth versus −1.5 ± 1.6 SDS in the group with catch-up growth. Overall, the mean final height was −2.4 ± 1.8 SDS and was strongly correlated with the mean height at prednisone discontinuation (fig. 2).

In a study of 65 patients with different forms of JIA [3], the final height SDS was found to be below −2 SDS in 11% of patients, all of whom had had polyarticular disease treated with GC therapy, and this polyarticular or systemic disease was associated with a final height shorter than the target height. In our own study [2], 41% of patients suffering from systemic forms of JIA had a final height below –2 SDS and 87% of patients had a final height below their target height. Altogether, these data suggest that polyarticular or systemic JIA treated with GCs is associated with an increased risk of reduced final height. The final height of these patients may vary from one patient to another, mainly depending on the severity of the disease and on their linear growth during and after prednisone therapy. Growth retardation during the active phase of JIA was mainly dependent on disease severity and duration, but worsened by high-dose GC therapy. We believe that this is a key period for any intervention aiming at improving final height.

Mechanism of Abnormal Growth Velocity and the Potential Role of Growth Hormone Treatment

Energy malnutrition contributes to growth failure in these children, and dietary intake may be inadequate because of chronic anorexia. However, chronic inflammation is probably the most important determinant of growth retardation in JIA. Indeed, impairment of linear growth is seen during periods of disease activity, with subsequent normalization of growth rate during remission. In addition, in patients with systemic JIA and growth retardation treated with growth hormone (GH), growth velocity during treatment appears inversely correlated with the intensity of inflammation.

In the last few years, progress in our understanding of inflammation, and especially of the role of cytokines, has opened up new fields of investigation. Three cytokines, interleukin (IL)-1, tumor necrosis factor-α and IL-6, possess a particularly intense pro-idiopathic activity and have, for this reason, been extensively investigated. Experimental work was carried out on a murine transgenic model in which an over-expression of IL-6 gene could be observed [4]. As a consequence, these animals had high circulating levels of IL-6, and interestingly, an important growth defect. The reduction in the growth rate led to an adult size which was about 30–50% smaller than that of non-transgenic littermates. Interestingly, the growth defect was completely abolished by immunoneutralisation of IL-6 which demonstrates the direct role of IL-6 over-expression in the growth defect. The exact mechanism remained to be determined, although a role of insulin-like growth factor 1 (IGF-1) binding protein 3 has been shown in transgenic animals which could result in a decreased half-life and clearance of IGF-1.

GCs have a general anti-anabolic and catabolic influence on bone and cartilage. Therefore, they have a direct action on the growth plate, suppressing multiple gene expression. GCs interfere with chondrocyte proliferation, matrix proteoglycan synthesis and increase the apoptotic rate of hypertrophic cells. In the tissues adjacent to the growth plate, GCs enhance osteoclastic activity and suppress osteoblast development and function. Thus, GC therapy started during childhood induces severe bone loss which may increase the risk of osteoporosis and fracture in early adulthood. In addition, GCs interfere with the GH-IGF-1 axis, and therefore, influence growth. Several factors influence the GH-IGF-1 axis, and thus, it is difficult to dissociate the responsibility of GC administration from other causes like malnutrition or chronic inflammation which also have distinct action on growth factor synthesis or secretion.

However, in JIA, pharmacological stimulation of GH and sleep-related GH secretion are normal, as well as IGF-1 plasma concentrations and circulating IGF binding protein. There is a wide heterogeneity among the patients, some having clearly abnormal values [5].

GH has linear growth, protein anabolic and bone-protective effects, and significant effects on

Table 1. Studies analysing GH therapy in JIA

References	Duration of GH Tt years	n	GV at baseline cm/year	GV after GH Tt cm/year	Height SDS at baseline	Height SDS after GH Tt	Prednisone dose mg/kg/day
Davies et al. [15], 1997[a]	1	10	2.4	4.5	–3.1	–1.1	5–11
	1	10	2.0	6.1	–2.9	+0.5	5–11
Touati et al. [5], 1998	1	15	1.9	5.4	–4.3	–4.3	0.38
Simon et al. [12], 2003[b]	3	13	2.1	6.0	–4.6	–4.5	0.39
				5.0		–4.5	
				4.1		–4.3	
Bechtold et al. [10], 2003	4	18 Tt	2.9	7.2	–3.3	–2.3	0.2
	0	20 C	2.6	3.3	–2.3	–3.0	0.2

Note the marked decrease in growth velocity (GV) and the severity of growth retardation before GH treatment. GH doses ranged from 0.33 to 0.46 mg/kg/week. Only the study by Bechtold et al. was controlled; all the others are uncontrolled open studies. Tt = treatment; C = control.
[a] Patients received 12 (line 1) and 24 IU/m^2/week (line 2) of GH. [b] The 1st, 2nd and 3rd lines indicate the growth velocity or height after 1, 2 or 3 years of treatment.

fat metabolism. GH increases nitrogen retention, protein synthesis and lean body mass. It decreases adiposity by increasing fat mobilisation and lipid oxidation. GH is important in the regulation of both bone formation and bone resorption.

Treatment with recombinant human GH (rhGH) has been tried in many catabolic situations such as in haemodialysis [6], in cystic fibrosis patients [7] or after surgery to improve protein metabolism and accelerate recovery [8]. Therefore, it was hypothesised that GH treatment may counteract the catabolic effects of GCs in children with JIA and improve their growth.

Results of Growth Hormone Treatment

Efficacy of GH Treatment
For the last 10 years, children with growth failure due to JIA have received a GH treatment (table 1). Different doses of rhGH were used, ranging from 0.33 to 0.46 mg/kg/week. Data from non-controlled short-term studies (1 year of rhGH treatment) were encouraging and showed that rhGH treatment improved growth velocity and induced favourable changes in body composition such as a gain in lean mass or fat-free mass, a decrease in adiposity, and an increase in bone calcium accretion and bone formation [5, 9]. Long-term studies, mainly of JIA children, were consistent with the short-term data. A 4-year controlled study reported a height gain of 1 SD in GH-treated patients, although the control group experienced a height loss of 0.7 SD [10]. Significant improvements in body composition, lean mass and bone mineralisation were observed in two rhGH therapy trials [11, 12]. This was recently confirmed in a controlled study showing that GH-treated children had higher muscle mass and bone mineral content, assessed by peripheral quantitative computed tomography, than control subjects [13]. Further analysis of adult height and body composition in these patients are needed to evaluate the overall beneficial effects of rhGH treatment in patients with chronic diseases.

However, there is great variability in the response to rhGH treatment among GC-treated children. In some cases, rhGH treatment can induce catch-up growth, but in others, it can only restore linear growth and prevent the height loss that usually occurs during the natural course of the disease. Children who exhibit the best growth response also have the most significant changes in body composition. This variability in the response to rhGH treatment is mainly due to the severity of the underlying disease. In JIA patients, marked differences in growth responses have been reported according to the type of the disease (polyarticular or systemic forms of JIA) [14], and negative correlations have been found between growth velocity and either prednisone dosage [5, 10/11, 12] or markers of inflammation (erythrocyte sedimentation rate, C-reactive protein) [10/11, 15]. The duration of exposure to GCs, which has deleterious effects on the growth plate and metabolism, might also influence the response to rhGH treatment. For severely growth-retarded children who have already had many years of GC exposure, severe osteoporosis and muscle wasting, subsequent rhGH treatment probably could not reverse the growth retardation and probably would not lead to the normalisation of their adult height and body composition. In non-GH-treated JIA children, the height at the end of steroid therapy is highly correlated with the final height, as it is clearly shown in figure 2. The prevention of severe growth and metabolic disturbances with early administration of GH therapy in GC-treated patients might be a better strategy than using rhGH to cure the problems caused by long-term GC treatment. A clinical trial is currently addressing this issue.

Safety of rhGH Therapy in GC-Treated Patients
Two important issues should be discussed concerning the safety of rhGH treatment in GC-treated patients: the potential impact of rhGH treatment on the course of the disease and the diabetogenic effect of high-dose rhGH treatment in GC-treated children.

In JIA patients, no significant changes in disease activity and/or joint scores have been reported during rhGH treatment [5, 10/11, 14]. In this respect, GH administration seems to be safe. However, a careful clinical follow-up, monitored by both the paediatric endocrinologist and the rheumatologist, is recommended to confirm the safety of rhGH treatment in these patients.

High-dose rhGH treatment appears to counteract the catabolic effects of GCs in severely ill children. However, chronic administration of rhGH induces insulin resistance in GH as well as non-GH-deficient patients. In GC-treated patients, chronic rhGH treatment should be used with caution, as GH and GCs have similar effects on carbohydrate metabolism, and these effects are enhanced during combined treatment [16]. In studies of rhGH treatment in GC-treated patients, glucose tolerance has been investigated by the monitoring of fasting glycaemia, insulinaemia, and glycosylated haemoglobin, or by the annual assessment of an oral glucose tolerance test. Surprisingly, glucose intolerance or overt diabetes mellitus is seldom reported in these patients. In short-term treatment (<2 years), subtle changes in either fasting glycaemia or in fasting or stimulated insulinaemia with variable changes in haemoglobin A_{1c} have been reported [5, 17]. In long-term studies, only a few patients experienced transient glucose intolerance [12] or overt diabetes mellitus requiring transient insulin therapy [17]. The consequences of long-term hyperinsulinaemia in GC-treated patients are unknown, and no data are available about glucose tolerance after discontinuation of rhGH treatment.

Conclusion

The effects of rhGH treatment in JIA children receiving GCs are promising, showing that GH treatment can improve growth velocity and increase lean mass and bone mineralisation with a reasonably good safety profile. Different variables can influence the response to rhGH therapy in these children: duration of GC treatment, height SDS at the start of the treatment, delayed or slow progression of puberty, severity of the disease and GC dose during rhGH treatment. Long-term studies are needed to evaluate the impact of rhGH treatment on adult height and body composition. Nevertheless, the present data are already very promising.

References

1 Still G: On a form of chronic joint disease in children. Med-chirurg Trans 1897;80:47–59.
2 Simon D, Fernando C, Czernichow P, Prieur AM: Linear growth and final height in patients with systemic juvenile idiopathic arthritis treated with long-term glucocorticoids. J Rheumatol 2002;29:1296–1300.
3 Zak M, Muller J, Pedersen FK: Final height, armspan, subischial leg length and body proportions in juvenile chronic arthritis: a long-term follow-up study. Horm Res 1999;52:80–86.
4 De Benedetti F, Alonzi T, Moretta A, et al: Interleukin-6 causes growth impairment in transgenic mice through a decrease in insulin-like growth factor-I. A model for stunted growth in children with chronic inflammation. J Clin Invest 1997;99:643–650.
5 Touati G, Prieur AM, Ruiz JC, Noel M, Czernichow P: Beneficial effects of one-year growth hormone administration to children with juvenile chronic arthritis on chronic steroid therapy. Effects on growth velocity and body composition. J Clin Endocrinol Metab 1998; 83:403–409.
6 Garibotto G, Barreca A, Russo R, Sofia A, Araghi P, Cesarone A, Malaspina M, Fiorini F, Minuto F, Tizianello A: Effects of recombinant human growth hormone on muscle protein turnover in malnourished hemodialysis patients. J Clin Invest 1997;99:97–105.
7 Hardin D, Ellis KJ, Dyson M, Rice J, McConnell R, Seilhemer D: Growth hormone decreases protein catabolism in children with cystic fibrosis. J Clin Endocrinol Metab 2001;86:4424–4428.
8 Wilmore DW: The use of growth hormone in severely ill patients. Adv Surg 1999;33:261–274.
9 Touati G, Ruiz JC, Porquet D, Kindermans C, Prieur AM, Czernichow P: Effects on bone metabolism of one year recombinant human growth hormone administration to children with juvenile chronic arthritis undergoing chronic steroid therapy. J Rheumatol 2000;27:1287–1293.
10 Bechtold S, Ripperger P, Häfner R, Said E, Schwartz HP: Growth hormone improves height in patients with juvenile idiopathic arthritis: 4-year data of a controlled study. J Pediatr 2004;143:512–519.
11 Bechtold S, Ripperger P, Bonfig W, Schmidt H, Bitterling H, Häfner R, Schwartz HP: Bone mass development and bone metabolism in juvenile idiopathic arthritis: treatment with growth hormone for 4 years. J Rheumatol 2003; 31:7–12.
12 Simon D, Lucidarme N, Ruiz JC, Prieur AM, Czernichow P: Effects on growth and body composition of growth hormone treatment in children with juvenile idiopathic arthritis requiring steroid therapy. J Rheumatol 2003;30:2492–2499.
13 Bechtold S, Ripperger P, Bonfig W, Dalla Pozza R, Häfner R, Schwartz HP: Growth hormone changes bone geometry and body composition in patients with juvenile idiopathic arthritis requiring glucocorticoid treatment: a controlled study using peripheral quantitative computed tomography. J Clin Endocrinol Metab 2005;90:3168–3173.
14 Davies UM, Rooney M, Preece MA, Ansell BM, Woo P: Treatment of growth retardation in juvenile chronic arthritis with recombinant human growth hormone. J Rheumatol 1994;21:153–158.
15 Davies UM, Jones J, Reeve J, Camacho-Hubner C, Charlett A, Ansell BM, Preece M, Woo P: Effects of disease activity and recombinant human growth hormone on insulin-like growth factor 1, insulin-like growth factor binding proteins 1 and 3, and osteocalcin. Arthritis Rheum 1997;40:332–340.
16 Horber FF, Marsh M, Haymond MW: Differential effects of prednisone and growth hormone on fuel metabolism and insulin antagonism in humans. Diabetes 1991;40:141–149.
17 Allen D, Julius J, Breen T, Attie K: Treatment of glucocorticoid-induced growth suppression with growth hormone. J Clin Endocrinol Metab 1998; 83:2824–2829.

The KIGS Experience with Growth Hormone Treatment of Juvenile Rheumatoid Arthritis

Edward O. Reiter

Poor growth is a characteristic feature of chronic inflammatory disease. Czernichow [this vol., pp. 286–291] has reviewed growth and growth hormone (GH) treatment in children with juvenile rheumatoid arthritis (JRA). De Benedetti et al. [1], studying JRA in humans and in a transgenic murine model expressing excessive interleukin-6, demonstrated an interleukin-6-mediated decrease in insulin-like growth factor 1 (IGF-1) production to be a credible mechanism by which chronic inflammatory disease could lead to poor growth. The close relationship of the GH receptor to that of multiple cytokines [2] makes this an interesting hypothesis. A complex cascade of cytokines, as part of the inflammatory response to acute and chronic infection, can impact the endocrine system at many levels [3, 4], impairing the mineral and nutrient metabolism and the growth and remodeling of bone [5], as well as IGF-1 production by diminishing the JAK2/STAT5 signal transduction pathway efficiency [6].

Multiple short- and long-term studies of GH treatment (as noted by Czernichow) have been reported [7–10], with the best data found in a 4-year study [10] in which the height standard deviation score (SDS) improved by 1.0 in the treated group, but fell by 0.7 in untreated children. Lean mass and bone mineral density improvements have been found [9].

KIGS Data on the Treatment of Juvenile Rheumatoid Arthritis with Growth Hormone

In the KIGS database, information regarding a modest number of patients with JRA, who have received GH treatment, is available. Responses to 1 year of GH treatment in 10 prepubertal children with JRA are shown in table 1. There is no gender-related preference. The median age of onset of GH therapy was 9.9 years; the children were small and slight, with a height SDS of –3.2 and a weight SDS of –2.6, showing markedly delayed bone age. The children's heights were far from the midparental target (–4.3 SDS). In the first year of

Baystate Children's Hospital, Tufts University School of Medicine
759 Chestnut Street, Springfield, MA 01199 (USA)

Table 1. Rheumatoid arthritis – prepubertal longitudinal growth in patients treated for the first year with GH

	n	Median	10th percentile	90th percentile
At GH start				
Age, years	10	9.9	7.0	13.7
Bone age, years	4	6.2	2.5	13.0
Height SDS (Prader)	10	−3.2	−5.4	−2.6
Height velocity, cm/year	5	4.0	2.5	7.8
Height velocity SDS (Prader)	5	−2.0	−4.1	4.0
BMI SDS	10	−0.6	−2.6	1.7
GH dose, mg/kg/week	10	0.26	0.13	0.35
After 1 year of GH treatment				
Age, years	10	10.9	8.0	14.8
Height SDS (Prader)	10	−3.1	−5.1	−2.4
Height velocity, cm/year	10	4.4	1.3	8.3
Height velocity SDS (Prader)	9	−1.2	−4.2	3.4
Δ height SDS (Prader)	10	0.0	−1.5	0.4
BMI SDS	10	−0.5	−2.3	1.4

BMI = Body mass index.

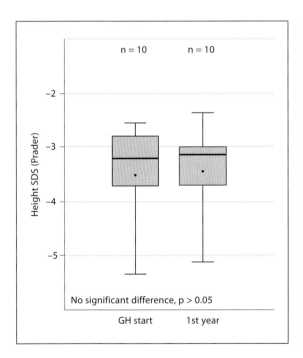

Fig. 1. Height SDS prior to and after 1 year of GH treatment in prepubertal children with JRA. The box plots represent medians and 25th and 75th percentiles, with whiskers at the 10th and 90th percentiles. The dot shows the mean.

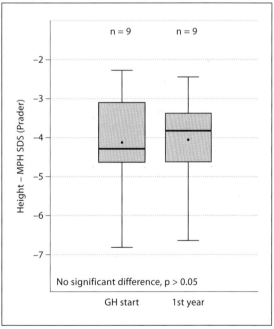

Fig. 2. Height SDS – midparental target height (MPH) prior to and after 1 year of GH treatment in prepubertal children with JRA. The box plots represent medians and 25th and 75th percentiles, with whiskers at the 10th and 90th percentiles. The dot shows the mean.

Table 2. Rheumatoid arthritis – cross-sectional data

	All				Females		Males	
	n	median	10th percentile	90th percentile	n	median	n	median
Background								
Birth weight SDS	34	–0.1	–1.1	1.2	21	–0.4	13	0.1
Birth length SDS	30	0.4	–1.8	2.3	18	0.1	12	0.4
MPH SDS (Prader)	33	–0.2	–1.2	1.1	21	–0.3	12	–0.1
Maximum GH, μg/l	24	12.7	4.7	28.6	16	14.2	8	11.3
IGF-1 SDS	11	–3.0	–3.6	–0.5	7	–2.1	4	–3.1
At GH start								
Age, years	37	11.7	8.1	13.9	23	11.4	14	11.7
Bone age, years	13	10.0	4.3	13.0	11	10.5	2	5.2
Height SDS (Prader)	37	–3.1	–5.7	–2.2	23	–3.2	14	–3.0
Height – MPH SDS (Prader)	33	–3.5	–5.3	–1.2	21	–4.0	12	–3.0
Height velocity, cm/year	17	3.2	1.4	5.9	10	2.0	7	3.3
Weight SDS	37	–2.3	–3.8	0.1	23	–2.3	14	–2.0
BMI SDS	37	–0.8	2.1	1.9	23	–1.0	14	0.6
GH dose, mg/kg/week	37	0.26	0.16	0.37	23	0.26	14	0.25
At latest visit								
Age, years	37	16.1	10.9	19.8	23	15.5	14	16.8
Height SDS (Prader)	37	–2.8	–4.9	–1.2	23	–2.8	14	–2.7
Height – MPH SDS (Prader)	33	–2.6	–4.7	0.8	21	–2.7	12	–2.5
Δ height (latest to start) SDS (Prader)	37	0.5	–0.6	2.0	23	0.9	14	0.0
Weight SDS	37	–1.9	–4.9	0.4	23	–2.6	14	–1.1
BMI SDS	37	–0.8	–2.8	1.2	23	–1.2	14	0.2
Years on GH	37	4.0	0.6	8.0	23	3.8	14	4.8
Mean total GH dose, mg/kg/week	37	0.30	0.19	0.45	23	0.31	14	0.27

MPH = Midparental height; BMI = body mass index.

treatment, height velocity increased inconsequentially from 4.0 to 4.4 cm/year, while neither the height SDS nor the approximation to the midparental target changed (fig. 1, 2). It should be noted that the weight SDS did not change either. These data, though limited in number, do not suggest that GH had an early benefit for the prepubertal children.

In a larger group of children, including those who were pubertal, there are data on 37 patients with JRA (approximately 60% females), with a median duration of GH treatment of 4 years (table 2). Onset of treatment was not until 11.7 years of age, with the height SDS being –3.1 and the weight SDS –2.3. There was a bone age delay of nearly 2 years in those patients in whom data were available. Basal IGF-1 SDS levels are below –3.0, along with the findings of diminished IGF production in chronic inflammatory diseases. The response to GH is characterized by a somewhat meager change over this 4-year period, as the height SDS only improved by 0.3 and the approximation to the midparental target height SDS by 0.9. There being no control group, one cannot ascertain whether the study group was simply prevented from drifting even lower than its pretreatment growth channel. Such data were reported in the longest study including a control group [10]. In both treatment groups, the GH dose, though generally higher than that utilized for GH deficiency in Europe, did not reach levels needed in patients in whom relative GH insensitivity is present. Utilization of IGF-1 determinations to give some suggestion as to the patients' biochemical responses to exogenous GH might be of great value in determining whether higher doses of GH are necessary to achieve the desired anabolic effects.

The use of GH in children with JRA remains experimental, though the data shown by Czernichow [this vol., pp 286–291] suggest the need for a longer and larger study. The value of anabolic therapy in children with a chronic inflammatory disease often receiving glucocorticoids does at least seem reasonable, demanding further careful study.

References

1 De Benedetti F, Alonzi T, Moretta A, Lazzaro D, Costa P, Poli V, Martini A, Ciliberto G, Fattori E: Interleukin 6 causes growth impairment in transgenic mice through a decrease in insulin-like growth factor-I. J Clin Invest 1997;99:643–650.

2 Bazan JF: Hemopoietic receptors and helical cytokines. Immunol Today 1990;11:350–354.

3 McCann SM, Lyson K, Karanth S, Gimeno M, Belova N, Kamat A, Rettori V: Role of cytokines in the endocrine system. Ann N Y Acad Sci 1994;741:50–63.

4 Vassilopoulou-Sellin R: Endocrine effects of cytokines. Oncology 1994;8:43–50.

5 Skerry TM: The effects of the inflammatory response on bone growth. Eur J Clin Nutr 1994;48(suppl 1):S190–S198.

6 Lang CH, Hong-Brown L, Frost RA: Cytokine inhibition of JAK-STAT signaling: a new mechanism of growth hormone resistance. Pediatr Nephrol 2005;20:306–312.

7 Saha MT, Haapasaari J, Hannula S, Sarna S, Lenko HL: Growth hormone is effective in the treatment of severe growth retardation in children with juvenile chronic arthritis. Double blind placebo-controlled follow-up study. J Rheumatol 2004;31:1413–1417.

8 Bechtold S, Ripperger P, Muhlbayer D, Truckenbrodt H, Hafner R, Butenandt O, Schwarz HP: GH therapy in juvenile chronic arthritis: results of a two-year controlled study on growth and bone. J Clin Endocrinol Metab 2001;86:5737–5744.

9 Simon D, Lucidarme N, Prieur AM, Ruiz JC, Czernichow P: Effects on growth and body composition of growth hormone treatment in children with juvenile idiopathic arthritis requiring steroid therapy. J Rheumatol 2003;30:2492–2499.

10 Bechtold S, Ripperger P, Hafner R, Said E, Schwarz HP: Growth hormone improves height in patients with juvenile idiopathic arthritis: 4-year data of a controlled study. J Pediatr 2003;143:512–519.

Cystic Fibrosis – Growth Hormone Treatment

Dirk Schnabel

Cystic fibrosis (CF) is the most common life-threatening autosomal recessive disease of the white population, affecting 1 in 2,500 live births. CF is caused by defects in a single gene on chromosome 7 encoding the protein CF transmembrane regulator, which functions as a cyclic adenosine monophosphate-regulated chloride channel. In homozygous affected individuals, the CF transmembrane regulator defect results in a multisystem disorder, with the dominant clinical features of chronic lung disease and exocrine pancreatic insufficiency.

Advances in medical treatment including aggressive oral nutrition (caloric intake >120% of the recommended daily allowance) with adequate pancreatic enzyme and vitamin supplementation, physiotherapy and antibiotics treatment have resulted in an improvement in prognosis and symptoms with increasing numbers of patients surviving into adult life [1].

Despite this progress in daily disease-specific therapy, sustained improvement in weight for height indices is not achieved in all patients.

Many patients with CF are malnourished (27.5% of the female patients aged 18–20 years, 53.5% of the males in this age group) [1], and catabolism has been recognized as a poor prognostic marker in these patients, as it is correlated with a reduced life expectancy [2].

In addition to poor nutritional status, many patients are growth retarded. The report of the German CF Foundation Registry 'Qualitätssicherung Mukoviszidose' demonstrates that 3% of women and 13% of men, aged 18–20 years, are below the 3rd percentile for height. CF patients are growth retarded compared with their familial genetic background, as most of them fail to achieve the midparental height range. Adult height is reduced and corresponds to the 25th–42nd percentiles for males and the 25th–44th percentiles for females [3].

Malnutrition is a major cause of growth retardation and results from loss of exocrine pancreatic function, elevated energy requirements, systemic anorexia in patients with severe pulmonary disease manifestation and temporarily during pulmonary exacerbation in all CF patients, chron-

Department of Pediatric Endocrinology and Diabetology
University Children's Hospital, Charité
Humboldt University Berlin
Augustenburger Platz 1
DE–13353 Berlin (Germany)

ic pulmonary disease, as well as increased energy expenditure. Chronically increased levels of inflammatory cytokines (tumor necrosis factor α, interleukins 1 and 6) cannot only affect the production and secretion of growth hormone (GH) or growth factors but can also inhibit growth at the tissue level.

CF patients are growth retarded, which is clinically relevant not only because it affects the quality of life, but also because the severity of growth retardation correlates with the severity of lung disease.

GH as an anabolic adjunct to stimulate growth, but also improving lung function and clinical status, was first used by Sackey et al. [4]. Since this initial report, 11 studies (table 1) of various designs (prospective without control, n = 4; retrospective without control, n = 1; retrospective with controls, n = 1; prospective randomized controlled, n = 3; prospective randomized crossover, n = 2) have been conducted. The first double-blind placebo-controlled trial has recently been completed [19].

Most studies included prepubertal patients, whereas two trials investigated pubertal [5] and young adults [6] and one study focused on GH effects in prepubertal patients additionally receiving enteral nutrition [7]. Because all published studies were conducted with a small number of patients (n = 5–24), most were defined as pilot studies.

The duration of GH treatment varied between 6 and 36 months. In all but one study which utilized a lower dose [4], GH dosages between 0.27 and 0.35 mg/kg body weight/week were administered. Except for one study [8], the dosing frequency used was 6–7 times per week.

Results

Growth/Growth Velocity

All published studies of GH treatment in children with CF demonstrated significant improvements in height, growth velocity and height standard deviation score (SDS). The growth response was dose dependent. In the first published study using a GH dose of 0.16 mg/kg body weight/week [4], growth velocity increased in 3 out of 4 patients. Huseman et al. [8] observed a higher mean growth rate with GH (given 3 times per week) than before treatment (7.7 vs. 5.7 cm/year). Hardin et al. [9] and Hütler et al. [10] evaluated growth-stimulating effects of GH given in comparable dosages in prepubertal patients and found increases in growth velocity in the same order of magnitude (fig. 1). The best growth response was reported by Hardin et al. [7] in patients receiving GH in combination with enteral nutrition by G tube (mean growth velocity with G tube, 3.3 ± 1.1 cm/year; GH only, 8.2 ± 1.3 cm/year; G tube + GH, 10.3 ± 2.0 cm/year).

Insulin-Like Growth Factor 1

Insulin-like growth factor 1 (IGF-1) as the metabolic mediator of GH increased with GH administration. Schnabel et al. [11] reported increases in IGF-1 (at baseline, –1.5 ± 0.8 SDS; at 3 months, 0.1 ± 0.6 SDS; at 6 months, –0.3 ± 0.4 SDS; p < 0.005) and sustained diminished IGF-1 levels during the control period (at baseline, –1.4 ± 0.7 SDS; at 3 months, –1.1 ± 0.5 SDS; at 6 months, –1.4 ± 0.7 SDS; n.s.).

Hardin et al. [9, 12] found significantly increased IGF-1 levels following GH treatment (at baseline, 0.9 ± 0.5 ng/ml; at 6 months, 3.3 ± 1.9 ng/ml; at 12 months, 2.6 ± 1.8 ng/ml; p < 0.044), while in the control group, IGF-1 levels did not change. Somatomedin C also significantly increased in the study of Huseman et al. [8] from a mean value of 0.6 ± 0.1 to 1.6 ± 0.6 U/ml after therapy (12 months).

Protein Metabolism

Healthy children need a positive net protein balance which is crucial for growth and development of puberty. In contrast, catabolism is common in malnourished CF patients. The anabolic

Table 1. Overview of the trials using GH in CF

Study	Study design	Patients	GH treatment	Results (control versus GH)
Sackey et al. [4], 1995	prospective, uncontrolled	n = 7 prepubertal	0.16 mg/kg/week 6–12 months	*GV:* 0.3 versus 4.1 cm/year *WV:* 5 +/2 – *FEV_1:* no decrease
Huseman et al. [8], 1996	prospective, uncontrolled	n = 8 prepubertal	0.27 mg/kg/week 12 months	*GV:* 5.8 ± 0.3 versus 7.7 ± 0.4 cm/year *WV:* 1.9 ± 0.1 versus 3.2 ± 0.3 kg/year *FEV_1:* no decrease *protein metabolism:* –0.6 ± 0.1 versus 0.3 ± 0.1 g protein/kg/day
Schnabel et al. [11], 1997	prospective, randomized, crossover	n = 12 prepubertal	0.33 mg/kg/week 6 months	*net protein balance:* –0.1 + 0.4 (at baseline) versus 0.5 + 0.3 g protein/kg/day (at 6 months of GH) *LBM:* 1.8 + 1.1 versus 5.4 + 0.9 kg/year
Hardin et al. [17], 1997	prospective, randomized, controlled	n = 24 prepubertal (n = 21) pubertal (n = 3)	0.29 mg/kg/week 12–36 months	*GV:* 3.7 ± 2.5 versus 7.7 ± 1.7 cm/year *weight:* –0.04 ± 1.2 versus 0.3 ± 0.7 SDS (after 2 years)
Alemzadeh et al. [18], 1998	prospective, uncontrolled	n = 5 prepubertal	0.30 mg/kg/week 24 months	*height:* –2.8 ± 0.3 versus –0.9 ± 0.2 SDS *body weight:* –2.0 ± 0.2 versus –0.1 ± 0.1 SDS (after 2 years)
Hardin et al. [12], 1998	prospective, uncontrolled	n = 9 prepubertal	0.35 mg/kg/week 12 months	*height:* –1.9 ± 0.7 versus –1.3 ± 0.9 SDS *BV:* 1.7 ± 1.0 versus 3.8 ± 1.6 kg/year increase in *LBM* and *muscle strength* *FEV_1:* no decrease *hemoglobin A_{1c}:* unaffected
Hardin et al. [9, 13], 2001	prospective, randomized, controlled	n = 19 prepubertal	0.3 mg/kg/week 12 months	*GV:* 3.8 + 1.4 versus 8.1 + 2.4 cm/year *WV:* 2.1 + 0.9 versus 4.5 + 1.1 kg/year *FVC > FEV_1:* improvement *LBM:* increase *glucose metabolism:* unaffected
Hütler et al. [10], 2002	prospective, randomized, crossover	n = 10 prepubertal	0.33 mg/kg/week 6 months	*GV:* 4.1 + 1.1 versus 8.7 + 0.9 cm/year *WV:* 1.1 + 0.8 versus 4.7 + 0.7 kg/year *FEV_1/FVC:* no decrease *exercise tolerance:* increase *glucose metabolism:* unaffected
Schibler et al. [6], 2003	prospective, randomized, controlled	n = 20 age 10–23 years	0.33 mg/kg/week 12 months	*GV:* 1.9 ± 2.2 versus 2.5 ± 2.0 kg/year *LBM:* increase *exercise tolerance:* increase *FEV_1:* no decrease
Hardin et al. [7], 2005	prospective, randomized, controlled	n = 18 prepubertal	0.3 mg/kg/week 12–24 months	*height:* –2.8 ± 0.3 versus –0.9 ± 0.2 SDS *body weight:* –2.0 ± 0.2 versus –0.1 ± 0.1 SDS (after 2 years)
Hardin et al. [5], 2005	retrospective, controlled	n = 13 pubertal	0.3 mg/kg/week 12 months	*mean GV:* 4.5 versus 8.3 cm/year *mean WV:* 1.4 versus 7.3 kg/year *FVC > FEV_1:* improvement *glucose metabolism:* unaffected

GV = Growth velocity; WV = weight velocity; LBM = lean body mass.

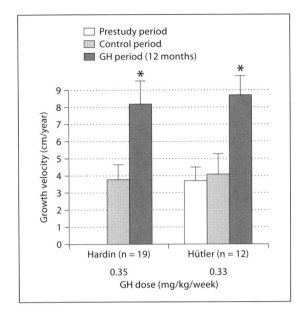

Fig. 1. Growth velocity for the control patients and the GH-treated group after 12 months in the trial by Hardin et al. [9]. Hütler et al. [10] compared the prestudy period with the periods of high caloric intake (control) and GH treatment of the same patients. Data are means ± SE. * p < 0.002 versus controls.

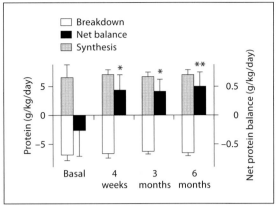

Fig. 2. Metabolic effects of GH on protein synthesis and breakdown and net protein measured by a stable isotope technique, using [^{15}N]glycine, in 12 dystrophic prepubertal CF patients. Data are means ± SE. * p < 0.01; ** p < 0.001 versus baseline values [11].

effects of exogenous GH were measured using a stable isotope technique. Huseman et al. [8] and Schnabel et al. [11] used [^{15}N]glycine, while Hardin et al. [13] used [1-^{13}C]leucine. Anabolic effects of GH treatment were found in 5 out of 9 subjects [8].

Schnabel et al. [11] reported a negative mean net protein balance at baseline (−0.1 ± 0.4 g protein/kg body weight/day) in 12 dystrophic CF children. With GH, the mean net protein balance turned positive after 4 weeks (0.6 ± 0.3 g protein/kg/day), an effect that was maintained after 6 months (0.5 ± 0.3 g protein/kg/day) (fig. 2). In the control group, the catabolic situation at baseline (−0.1 ± 0.4 g protein/kg/day) did not change despite high caloric intake in the following 6 months (−0.2 + 0.3 g protein/kg/day).

Hardin et al. [13] observed a reduction in whole-body protein breakdown measured by the leucine rate of appearance with no change in protein synthesis after 6 and 12 months of GH therapy (at baseline, 181 ± 24 μmol/kg/h; at 6 months, 135 ± 26 μmol/kg/h; at 12 months, 140 ± 20 μmol/kg/h). In the control group, the catabolic situation remained unchanged.

The positive net protein balance is thought to result from a GH-induced decrease in protein breakdown, thereby improving growth and weight velocity as well as increasing lean tissue mass.

Darmaun et al. [14] analyzed the effects of the nonessential amino acid glutamine in combination with GH over 4 weeks on protein metabolism. The short course of GH had a potent anabolic effect that is mediated by stimulation of protein synthesis, but did not influence glutamine kinetics. The combined glutamine and GH regimen had no stronger anabolic effect than GH alone.

Body Weight/Body Composition
All but one study, in which GH was given only 3 times per week, have demonstrated significant improvements in weight velocity.

Mean weight velocity compared with baseline in the GH group increased between 3.2 [8], 4.2 [9] and 5.0 kg/year [10], while in the control periods/control groups, weight velocity did not change significantly (fig. 3).

Body composition was assessed by various techniques (skin fold thickness, bioelectrical impedance, dual-energy X-ray absorptiometry). Hardin et al. [12] described decreased skin fold thickness despite increased body weight and suggested improved lean tissue mass as a result of GH intervention. Schnabel et al. [11] found body composition unchanged during the control period (Δ 1.8 ± 1.1 kg/year), whereas GH increased lean body mass (Δ 5.4 ± 0.9 kg/year) (fig. 4). The lipolytic effect of GH was only modest.

Lean tissue mass also improved in the study by Hardin et al. [9] (4.7 ± 1.7 kg/year with GH vs. 2.1 ± 1.6 kg/year in the control group).

Pulmonary Function

Pulmonary function is most commonly studied using the following parameters: forced expiratory volume in 1 s (FEV_1) and forced vital capacity (FVC). Both can be expressed as absolute values or as percent predicted. Sackey et al. [4] and Huseman et al. [8] did not find significant changes in lung function. In a nonrandomized study, Hardin et al. [12] found that FEV_1 and FVC (expressed as percent predicted) increased during the 12 months of GH treatment in all but 2 patients. Hütler et al. [10] observed no change in either lung function parameter in the control period, while in the GH period, both parameters increased. However, due to the small number of patients, this change was not significant. In their adolescent trial, Hardin et al. [5] found a significant improvement in FVC (expressed in absolute values) with GH.

Hardin et al. [5] postulates increases in absolute values as an improvement in lung function, because untreated CF patients did not achieve the same degree of improvement in linear growth without GH. Whereas this is debatable, all authors found at least a trend toward improvement reflecting stabilization of FEV_1 (percent predicted) during the GH period. This can be interpreted to reflect treatment benefit, since CF is characterized by a disease-specific decline in FEV_1 of approximately 3–5% per year.

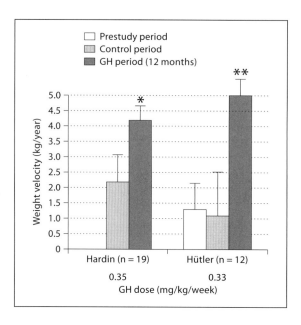

Fig. 3. Weight velocity for the control group and the GH-treated group after 12 months in the trial by Hardin et al. [9]. Hütler et al. [10] compared the prestudy period with the periods of high caloric intake (control) and GH treatment of the same patients. Data are means ± SE. * p < 0.004; ** p < 0.002 versus controls.

Days off School/Work

Hardin et al. [9] documented the effect of GH on the clinical status by recording the number of hospitalizations and outpatient intravenous antibiotic courses for each subgroup as compared with the year prior to the study. The group receiving GH demonstrated a significant reduction in both, while there was a slight increase in hospitalizations in the control group.

Sackey et al. [4] demonstrated a decrease in the number of courses of antibiotic therapy during GH treatment compared with pretreatment data.

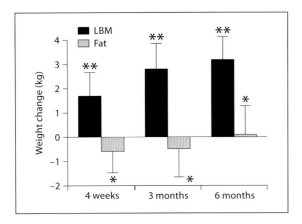

Fig. 4. Body composition was analyzed using bioelectrical impedance. Changes of lean body mass (LBM) and fat mass (FM) during GH treatment compared with baseline [11]. Data are means ± SE. * p < 0.05; ** p < 0.005.

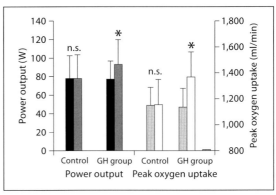

Fig. 5. Exercise testing performed by an incremental test on an electronically braked cycle ergometer at baseline, after the 6-month control and the 6-month GH period [10]. Data are means ± SE. * p < 0.01 versus baseline of the control or GH period.

Exercise Capacity

Exercise capacity was used as a parameter reflecting clinical status. Hütler et al. [10] assessed exercise tolerance in terms of peak power output and peak oxygen uptake measured during cycle ergometry in prepubertal underweight CF patients. They found a significant improvement in peak power output (77 vs. 91 W; p < 0.01) and peak oxygen uptake (1,150 vs. 1,350 ml/min; p < 0.01) (fig. 5). Schibler et al. [6] included older patients (mean age 15.4 years in the GH group, 16.8 years in the control group) in their study, but also found a significant improvement in peak power output (Δ +21 W), while the control group lost peak power output (Δ −11 W). In a prospective, uncontrolled study by Sackey et al. [4], treadmill endurance capacity was found to be decreased after 6 months (11.3 vs. 10.0 min; p < 0.015), but was unchanged compared with baseline after 12 months of GH therapy (11.5 vs. 11.2 min).

Isokinetic muscle strength of the knee flexors/extensors, measured by a Cybex dynamometer, was found improved after 12 [12] but also after 6 months of GH treatment [10].

Hardin et al. [9] observed increases in respiratory muscle strength (maximum inspiratory pressure −59 vs. −89 mm Hg, p < 0.039; maximum expiratory pressure 62 vs. 92 mm Hg, p < 0.042).

Bone Metabolism

Schnabel et al. [15, 20] observed diminished bone formation rate (measured by bone alkaline phosphatase, BALP) and bone resorption (investigated by deoxypyridinoline, DPD/Cr). While BALP and DPD/Cr did not change significantly in the control group, GH treatment significantly improved BALP (at baseline, −0.9 ± 0.6 SDS; at 6 months, 0.9 ± 0.7; p < 0.005) and DPD/Cr (at baseline, −2.0 ± 0.9 SDS; at 6 months, 0.1 ± 1.1 SDS; p < 0.005). Bone mineral density assessed by peripheral quantitative computerized tomography of the radius revealed total and spongiosa bone density within the normal range in both groups (GH, control) at baseline, with no significant changes in the following 6 months. The increased bone turnover did not result in a net gain of bone mineral density, but seemed to reflect the changes in growth velocity. Hardin et al. [16] reported an improvement in bone mineral content measured by dual-energy X-ray absorptiometry with GH in short CF patients. These data have to be interpreted with caution, since bone mineral content was not related to height.

Side Effects

No serious adverse effects of GH have been reported in any of the studies mentioned above (fig. 6). Studies in CF patients using GH in pharmacological dosages should incorporate glucose tolerance testing, because disturbances in glucose metabolism are common in CF and become a greater clinical concern with increasing age. Random blood glucose levels or hemoglobin A_{1c} concentrations are not sufficient to diagnose abnormal glucose metabolism. None of the patients developed glucose impairment investigated by oral glucose tolerance test [9]. Only the retrospective study by Hardin et al. [17] reported impaired glucose tolerance in 2 out of 24 CF patients receiving GH. These patients were pubertal and did not receive glucose testing before initiating GH treatment.

GH treatment did not result in appropriate bone age maturation [9]. After 12 months, the change in bone age divided by the chronological age was 0.9 ± 1.2 in the control group and 1.1 ± 0.9 in the GH-treated group (n.s.).

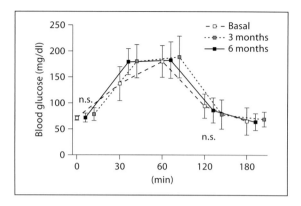

Fig. 6. Glucose metabolism during the study in the GH-treated group assessed by glucose tolerance testing (1.75 g glucose/kg body weight; maximum 75 g). Data are means ± SE [Schnabel, unpubl. data].

Conclusions

All published trials of GH treatment in patients with CF, mostly done in prepubertal children, have demonstrated significant improvements in growth velocity.

Clear-cut clinical benefits were also observed with an improvement in the increase in pulmonary function (FVC, FEV_1), a reduced number of hospitalizations and days off school and work in some trials.

The studies investigating severely malnourished patients suggest a potential role for GH as an adjunct to overcome dystrophy. In these patients, before starting GH treatment, nutrition was optimized according to the individual needs of the patient, and intensive pulmonary therapy and physiotherapy were provided.

In these patients, improved anabolism provided the basis for increased growth and weight gain, an increased lean body mass and, consequently, an improvement in exercise capacity.

The data suggest that GH, given for a limited period of time, provides an effective and safe treatment in patients with CF, especially in prepubertal children.

Further studies are needed to confirm these data in a higher number of patients, especially addressing potential long-term benefits of GH treatment on clinical status and well-being. Safety aspects, for example the effects on glucose metabolism, have to be evaluated in detail.

In addition, it would be very interesting to assess if the gain in growth and weight velocity and the increase in exercise capacity has an impact on the patient's quality of life.

References

1 Stern M, Ballmann M: Qualitätssicherung Mukoviszidose. Überblick über den Gesundheitszustand der Patienten in Deutschland 1999. Hannover, Zentrum für Qualitätsmanagement im Gesundheitswesen, 2000.
2 Sharma R, Florea VG, Bolger AP, Doehner W, Florea ND, Coats AJS, Hodson ME, Anker SD, Henein MY: Wasting as an independent predictor of mortality in patients with cystic fibrosis. Thorax 2001;56:746–750.
3 Schnabel D, Staab D: Wachstum und Pubertät bei Patienten mit zystischer Fibrose. Monatsschr Kinderheilkd 1999; 147(suppl 2):S44.
4 Sackey AH, Taylor CJ, Barraclough M, Wales JKH, Pickering M: Growth hormone as a nutritional adjunct in cystic fibrosis: results of a pilot study. J Hum Nutr Diet 1995;8:185–191.
5 Hardin DS, Ferkol T, Ahn C, Dreimane D, Dyson M, Morse M, Prestidge C, Rice J, Seilheimer DK: A retrospective study of growth hormone use in adolescents with cystic fibrosis. Clin Endocrinol 2005;62:560–566.
6 Schibler A, von der Heiden R, Birrer P, Mullis PE: Prospective randomised treatment with recombinant human growth hormone in cystic fibrosis. Arch Dis Child 2003;88:1078–1081.
7 Hardin DS, Rice J, Ahn C, Ferkol T, Howenstine M, Spears S, Prestidge C, Seilheimer DK, Shepard R: Growth hormone treatment enhances nutrition and growth in children with cystic fibrosis receiving enteral nutrition. J Pediatr 2005;146:324–328.
8 Huseman CA, Colombo JL, Brooks MA, Smay JR, Greger NG, Sammut PH, Bier DM: Anabolic effect of biosynthetic growth hormone in cystic fibrosis patients. Pediatr Pulmonol 1996;22:90–95.
9 Hardin DS, Ellis KJ, Dyson M, Rice J, McConnell R, Seilheimer DK: Growth hormone improves clinical status in prepubertal children with cystic fibrosis: results of a randomized controlled trial. J Pediatr 2001;139:636–642.
10 Hütler M, Schnabel D, Staab D, Tacke A, Wahn U, Böning D, Beneke R: Effect of growth hormone on exercise tolerance in children with cystic fibrosis. Med Sci Sports Exerc 2002;34:567–572.
11 Schnabel D, Staab D, Tacke A, Brösicke H, Wahn U, Grüters A: Effects of growth hormone treatment (hGH) on whole body protein turnover and body composition in patients with cystic fibrosis (CF). Horm Res 1997;48(suppl 2):71.
12 Hardin DS, Stratton R, Kramer JC, Reyes de la Rocha S, Govaerts K, Wilson DP: Growth hormone improves weight velocity and height velocity in prepubertal children with cystic fibrosis. Horm Metab Res 1998;30:636–641.
13 Hardin DS, Ellis KJ, Dyson M, Rice J, McConnell R, Seilheimer DK: Growth hormone decreases protein catabolism in children with cystic fibrosis. J Clin Endocrinol Metab 2001;86:4424–4428.
14 Darmaun D, Hayes V, Schaeffer D, Welch S, Mauras N: Effects of glutamine and recombinant human growth hormone on protein metabolism in prepubertal children with cystic fibrosis. J Clin Endocrinol Metab 2004;89:1146–1152.
15 Schnabel D, Schönau E, Staab D, Tacke A, Felsenberg D, Wahn U, Grüters A: Effects of growth hormone therapy on bone metabolism in patients with cystic fibrosis; in Schönau E, Matkovic V (eds): Pediatric Osteology: Prevention of Osteoporosis – A Pediatric Task? Singapore, Elsevier Science, 1998, pp 209–217.
16 Hardin DS, Ahn C, Prestidge C, Seilheimer DK, Ellis KJ: Growth hormone improves bone mineral content in children with cystic fibrosis. J Pediatr Endocrinol Metab 2005;18:589–595.
17 Hardin DS, Sy JP: Effects of growth hormone treatment in children with cystic fibrosis: the National Cooperative Growth Study experience. J Pediatr 1997;131:65–69.
18 Alemzadeh R, Upchurch L, McCarthy V: Anabolic effects of growth hormone treatment in young children with cystic fibrosis. J Am Coll Nutr 1998;17:419–424.
19 Schnabel D, Grasemann C, Staab D, Wollmann H, Ratjen F for the German CF Growth Hormone study group: A multi-center, randomized, double-blind placebo-controlled trial evaluating the metabolic and respiratory effects of growth hormone in children with cystic fibrosis. Pediatrics 2007, in press.
20 Schnabel D, Schönau E, Staab D, Tacke A, Wahn U, Felsenberg D, Grüters A: Effects of growth hormone therapy on bone metabolism in patients with cystic fibrosis. Horm Res 1998;50(suppl 3):61.

The KIGS Experience with Growth Hormone Treatment of Cystic Fibrosis

Edward O. Reiter

In patients with cystic fibrosis (CF), chronic pulmonary infection with bronchiectasis, pancreatic insufficiency with exocrine and endocrine inadequacy, malabsorption and malnutrition [1–7] all contribute to decreased growth and late sexual maturation. In 17,857 patients with CF, mean height was at the 21st percentile and mean weight at the 9th percentile [8]. Early impairment of height and weight growth and retardation of skeletal maturation may progress or plateau during mid-childhood years but become most marked in the preadolescent period when growth and maturational changes are frequently delayed [1, 8–11]. The degree of growth retardation is most closely related to the severity and variability of the pulmonary disease rather than to pancreatic dysfunction [2, 4, 5]. The degree of steatorrhea does not correlate well with growth impairment, though improved nutrition programs enhance the overall clinical picture [6, 7]. Adult heights in surviving patients with CF approach the normal range [2]. Endocrine abnormalities, such as failure of both α and β islet cells with decreased glucagon and insulin production do not seem to influence prepubertal growth patterns in children with CF. The incidence of diabetes mellitus increases as patients live beyond the second decade [8]. Alterations in vitamin D metabolism, while potentially affecting skeletal mineralization, do not diminish growth [12]. Delayed sexual maturation in which gonadotropin-releasing hormone administration evokes a prepubertal pattern of pituitary gonadotropin secretion in adolescent patients is similar to that in the constitutional delay of growth and maturation [10, 11, 13].

The growth hormone (GH)/insulin-like growth factor (IGF) axis shows evidence of some degree of acquired GH insensitivity with lowered mean IGF-1 and elevated GH levels [14, 15]. Schnabel [this vol., pp. 296–303] has extensively updated the issues surrounding GH treatment of children with CF for this KIGS 20th Anniversary volume. A modest literature has been developed regarding this subject. Treatment of prepubertal CF children with GH for 1 year resulted in an anabolic effect, with greater growth velocity and nitrogen retention and increased protein and decreased fat stores [16, 17]. In a 2-year GH treatment program of CF patients who received enteral nutrition prior to and during GH therapy, auxological parameters continued to improve

Baystate Children's Hospital, Tufts University School of Medicine
759 Chestnut Street, Springfield, MA 01199 (USA)

Table 1. Prepubertal CF patients treated for the first year with GH

	n	Median	10th percentile	90th percentile
At GH start				
Age, years	19	10.4	3.6	14.0
Bone age, years	6	6.2	4.2	11.0
Height SDS (Prader)	19	–3.2	–4.7	–1.2
Height velocity, cm/year	6	4.8	2.3	5.6
Height velocity SDS (Prader)	6	–1.5	–5.5	0.6
BMI SDS	19	–1.6	–2.5	0.0
GH dose, mg/kg/week	19	0.29	0.10	0.49
After 1 year on GH				
Age, years	19	11.4	4.7	15.1
Height SDS (Prader)	19	–2.4	–4.2	–1.2
Height velocity, cm/year	19	7.5	4.3	9.5
Height velocity SDS (Prader)	19	1.1	–4.0	4.7
Δ height SDS (Prader)	19	.3	–0.7	1.1
Studentized residual SDS	10	–0.9	–2.4	0.1
BMI SDS	19	–0.9	–2.4	0.6

BMI = Body mass index.

[18]. Pulmonary function improved in most patients. A 4-year longitudinal study utilizing the National CF Foundation Registry found that improved nutrition status and growth were associated with a slower age-related decrement of pulmonary function [19]. The current perspective would suggest that GH treatment should be adjunctive to an aggressive nutritional program, appropriate pulmonary care without glucocorticoid administration, and careful assessment of carbohydrate metabolism [20].

KIGS Data on the Treatment of Patients with Cystic Fibrosis

In the KIGS database, information regarding a modest number of patients with CF who have received GH treatment is available. Responses to 1 year of GH treatment in 19 prepubertal children with CF are shown in table 1. Over 70% are males, with the median age at onset of GH therapy being 10.4 years; the children are small and slight, with a height standard deviation score (SDS) of –3.2 and a weight SDS of –2.9, as well as a markedly delayed bone age. The children's heights were far from the midparental target (–2.5 SDS). In the first year of treatment, height velocity increased from 4.8 to 7.5 cm/year, though neither the height SDS nor the approximation to the midparental target rose significantly, as the range of response was large (fig. 1, 2). One year is a short period of time, but nonetheless, it should be noted that the weight SDS did increase by 0.6 units, certainly a major increment and a very important finding in view of the relationship of nutritional status with pulmonary function [21] and bone mineral density [22]. It should be noted that there is a reasonably large studentized residual, as the predicted growth for 1 year exceeded the actual growth by 2.3 cm.

In a larger group of children, including those who were pubertal, there are data on 43 patients with CF (again approximately 70% males), with a median duration of GH treatment of 2.3 years

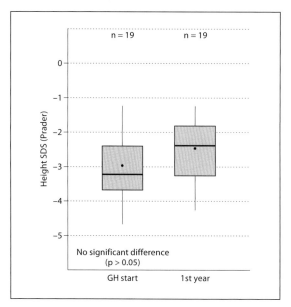

Fig. 1. Height SDS prior to and after 1 year of GH treatment in prepubertal children with CF. The box plots represent the medians and 25th and 75th percentiles, with whiskers at the 10th and 90th percentiles. The dot shows the mean.

Fig. 2. Height SDS – midparental target height (MPH) prior to and after 1 year of GH treatment in prepubertal children with CF. The box plots represent the medians and 25th and 75th percentiles, with whiskers at the 10th and 90th percentiles. The dot shows the mean.

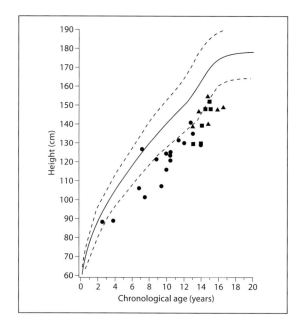

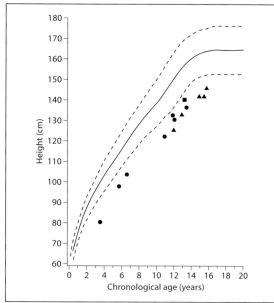

Fig. 3. Height at GH start in boys. Dashed lines = 10th and 90th percentiles; solid line = median; ■ = no information on puberty; ▲ = pubertal; ● = prepubertal.

Fig. 4. Height at GH start in girls. Dashed lines = 10th and 90th percentiles; solid line = median; ■ = no information on puberty; ▲ = pubertal; ● = prepubertal.

Table 2. Cross-sectional data

	All				Females		Males	
	n	median	10th percentile	90th percentile	n	median	n	median
Background								
Birth weight SDS	35	−0.7	−2.7	1.8	13	−1.2	23	−0.5
Birth length SDS	21	−1.3	−2.4	0.8	9	−1.5	12	−0.7
MPH SDS (Prader)	36	−0.8	−2.3	0.8	12	−0.5	24	−0.8
Maximum GH, μg/l	31	8.1	3.1	17.8	10	8.4	21	8.1
IGF-1 SDS	14	−1.4	−3.0	0.5	4	−1.6	10	−1.3
At GH start								
Age, years	43	12.8	6.6	15.1	13	12.1	30	12.9
Bone age, years	11	10.0	5.0	13.5	4	7.7	7	11.0
Height SDS (Prader)	43	−3.1	−3.9	−1.7	13	−3.5	30	−2.8
Height − MPH SDS (Prader)	36	−2.2	−3.9	−1.1	12	−3.2	24	−2.1
Height velocity, cm/year	16	3.7	2.2	6.5	3	2.6	13	4.6
Weight SDS	43	−2.4	−4.1	−1.1	13	−2.4	30	−2.4
BMI SDS	43	−0.8	−2.4	0.1	13	−0.8	30	−0.8
GH dose, mg/kg/week	43	0.29	0.16	0.46	13	0.27	30	0.30
At the latest visit								
Age, years	43	15.4	8.1	18.3	13	15.3	30	15.5
Height SDS (Prader)	43	−2.1	−3.7	−0.7	13	−3.0	30	−1.8
Height − MPH SDS (Prader)	36	−1.7	−3.1	0.1	12	−2.1	24	−1.2
Δ height SDS between GH start and latest visit (Prader)	43	0.7	−0.1	2.1	13	0.4	30	0.7
Weight SDS	43	−1.5	−3.7	0.5	13	−1.5	30	−1.6
BMI SDS	43	−0.6	−2.6	1.2	13	−0.5	30	−0.7
Years on GH	43	2.3	0.6	5.8	13	2.3	30	2.2
Mean total GH dose, mg/kg/week	42	0.30	0.19	0.41	13	0.31	29	0.30

MPH = Midparental target height.

(table 2). The onset of treatment was not until 12.8 years of age, with the height SDS being −3.1 (fig. 3, 4) and the weight SDS −2.4. Bone ages were delayed by nearly 3 years in those patients in whom data were available. The response to GH is characterized by an increase in about 1 SDS both in height and weight. In both treatment groups, the GH dose, though generally higher than that utilized for GH deficiency in Europe, did not reach levels that might be needed in patients in whom relative GH insensitivity was present. Utilization of IGF-1 determinations to give some suggestion as to the patients' biochemical responses to exogenous GH might be of great value in determining whether higher doses of GH are needed to achieve the desired anabolic effects.

These KIGS data generally suggest that GH treatment in patients with CF does increase height and weight growth, but do not provide information on other more critical matters. Important criteria for success would include positive anabolic measures, evidence of slowing of the inexorable decrement of pulmonary function (and its tests), bone mineral density assessments and improved quality of life indicators. Such data are not readily available in the database, but are found in many of the investigator-initiated studies described by Schnabel [this vol., pp. 296–303] and in the references given in his and in this chapter.

References

1 Landon C, Rosenfeld RG: Short stature and pubertal delay in male adolescents with cystic fibrosis. Am J Dis Child 1984;138:388–391.
2 Preece MA, Law CM, Davies PSW: The growth of children with chronic paediatric disease. Clin Endocrinol Metab 1986;15:453–477.
3 Sproul A, Huang N: Growth patterns in children with cystic fibrosis. J Pediatr 1964;65:664–676.
4 Lapey A, Kattwinkel J, Di Sant'Agnese PA, Laster L: Steatorrhea and azotorrhea and their relation to growth and nutrition in adolescents and young adults with cystic fibrosis. J Pediatr 1974;84:328–334.
5 Mearns M: Growth and development; in Hodson E, Norman A, Batten J (eds): Cystic Fibrosis. London, Bailliere Tindall, 1983, pp 183–196.
6 Shepherd RW, Holt TL, Thomas BJ, Kay L, Isles A, Francis PJ, Ward LC: Nutritional rehabilitation in cystic fibrosis: controlled studies of effects on nutritional growth retardation, body protein turnover, and course of pulmonary disease. J Pediatr 1986;109:788–794.
7 Reiter EO, Gerstle RS: Cystic fibrosis in puberty and adolescence; in Lerner RM, Petersen AC, Brooks-Gunn J (eds): Encyclopedia of Adolescence. New York, Garland, 1991, pp 187–195.
8 FitzSimmons SC: The changing epidemiology of cystic fibrosis. J Pediatr 1993;122:1–9.
9 Karlberg J, Kjellmer I, Kristiansson B: Linear growth in children with cystic fibrosis. 1. Birth to 8 years of age. Acta Paediatr Scand 1991;80:508–514.
10 Reiter EO, Stern RC, Root AW: The reproductive system in cystic fibrosis. 1. Basal gonadotropin and sex steroid levels. Am J Dis Child 1981;135:422–426.
11 Reiter EO, Stern RC, Root AW: The reproductive system in cystic fibrosis. 2. Changes in gonadotrophins and sex steroids following LHRH. Clin Endocrinol 1982;16:127–137.
12 Reiter EO, Brugman SM, Pike JW, Pitt M, Dokoh S, Haussler MR, Gerstle RS, Taussig LM: Vitamin D metabolites in adolescents and young adults with cystic fibrosis: effects of sun and season. J Pediatr 1985;106:21–26.
13 Aswani N, Taylor CJ, McGaw J, Pickering M, Rigby AS: Pubertal growth and development in cystic fibrosis: a retrospective review. Acta Paediatr 2003;92:1029–1032.
14 Laursen EM, Juul A, Lanng S, Hoiby N, Koch C, Muller J, Skakkebaek NE: Diminished concentrations of insulin-like growth factor I in cystic fibrosis. Arch Dis Child 1995;72:494–497.
15 Street ME, Ziveri MA, Spaggiari C, Via-ani I, Volta C, Grzincich GL, Virdis R, Bernasconi S: Inflammation is a modulator of the insulin-like growth factor (IGF)/IGF-binding protein system inducing reduced bioactivity of IGFs in cystic fibrosis. Eur J Endocrinol 2006;154:47–52.
16 Huseman CA, Columbo JL, Brooks MA, Smay JR, Greger NG, Sammut PH, Bier DM: Anabolic effect of biosynthetic growth hormone in cystic fibrosis. Pediatr Pulmonol 1996;22:90–95.
17 Hardin DS, Stratton R, Kramer JC, Reyes de la Rocha S, Govaerts K, Wilson DP: Growth hormone improves weight velocity and height velocity in prepubertal children with cystic fibrosis. Horm Metab Res 1998;30:636–641.
18 Hardin DS, Rice J, Ahn C, Ferkol T, Howenstine M, Spears S, Prestidge C, Seilheimer DK, Shepherd R: Growth hormone treatment enhances nutrition and growth in children with cystic fibrosis receiving enteral nutrition. J Pediatr 2005;146:324–328.
19 Zemel BS, Jawad AF, FitzSimmons S, Stallings VA: Longitudinal relationship among growth, nutritional status, and pulmonary function in children with cystic fibrosis: analysis of the Cystic Fibrosis Foundation National CF Patient Registry. J Pediatr 2000;137:374–380.
20 Colombo C, Battezzati A: Growth failure in cystic fibrosis: a true need for anabolic agents? J Pediatr 2005;146:303–305.
21 Taylor AM, Bush A, Thomson A, Oades PJ, Marchant JL, Bruce-Morgan C, Holly J, Ahmed L, Dunger DB: Relation between insulin-like growth factor-I, body mass index, and clinical status in cystic fibrosis. Arch Dis Child 1997;76:304–309.
22 Street ME, Spaggiari C, Ziveri MA, Volta C, Federico G, Baroncelli GI, Bernasconi S, Saggese G: Analysis of bone mineral density and turnover in patients with cystic fibrosis: associations between the IGF system and inflammatory cytokines. Horm Res 2006;66:162–168.

Idiopathic Short Stature: Definition, Spontaneous Growth and Response to Treatment

Jan M. Wit

Idiopathic short stature (ISS) is a purely descriptive term that refers to a child, adolescent or adult with a height below the age reference for population and sex, in whom, with current diagnostic tools, no etiological diagnosis is made. In this paper, four topics will be discussed: (1) definition, including the possible pathophysiology; (2) spontaneous growth and height prognosis; (3) the effects of growth hormone (GH) treatment on growth, either alone or in combination with a gonadotropin-releasing hormone analogue (GnRHa) or aromatase inhibitors, and (4) future prospects. The psychosocial aspects of being short, effects of therapy on quality of life, potential side effects and ethical and economical aspects will not be discussed.

Department of Paediatrics, J6S
Leiden University Medical Center
Albinusdreef 2
PO Box 9600
NL–2300 RC Leiden (The Netherlands)

Definition and Possible Pathophysiology

According to an expert workshop [1], ISS is defined as a condition in which the height of the individual is more than 2 standard deviations (SD) below the corresponding mean height for a given age, sex and population group, and in which no identifiable disorder is present. ISS is subclassified into familial short stature (FSS; the child is short compared with the relevant population, but remains within the expected target range for his or her family) or non-FSS (NFSS; the child is short for the population as well as for the familial target range). While this definition is useful, there are still several open ends. In a recent paper [2], I reviewed some of these.

One of the important issues is that at present, there is no consensus about which disorder should be excluded, and how, before the 'diagnosis' ISS is made [3]. It obviously depends on the skills of the clinician whether he or she performs a thorough medical history, physical examination and laboratory screening to exclude known causes of short stature. In the absence of abnormalities in the history and physical examination,

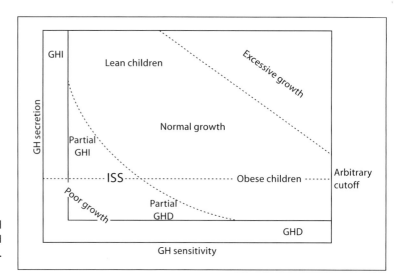

Fig. 1. Hypothetical 2-dimensial model of growth as a resultant of GH secretion and GH sensitivity [81]. GHI = GH insufficiency.

laboratory screening should at least include screening for celiac disease (through antiendomysial or antitissue glutaminase antibodies) [4], Turner syndrome, hypothyroidism, anemia, chronic inflammatory diseases [5], and possibly, also renal acidosis [6].

If one accepts that the GH/insulin-like growth factor 1 (IGF-1) axis is the most important axis involved in growth regulation, one could make a rough subclassification of the likely causes of what we now call ISS: (1) subtle disorders of GH secretion, (2) subtle disorders of GH sensitivity, and (3) a combination of genetic factors directly influencing growth plate biology leading to short stature (fig. 1). Alternatively, one could distinguish 3 main classes: IGF deficiency (primary or secondary), IGF resistance [7] and other causes. However, one should remember that GH acts not only through IGF-1 generation, but has a direct effect on bone and cartilage as well.

Subtle Disorders of GH Secretion

ISS is a condition that remains after exclusion of other conditions, but the difficulty of diagnosing or excluding GH deficiency (GHD) is well known [8, 9]. The distinction between isolated partial GHD and ISS is, to a great extent, arbitrary. There is no gold standard for GHD, as all parameters have arbitrary cutoff levels and a low accuracy. In particular, GH provocation test is an unreliable tool for the diagnosis of GHD, because of high intertest variation, high interassay variation, divergent standards, the effect of age and body mass index on maximal serum GH levels, and the arbitrary age limits beyond which sex steroid priming is advocated [10].

This situation implies that quite a number of children diagnosed with 'partial GHD' may in fact not really have a diminished GH secretion. Studies which retested cases diagnosed with GHD in childhood when they were adults have shown that a substantial portion of them have a normal GH peak after provocation [11]. I believe that this reflects false-positive results of the initial GH provocation tests rather than 'transient' GHD, but there is no formal proof of this assumption. On the other hand, there is little reason to think that there are no false-negative results which are now labeled ISS but in reality may have restricted growth because of a diminished GH secretion (for a given GH sensitivity).

This situation highlights that in some children diagnosed with GHD, GH secretion may in fact not be the rate-limiting step, while in others considered as non-GH deficient (and thus labeled ISS), a limited GH secretion may well be involved. One example is the recent discovery of a range of haplotypes of the GH promoter, with 3 times lower to 3 times higher functionality than that of the most frequent (wild-type) promoter [12, 13]. Many of these children have a normal GH peak after provocation; thus, they may be examples of the hypothetical neurosecretory dysfunction that has been postulated on the basis of 24-hour profiles [14].

Obviously, it is dependent on the decision of the clinician whether subtle disorders of GH secretion will be sought. If clinicians decide to perform a 12- or 24-hour GH profile in all children with a low IGF-1 and IGF binding protein 3 (IGFBP-3; below an arbitrary cutoff limit) and a normal GH peak in the provocation test, there will certainly be children who show a low spontaneous secretion (again, below an arbitrary cutoff) [15, 16]. These children will be labeled 'GH insufficient' (neurosecretory dysfunction), while a similar child who is not tested will be labeled ISS.

An experimental finding that lends support to the notion that part of the children with ISS may have subtle disorders of GH secretion is that on a low dosage of GH (0.5 mg/m^2 body surface/day, corresponding to 0.12 mg/kg/week, if the body surface is close to 1 m^2), mean plasma IGF-1 rises from –1 to 0 SD score (SDS) [17] (table 1).

Subtle Disorders of GH Sensitivity
Several forms of abnormalities of the GH receptor (GHR) have been identified, either resulting in abnormal GH binding, defective receptor dimerization, defective anchoring in the cell membrane, or defective signal transduction [18]. It is uncertain whether heterozygous mutations in the GHR play a role [19, 20]. Also, abnormalities downstream of the GHR have been found, such as a mutation of STAT5B [21], IκB [22], acid-labile subunit [23], IGF-1 [24, 25] and the IGF-1 receptor (IGF1R) [26]. Most cases with disorders of IGF-1 and IGF1R described so far are associated with a low birth size [for a review, see ref. 27]. We have also shown that heterozygous carriers of the IGF-1 mutation are significantly shorter at birth (but still within the normal range) and postnatally compared with noncarrier family members [25]. Thus, some cases with apparent ISS may in fact have heterozygous IGF-1 deletions or mutations. For further details, the reader is referred to recent reviews on this topic [18, 27].

It is up to the clinician to decide whether he or she will perform an IGF-1 generation test in children with a combination of high GH peak in the provocation test and low IGF-1 and IGFBP-3. This should theoretically distinguish between mutations in the translated part of the GH gene on the one hand and GHR or postreceptor defects on the other, although there is uncertainty about the cutoff limits of the test and the predictive power. So far, the prevalence of such disorders appears very low [28–33], and these investigations were only carried out in few potential candidates.

Experimental evidence in children with ISS lends support to the hypothesis that part of these children have a diminished sensitivity to GH and/or IGF-1, as no increase in growth velocity was observed at a low substitution dosage (0.5 mg/m^2/day), in spite of the normalization of plasma IGF-1 [17] (table 1). This also suggests that the change in plasma IGF-1 does not always run parallel with an increase in growth velocity.

Table 1. Estimated GH dose effect relations

GH dose mg/kg/week	IGF-1 SDS	Δ first-year HV cm/year	Δ BA/age	FH gain cm
0	–1.0			
0.12	0.0	+1		
0.25	0.0	+4	1.0	+4.5
0.35		+5	1.0	+7.2
0.50	+0.8	+5	1.8	0?

HV = Height velocity; BA = bone age; FH = final height. Data are based on Kamp et al. [17, 53] and Wit et al. [50].

Genetic Disorders Not Directly Associated with the GH-IGF-1 Axis

An important additional dimension is how far genetic testing should go before one is sufficiently sure that the condition is idiopathic [34]. For example, a heterozygous deletion or mutation of SHOX has been described in about 2.5% of ISS children (although it is uncertain whether all had normal body proportions) [35, 36], but in many cases, this was not tested in children considered to have ISS. Similar considerations apply to testing for chromosomal disorders such as XY/XO mosaicism [37]. Recently, it was reported that heterozygous mutations in the natriuretic peptide receptor B *(NPR2)* cause short stature [38]. As body stature is a polygenic trait, I speculate that in the majority of short individuals, shortness is the net result of a combination of various mutations and polymorphisms in a multitude of genes.

Spontaneous Growth and Height Prognosis

Over the last 20 years, several studies on the spontaneous growth pattern of ISS have been published [39–43]. In one of these studies, the classification, as proposed by the expert panel [1], was used, subdividing children into FSS and NFSS, with 2 further subdivisions each, according to puberty onset. Male and female subjects with FSS had a mean final height of 2.1 and 0.6 cm less than the target height. The final height SDS was very similar to the prepubertal height SDS. For male and female subjects with NFSS, the mean final height was 8.3 and 6.8 cm less than the target height, but substantially higher than the initial height SDS [43]. The mean final height was a few centimeters less than the predicted adult height (based on bone age readings) in most studies [41]. In a later study, we observed that while the mean final height is quite similar to the mean predicted height in ISS, there is a large interindividual variation that is primarily correlated with bone age delay; a large delay leads to a large overprediction, and a small delay to underprediction [44], suggesting that present bone age-based height prediction algorithms are inaccurate. In a recent review, I discussed this topic in more detail [2].

Effect of Growth Hormone Therapy

The Effect of GH on Growth
Since 1985, many clinical trials have been performed to study the efficacy of GH treatment in ISS; however, many of these do not comply with the strict rules that can be applied to clinical trials [45, 46]. In most instances, the design was to administer a fixed dose per kilogram body weight or square meter body surface from childhood up to near final height. Other designs include regimens of a dose increment after the first year of treatment, a high dose of GH restricted to the prepubertal period and a combination of GH with a GnRHa in adolescence. Outcome measures are height velocity (as change in height SDS, or as velocity per se in centimeters/year or SDS), bone age advance, final height and measures of psychosocial adjustment.

As expected, there is a dose-response relationship between GH and short-term growth velocity response in children with ISS. At the lowest dosage given in our diagnostic dose-response study (corresponding to 0.12 mg/kg body weight/week), there was virtually no change in growth velocity, in spite of a normalization of plasma IGF-1 [17]. The acceleration of growth velocity is already substantial at a dosage close to a substitution dosage (0.66 mg/m^2 body surface/day, approximately equivalent to 0.17 mg/kg/week) [47, 48], and slightly more at a dosage of 0.25–0.35 mg/kg/week [49]. Height velocity at a dosage of 0.50 mg/kg/week was equal to that of 0.25 mg/kg/week [17]. In other studies, similar findings have been reported. These results indicate that in a majority of children, either the endogenous GH secretion is suboptimal for normal growth, or the GH sensitivity is only slightly decreased and can be overcome by administration of GH substitution doses on top of the spontaneous GH secretion.

Similar to all other indications for GH treatment, after the first year, height velocity gradually tapers off in subsequent years. Increasing the dosage after the first year would then seem to be a rational step. Indeed, such a step-up regimen has been tried [47–49], but in spite of some effect on height velocity, final height did not or hardly show any improvement [44, 50]. Thus, the initial dosage appears the key to a good final height gain.

With regard to the influence of GH on the rate of bone age advancement and the onset and pace of puberty, a dose-response relationship is apparent. In a randomized placebo-controlled study with a dosage of 0.22 mg/kg/week [51] and in a British randomized controlled study using approximately 0.33 mg/kg/week [52], no effect was observed, while in a randomized controlled study with a dosage of 0.50 mg/kg/week, a significant advancement of bone age and onset of puberty was seen [53]. In another study using a high dose of GH (0.7 mg/kg/week), height velocity strongly increased, and this was not associated with accelerated bone age [54].

In the last years, several cohorts have reached final height, so that a global picture has emerged of long-term efficacy. However, final height, usually expressed as the SDS for the population and sex, is correlated with the initial height SDS and bone age delay at start [44]. The parameter which is used most is the difference between final height and predicted adult height, but there is a marked intra- and interobserver error in bone age readings, i.e. different bone age methods yield different results [55], and the accuracy of the prediction is strongly dependent on the severity of bone age advancement [44].

While the dose effect with respect to short-term growth response is of modest size, there appears to be a stronger dose-response relationship if final height is taken as outcome measure. At an initial dosage range between 0.17 and 0.25 mg/kg/week, even if the dosage is increased in later years [44], the average effect on final height is approximately 3–4 cm. This was found in the only placebo-controlled trial in which GH was administered 3 times per week in a weekly dosage of 0.22 mg/kg [51], as well as in studies using historical controls, or in controlled trials [for a review, see ref. 41, 44, 56, 57]. All studies using a dosage of approximately 0.35 mg/kg/week from start until near final height have shown an average final height gain of about 7 cm [50, 56, 58]. The Food and Drug Administration has registered ISS as an indication for two of the GH preparations. The first was based on the combination of a placebo-controlled study with a relatively low dose, administered at low frequency [51], having an effect of approximately 3 cm, and a long-term dose-response study showing that the high dosage was significantly more efficacious than the lower dosage regimens [44, 50]. The second was based on an earlier study where growth of GH-treated children was compared with historical controls [59].

One could speculate whether a still higher dosage would lead to better short-term growth and better final height. Indeed, one short-term study provided provisional data supporting this hypothesis [54]. However, in our studies, high-dose GH treatment (approximately 0.50 mg/kg/week) limited to the prepubertal period [17, 53] indeed increased the height SDS, but also accelerated bone maturation and puberty. After 5 years, the height SDS for bone age and predicted adult height has not changed in comparison with untreated controls. Final heights are not yet available. Thus, it may well be that the dosage of 0.35 mg/kg/week is close to the optimum dosage for this condition. An alternative regimen may be to titrate GH dosage with the initial goal of keeping IGF-1 in the range of +2 to +3 to optimize growth velocity, followed by a maintenance phase aiming at IGF-1 levels in the middle of the normal range [60].

In all studies, it has been observed that there is quite some interindividual variation in the long-term growth response. Probably, this is also the case for the effect on final height, but it is difficult to prove due to the uncertainty about the best outcome measure. GH peak during the GH stimulation test has a low predictive value [61]. Several variables at the onset of therapy are correlated with the outcome, including age, initial height SDS, pretreatment growth velocity, target height minus initial height SDS, integrated concentration of GH, serum IGF-1 and IGFBP-3, and bone age delay [48, 62–66]. However, the predictive power is too low for clinical purposes. The same applies to the IGF-1 generation test [17, 33, 67–69]. Children with the polymorphism in the GHR that leads to a GHR molecule of which exon 3 is skipped (d3) appear to show a better response to GH than to the full-length variant [70].

The Effect of Concomitant Therapies in Combination with GH on Growth
It is generally believed that GH alone may not be effective when started in puberty, although formal proof has not been presented. Therefore, it was postulated that the effect of GH might be improved by adding a GnRHa or another inhibitor of the sex steroid effect on the growth plate.

We recently summarized the effects of adding GnRHa to GH in several conditions [71]. More recently, in a randomized controlled trial, we showed that the effect of a 3-year therapy of GH and GnRHa versus no treatment in children with ISS or intrauterine growth retardation [72] was approximately 4 cm, 50% of the estimated effect on predicted adult height [Van Gool et al., submitted]. From the accumulated evidence, it is apparent that the duration of the treatment period is important with regard to the effect on final height [73, 74]. It may also be important that GH is continued after discontinuation of the GnRHa, but this has not yet been formally tested.

The aim of this form of treatment is not to increase height in the first year of therapy, as the height SDS remains the same in comparison with untreated controls. This regimen only aims at extending the available time for growth by several years, which should enable the body to reach a taller final height. This obviously has an effect on the balance of pros and cons: one advantage of GH treatment (short-term growth acceleration) is taken away, and a disadvantage is added (postponement of pubertal development) [75]. As an alternative to the combination of GH + GnRHa, aromatase inhibitors have been administered, and preliminary results indicate that this may increase the final height [76, 77]. Previously, the combination of GH and cyproterone acetate was studied, which did not have a positive effect on final height [78].

Future Prospects

It is reasonable to predict that the pathophysiology of ISS will gradually be unraveled in the coming decades by the development of new genetic tools. Genomic arrays and new techniques to assess the number of alleles will certainly become available, which will lead to the discovery of new genetic causes of short stature. In the subsequent phase, computer models may become available to assess the effects of combinations of genetic variants. Thus, it may be predicted that step by step, the range of ISS will be made smaller. Possibly, at the same time, the genetic factors of the tempo of growth and the onset and tempo of puberty will be elucidated so that more accurate predictions of final height may become available.

With respect to therapy, GH may well remain the mainstay of management of short stature, despite the fact that in many cases GH insufficiency is not the rate-limiting element, analogous to the situation for Turner syndrome, chronic renal insufficiency and short children born small for gestational age. In children with disorders in the GHR and GH signaling pathway, treatment with IGF-1 may become a logical alternative, although

GH therapy has a positive effect on growth in children with heterozygous IGF1R mutations [79]. In those children in whom GH has not been proven to be effective, including achondroplasia, hypochondroplasia and other forms of osteochondrodystrophy, new insights into the effect of fibroblast growth factor on the growth plate may lead to the development of drugs that directly block the effect of the constitutively active fibroblast growth factor receptor 3. Along similar lines, it is not unlikely that the effects of SHOX haploinsufficiency on growth can be approached more directly than the relatively crude therapy with supraphysiologic GH dosages. Further elucidation of the physiological role of the C-type natriuretic peptide and its receptor *NPR2* may lead to the development of drugs that have an effect on the signaling cascade. Analogous speculations can be made about the role of the mitogen-activated protein kinase pathway of GH that appears to be affected in children with Noonan syndrome and Costello syndrome [80].

The decision to start GH treatment in a child with ISS, as well as in children with many other conditions where GH secretion appears normal, will depend on carefully weighing the various advantages and disadvantages of treatment, including the degree of shortness or the psychosocial stress the child appears to have (table 2). Still, in a global perspective, the treatment of short stature, whatever its cause, will always remain a relatively small issue in comparison with the gigantic challenges that mankind faces and will continue to face in the future, with respect to overpopulation, pollution, extreme differences in economical welfare, shortages of water and energy.

Table 2. Arguments in favor of and against GH therapy in children with ISS, adapted from Wit [82]

Points arguing in favor of GH therapy
1. GH in a supraphysiological dosage generally increases height velocity in childhood, leads to less height deficit in childhood and adolescence, and to an adult height which is on average 7 cm higher
2. GH administration can be felt to be rewarding for the child, parents and clinician because they feel that something is being done
3. GH injections are generally well tolerated
4. Significant adverse events have not been observed
5. GH may increase bone mass density
6. Some children labeled ISS may have a form of GH insufficiency (e.g., neurosecretory dysfunction, abnormal GH molecule, inactive GH promoter)

Points arguing against GH therapy
1. Even with a supraphysiological dosage, the average effect on final height is modest (final height is still below or in the lower half of the normal distribution of the population and lower than target height)
2. The growth response is variable and cannot be predicted with acceptable accuracy
3. Most studies on psychosocial adjustment in short children and adults have failed to demonstrate a significant negative effect of shortness and significant changes during therapy
4. GH treatment leads to medicalization (daily injections, regular clinic visits)
5. Theoretical risk of unwanted long-term sequelae of elevated serum GH and IGF-1
6. Large-scale use at the present price would consume an important part of the health budget
7. Ethical considerations that GH treatment in allegedly short 'normal' children may be considered as an unacceptable form of cosmetic medicine

Conclusion

ISS is a heterogeneous condition, whose frequency will decrease with expanding knowledge. GH in supraphysiologic dosage increases the final height by about 7 cm, but for the individual child, the height gain is difficult to predict. Future elucidation of genetic factors involved in growth and maturation may lead to alternative therapeutic approaches.

References

1 Ranke MB: Towards a consensus on the definition of idiopathic short stature. Summary. Horm Res 1996;45(suppl 2):64–66.
2 Wit JM: Idiopathic short stature: reflections about definition and spontaneous growth. Horm Res, in press.
3 Grote FK, Oostdijk W, De Muinck Keizer-Schrama SM, Dekker FW, Verkerk PH, Wit JM: Growth monitoring and diagnostic work-up of short stature: an international inventorization. J Pediatr Endocrinol Metab 2005;18:1031–1038.
4 van Rijn JC, Grote FK, Oostdijk W, Wit JM: Short stature and the probability of coeliac disease, in the absence of gastrointestinal symptoms. Arch Dis Child 2004;89:882–883.
5 Donaldson MDC, Paterson W: Abnormal growth: definition, pathogenesis and practical assessment; in Kelnar CJH, Savage MO, Stirling H, Saenger P (eds): Growth Disorders. Pathophysiology and Treatment. London, Chapman and Hall, 1998, pp 197–224.
6 Adedoyin O, Gottlieb B, Frank R, et al: Evaluation of failure to thrive: diagnostic yield of testing for renal tubular acidosis. Pediatrics 2003;112:e463.
7 Rosenfeld RG: The molecular basis of idiopathic short stature. Growth Horm IGF Res 2005;15:S3–S5.
8 Rosenfeld RG, Albertsson-Wikland K, Cassorla F, et al: Diagnostic controversy: the diagnosis of childhood growth hormone deficiency revisited. J Clin Endocrinol Metab 1995;80:1532–1540.
9 Consensus guidelines for the diagnosis and treatment of growth hormone (GH) deficiency in childhood and adolescence: summary statement of the GH Research Society. GH Research Society. J Clin Endocrinol Metab 2000;85:3990–3993.
10 Marin G, Domene HM, Barnes KM, Blackwell BJ, Cassorla FG, Cutler GB Jr: The effects of estrogen priming and puberty on the growth hormone response to standardized treadmill exercise and arginine-insulin in normal girls and boys. J Clin Endocrinol Metab 1994;79:537–541.
11 Tauber M, Moulin P, Pienkowski C, Jouret B, Rochiccioli P: Growth hormone (GH) retesting and auxological data in 131 GH-deficient patients after completion of treatment. J Clin Endocrinol Metab 1997;82:352–356.
12 Millar DS, Lewis MD, Horan M, et al: Novel mutations of the growth hormone 1 (GH1) gene disclosed by modulation of the clinical selection criteria for individuals with short stature. Hum Mutat 2003;21:424–440.
13 Horan M, Millar DS, Hedderich J, et al: Human growth hormone 1 (GH1) gene expression: complex haplotype-dependent influence of polymorphic variation in the proximal promoter and locus control region. Hum Mutat 2003;21:408–423.
14 Spiliotis BE, August GP, Hung W, Sonis W, Mendelson W, Bercu BB: Growth hormone neurosecretory dysfunction. A treatable cause of short stature. JAMA 1984;251:2223–2230.
15 Dammacco F, Boghen MF, Camanni F, et al: Somatotropic function in short stature: evaluation by integrated auxological and hormonal indices in 214 children. J Clin Endocrinol Metab 1993;77:68–72.
16 Rogol AD, Blethen SL, Sy JP, Veldhuis JD: Do growth hormone (GH) serial sampling, insulin-like growth factor-I (IGF-I) or auxological measurements have an advantage over GH stimulation testing in predicting the linear growth response to GH therapy? Clin Endocrinol (Oxf) 2003;58:229–237.
17 Kamp GA, Zwinderman AH, van Doorn J, et al: Biochemical markers of growth hormone (GH) sensitivity in children with idiopathic short stature: individual capacity of IGF-I generation after high-dose GH treatment determines the growth response to GH. Clin Endocrinol (Oxf) 2002;57:315–325.
18 Rosenfeld RG: Molecular mechanisms of IGF-I deficiency. Horm Res 2006;65(suppl 1):15–20.
19 Goddard AD, Dowd P, Chernausek S, et al: Partial growth-hormone insensitivity: the role of growth-hormone receptor mutations in idiopathic short stature. J Pediatr 1997;131:S51–S55.
20 Hujeirat Y, Hess O, Shalev S, Tenenbaum-Rakover Y: Growth hormone receptor sequence changes do not play a role in determining height in children with idiopathic short stature. Horm Res 2006;65:210–216.
21 Kofoed EM, Hwa V, Little B, et al: Growth hormone insensitivity associated with a STAT5b mutation. N Engl J Med 2003;349:1139–1147.
22 Janssen R, van Wengen A, Hoeve MA, et al: The same IκBα mutation in two related individuals leads to completely different clinical syndromes. J Exp Med 2004;200:559–568.
23 Domene HM, Bengolea SV, Martinez AS, et al: Deficiency of the circulating insulin-like growth factor system associated with inactivation of the acid-labile subunit gene. N Engl J Med 2004;350:570–577.
24 Woods KA, Camacho-Hubner C, Savage MO, Clark AJ: Intrauterine growth retardation and postnatal growth failure associated with deletion of the insulin-like growth factor I gene. N Engl J Med 1996;335:1363–1367.
25 Walenkamp MJ, Karperien M, Pereira AM, et al: Homozygous and heterozygous expression of a novel insulin-like growth factor-I mutation. J Clin Endocrinol Metab 2005;90:2855–2864.
26 Abuzzahab MJ, Schneider A, Goddard A, et al: IGF-I receptor mutations resulting in intrauterine and postnatal growth retardation. N Engl J Med 2003;349:2211–2222.
27 Walenkamp MJE, Wit JM: Genetic disorders in the growth hormone-IGF-I axis. Horm Res 2006;66:221–230.
28 Cotterill AM, Camacho-Hubner C, Duquesnoy P, Savage MO: Changes in serum IGF-I and IGFBP-3 concentrations during the IGF-I generation test performed prospectively in children with short stature. Clin Endocrinol (Oxf) 1998;48:719–724.
29 Lopez-Bermejo A, Buckway CK, Rosenfeld RG: Genetic defects of the growth hormone-insulin-like growth factor axis. Trends Endocrinol Metab 2000;11:39–49.
30 Buckway CK, Guevara-Aguirre J, Pratt KL, Burren CP, Rosenfeld RG: The IGF-I generation test revisited: a marker of GH sensitivity. J Clin Endocrinol Metab 2001;86:5176–5183.
31 Buckway CK, Selva KA, Pratt KL, Tjoeng E, Guevara-Aguirre J, Rosenfeld RG: Insulin-like growth factor binding protein-3 generation as a measure of GH sensitivity. J Clin Endocrinol Metab 2002;87:4754–4765.
32 Selva KA, Buckway CK, Sexton G, et al: Reproducibility in patterns of IGF generation with special reference to idiopathic short stature. Horm Res 2003;60:237–246.

33 Rosenfeld RG, Buckway C, Selva K, Pratt KL, Guevara-Aguirre J: Insulin-like growth factor (IGF) parameters and tools for efficacy: the IGF-I generation test in children. Horm Res 2004; 62(suppl 1):37–43.
34 Kant SG, Wit JM, Breuning MH: Genetic analysis of short stature. Horm Res 2003;60:157–165.
35 Rappold GA, Fukami M, Niesler B, et al: Deletions of the homeobox gene SHOX (short stature homeobox) are an important cause of growth failure in children with short stature. J Clin Endocrinol Metab 2002;87:1402–1406.
36 Munns CF, Glass IA, Flanagan S, et al: Familial growth and skeletal features associated with SHOX haploinsufficiency. J Pediatr Endocrinol Metab 2003;16:987–996.
37 Richter-Unruh A, Knauer-Fischer S, Kaspers S, Albrecht B, Gillessen-Kaesbach G, Hauffa BP: Short stature in children with an apparently normal male phenotype can be caused by 45,X/46,XY mosaicism and is susceptible to growth hormone treatment. Eur J Pediatr 2004;163:251–256.
38 Olney RC, Bukulmez H, Bartels CF, et al: Heterozygous mutations in natriuretic peptide receptor-B *(NPR2)* are associated with short stature. J Clin Endocrinol Metab 2006;91:1229–1232.
39 Heitmann BL, Sorensen TIA, Keiding N, Skakkebaek NE: Predicting the adult height of short children. Br Med J 1994; 308:360.
40 Ranke MB, Grauer ML, Kistner K, Blum WF, Wollmann HA: Spontaneous adult height in idiopathic short stature. Horm Res 1995;44:152–157.
41 Wit JM, Kamp GA, Rikken B: Spontaneous growth and response to growth hormone treatment in children with growth hormone deficiency and idiopathic short stature. Pediatr Res 1996; 39:295–302.
42 Price DA: Spontaneous adult height in patients with idiopathic short stature. Horm Res 1996;45(suppl 2):59–63.
43 Rekers-Mombarg LTM, Wit JM, Massa GG, et al: Spontaneous growth in idiopathic short stature. Arch Dis Child 1996;75:175–180.
44 Wit JM, Rekers-Mombarg LT: Final height gain by GH therapy in children with idiopathic short stature is dose dependent. J Clin Endocrinol Metab 2002;87:604–611.
45 Hindmarsh PC: Evidence-based decisions in growth hormone therapy; in Hindmarsh PC (ed): Current Indications for Growth Hormone Therapy. Basel, Karger, 1999, pp 1–12.
46 Farewell VT, Cook RJ: Methodological issues for clinical trials in growth hormone therapy; in Hindmarsh PC (ed): Current Indications for Growth Hormone Therapy. Basel, Karger, 1999, pp 13–32.
47 Wit JM, Rietveld DH, Drop SL, et al: A controlled trial of methionyl growth hormone therapy in prepubertal children with short stature, subnormal growth rate and normal growth hormone response to secretagogues. Acta Paediatr Scand 1989;78:426–435.
48 Wit JM, Fokker MH, de Muinck Keizer-Schrama SMPF, et al: Effects of two years of methionyl growth hormone therapy in two dosage regimens in prepubertal children with short stature, subnormal growth rate and normal growth hormone response to secretagogues. J Pediatr 1989;115:720–725.
49 Rekers-Mombarg LT, Massa GG, Wit JM, et al: Growth hormone therapy with three dosage regimens in children with idiopathic short stature. European Study Group Participating Investigators. J Pediatr 1998;132:455–460.
50 Wit JM, Rekers-Mombarg LT, Cutler GB, et al: Growth hormone (GH) treatment to final height in children with idiopathic short stature: evidence for a dose effect. J Pediatr 2005;146:45–53.
51 Leschek EW, Rose SR, Yanovski JA, et al: Effect of growth hormone treatment on adult height in peripubertal children with idiopathic short stature: a randomized, double-blind, placebo-controlled trial. J Clin Endocrinol Metab 2004;89:3140–3148.
52 McCaughey ES, Mulligan J, Voss LD, Betts PR: Randomised trial of growth hormone in short normal girls. Lancet 1998;351:940–944.
53 Kamp GA, Waelkens JJ, De Muinck Keizer-Schrama SM, et al: High dose growth hormone treatment induces acceleration of skeletal maturation and an earlier onset of puberty in children with idiopathic short stature. Arch Dis Child 2002;87:215–220.
54 Lesage C, Walker J, Landier F, Chatelain P, Chaussain JL, Bougneres PF: Near normalization of adolescent height with growth hormone therapy in very short children without growth hormone deficiency. J Pediatr 1991;119: 29–34.
55 Brämswig JH, Fasse M, Holthoff ML, von Lengerke HJ, von Petrykowski W, Schellong G: Adult height in boys and girls with untreated short stature and constitutional delay of growth and puberty: Accuracy of five different methods of height prediction. J Pediatr 1990; 117:886–891.
56 Finkelstein BS, Imperiale TF, Speroff T, Marrero U, Radcliffe DJ, Cuttler L: Effect of growth hormone therapy on height in children with idiopathic short stature: a meta-analysis. Arch Pediatr Adolesc Med 2002;156:230–240.
57 Bryant J, Cave C, Milne R: Recombinant growth hormone for idiopathic short stature in children and adolescents. Cochrane Database Syst Rev 2003;(2):CD0044440. DOI: 10.1002/14651858.CD004440.
58 Kemp SF, Kuntze J, Attie KM, et al: Efficacy and safety results of long-term growth hormone treatment of idiopathic short stature. J Clin Endocrinol Metab 2005;90:5247–5253.
59 Hintz RL, Attie KM, Baptista J, Roche A: Effect of growth hormone treatment on adult height of children with idiopathic short stature. Genentech Collaborative Group. N Engl J Med 1999;340: 502–507.
60 Park P, Cohen P: The role of insulin-like growth factor I monitoring in growth hormone-treated children. Horm Res 2004;62(suppl 1):59–65.
61 Bright GM, Julius JR, Lima J, Blethen SL: Growth hormone stimulation test results as predictors of recombinant human growth hormone treatment outcomes: preliminary analysis of the national cooperative growth study database. Pediatrics 1999;104:1028–1031.
62 Zadik Z, Landau H, Limoni Y, Lieberman E: Predictors of growth response to growth hormone in otherwise normal short children. J Pediatr 1992;121: 44–48.

63 Kristrom B, Jansson C, Rosberg S, Albertsson-Wikland K: Growth response to growth hormone (GH) treatment relates to serum insulin-like growth factor I (IGF-I) and IGF-binding protein-3 in short children with various GH secretion capacities. Swedish Study Group for Growth Hormone Treatment. J Clin Endocrinol Metab 1997;82:2889–2898.

64 Rikken B, van Doorn J, Ringeling A, Van den Brande JL, Massa G, Wit JM: Plasma levels of insulin-like growth factor (IGF)-I, IGF-II and IGF-binding protein-3 in the evaluation of childhood growth hormone deficiency. Horm Res 1998;50:166–176.

65 Ranke MB, Guilbaud O, Lindberg A, Cole T: Prediction of the growth response in children with various growth disorders treated with growth hormone: analyses of data from the Kabi Pharmacia International Growth Study. International Board of the Kabi Pharmacia International Growth Study. Acta Paediatr Suppl 1993;82(suppl 391):82–88.

66 Coutant R, de Casson FB, Rouleau S, et al: Divergent effect of endogenous and exogenous sex steroids on the insulin-like growth factor I response to growth hormone in short normal adolescents. J Clin Endocrinol Metab 2004;89:6185–6192.

67 Thalange NK, Price DA, Gill MS, Whatmore AJ, Addison GM, Clayton PE: Insulin-like growth factor binding protein-3 generation: an index of growth hormone insensitivity. Pediatr Res 1996;39:849–855.

68 Attie KM, Carlsson LM, Rundle AC, Sherman BM: Evidence for partial growth hormone insensitivity among patients with idiopathic short stature. The National Cooperative Growth Study. J Pediatr 1995;127:244–250.

69 Darendeliler F, Ocal C, Bas F: Evaluation of insulin-like growth factor (IGF)-I and IGF binding protein-3 generation test in short stature. J Pediatr Endocrinol Metab 2005;18:443–452.

70 Dos SC, Essioux L, Teinturier C, Tauber M, Goffin V, Bougneres P: A common polymorphism of the growth hormone receptor is associated with increased responsiveness to growth hormone. Nat Genet 2004;36:720–724.

71 Wit JM, Balen HV, Kamp GA, Oostdijk W: Benefit of postponing normal puberty for improving final height. Eur J Endocrinol 2004;151(suppl 1):S41–S45.

72 Kamp GA, Mul D, Waelkens JJ, et al: A randomized controlled trial of three years growth hormone and gonadotropin-releasing hormone agonist treatment in children with idiopathic short stature and intrauterine growth retardation. J Clin Endocrinol Metab 2001; 86:2969–2975.

73 Balducci R, Toscano V, Mangiantini A, et al: Adult height in short normal adolescent girls treated with gonadotropin-releasing hormone analog and growth hormone. J Clin Endocrinol Metab 1995;80:3596–3600.

74 Pasquino AM, Pucarelli I, Roggini M, Segni M: Adult height in short normal girls treated with gonadotropin-releasing hormone analogs and growth hormone. J Clin Endocrinol Metab 2000; 85:619–622.

75 Kaplowitz PB: If gonadotropin-releasing hormone plus growth hormone (GH) really improves growth outcomes in short non-GH-deficient children, then what? J Clin Endocrinol Metab 2001;86:2965–2968.

76 Dunkel L: Use of aromatase inhibitors to increase final height. Mol Cell Endocrinol 2006;254–255:207–216.

77 Hero M, Wickman S, Dunkel L: Treatment with the aromatase inhibitor letrozole during adolescence increases near-final height in boys with constitutional delay of puberty. Clin Endocrinol (Oxf) 2006;64:510–513.

78 Kawai M, Momoi T, Yorifuji T, et al: Combination therapy with GH and cyproterone acetate does not improve final height in boys with non-GH-deficient short stature. Clin Endocrinol (Oxf) 1998;48:53–57.

79 Raile K, Klammt J, Schneider A, et al: Clinical and functional characteristics of the human Arg59Ter insulin-like growth factor 1 receptor (IGF1R) mutation: implications for a gene dosage effect of the human IGF1R. J Clin Endocrinol Metab 2006;91:2264–2271.

80 Schubbert S, Zenker M, Rowe SL, et al: Germline KRAS mutations cause Noonan syndrome. Nat Genet 2006;38: 331–336.

81 Kamp GA: Growth hormone secretion, sensitivity and treatment in short children. Academic thesis. Leiden University, 2000.

82 Wit JM: Growth hormone therapy. Best Pract Res Clin Endocrinol Metab 2002; 16:483–503.

Short- and Long-Term Response to Growth Hormone in Idiopathic Short Stature: KIGS Analysis of Factors Predicting Growth

Michael B. Ranke[a]   Anders Lindberg[b]   David A. Price[c]   Feyza Darendeliler[d]
Kerstin Albertsson-Wikland[e]   Patrick Wilton[f]   Edward O. Reiter[g]

Inclusion Criteria and Patient Cohorts

Our study included patients classified by investigators as having idiopathic short stature (ISS) or idiopathic growth hormone deficiency (GHD) as defined by the KIGS Aetiology Classification List (diagnostic code Nos. 3.1 and 1.1), in whom the results of GH provocation tests showed peak values that exceeded 10 μg/l. An exclusion criterion for this study was a birth weight standard deviation score (SDS) below −2.0 for gestational age. A total of 5,246 children with ISS were documented in the KIGS database by January 2006. Information about all ISS patients included in KIGS before and at the start of GH treatment is listed in table 1.

A total of 2,875 prepubertal patients were treated for a full year. Information about these patients at the start of GH treatment and after 1 year on GH is listed in table 2.

Two cohorts were analyzed in our study: the first comprised the final height group (n = 327), synonymous with near adult height (NAH), and the second group (n = 657) served as the prediction model cohort. Patients in the NAH group had received at least 4 years of GH therapy, of which at least 1 year was before the onset of puberty (puberty was defined as a max testes volume >3 ml, or Tanner breast stage B2+). Height measurements were recorded at intervals of 9–15 months and used to calculate height velocity (centimeters per year). The only patients considered were those receiving more than 5 injections of GH per week. The end of growth was taken to be ≥16 years in boys and ≥14 years in girls, as well as when the height velocity during the preceding years was <2 cm/year, or when the growth curve showed an asymptotic pattern indicating the end of growth. The GH dosage remained ap-

[a]Paediatric Endocrinology Section
University Children's Hospital, University of Tübingen
Hoppe-Seyler-Strasse 1, DE–72076 Tübingen (Germany)
[b]Pfizer Endocrine Care
KIGS/KIMS/ACROSTUDY Medical Outcomes
Vetenskapsvägen 10, SE–191 90 Sollentuna (Sweden)
[c]Royal Manchester Children's Hospital, Hospital Road
Pendlebury, Swinton, Manchester M27 4HA (UK)
[d]Department of Pediatrics, Istanbul Faculty of Medicine
Istanbul University, TR–34390 Capa–Istanbul (Turkey)
[e]Paediatric Growth Research Centre, Department of Paediatrics
Queen Silvia Children's Hospital, Sahlgrenska, Academy of
Gothenburg University, SE–416 85 Gothenburg (Sweden)
[f]Pfizer Inc., 235 East 42nd Street, New York, NY 10017-15515 (USA)
[g]Baystate Children's Hospital, Tufts University School of Medicine
759 Chestnut Street, Springfield, MA 01199 (USA)

Table 1. All ISS patients documented at the start of GH therapy

	All				Females		Males	
	n	median	10th centile	90th centile	n	median	n	median
Background								
Birth weight SDS	4,602	−0.7	−1.6	0.6	1,555	−0.7	3,047	−0.7
Birth length SDS	3,204	−0.4	−1.5	0.9	1,108	−0.5	2,096	−0.4
MPH SDS (Prader)	4,961	−1.9	−3.1	−0.2	1,674	−1.9	3,287	−1.8
Maximum GH, µg/l	5,246	14.4	10.7	28.0	1,776	14.4	3,470	14.5
IGF-1 SDS	1,170	−1.8	−3.0	−0.4	370	−1.8	800	−1.8
At GH start								
Age, years	5,246	10.8	5.5	14.3	1,776	10.6	3,470	10.9
Bone age, years	2,265	8.5	3.0	12.5	764	8.5	1,501	8.5
Height SDS (Prader)	5,246	−3.0	−4.1	−2.1	1,776	−3.2	3,470	−2.9
Height velocity, cm/year	2,389	4.5	2.9	0.2	818	4.6	1,571	4.5
BMI SDS	5,246	−0.5	−1.9	0.9	1,776	−0.6	3,470	−0.5
GH dose, mg/kg/week	5,246	0.19	0.15	0.30	1,776	0.19	3,470	0.19

IGF-1 = Insulin-like growth factor 1; BMI = body mass index.

Table 2. Prepubertal ISS patients treated for the first year with GH

	All				Females		Males	
	n	median	10th centile	90th centile	n	median	n	median
At GH start								
Age, years	2,875	9.1	5.1	12.9	856	8.6	2,019	9.4
Bone age, years	1,300	6.8	2.8	11.0	380	6.5	920	7.0
Height SDS (Prader)	2,875	−3.1	−4.1	−2.2	856	3.4	2,019	−3.0
Height velocity, cm/year	1,409	4.6	3.0	6.3	443	4.6	966	4.6
Height velocity SDS (Prader)	1,405	−1.5	−3.8	0.5	443	−1.6	962	−1.4
BMI SDS	2,875	−0.5	−1.8	0.8	856	−0.6	2,019	−0.4
GH dose, mg/kg/week	2,875	0.19	0.16	0.30	856	0.19	2,019	0.19
After 1 year								
Age, years	2,875	10.1	6.0	13.9	856	9.5	2,019	10.4
Height SDS (Prader)	2,875	−2.5	−3.5	−1.5	856	−2.6	2,019	−2.4
Height velocity, cm/year	2,875	7.7	5.7	10.1	856	7.6	2,019	7.7
Height velocity SDS (Prader)	2,871	2.7	−0.4	6.1	855	2.3	2,016	2.9
Δ height SDS (Prader)	2,875	0.5	−0.2	0.9	856	0.5	2,019	0.5
Studentized residual (2) SDS	962	−0.5	−1.6	0.6	251	−0.6	711	−0.4
BMI SDS	2,857	−0.5	−0.5	−1.8	848	−0.7	2,009	−0.4

BMI = Body mass index; studentized residual (2) = applying the model for IGHD without maxGH.

proximately constant during the total period of treatment.

Analysis of Factors Predicting the First Prepubertal Year on Growth Hormone

Data of 657 prepubertal children treated for at least 1 prepubertal year and for whom data are available for all the parameters relevant to the prediction analysis were used for an analysis of first-year height velocity, as described before. Through this multiple linear regression analysis, we found 4 variables predictive of the growth response: age, GH dose, height – midparental (MPH) SDS, and weight SDS. All single predictors were significant ($p < 0.0001$). The equation describing the predicted height velocity for the first year of GH therapy is as follows: predicted height velocity (cm/year) = 9.11 + [–0.29 × age at GH start (years)] + [0.31 × weight SDS at GH start] + [7.28 × GH dose (mg/kg/week)] + [–0.33 × (height – MPH) SDS]; error SD = ±1.2 cm/year. By means of this 4-parameter model, 39% of the variability of the growth response could be explained. Age was the most important of the 4 identified predictors, accounting for 21% of the variability, followed by GH dosage (11%), weight SDS (4%) and height deficit (height – MPH SDS, 4%). We did not include the height SDS in the model because it correlated highly with the weight SDS ($R^2 = 0.93$; $p < 0.0001$) and also because its predictive value was lower. Our results clearly show that the strongest response to treatment during the first year occurs in younger children on higher doses of GH.

Determinants of Response to Growth Hormone Leading to Adult Height

A multiple linear regression analysis was conducted based on 256 (148 male) individuals who had reached NAH on GH in order to determine the factors influencing the adult height reached and the change in height, respectively. The characteristics of these patients at GH start, at puberty onset and at NAH are listed in table 3. The height at the start of GH treatment and NAH are illustrated in figure 1 in comparison with the normal reference ranges of Prader. The height SDS and the height SDS corrected for MPH at GH start, after the first year on GH, at puberty onset and at NAH are illustrated in figure 2.

The regression equation for the NAH height SDS was: final height SDS = 1.26 + [0.37 × MPH SDS] + [–0.05 × age (years)] + [0.70 × height SDS] + [0.24 × studentized residual during the first year of GH therapy]. This equation explains 64% of the variability, with an error of 0.6 SD. Thus, the height achieved depends on the height at the time GH therapy starts (the taller, the better), the age at GH start (the younger, the better), the stature of the parents (the taller, the better), and the first-year responsiveness to GH (the greater, the better). Simple linear regression between the NAH height SDS and the height SDS at GH start as well as the studentized residuals for the first year on GH therapy is illustrated in figure 3.

The regression equation for the change in the height SDS from GH start to final height was: Δ height SDS = 1.13 + [–0.36 × (height – MPH) SDS] + [–0.05 × age (years)] + [0.24 × studentized residual during the first year]. This equation explains 39% of the variability, with an error of 0.6 SD. The gain in the height SDS is associated with the distance between the height at GH start and the target height (the smaller the patient, the better), the age at GH start (the younger, the better) and the responsiveness to GH during the first year (the greater, the better). Simple linear regression between the Δ height SDS (total gain in height) and the height – MPH SDS as well as the first-year studentized residuals is illustrated in figure 4. Thus, the responsiveness during the first year is related to both the absolute final height as well as the gain in height.

Table 3. ISS patients treated to final height with GH

	All				Females		Males	
	n	median	10th centile	90th centile	n	median	n	median
At GH start								
Age, years	327	9.6	6.0	12.5	137	9.0	190	10.1
Bone age, years	168	7.3	3.5	10.0	64	7.0	104	7.5
Height SDS (Prader)	327	−3.1	−4.2	−2.2	137	−3.4	190	−2.9
Height velocity, cm/year	175	4.6	3.1	6.0	76	4.4	99	4.6
Height velocity SDS (Prader)	175	−1.3	−3.7	0.4	76	−1.4	99	−1.2
BMI SDS	327	−0.5	−1.7	0.6	137	−0.6	190	−0.5
GH dose, mg/kg/week	327	0.19	0.15	0.27	137	0.19	190	0.19
At puberty								
Age, years	126	12.4	10.6	14.3	52	11.9	74	12.6
Height SDS (Prader)	126	−1.6	−2.5	−0.7	52	−1.7	74	−1.6
Δ height SDS between GH start and puberty (Prader)	126	1.4	0.7	2.5	52	1.6	74	1.2
BMI SDS	126	−0.5	−2.0	0.7	52	−0.5	74	−0.5
NAH								
Age, years	327	17.1	15.0	19.0	137	15.8	190	17.7
Height SDS (Prader)	327	−1.7	−3.1	−0.6	137	−2.1	190	−1.6
Δ height SDS between puberty and the end of GH treatment (Prader)	126	0.1	−0.8	0.8	52	0.1	74	0.1
BMI SDS	321	−0.2	−1.5	1.0	133	−0.2	188	−0.2
Years of puberty on GH	126	4.0	2.5	5.7	52	3.7	74	4.2
Total years on GH	327	6.6	4.6	10.0	137	6.3	190	7.0

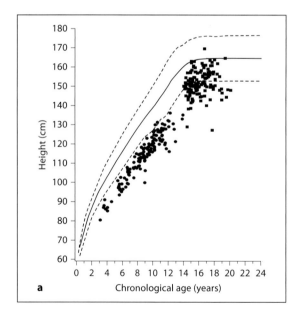
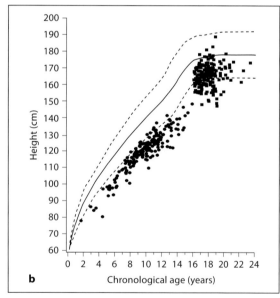

Fig. 1. Height at GH start in boys (**a**) and girls (**b**) with ISS who have reached NAH, compared with references of Prader. Dashed lines = −2 and +2 SD of normal references; solid line = 0 SD of normal references.

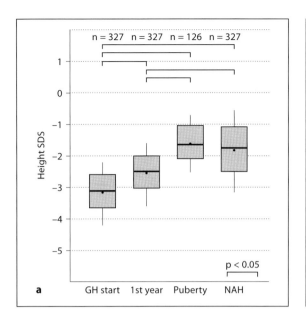
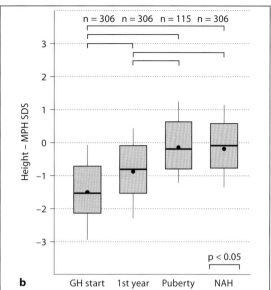

Fig. 2. Height SDS (**a**) and height – MPH SDS (**b**) in children with ISS treated to NAH at GH start, after 1 year, at puberty onset and at NAH.

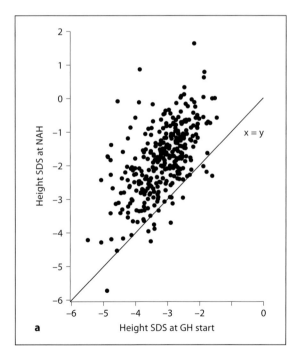
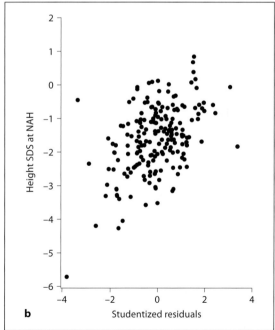

Fig. 3. Simple linear correlations between the NAH SDS and the height SDS at GH start (**a**), as well as the studentized residuals of the first prepubertal year on GH (**b**).

KIGS Analysis of Short- and Long-Term Response to GH in ISS 323

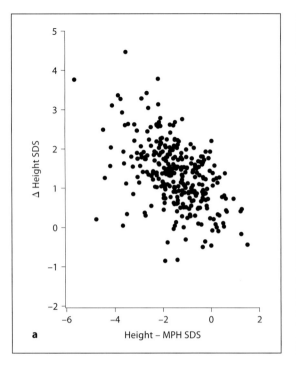 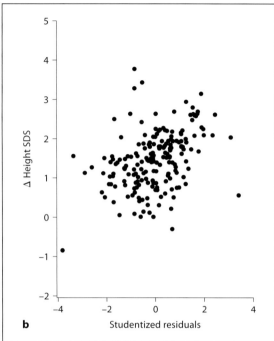

Fig. 4. Simple linear correlations between the gain in the total height SDS (from the start of GH treatment to NAH) and the height SDS corrected for the MPH SDS (**a**), as well as the studentized residuals of the first prepubertal year on GH (**b**).

Discussion

The issues related to the treatment of ISS patients with GH are discussed in great detail by Jan Maarten Wit [this vol., pp. 309–318].

For the NAH analysis, we only included the data of children (1) who had received at least 4 years of recombinant human GH treatment, including 1 year preceding puberty, (2) who had reached NAH, and (3) whose height velocity during the first year of GH treatment could be accurately calculated within a time frame of 9–15 months. The limitations of pharmacoepidemiological studies are chiefly related to the fact that (1) there is no built-in control for reporting to the databases, (2) the information is voluntarily provided by a multitude of investigators, and (3) no untreated patients are available as a control group.

However, analyses from the KIGS database have shown that the anthropometrical data available are not qualitatively inferior than those of formal studies and that there is no bias in reporting.

The patients in the KIGS cohort were treated with variable doses of GH within a relatively narrow dosage range which was of the same magnitude as GH replacement dosages for patients with idiopathic GHD. The total gain in height, from the beginning to the end of GH therapy, amounted to 1.4 SDS in males and 1.3 SDS in females. These figures do not differ statistically. We found no indication of an earlier onset of puberty in the cohort; instead, there was a delay in the age of pubertal onset.

In view of observations reported in studies of idiopathic GHD, which showed that high GH doses applied during puberty only led to minor height gain, we decided to focus our analysis on patients with a long phase of prepubertal treatment. It can also be assumed that any height gain in young children is of great psychological benefit, and that treatment is more cost-effective in younger/smaller individuals. Prepubertal treatment in these patients is undoubtedly efficacious.

The analysis of our data shows that the NAH SDS correlates positively with the height SDS at the start of GH therapy (the taller, the better); it correlates negatively with the age at GH start and positively with the first-year response (data not shown), the Δ height SDS and the responsiveness (studentized residual) (fig. 4). The overall gain in the height SDS correlates positively with the height deviation from the target height (the smaller, the better), the GH dose and the gain in height during the first year of treatment (both response and responsiveness). This relationship between the short- and the long-term response suggests that the individual responsiveness to GH is a major determinant of the efficacy of GH treatment. The fact that less variability of the response could be explained, as compared with idiopathic GHD, Turner syndrome and small for gestational age children, suggests that ISS involves a more heterogeneous group in terms of the underlying pathogenesis of the growth disorder.

This analysis shows that severely short, prepubertal children who face the risk of remaining short do have a good chance to benefit from long-term GH treatment if they are young. Both the absolute final height as well as the gain in height are positively correlated with responsiveness to exogenous GH. This responsiveness to GH can be deduced from the first-year growth during GH treatment. Conversely, this information can subsequently be used to assess whether the continuation of GH treatment is appropriate in terms of individual benefits as well as in terms of cost-effectiveness.

Turner Syndrome – Growth Hormone Treatment

Ron G. Rosenfeld

As first described by Henry Turner [1] almost 60 years ago, the Turner syndrome (TS) was defined by phenotype, specifically the combination of cubitus valgus, webbing of the neck, sexual infantilism and short stature. With the development of karyotypic analysis 20 years later, a chromosomal definition of TS was advanced. However, it soon became apparent that monosomy for the X chromosome only accounted for approximately half of patients meeting the phenotypic criteria for TS, the balance proving to have either deletions of critical components of one X chromosome, or mosaicism involving an absent or deleted X chromosome. It is now clear that multiple genes are likely to be involved in the TS phenotype, explaining, at least in part, the phenotypic variability observed when patients with X chromosome monosomy, X chromosome deletions and mosaicism are compared. At least one such gene has been identified on Xp22.33 and termed 'SHOX' (short stature homeobox) [2]. Located on the pseudoautosomal region of the X and Y chromosomes, SHOX normally escapes X inactivation; haploinsufficiency of SHOX results in short stature in TS, as well as contributing to many of the characteristic skeletal deformities, such as micrognathia, mesomelia, cubitus valgus, short metacarpals, high-arched palate and Madelung deformity. Isolated heterozygosity for the SHOX gene is associated with Leri-Weil dyschondrosteosis, while the homozygous defect causes Langer's osteodysplasia. However, it is of note that the degree of short stature observed with simple haploinsufficiency for SHOX is, typically, not as severe as that observed with TS, suggesting that haploinsufficiency for additional genes located on the short arm of the X chromosome contributes to the growth retardation characteristic of TS [3, 4]. It is likely that some of these genes also play a role in the lymphatic hypoplasia and ovarian failure typical of TS. Thus, TS should not be equated with a mere SHOX deficiency. Rather, it is best defined as a constellation of physical features resulting from haploinsufficiency of a number of specific genes on the short arm of the X chromosome which normally escape X inactivation. Indeed, it is likely that a full spectrum of disorders exists, defined by the number of critical Xp genes that have been lost, and, consequently, no single definition of TS may ever be definitively identified.

Lucile Packard Foundation for Children's Health
(Stanford University), 400 Hamilton Avenue, Suite 340
Palo Alto, CA 94301 (USA)

Spontaneous Growth

Of all of the phenotypic features of TS, it is short stature which is both most common and the most frequent cause for referral to pediatric endocrinology centers. In most studies, >95% of TS patients seen in endocrinology clinics have some degree of growth retardation [5, 6]. While this observation undoubtedly reflects a degree of ascertainment bias, it is of note that even when evaluation is restricted to prenatally diagnosed TS, short stature remains a characteristic and highly frequent finding. In many cases, the growth retardation begins prenatally (although severe intrauterine growth retardation of liveborn TS patients is uncommon) and persists through early childhood [7]. Davenport et al. [8] reported that the mean height of TS patients fell from –0.7 standard deviations (SD) at birth, to –1.6, –1.8 and –2 SD at 1, 2 and 3 years, respectively. Growth attenuation was attributed to (1) a slow infancy growth component, (2) a slow childhood growth component, and (3) a delayed onset of the childhood growth component.

From early childhood on, height velocity typically hovers near the bottom of the normal range or slightly below, resulting in a gradual deviation from the normal growth curve. Thus, some TS patients remain within the lower part of the normal range until mid- or even late childhood, although >95% eventually fall below the –2 SD range for age. Added to the slow childhood growth is a delayed and frequently blunted adolescent growth spurt. While this may add some compensatory growth during late adolescence, it is generally insufficient to allow attainment of normal adult stature. As a result, TS patients end up with adult heights which are, typically, approximately 20 cm below the mean for females of their respective ethnic group. Although it has not been studied carefully, it does appear that the secular trend in height increase observed during the 20th century has affected the Turner population as well, although clearly not sufficiently to narrow the deficit with the normal population.

There are important diagnostic implications of the growth characteristics of TS. Growth failure is frequently subtle and cumulative, often resulting in a delayed diagnosis of TS. A cardinal rule of thumb should be that the diagnosis of TS should be considered in any girl with unexplained growth retardation, regardless of the presence or absence of dysmorphic features.

Height Prognosis

The construction of growth charts based upon the natural history of observed growth in TS has greatly aided our understanding of spontaneous growth in TS, as well as providing a tool for prognosis of adult height in individual TS patients. The earliest well-documented growth charts for TS girls were constructed by Lyon et al. [9], and these curves have provided a reasonable historical basis for assessing the effects of growth-promoting therapy. Furthermore, extensive analysis of growth of TS girls in the first 24 months of life has facilitated the development of growth curves for affected infants and young children [8]. Many individual countries have now established TS growth curves based upon their own indigenous populations of TS and normal females, and growth patterns for TS girls in different nations have been shown to reflect the genetic background of the population at hand [10]. Where possible and appropriate, ethnic-specific TS growth curves appear to be most suitable.

Prediction Models

Ranke et al. [11] have pioneered the development of prediction models for both short- and long-term height gains in TS patients treated with growth hormone (GH). In a follow-up to adult height of 188 GH-treated TS patients, the total

Δ height correlated negatively with bone age and the height SD score at the start of GH therapy, but positively with the Δ height after the first year of treatment and at the onset of puberty, as well as with the duration of GH treatment. The final height correlated positively with the height at the initiation of GH, the first-year Δ height and the height at the onset of puberty. Using a previously published predictive model [12], it was found that the height observed at follow-up and the height predicted at the start of therapy were highly correlated.

Review of the Literature on Growth Hormone Treatment

It is of historical note that Henry Turner [1], in his 1938 paper, first commented on the use of GH in TS: 'Anterior pituitary growth hormone, 2 cc three times daily, was prescribed, and injections were continued for approximately five months, without any appreciable increase in her height.' It is not entirely clear what Dr. Turner actually administered to this patient, as human cadaveric GH was not available until 20 years later. One must presume that at best, Dr. Turner prescribed a crude bovine or ovine pituitary extract, which never was likely to stimulate growth, even in children with GH deficiency. Nevertheless, the perceived inability of GH to stimulate growth in TS remained engrained for the next 40–50 years. This position was seemingly supported by observations that GH secretion was within the broad normal range, at least in prepubertal TS patients, who also tended to have normal serum concentrations of insulin-like growth factor 1.

However, by the 1970s, isolated case reports and clinical investigations began to suggest that GH might have some efficacy in TS [13, 14]. These studies had a number of important limitations: (1) the number of subjects studied was limited; (2) doses of GH employed were generally low; (3) duration of therapy was brief, often less than 1 year, and (4) studies were uncontrolled. Unfortunately, the first large-scale, partially controlled study was prematurely terminated by the removal of pituitary-derived human GH (hGH) from distribution in the United States [15].

One other study employing pituitary-derived hGH deserves comment. Rudman et al. [16] administered hGH, either alone or in combination with oxandolone, to 6 TS patients, with improvement in growth rates from a reported pretreatment value of 2.0 cm/year to 3.8 and 7.6 cm/year, respectively. These observations were extended in the first prospective, large-scale, randomized study of the use of recombinant hGH in TS [17, 18]. After an initial phase lasting 12–24 months, 70 prepubertal TS patients were randomly assigned to 1 of 4 groups: (group 1) observation, (group 2) oxandrolone 0.125 mg/kg/day, (group 3) hGH 0.125 mg/kg 3 times per week, or (group 4) combination GH plus oxandrolone at the dosages stated above. After 1–2 years in this first phase of the study, subjects receiving GH alone (group 3) continued to receive GH alone at the above dosage, which, after 2 years, was changed to the same weekly dosage but distributed over 7 daily administrations. Subjects in the other 3 arms were placed on combination GH plus oxandrolone (0.0625 mg/kg/day). The 17 subjects receiving GH alone all completed the trial and reached an adult height of 150.4 ± 5.5 cm (mean ± SD), 8.4 cm taller than their mean projected adult height, based on the TS growth curves of Lyon et al. [9]. The 43 subjects receiving GH plus oxandrolone attained a mean adult height of 152.1 ± 5.9 cm, 10.3 cm taller than their mean projected adult height. Although this study did not include a parallel control group not receiving treatment until adult height, a historical control group of TS patients attained a mean adult height of 144.2 cm, precisely matching their projected adult height and significantly shorter than either the GH alone or GH plus oxandrolone groups.

Although this study appeared to convincingly demonstrate the ability of GH to stimulate growth and enhance adult height in patients with TS, a few subsequent studies seemed to give less encouraging results [19–21]. However, in general, such studies were characterized by a relatively late age for the onset of GH therapy, a more modest GH dosage and/or early introduction of estrogen replacement. A major prospective Dutch study strongly supported the conclusions of the original American study and, indeed, extended these observations [22]. Employing several different GH regimens and a relatively late age for the onset of estrogen replacement, mean final heights ranging from 157.6 to 163.6 cm were achieved. Fifty of the 60 girls (83%) reached a final height within the normal range for women (i.e. above –2 SD). Depending upon the treatment protocol, the mean gain in height over the projected adult height ranged from 11.9 to 16.9 cm. The factors found to be most predictive of final height were the GH dosage, the height SD prior to treatment, the chronological age at the start of treatment and the height velocity during the first year of GH therapy. In both the American and Dutch studies, GH was well tolerated, with no significant adverse effects and no evidence of a diabetogenic effect.

A recently completed multicenter French study, employing GH at a mean dosage of 0.26 ± 0.06 mg/kg/week for a mean of 5.0 ± 2.2 years, and with a late introduction of estrogens (at a mean of 15 years of age), resulted in a mean adult height of 149.9 ± 6.1 cm, 8.5 cm above the mean projected adult height [23]. However, only a multicenter Canadian study employed a parallel, randomized control group that received no GH and was followed to adult height [24]. In this investigation, GH was administered 6 times per week at a dosage of 0.30 mg/kg/week, and both GH-treated and control subjects received estrogen replacement at 13 years of age. Interpretation of results is impacted, to some degree, by a relatively high dropout rate, especially in the control group. Of those completing the protocol, GH-treated subjects attained a mean adult height of 149 ± 6.4 cm, compared with 142.2 ± 6.6 cm in the control group. Analysis of covariance suggested a mean height gain due to GH of +7.2 cm.

Given the role of estrogen in epiphyseal maturation, it is not surprising that the age at which estrogen replacement commences impacts adult height (both in the presence and absence of GH treatment). While early studies indicated that delaying estrogen replacement could improve final height outcomes in TS patients receiving GH, such an approach is not always to be recommended, as delaying estrogen not only has the psychosocial disadvantage of delaying puberty in individuals who may already be suffering from a poor self-image, but may have a negative impact on bone mineral accretion and subsequent risk of osteoporosis [25]. These factors support the importance of early introduction of GH therapy, which will not only permit maximization of adult height, but allow for estrogen replacement at an age-appropriate time [26].

Outlook

As described above, studies from multiple countries, employing a variety of GH regimens, have established and confirmed the efficacy of GH therapy in stimulating growth in girls with TS. The general conclusions of these investigations may be summarized as follows.

1 GH treatment is capable of both stimulating short-term growth and enhancing adult stature in TS.
2 Early initiation of GH permits most TS girls to enter into the normal height range during childhood, thereby minimizing the period of short stature. It has become a not uncommon phenomenon to see TS girls who can never recall having been short, because treatment was begun at an early age.
3 Furthermore, early initiation of GH permits most TS girls to begin estrogen replacement (if necessary) at an age-appropriate time.

4 The response of TS patients to GH is not of the same magnitude as that observed in GH deficiency. Such observations support the realization that the growth failure of TS is not due to a perturbation of the GH/insulin-like growth factor axis, but rather reflects an underlying skeletal dysplasia resulting from *SHOX* deficiency, as well as haploinsufficiency of other critical genes located on the short arm of the X chromosome.
5 The response of TS patients to GH is, at least in part, dose dependent. Flexible GH dosing schedules should allow optimization of growth in individual patients.
6 GH has proven to be safe in TS. Early concerns about GH enhancing the risk of glucose intolerance or cardiac disease in TS have not been supported to date.

A major benefit of the availability of GH for TS, which, perhaps, would not have been predicted 20 years ago, has been the ability to bring large numbers of TS girls under the care of pediatric endocrinologists, often at much earlier ages than had been the case previously. Up through the 1970s, girls with TS had been scattered among cardiology, nephrology, genetics or general clinics, frequently never being referred for endocrine evaluation or not until pubertal delay or amenorrhea prompted endocrine consultation. The ability to follow large numbers of TS patients in endocrine clinics has resulted in a much greater appreciation of the natural history of TS, as well as an opportunity to develop protocols for integrated care. This has, in turn, led to investigations of the specific healthcare needs of adult TS women and to the emergence of clinics dedicated to such patients.

Despite this impressive progress, important issues remain [27].
1 How can the identification of TS patients at the earliest possible age be facilitated?
2 At what age should GH therapy be initiated? Options that have been recommended include: (1) as soon as the diagnosis has been made, (2) as soon as the patient falls below the 5th percentile of the normal female growth curve, and (3) at the age of 2 (or 4 years), but comparative data are lacking.
3 What GH regimen will simultaneously optimize growth and be most cost-effective?
4 Will prediction models help us address the question above?
5 Are there special characteristics of some TS patients which would render them more (or less) responsive to GH? Possible candidates that require further exploration include karyotype and polymorphisms of the GH receptor gene [28].
6 How does one ideally balance the need for growth and estrogen replacement?
7 Are there any long-term risks of GH therapy that have not been identified to date?
8 What genes, besides *SHOX*, contribute to the growth failure of TS?
9 What impact will growth-promoting therapy have on psychosocial well-being of individuals with TS?
10 How do we integrate GH therapy into a model of lifetime healthcare for TS patients?

As we assess the progress that has been made over the last 20 years in both the understanding of TS and in its treatment, it is all the more rewarding to note that these questions are addressable and that future years should lead to further improvements in the care for both girls and women with TS.

References

1 Turner H: A syndrome of infantilism, congenital webbed neck, and cubitus valgus. Endocrinology 1938;28:566–574.
2 Rao E, Weiss B, Fukami M, Rump A, Niesler B, Mertz A, Muroya K, Binder G, Kirsch S, Winkelmann M, Nordsiek G, Heinrich U, Breuning MH, Ranke MB, Rosenthal A, Ogata T, Rappold GA: Pseudoatosomal deletions encompassing a novel homeobox gene causes growth failure in idiopathic short stature and Turner syndrome. Nat Genet 1997;16:54–63.
3 Ogata T, Matsuo N: Sex chromosome aberrations and stature: deduction of the principal factors involved in the determination of adult height. Hum Genet 1993;91:551–562.
4 Zinn AR, Ross JL: Critical regions for Turner syndrome phenotypes on the X chromosome; in Saenger P, Pasquino AM (eds): Optimizing Health Care for Turner Patients in the 21st Century. Amsterdam, Elsevier, 2000, pp 19–28.
5 Palmer CG, Reichmann A: Chromosomal and clinical findings in 110 females with Turner syndrome. Hum Genet 1976;35:35–49.
6 Park E, Bailey JD, Ciwell CA: Growth and maturation of patients with Turner's syndrome. Pediatr Res 1983;17:1–7.
7 Ranke MB, Stubbe P, Majewski F, Bierich JR: Spontaneous growth in Turner's syndrome. Acta Paediatr Suppl 1988;343:22–30.
8 Davenport ML, Punyasavatstut N, Gunther D, Savendahl L, Stewart PW: Turner syndrome: a pattern of early growth failure. Acta Paediatr Suppl 1999;88:118–121.
9 Lyon AL, Preece MA, Grant DB: Growth curves for girls with Turner syndrome. Arch Dis Child 1985;60:932–935.
10 Ranke MB, Grauer ML: Adult height in Turner syndrome: results of a multinational study 1993. Horm Res 1994;42:90–94.
11 Ranke MB, Partsch CJ, Lindberg A, Dörr HG, Bettendorf M, Hauffa BP, Schwartz HP, Mehls O, Sander S, Stahnke N, Steinkamp H, Said E, Sippell W: Adult height after GH therapy in 188 Ullrich-Turner syndrome patients: results of the German IGLU follow-up study 2001. Eur J Endocrinol 2002;147:625–633.
12 Ranke M, Lindberg A, Chatelain P, Wilton P, Cutfield W, Albertsson-Wikland K, Price DA: Prediction of long-term response to recombinant human growth hormone in Turner syndrome: development and validation of mathematical models. J Clin Endocrinol Metab 2000;85:4212–4218.
13 Hutchings JJ, Escamilla RF, Li CH, Forsham PH: Human growth hormone administration in Turner's syndrome. Am J Dis Child 1965;109:318–321.
14 Tzagournis M: Response to long-term administration of human growth hormone in Turner's syndrome. JAMA 1969;210:2373–2376.
15 Raiti S, Moore WV, Van Vliet G, Kaplan S: Growth-stimulating effects of human growth hormone therapy in patients with Turner syndrome. J Pediatr 1986;109:944–949.
16 Rudman D, Goldsmith M, Kutner M, Blackston D: Effect of growth hormone and oxandrolone singly and together on growth rate in girls with X chromosome abnormalities. J Pediatr 1980;96:132–135.
17 Rosenfeld RG, Hintz RL, Johanson AJ, Brasel JA, Burstein S, Chernausek SD, Clabots T, Frane J, Gotlin RW, Kuntze J, Lippe BM, Mahoney PC, Moore WV, New MI, Saenger P, Stoner E, Sybert V: Methionyl human growth hormone and oxandrolone in Turner syndrome: preliminary results of a prospective randomized trial. J Pediatr 1986;109:936–943.
18 Rosenfeld RG, Attie KM, Frane J, Brasel JA, Burstein S, Cara JF, Chernausek S, Gotlin RW, Kuntze J, Lippe BM, Mahoney CP, Moore WV, Saenger P, Johanson AJ: Growth hormone therapy of Turner's syndrome: beneficial effect on adult height. J Pediatr 1998;132:319–324.
19 Van den Broeck J, Massa GG, Attanasio A, Matranga A, Chaussain JL, Price DA, Arskog D, Wit JM: Final height after long-term growth hormone treatment in Turner syndrome. European Study Group. J Pediatr 1995;127:729–735.
20 Chu CE, Paterson WF, Kelnar CJ, Smail PJ, Greene SA, Donaldson MD: Variable effect of growth hormone on growth and final adult height in Scottish patients with Turner's syndrome. Acta Paediatr 1997;86:160–164.
21 Taback SP, Collu R, Deal CL, Guyda HJ, Salisbury S, Dean HJ, Van Vliet G: Does growth hormone supplementation affect adult height in Turner's syndrome? Lancet 1996;348:25–27.
22 van Parenen YK, de Muinck Keizer-Schrama SMPF, Stijnen T, Sas TCJ, Jansen M, Otten BJ, Hoorwed-Nijman JJG, Vulsma T, Stokvis-Brantsma WH, Rouwe CW, Reeser HM, Gerver WJ, Gosen JJ, Rongen-Westerlaken C, Drop SLS: Final height in girls with Turner syndrome after long-term growth hormone treatment in three dosages and low dose estrogens. J Clin Endocrinol Metab 2003;88:1119–1125.
23 Soriano-Guillen L, Coste J, Ecosse E, Leger J, Tauber M, Cabrol S, Nicolio M, Brauner R, Chaussain JL, Carel JC: Adult height and pubertal growth in Turner syndrome after treatment with recombinant growth hormone. J Clin Endocrinol Metab 2005;90:5197–5204.
24 Canadian Growth Hormone Advisory Committee: Impact of growth hormone supplementation on adult height in Turner syndrome: results of the Canadian randomized controlled trial. J Clin Endocrinol Metab 2005;90:3360–3366.
25 Chernausek SD, Attie KM, Cara JF, Rosenfeld RG, Frane J: Growth hormone therapy of Turner syndrome: the impact of age of estrogen replacement on final height. J Clin Endocrinol Metab 2000;85:2439–2445.
26 Reiter EO, Blethen SL, Baptista J, Price L: Early initiation of growth hormone treatment allows age-appropriate estrogen use in Turner's syndrome. J Clin Endocrinol Metab 2001;86:1936–1941.
27 Carel JC: Editorial: growth hormone in Turner syndrome: twenty years after, what can we tell our patients? J Clin Endocrinol Metab 2005;90:3793–3794.
28 Binder G, Baur F, Schweizer R, Ranke MB: The d3-growth hormone (GH) receptor polymorphism is associated with increased responsiveness to GH in Turner syndrome and short small-for-gestational age children. J Clin Endocrinol Metab 2006;91:659–664.

Turner Syndrome within KIGS Including an Analysis of 1146 Patients Grown to Near Adult Height

Michael B. Ranke[a] Anders Lindberg[b]

Patients with Turner syndrome (TS) were included in the second group of patients where recombinant human growth hormone (GH) was approved for the treatment of short stature. Presently, more than 5,500 Turner patients are included in the KIGS database. More than 1,000 patients were treated to adult height, thus offering the unique opportunity to analyse the factors affecting height outcomes. This can be utilised to treat short girls with TS more effectively and efficaciously.

Methods

For consistency with other KIGS chapters, we used the height standards of Prader et al. [1] for normal children and the weight standards of Freeman et al. [2]. The height references for Turner individuals by Ranke et al. [3] were also applied. Projected adult height was calculated according to Lyon et al. [4]. Birth weight for gestational age was transformed into a standard deviation score (SDS) based on the standards of Niklasson et al. [5]. The midparental height (MPH) SDS was calculated as follows: (father's height SDS + mother's height SDS)/1.61. Bone age determinations were done by the treating physician and calculated according to the method of Greulich and Pyle [6]. In order to calculate and analyse the extent of the observed growth during the first year of GH treatment, the height velocity was predicted according to the KIGS model for Turner patients by Ranke et al. [7], and the studentised residual was calculated.

Analysis of Factors Influencing Near Adult Height and Height Gain
A multiple regression analysis was performed in order to study the factors influencing height outcomes in response to GH treatment. The dependent variable chosen was height measured in centimetres and SDS based on Turner references, or change in height from the start of GH treatment to near adult height (NAH) measured in centimetres and SDS based on Turner references.

The following independent variables were tested: (1) status at birth: weight SDS, length SDS and ponderal index; (2) genetic background: mother's height SDS, father's height SDS, MPH SDS and karyotype; (3) treatment modality: GH dosage [per kilogram body weight and per kilogram ideal body weight (weight for height)], frequency of GH injections, and accumulated years of GH treatment; (4) variables at the start of treatment: age, bone age, height SDS, weight SDS, height SDS minus

[a] Paediatric Endocrinology Section
University Children's Hospital, University of Tübingen
Hoppe-Seyler-Strasse 1, DE–72076 Tübingen (Germany)
[b] Pfizer Endocrine Care
KIGS/KIMS/ACROSTUDY Medical Outcomes
Vetenskapsvägen 10, SE–191 90 Sollentuna (Sweden)

MPH SDS, and peak GH concentration in serum during stimulation testing; (5) variables at puberty onset: age, bone age, height SDS, weight SDS, and height SDS minus MPH SDS. The SDS was calculated as follows: SDS = (patient value minus mean value for age- and sex-matched normal subjects)/SD of the value for age- and sex-matched normal subjects.

Results

Karyotype

The relative frequency of the documented karyotypes is listed in table 1.

Start of Treatment

The characteristics of all Turner patients at the start of GH therapy are listed in table 2.

First Prepubertal Year on GH

The characteristics of patients treated for 1 prepubertal year are listed in table 3. Height velocity during the first year on GH in relation to normal and Turner references are illustrated in figure 1.

Treatment to NAH

In 1,146 individuals, NAH had been reached. The characteristics of the individuals at GH onset, at onset of puberty and at NAH are listed in table 4. The relationship between patients who reached NAH and karyotypes is listed in table 5. Height at GH start and NAH are illustrated in figure 2 in relation to normal and Turner references. The height SDS of the patient cohort treated to NAH at GH start, after 1 year of treatment, at puberty onset and at NAH are illustrated in figure 3.

Analysis of Factors Influencing NAH and Height Gain

NAH was found to be related to (1) MPH (positive), (2) height at GH start (positive), (3) studentised residual ('index of responsiveness') during the 1st year on GH (positive), (4) mean dose of GH per week (positive), and (5) age at the start of puberty (positive). All parameters were significant at a probability level of $p < 0.01$.

The regression equation is as follows: NAH (cm) = 142.9 + [MPH SDS × 1.37] + [height at GH start SDS (TS) × 4.11] + [studentised residual during the 1st year of treatment × 1.99] + [mean GH dose (mg/kg/week) × 4.82] + [age at the start of puberty (years) × 0.74]. This equation explains 67% of the variability of NAH with an error SD of 3.6 cm.

The gain in height from GH start to NAH was found to be related to (1) MPH (positive), (2) height at GH start (negative), (3) studentised residual (index of responsiveness) during the 1st year of GH treatment (positive), (4) mean dose of GH per week (positive), (5) age at the start of puberty (positive), (6) age at GH start (negative), and (7) birth weight (positive). All parameters were significant at a probability level of $p < 0.01$.

The regression equation is as follows: Δ height (cm) = 64.0 + [MPH SDS × 1.37] + [height at GH start SDS (TS) × −0.70] + [studentised residual during the 1st year of treatment × 2.08] + [mean GH dose (mg/kg/week) × 6.73] + [age at puberty

Table 1. Distribution of karyotypes in KIGS patients with TS

Karyotype	All (n = 4,816)	Prenatal (n = 231)	NAH (n = 1,050)
45,X	50.4	46.8	57.1
46,X,Xp–	1.1	0.9	1.1
46,X,Xq–	0.6	0.9	0.6
46,X,iXq	7.4	7.4	6.6
46,X,Xr	0.2	–	0.3
45,X/46,XX	11.3	16.0	8.9
45,X/46,X,Xr	4.2	2.6	3.4
45,X/46,XiXq	10.7	11.7	10.7
45,X/47,XXX	4.4	4.3	3.8
Other 45,X, mosaic, variant	9.0	9.5	7.1
45,X/46,XY	0.8	–	0.4

Data are given as percentages.

Table 2. Characteristics of patients at the start of GH therapy

Variables	n	Median	10th centile	90th centile	Mean ± SD
Background					
Birth weight SDS	5,216	−1.1	−2.6	0.4	−1.1 ± 1.2
Birth length SDS	3,732	−0.9	−2.5	0.9	−0.8 ± 1.4
MPH SDS (Prader)	5,361	−0.5	−2.1	1.0	−0.6 ± 1.2
Maximum GH, µg/l	2,794	11.9	4.3	28.2	14.5 ± 11.6
IGF-1 SDS	960	−1.6	−3.0	0.3	−1.5 ± 1.6
At GH start					
Age, years	5,829	10.0	4.6	14.3	9.7 ± 3.7
Bone age, years	2,286	9.5	3.5	12.5	8.7 ± 3.2
Height, cm	5,829	129.0	94.0	138.8	117.8 ± 17.2
Height SDS (Prader)	5,829	−3.3	−4.6	−2.2	−3.4 ± 1.0
Height SDS (TS)	5,771	0.1	−1.2	1.4	0.1 ± 1.1
Projected height, cm	5,771	146.9	138.7	154.8	146.8 ± 6.4
Height velocity, cm/year	2,039	4.4	2.5	6.6	4.6 ± 1.9
Body mass index SDS	5,828	0.3	0.2	0.4	0.4 ± 1.1
GH dose, mg/kg/week	5,829	0.30	0.17	0.38	0.29 ± 0.09

IGF-1 = Insulin-like growth factor 1.

Table 3. Pre-pubertal patients treated for the first year with GH

Variables	n	Median	10th centile	90th centile	Mean ± SD
At GH start					
Age, years	3,562	8.7	4.3	13.0	8.6 ± 3.4
Bone age, years	1,399	8.0	3.1	11.5	7.7 ± 3.1
Height, cm	3,562	114.4	91.9	132.9	112.9 ± 15.9
Height SDS (Prader)	3,562	−3.1	−4.3	−2.0	−3.1 ± 0.9
Height SDS (TS)	3,516	0.0	−1.3	1.2	0.0 ± 1.0
Height velocity, cm/year	1,326	4.5	2.8	6.7	4.7 ± 1.9
Height velocity SDS (Prader)	1,322	−1.7	−3.9	0.5	−1.7 ± 1.8
BMI SDS	3,561	0.2	−1.1	1.7	0.3 ± 1.1
GH dose, mg/kg/week	3,562	0.30	0.18	0.38	0.29 ± 0.09
After 1 year					
Age, years	3,562	9.7	5.2	14.0	9.6 ± 3.4
Height SDS (Prader)	3,562	−2.5	−3.7	−1.3	−2.5 ± 1.0
Height velocity, cm/year	3,562	7.6	5.3	9.9	7.6 ± 1.9
Height velocity SDS (Prader)	3,557	2.4	−0.5	5.8	2.6 ± 2.8
Δ height SDS (Prader)	3,562	0.5	−0.8	1.0	0.3 ± 0.7
Δ height SDS (TS)	3,516	0.7	0.3	1.1	0.7 ± 0.4
Studentised residual SDS	2,705	−0.2	−1.6	1.2	−0.2 ± 1.2
Body mass index SDS	3,541	0.2	−1.1	1.6	0.2 ± 1.1

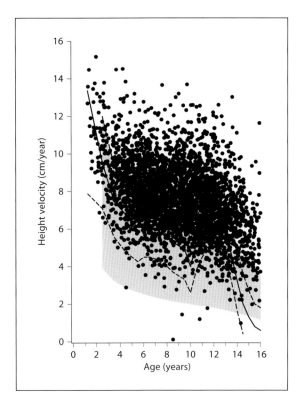
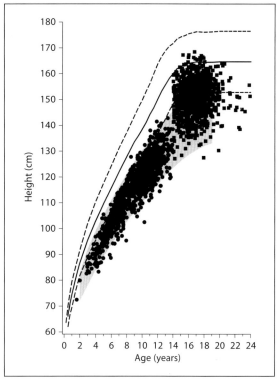

Fig. 1. Height velocity during the first prepubertal year of GH treatment in girls with TS compared with references of Prader et al. [1] and disease-specific references [3]. Dashed lines = ± 2 SD of normal references; solid line = 0 SD of normal references; shaded area = range for Turner references.

Fig. 2. Height compared with age for girls with TS who have reached NAH imposed on the references of Prader et al. [1] and Turner disease-specific references [3]. Dashed lines = ± 2 SD of normal references; solid line = 0 SD of normal references; shaded area = range for Turner references.

start (years) × 0.97] + [age at GH start (years) × −4.76] + [birth weight SDS × 0.34]. This equation explains 90% of the variability of Δ height (cm) with an error SD of 3.6 cm.

Commentary

The patients enrolled in KIGS reflect the worldwide development of TS and the great variability in patient characteristics. In all respects, the characteristics of this patient cohort resemble those observed in other large series initiated in the late 1980s at GH doses slightly higher than those used in GH deficiency, with an induction of puberty usually after the age of 13 years. Consequently, the height gain observed was similar to other studies. Our descriptive data show that after the onset of puberty, there is only little or no further gain in height, which is probably not surprising in the light of the dose-response relationship between height gain and GH during puberty [see chapter by Rosenfeld, this vol., pp. 326–331].

It seems to be against intuition that the height outcomes in our cohort were not affected by the

Table 4. Patients treated with GH to near final height

Variables	n	Median	10th centile	90th centile	Mean ± SD
At GH start					
Age, years	1,146	9.4	5.5	12.1	9.0 ± 2.5
Bone age, years	544	8.1	4.0	10.5	7.9 ± 2.4
Height SDS (Prader)	1,146	−3.1	−4.2	−2.0	−3.1 ± 0.9
Height SDS (TS)	1,144	0.0	−1.3	1.1	0.0 ± 1.0
Height velocity, cm/year	457	4.4	2.7	6.2	4.4 ± 1.5
Height velocity SDS (Prader)	456	−1.7	−4.1	0.4	−1.7 ± 1.8
Body mass index SDS	1,146	0.2	−1.1	1.6	0.2 ± 1.1
GH dose, mg/kg/week	1,146	0.28	0.17	0.37	0.28 ± 0.08
At puberty					
Age, years	633	13.3	11.5	15.4	13.4 ± 1.6
Height SDS (Prader)	633	−1.5	−2.7	−0.4	−1.6 ± 0.9
Height SDS (TS)	633	1.7	0.1	3.1	1.6 ± 1.2
Δ height from start to puberty SDS (Prader)	633	1.5	0.6	2.5	1.5 ± 0.8
Δ height from start to puberty SDS (TS)	632	1.5	0.8	2.7	1.6 ± 0.8
Body mass index SDS	628	0.4	−0.9	1.7	0.4 ± 1.1
At adult height					
Age, years	1,146	16.7	15.0	18.6	16.8 ± 1.5
Height SDS (Prader)	1,146	−2.3	−3.7	−0.9	−2.3 ± 1.1
Height SDS (TS)	1,146	1.6	0.1	3.0	1.6 ± 1.2
Δ height from puberty to end of treatment SDS (Prader)	633	−0.7	−1.4	0.1	−0.7 ± 0.6
ΔHeight from puberty to end of treatment SDS (TS)	633	0.0	−0.6	0.7	0.0 ± 0.5
Body mass index SDS	1,125	0.7	−0.7	2.1	0.7 ± 1.1
GH treatment during puberty, years	633	2.8	1.2	4.4	2.8 ± 1.3
Total GH treatment, years	1,146	6.7	4.6	10.6	7.1 ± 2.2

Table 5. Characteristics (medians) in Turner patients treated to NAH in relation to karyotype

Karyotype	n	Age at start of treatment, years	Height at start of treatment, cm	Projected adult height, cm	Age at NAH years	NAH cm
45,X	525	9.3	117.5	146.9	16.9	151.7
45,X,iXq	59	10.5	119.2	144.9	17.0	149.2
45,X/46,XX	76	10.2	119.0	145.9	16.6	149.6
45,X/46,X,Xr	34	9.8	115.6	144.4	16.7	148.5
45,X/46,X,iXq	99	9.7	118.9	144.7	16.9	150.3
45,X/47,XXX	25	10.3	121.4	146.3	16.1	152.3
All karyotypes	987	9.8	118.0	146.1	16.9	151.0

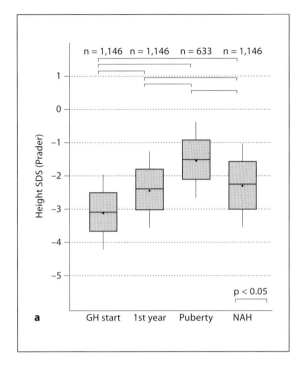
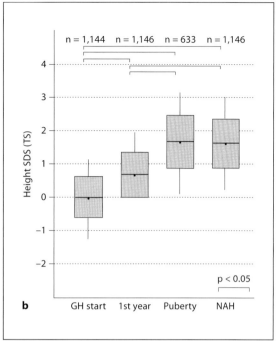

Fig. 3. Height SDS using Prader references (**a**) and disease-specific references (**b**) in children with TS treated to NAH at GH start, after 1 year of treatment, at puberty onset and at NAH.

karyotype of the individuals, which mirrors the situation of spontaneous growth, which is not essentially unaffected by karyotype either [8]. However, the reason for this is probably the common genetic basis for growth disorder in TS (*SHOX* haploinsufficiency) [9]. Likewise, it must be assumed that the long-term response to GH in TS is the result of a factor common to all patients.

We have shown that GH dose and the responsiveness to GH are the main determinants for the first prepubertal years in TS [7]. In a recent study, we have been able to show that the short- and long-term gain in height in TS is a function of the polymorphism of the GH receptor gene [10], which was originally found to affect short-term growth in GH deficiency [11]. This verifies and expands the concept of responsiveness to GH as the determinant of response which has resulted in prediction models which were based on easily accessible auxological parameters [7]. The role of insulin-like growth factor 1 measurements as a diagnostic tool for short stature and as a parameter to evaluate the safety and efficacy of GH treatment is discussed in detail in the chapter by Ranke [this vol., pp. 83–92]. Within the context of TS, we have illustrated the data of 791 cases before GH treatment was started (fig. 4). Further data from 206 patients illustrate insulin-like growth factor 1 levels during the first year of treatment (fig. 5). It can be seen that the levels tend to be low before the start of GH therapy; however, during treatment (before and during puberty), the insulin-like growth factor 1 levels exceeded the upper normal range in about one third of cases.

The current analysis of patients treated to NAH was initiated in an attempt to individualise

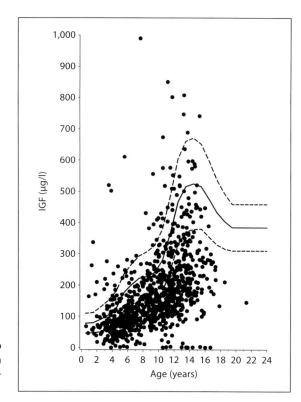

Fig. 4. Insulin-like growth factor 1 levels (IGF) related to age in TS patients before GH treatment; references from Juul et al. [12]. Dashed lines = ± 2 SD of normal references; solid line = 0 SD of normal references.

and optimise GH treatment in children with TS both in terms of efficacy and cost-effectiveness. The regression equations derived from a very large cohort of patients support the principal concepts of treatment in TS and, additionally, provide a numerical structure. The same parameters emerged to be instrumental in affecting adult height as well as gain in height. Both response parameters are affected by MPH (positive), GH dose (positive), responsiveness to GH (positive), age at GH start (negative) and age at puberty onset (positive). Paradoxically, absolute height is greater when the patient is relatively tall at GH start, while the gain in height is greater when the patient is relatively small. The magnitude of the explained variability of the outcome variable (67 and 90%) as well as the magnitude of the errors suggest that these regression equations can be used as guidelines in daily practice. Thus, the GH dose (and the timing of puberty onset) can be adapted to the patients' needs and responsiveness to GH treatment. This also means that lower doses of GH – or possibly even no treatment at all – can be elected. One of the remaining issues of great practical concern is the optimal treatment regime during puberty. This will require studies comparing Turner adolescents on GH treatment and controls, a modality which is ethically justified once proper prepubertal treatment has been conducted.

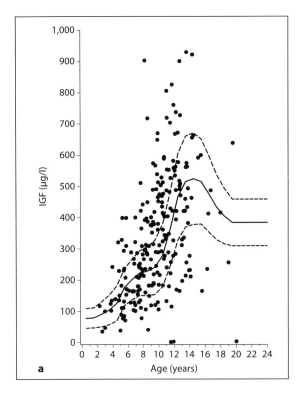 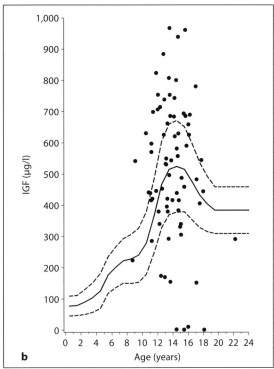

Fig. 5. Insulin-like growth factor 1 levels (IGF) related to age in TS patients on GH treatment before puberty (**a**) and during spontaneous or induced puberty (**b**); references from Juul et al. [12]. Dashed lines = ± 2 SD of normal references; solid line = 0 SD of normal references.

References

1 Prader A, Largo RH, Molinari L, Issler C: Physical growth of Swiss children from birth to 20 years of age. Helv Paediatr Acta 1989;43(suppl 52):1–125.
2 Freeman JV, Cole TJ, Chinn S, Jones PR, White EM, Preece MA: Cross-sectional stature and weight reference curves for the UK, 1990. Arch Dis Child 1995;73:17–24.
3 Ranke MB, Stubbe P, Majewski F, Bierich JR: Spontaneous growth in Turner's syndrome. Acta Paediatr Scand Suppl 1988;343:22–30.
4 Lyon AJ, Preece MA, Grant DB: Growth curve for girls with Turner syndrome. Arch Dis Child 1985;60:932–935.
5 Niklasson A, Ericson A, Fryer JG, Karlberg J, Lawrence C, Karlberg P: An update of the Swedish reference standards for weight, length and head circumference at birth for given gestational age (1977–1981). Acta Paediatr Scand 1991; 80:756–762.
6 Greulich WW, Pyle SI: Radiographic Atlas of the Skeletal Development of the Hand and Wrist. Stanford, Stanford University Press, 1952.
7 Ranke MB, Lindberg A, Chatelain P, et al: Prediction of long-term response to recombinant human growth hormone in Turner syndrome: development and validation of mathematical models. KIGS International Board. Kabi International Growth Study. J Clin Endocrinol Metab 2000;85:4212–4218.
8 Ranke MB, Grauer ML: Adult height in Turner syndrome: results of a multinational survey 1993. Horm Res 1994;42: 90–94.
9 Rao E, Weiss B, Fukami M, et al: Pseudoautosomal deletions encompassing a novel homeobox gene cause growth failure in idiopathic short stature and Turner syndrome. Nat Genet 1997;16: 54–63.
10 Binder G, Baur F, Schweizer R, Ranke MB: The d3-growth hormone receptor polymorphism is associated with increased responsiveness to GH in Turner syndrome and short small-for-gestational-age children. J Clin Endocrinol Metab 2006;91:659–664.
11 Dos Santos C, Essioux L, Teinturier C, Tauber M, Goffin V, Bougneres P: A common polymorphism of the growth hormone receptor is associated with increased responsiveness to growth hormone. Nat Genet 2004;36:720–724.
12 Juul A, Dalgaard P, Blum WF, Bang P, Hall K, Michaelsen KF, Müller J, Skakkebaek NE: Serum levels of insulin-like growth factor (IGF)-binding protein-3 (IGFBP-3) in healthy infants, children, and adolescents: the relation to IGF-I, IGF-II, IGFBP-1, IGFBP-2, age, sex, body mass index, and pubertal maturation. J Clin Endocrinol Metab 1995;80: 2534–2542.

Noonan Syndrome

Christopher J.H. Kelnar

Noonan syndrome (NS) is a rather frequent (incidence of 1 in 1,000–2,500 live births), genetic syndrome, with a variable phenotype, with many features similar to Turner syndrome. In addition to the characteristic pattern of dysmorphic features, affecting face, trunk and extremities, frequently, there is cryptorchidism with variable hypogonadism associated with features such as pulmonary valvular stenosis and other cardiac abnormalities, deafness, visual problems, clotting disorders and short stature [1]. However, these signs are inconstant, and therefore, the diagnosis is clinical, based on the presence of typical facial features and at least two others [2, 3]. Clinical diagnosis may be complicated, as the phenotype is variable and becomes milder with age.

Puberty generally occurs spontaneously but is typically delayed. The mean growth curves for children with NS follow the third percentile through childhood, but subsequently, there is a fall below the 'normal' range, consequent upon the typical finding of an average of 2 years of pubertal delay [4]. Final height is typically not achieved until the end of the second decade. Mean adult height is approximately 162.5 cm for males and 153 cm for females [5], although these standards are mostly based on cross-sectional studies involving relatively small samples, which exhibited bias in ascertainment towards shorter children with NS and those with cardiac defects or more obvious dysmorphic features.

NS has recently been found to be caused by mutations in the PTPN11 gene on the long arm of chromosome 12 (12q24.1) which encodes the protein tyrosine phosphatase SHP-2, a protein that controls cardiac semilunar valvulogenesis and that has other diverse effects on cell proliferation, differentiation and migration [6]. Phenotype-genotype correlations are poor [7], and so far, the molecular genetic abnormalities identified have only been found in 50% or fewer of those with the clinical diagnosis of NS [7, 8].

The Growth Hormone Axis

Defining the spectrum of growth hormone (GH) secretory ability in the general population is difficult, and even more so in persons with syn-

Department of Paediatric Endocrinology
Section of Child Life and Health
University of Edinburgh, 20 Sylvan Place
Edinburgh EH9 1UW (UK)

dromes [9]. Establishing a reasonable assessment of GH secretory ability or a firm diagnosis of GH deficiency can be challenging for several reasons [10]: (1) the pulsatile, and predominantly nocturnal, nature of GH secretion, (2) GH assay characteristics, and (3) the complexity of the control of GH secretion and the GH/insulin-like growth factor 1 (IGF-1) metabolic pathways that are central to the growth process [11].

The literature suggests that children with NS are typically not GH deficient [12]. However, there have been reports of impairment of the GH/IGF axis [13–16] and, in some cases, low mean overnight GH concentrations or high trough levels, which is suggestive of possible neurosecretory dysfunction [12, 15]. Further, it appears that 10–45% of patients with NS have suboptimal (<20 mU/l) GH levels in response to standard GH stimulation tests [12, 17, 18], and levels of markers of GH action, i.e. IGF-1 and IGF binding protein 3 (IGFBP-3), are characteristically low and rise with GH therapy [15, 18].

There is no evidence of clinically significant GH resistance, but GH insensitivity may play a role. This clinically based assumption seems to be supported by results from molecular genetic studies [19], which suggest that PTPN11/SHP-2 mutations in NS cause mild GH resistance by a postreceptor signalling defect.

It is unclear to what extent the 'low to normal' spontaneous GH levels simply reflect a spectrum of GH secretory ability among children with NS who are destined to be at the upper or lower ends of the NS height spectrum, or whether the apparently dysfunctional pattern of GH secretion represents a specific NS-related problem in some cases [20]. However, it is important to realize that in many syndromes, including NS, additional factors such as autoimmune hypothyroidism may impinge on growth [21] and that despite their limitations, syndrome-specific growth charts are often valuable for recognizing additional causes of poor growth for which specific treatment may be given.

Rationale for Growth Hormone Therapy in Noonan Syndrome

Possible reasons for treating NS patients with GH include correcting the often substantially shorter stature – although approximately half of the patients will reach an adult height within 2 standard deviations (SD) of the population mean, albeit at an older age – and the possible impairment/dysfunction of the GH/IGF-1 axis.

Although there are now a number of studies on the use of GH therapy in NS [12, 15, 17–19, 22–32], careful interpretation of their results is necessary to assess the clinical relevance of their findings, particularly the most appropriate outcomes by which to measure treatment efficacy.

In their report of 4-year data in a cohort of Dutch patients with NS, Noordam et al. [33] found a positive effect of GH therapy, as reflected by a greater increase in linear growth in the first year. Although skeletal maturation accelerated in the GH-treated group, the positive effect of therapy waned over the second year. After 3 years, in patients in whom GH therapy was discontinued after 2 years, there was notable 'catch-down' growth, with continued bone age maturation resulting in a lower height SD score (Ht-SDS) for bone age, compared with patients who had remained on GH therapy.

The Ht-SDS for bone age should be interpreted with caution for final height prediction. Catch-down growth is a well-recognized phenomenon after cessation of GH therapy in children with idiopathic short stature and has been hypothesized as being due to tolerance at target organ level [34]. In those with short stature who are not GH deficient, catch-down growth may be prevented by alternate daily (rather than daily) GH injections, allowing alternate-day physiological GH secretion [34].

In a recent Swedish study [30], 25 prepubertal children (age at treatment start 3.1–13.8 years) were randomized to receive GH at a dose of 33 or 66 μg/kg/day. In the 18 patients who reached final height, an improvement of 1.7 SDS was observed (equivalent to 10.4 cm compared with pretreatment height). No difference was seen between the two GH doses. Prepubertal height gain was maintained to final height, and the children achieved a height close to their midparental height.

Studies have also been carried out to examine the influence of the PTPN11 mutation status and the GH axis and response to GH therapy in children with NS. In a retrospective analysis of 3 years of human GH (hGH) treatment (47 μg/kg/day) and genotyping of PTPN11 in 14 patients with NS (50% with the mutation), Ferreira et al. [32] found that although hGH treatment significantly improved growth velocity in both groups, slightly better results were found in patients without mutations (mean ± SD changes in the Ht-SDS from baseline: 1.7 ± 0.1 vs. 0.8 ± 0.4; p < 0.01). This was associated with patients with mutations in PTPN11 achieving significantly smaller increments in IGF-1 levels during treatment compared with patients without mutations (86 ± 67 vs. 202 ± 93 μg/l; p = 0.03).

In a study by Binder et al. [31], who compared GH secretion and IGF-1/IGFBP-3 levels in children who had the SHP-2 mutation (M+ group) with those in mutation-negative individuals (M– group), levels of IGF-1 (–2.0 ± 0.7 vs. –1.1 ± 0.9 SDS; p = 0.005) and IGFBP-3 (–0.9 ± 1.3 vs. 0.4 ± 1.1 SDS; p = 0.006) were found to be lower in the M+ group, whereas GH levels tended to be higher in the M+ group during spontaneous secretion at night and on arginine stimulation (p ≥ 0.08). In a prepubertal subgroup that also received recombinant hGH, the mean change in the Ht-SDS after 1 year of therapy (0.043 mg/kg/day) was 0.7 ± 0.2 in the M+ group (n = 8), compared with +1.3 ± 0.4 in the M– group (n = 3; p = 0.007). These data suggest that SHP-2 mutations in NS cause mild GH resistance by a postreceptor signalling defect, which seems to be partially compensated for by elevated GH secretion. This defect may contribute to the short stature phenotype in children with SHP-2 mutations and their relatively poor response to recombinant hGH.

In a comparable retrospective multicentre study in NS patients with growth retardation [19], the mean peak GH level was 15.4 ± 6.5 ng/ml for the 35 patients. The mean blood IGF-1 concentration in 19 patients (11 M+) was low for age, sex and puberty (–1.6 ± 1.0 SDS), especially among M+ patients, but normalized after 1 year of GH therapy (p < 0.001), without any difference between M+ and M– patients. Acid-labile subunit levels were very low in 10 patients. By contrast, mean basal IGFBP-3 values were normal in 19 patients. GH therapy resulted in catch-up growth with improvement in the Ht-SDS, which was lower after 2 years in M+ patients (p<0.03). The authors concluded that the growth of M+ patients is reduced and responds less efficiently to GH than that of M– patients. Growth impairment in M+ children could be explained by an association of low IGF-1 and acid-labile subunit levels with normal IGFBP-3 levels with reduced free IGF-1, in addition to a possible GH resistance by a late postreceptor signalling defect.

Other outcomes that have been studied include bone mineral density (BMD), body composition and other metabolic data. Noordam et al. [29] found pretreatment trabecular volumetric BMD to be normal, but baseline cortical BMD was in the low-normal range and increased over 2 years of GH therapy. Fat-free mass and total body water were low before treatment and increased during the first 3 months of GH therapy, with only a slight subsequent increase. The percentage of fat mass fell over the first 6 months and then increased. The authors concluded that there are no major problems with BMD in prepubertal children with NS and that the changes in BMD and body composition during GH therapy are compatible with the known (e.g., lipolytic) effects of GH in situations such as GH deficiency and idiopathic short stature.

Limitations of Studies of GH Therapy in NS

Most current studies are potentially biased in their conclusions, and available 'outcomes' should be treated with caution. In general, studies have had small samples and have been observational with no randomization or placebo or other control groups. There has been inconsistent validation of the diagnosis of NS, particularly in the larger multicentre studies, which may have used pre-existing database records that in turn may have included patients with other conditions. There is also likely to be ascertainment bias in subjects recruited (towards those who are most dysmorphic, are shortest or have obvious cardiac abnormalities).

Many of these studies are short-term studies. As a result, surrogate markers (e.g., predicted adult height and target height), which are notoriously unreliable, are used for final height prediction, and thus, to determine the efficacy of GH therapy. Further, the confounding effects of puberty on growth velocity are poorly accounted for in some studies. Optimal GH regimens during puberty have not been established, although there is some evidence that in GH deficiency, mimicking the increases in endogenous GH secretion at the pubertal growth spurt, is associated with a better height outcome [35]. Issues surrounding GH or sex steroid regimens in pubertal-aged children with NS have not been addressed systematically, and the largely cross-sectional nature of the reference growth data is particularly problematic when looking at pubertal growth [9, 36, 37]. In spite of these limitations, GH treatment in the majority of reports induced catch-up growth in most of the NS patients. First data on long-term outcome demonstrate an effect comparable with or even better than in Turner syndrome [19].

Safety of Growth Hormone Treatment in Noonan Syndrome

Only a few studies have looked systematically at the cardiac and other potential adverse effects of GH therapy [18, 27, 28, 38]. An important consideration when deciding on the use of GH therapy to enhance growth in children with NS concerns the nature of cardiac defects and the potentially deleterious effect of GH on their progression in patients with dilatative cardiomyopathy [39]. More frequent, characteristic cardiac anomalies in children with NS include pulmonary valve stenosis (62%), unexplained left ventricular hypertrophy (20%) and secundum atrial septal defects [40–45].

Patients with a mean maximal left ventricular wall thickness >1 cm or other echocardiographic features of hypertrophic cardiomyopathy (which is not usually apparent clinically) [18, 41] could be at particular risk because of the known effects of GH on cardiac muscle mass in other situations, such as acromegaly [39], and patients with NS who have hypertrophic cardiomyopathy have generally been excluded from GH trials.

Still, current data are reassuring. Several studies concluded that after 4 years of GH treatment, there were no major adverse effects on left ventricular dimensions [18, 27, 38]. There is also evidence that patients with (non-cardiomyopathic) heart disease respond as well as those without heart disease in short- to medium-term growth [28].

However, there are virtually no data on the safety of GH therapy in children with pre-existing hypertrophic cardiomyopathy. In the present state of knowledge, although non-cardiomyopathic coronary heart disease does not adversely affect growth improvement and is not associated with any cardiac deterioration in patients undergoing GH therapy [28], the presence of hypertrophic cardiomyopathy should be excluded by echocardiography before considering GH therapy, and all patients with NS who are undergoing

GH therapy should be followed with annual echocardiography to monitor its development.

Benefits of Growth Hormone Therapy

By what criteria is GH therapy beneficial? Are short children disadvantaged psychologically before treatment and does treatment confer benefit? Final (adult) height has been taken as the most important endpoint, but this in itself is of limited relevance. Children (or adults) with severe short stature will have practical difficulties in daily living, but for the majority of individuals with NS, what matters is their height in comparison with others and how they function psychosocially [46, 47].

Despite methodological problems in assessing possible psychological disadvantage from short stature in childhood [48–50], it seems likely that there are genuine cultural differences in the psychological effects of short stature among developed countries [51, 52]. Nevertheless, although short children may show psychological stress individually, as groups (statistically), they do not appear to have clinically significant behavioural or emotional problems, and it needs to be established whether being made taller produces measurable benefit in terms of improved quality of life (QoL). Currently, there is no strong evidence that GH therapy improves psychological adaptation in short children [53, 54].

Intuitively, the value of a gain in height should relate to improvement in QoL. Unfortunately, evaluating QoL in children is complicated by methodological problems. QoL measures selected may be work, life or social success related, or predominantly psychometric, and often reflect the researcher's domain of interest rather than any shared understanding of QoL definitions or impact [50].

Indeed, height at and through puberty may be a better predictor of some aspects of QoL than adult height [55]. It is thus possible that there could be psychological [56] and economic benefits in being taller at adolescence, even if subsequent adult height is not increased [46, 50].

Conclusions

Many studies of the use of GH therapy in subjects with NS suffer from a number of methodological defects. Nevertheless, taken together, the available evidence suggests that there may be disturbance of the GH/IGF axis in at least some children with NS, probably at a post-GH receptor signalling level, and that GH therapy benefits growth in the short to medium term. Some studies indicate that adult height is significantly increased by long-term treatment.

NS (identified on a molecular genetic basis) comprises individuals with heterogeneous phenotypes, and individuals diagnosed clinically as having NS comprise heterogeneous molecular genetic groups – genotype-phenotype associations are still poorly understood. Nevertheless, the discovery of the NS gene is facilitating knowledge of the true incidence, and phenotypic diversity of NS will provide an opportunity for prospective randomized studies of GH therapy in better-defined populations that are less subject to ascertainment bias.

Better-quality, unbiased evidence of the efficacy and safety of GH therapy in NS will only come from appropriately controlled studies of sufficiently large numbers of subjects defined on such a basis and followed to final height. This is now possible but will require international cooperation. Improvement in final height is not an end in itself, and disease-specific and age-validated psychological and QoL tools and better modelling for health economic outcomes are still needed before the value of GH therapy in NS and other groups of children with short stature can be assessed.

References

1 Noonan JA: Hypertelorism with Turner phenotype. A new syndrome with associated congenital heart disease. Am J Dis Child 1968;116:373–380.
2 Duncan WJ, Fowler RS, Farkas LG, Ross RB, Wright AW, Bloom KR, Huot DJ, Sondheimer HM, Rowe RD: A comprehensive scoring system for evaluating Noonan syndrome. Am J Med Genet 1981;10:37–50.
3 van der Burgt I, Berends E, Lommen E, van Beersum S, Hamel B, Mariman E: Clinical and molecular studies in a large Dutch family with Noonan syndrome. Am J Med Genet 1994;53:187–191.
4 Ranke MB: Turner and Noonan syndromes; in Kelnar CJH, Savage MO, Stirling HF, Saenger P (eds): Growth Disorders – Pathophysiology and Treatment. London, Chapman and Hall, 1998, pp 623–639.
5 Ranke M, Heidemann P, Knupfer C, Enders H, Schmaltz AA, Bierich JR: Noonan syndrome: growth and clinical manifestations in 144 cases. Eur J Pediatr 1988;148:220–227.
6 Tartaglia M, Mehler EL, Goldberg R, Zampino G, Brunner HG, Kremer H, van Der Burgt I, Crosby AH, Ion A, Jeffery S, Kalidas K, Patton MA, Kucherlapati RS, Gelb BD: Mutations in PTPN11, encoding the protein tyrosine phosphatase SHP-2, cause Noonan syndrome. Nat Genet 2001;29:465–468.
7 Tartaglia M, Kamini K, Shaw A: PTPN11 mutations in Noonan syndrome: molecular spectrum, genotype-phenotype correlation, and phenotypic heterogeneity. Am J Hum Genet 2002; 70:1555–1563.
8 Kosaki K, Suzuki T, Muroya K, et al: PTPN11 (protein-tyrosine phosphatase, nonreceptor-type 11) mutations in seven Japanese patients with Noonan syndrome. J Clin Endocrinol Metab 2002; 87:3529–3533.
9 Kelnar CJH: Growth hormone therapy for syndromic disorders. Clin Endocrinol 2003;59:2–21.
10 Rosenfeld RG: Broadening the growth hormone insensitivity syndrome. N Engl J Med 1995;333:1145–1146.
11 Ranke MB, Haber P: Growth hormone stimulation tests; in Ranke M (ed): Diagnostics of Endocrine Function in Children and Adolescents, ed 2. Heidelberg, Barth, 1996, pp 134–148.
12 Noordam C, van der Burgt I, Sweep CG, Delemarre-van de Waal HA, Sengers RC, Otten BJ: Growth hormone (GH) secretion in children with Noonan syndrome: frequently abnormal without consequences for growth or response to GH treatment. Clin Endocrinol (Oxf) 2001;54:53–59.
13 Elders MJ, Char F: Possible etiologic mechanisms of the short stature in the Noonan syndrome. Birth Defects Orig Artic Ser 1976;12:127–133.
14 Spandoni GL, Bernardini S, Cianfarani S: Spontaneous growth hormone secretion in Noonan syndrome. Acta Paediatr Scand 1990;367(suppl):157.
15 Ahmed ML, Foot AB, Edge JA, Lamkin VA, Savage MO, Dunger DB: Noonan syndrome: abnormalities of the growth hormone/IGF-I axis and the response to treatment with human biosynthetic growth hormone. Acta Paediatr Scand 1991;80(suppl):446–450.
16 Tanaka K, Sato A, Naito T, Kuramochi K, Itabashi H, Takemura Y: Noonan syndrome presenting with growth hormone neurosecretory dysfunction. Intern Med 1992;31:908–911.
17 Romano AA, Blethen SL, Dana K, Noto RA: Growth hormone treatment in Noonan syndrome: the National Cooperative Growth Study experience. J Pediatr 1996;128:S18–S21.
18 Cotterill AM, McKenna WJ, Brady AF, Sharland M, Elsawi M, Yamada M, Camacho-Hübner C, Kelnar CJH, Dunger DB, Patton MA, Savage MO: The short-term effects of growth hormone therapy on height velocity and cardiac ventricular wall thickness in children with Noonan syndrome. J Clin Endocrinol Metab 1996;81:2291–2297.
19 Limal JM, Parfait B, Cabrol S, et al: Noonan syndrome: relationships between genotype, growth and growth factors. J Clin Endocrinol Metab 2006; 91:300–306.
20 Albertsson-Wikland K, Rosberg S, Isaksson O, Westphal O: Secretory pattern of growth hormone in children of differing growth rates. Acta Endocrinologica 1983;103(suppl 256):72.
21 Kelnar CJH: Thyroid disturbances in cytogenetic diseases. Dev Med Child Neurol 1989;31:400–404.
22 Thomas BC, Stanhope R: Long-term treatment with growth hormone in Noonan's syndrome. Acta Paediatr 1993;82:853–855.
23 Otten BJ: Short stature in Noonan syndrome: demography and response to growth hormone treatment in the Kabi International Growth Study; in Ranke MB, Gunnarsson R (eds): Progress in Growth Hormone Therapy – 5 Years of KIGS. Mannheim, J & J Verlag, 1996, pp 206–215.
24 de Schepper J, Otten BJ, Francois I, Bourguignon JP, Craen M, Van der Burgt I, Massa GC: Growth hormone therapy in pre-pubertal children with Noonan syndrome – first year growth response and comparison with Turner syndrome. Acta Paediatr 1997;86:943–946.
25 Municchi G, Pasquino AM, Pucarelli I, Cianfarani S, Passeri F: Growth hormone treatment in Noonan syndrome: report of four cases who reached final height. Horm Res 1995;44:164–167.
26 Kirk JMW, Betts PR, Donaldson MDC, Dunger DB, Johnston DI, Kelnar CJH, Price DA, Wilton P: Short stature in Noonan syndrome: response to growth hormone therapy. Arch Dis Child 2001; 84:440–443.
27 Macfarlane CE, Brown DC, Johnston LB, Patton MA, Dunger DB, Savage MO, McKenna WJ, Kelnar CJH: Growth hormone therapy and growth in children with Noonan syndrome: results of 3 years' follow-up. J Clin Endocrinol Metab 2001;86:1953–1956.
28 Brown DC, Macfarlane CE, McKenna WJ, Patton MJ, Dunger DB, Savage MO, Kelnar CJH: Growth hormone therapy in Noonan syndrome: non-cardiomyopathic congenital heart disease does not adversely affect growth improvement. J Pediatr Endocrinol Metab 2002; 15:851–852.
29 Noordam C, Span J, van Rijn RR, Gomes-Jardin E, van Kuijk C, Otten BJ: Bone mineral density and body composition in Noonan's syndrome: effects of growth hormone treatment J Pediatr Endocrinol Metab 2002;15:81–87.
30 Osio D, Dahlgren J, Wikland KA, Westphal O: Improved final height with long-term growth hormone treatment in Noonan syndrome. Acta Paediatr 2005;94:1232–1237.

31 Binder G, Neuer K, Ranke MB, Wittekindt NE: PTPN11 mutations are associated with mild growth hormone resistance in individuals with Noonan syndrome. J Clin Endocrinol Metab 2005;90:5377–5381.

32 Ferreira LV, Souza SA, Arnhold LI, Mendonca BB, Jorge AA: PTPN11 mutations and response to GH therapy in children with NS. J Clin Endocrinol Metab 2005;90:5156–5160.

33 Noordam C, Van der Burgt I, Sengers RC, Delemarre-van de Waal HA, Otten BJ: Growth hormone treatment in children with Noonan's syndrome: four year results of a partly controlled trial. Acta Paediatr 2001;90:889–894.

34 Lampit M, Hochberg Z: Prevention of growth deceleration after withdrawal of growth hormone therapy in idiopathic short stature. J Clin Endocrinol Metab 2002;87:3573–3577.

35 Mauras N, Attie KM, Reiter EO, Saenger P, Baptista J: High dose recombinant human growth hormone (GH) treatment of GH-deficient patients in puberty increases near-final height: a randomized, multicenter trial. Genentech, Inc, Cooperative Study Group. J Clin Endocrinol Metab 2000;85:3653–3660.

36 Buckler JMH: A Longitudinal Study of Adolescent Growth. London, Springer, 1990.

37 Kelnar CJH, Stanhope R: Height prognosis in girls with central precocious puberty treated with GnRH analogues. Clin Endocrinol 2002;56:295–296.

38 Noordam C, Draaisma JM, van den Nieuwenhof J, van der Burgt I, Otten BJ, Daniels O: Effects of growth hormone treatment on left ventricular dimensions in children with Noonan's syndrome. Horm Res 2001;56:110–113.

39 Osterzeil KJ, Strohm O, Schuler J, Mussolini F, Hanlein D, Willenbrock R, Anker SD, Peole-Wilson PA, Ranke MB, Dietz R: Randomised, double-blind, placebo-controlled trial of human recombinant growth hormone in patients with chronic heart failure due to dilated cardiomyopathy. Lancet 1998;351:1233–1237.

40 Caralis DG, Char F, Graber JD, Voigt GC: Delineation of multiple cardiac anomalies associated with Noonan syndrome in an adult and review of the literature. Johns Hopkins Med J 1974; 134:346–353.

41 Burch M, Mann JM, Sharland M, Shinebourne EA, Patton MA, McKenna WJ: Myocardial disarray in Noonan syndrome. Br Heart J 1992;68:586–588.

42 Wilmshurst PT, Katritsis D: Restrictive and hypertrophic cardiomyopathies in Noonan syndrome: the overlap syndromes. Heart 1996;75:94–97.

43 Cooke RA, Chambers JB, Curry PV: Noonan's cardiomyopathy: a non-hypertrophic variant. Br Heart J 1994;71:561–565.

44 Nishikawa T, Ishiyama S, Shimojo T, Takeda K, Kasajima T, Momma K: Hypertrophic cardiomyopathy in Noonan syndrome. Acta Paediatr Jpn 1996;38:91–98.

45 Ishizawa A, Oho S, Dodo H, Katori T, Homma S: Cardiovascular abnormalities in Noonan syndrome: the clinical findings and treatments. Acta Paediatr Jpn 1996;38:84–90.

46 Kelnar CJH: Pride and prejudice – stature in perspective. Acta Paediatr Scand Suppl 1990;370:5–15.

47 Skuse DH, Gilmour J, Tian CS, Hindmarsh PC: Psychosocial assessment of children with short stature: a preliminary report. Acta Paediatr Scand 1994; 406:11–16.

48 Frank NC, Stabler B: Psychological assessment of children with growth deficiency; in Kelnar CJH, Savage MO, Stirling HF, Saenger P (eds): Growth Disorders – Pathophysiology and Treatment. London, Chapman and Hall, 1998, pp 265–277.

49 Kranzler JH, Rosenbloom AL, Proctor B, Diamond FB Jr, Watson M: Is short stature a handicap? A comparison of the psychosocial functioning of referred and nonreferred children with normal short stature and children with normal stature. J Pediatr 2000;136:96–102.

50 Radcliffe DJ, Pliskin JS, Silvers JB, Cuttler L: Growth hormone therapy and quality of life in adults and children. Pharmacoeconomics 2004;22:499–524.

51 Stabler B, Clopper RR, Siegel PT, Stoppani C, Compton PG, Underwood LE: Academic achievement and psychological adjustment in short children. The National Cooperative Growth Study. J Dev Behav Pediatr 1994;15:1–6.

52 Skuse DH, Gilmour J: Psychological disorders; in Kelnar CJH, Savage MO, Stirling HF, Saenger P (eds): Growth Disorders – Pathophysiology and Treatment. London, Chapman and Hall, 1998, pp 483–496.

53 Sandberg DE, Brook AE, Campos SP: Short stature: a psychosocial burden requiring growth hormone therapy? Pediatrics 1994;94:832–840.

54 Sandberg DE: Should short children who are not growth hormone deficient be treated? West J Med 2000;172:186–189.

55 Persico N, Postlethwaite A, Silverman D: The Effect of Adolescent Experience on Labor Market Outcomes: the Case of Height. Philadelphia, University of Pennsylvania, 2002.

56 Mussen PH, Jones MC: Self-conceptions, motivations and interpersonal attitudes of late- and early-maturing boys. Child Dev 1957;28:243–256.

Short Stature in Noonan Syndrome: Results of Growth Hormone Treatment in KIGS

Barto J. Otten   Kees Noordam

Noonan syndrome (NS) is a condition affecting both sexes, with an incidence of about 1 in 2,000 births [1, 2]. Characteristic features of NS include short stature, a distinctive facial appearance, congenital heart defects (most frequently pulmonary valve stenosis or hypertrophic cardiomyopathy), thoracic deformities, bleeding diathesis and cryptorchidism in male patients [3].

In contrast to Turner syndrome, in NS, there is no definitive diagnostic test available. Over the last few years, mutations in the PTPN11 gene [4] and in KRAS [5] have been found in children with NS. It is estimated that in about 50% of the patients, such mutations can be found [6]. Therefore, NS remains mainly a clinical diagnosis. Establishing the diagnosis can be very difficult, especially in adulthood. There is great variability in expression, and the phenotype becomes less pronounced with increasing age [7]. Several scoring systems to help the diagnostic process have been developed. The most recent and useful scoring system was described in 1994 by Van der Burgt et al. [8].

Children with NS show a typical growth pattern [9, 10]: they are of normal size at birth, grow slowly during prepuberty and have a slightly delayed and decreased pubertal growth spurt. The median height in relation to the chronological age of subjects with NS is around the 3rd percentile for normal children, and they reach a mean adult height of 162.5 cm for men and 152.7 cm for women [10].

Patients and Methods

A group of 429 patients (288 males, 141 females) classified by the investigators as NS enrolled in the KIGS database was investigated. In addition to the Prader references, Noonan-specific growth standards [10] were used.

In a subset of children that stayed prepubertal during growth hormone (GH) treatment for at least 3 years, a 3-year longitudinal follow-up study was performed. This longitudinal cohort consisted of 85 patients, 61 boys and 24 girls.

Near adult height (NAH) was reached in a cohort of 38 patients (19 boys, 19 girls).

Department of Metabolic and Endocrine Disorders
Radboud University Medical Centre
PO Box 91-01, NL–6500 HB Nijmegen (The Netherlands)

Table 1. Background data and auxological characteristics of NS patients

	Both sexes				Females		Males	
	n	median	10th percentile	90th percentile	n	median	n	median
Background								
Birth weight SDS	393	−0.4	−2.1	1.0	133	−0.6	260	−0.4
Birth length SDS	269	−0.7	−2.6	1.4	99	−1.0	170	−0.7
MPH SDS (Prader)	394	−1.0	−2.6	0.7	132	−1.1	262	−0.9
Maximum GH, μg/l	321	10.1	4.8	27.3	111	11.4	210	9.9
IGF-1 SDS	121	−2.0	−3.4	−0.7	43	−2.1	78	−2.0
At start of GH treatment								
Age, years	429	9.7	4.3	14.4	141	9.7	288	9.7
Bone age, years	120	7.2	2.3	11.7	39	7.3	81	7.0
Height, cm					141	116.5	288	117.0
Height SDS (Prader)	429	−3.6	−4.9	−1.9	141	−3.8	288	−3.5
Height SDS (Noonan)	423	−1.1	−2.4	0.0	140	−1.0	283	−1.1
Height velocity, cm/year	193	4.4	2.9	6.5	62	4.3	131	4.4
BMI SDS	429	−0.5	−1.9	1.1	141	−0.6	288	−0.4
GH dose, mg/kg/week	429	0.25	0.16	0.36	141	0.26	288	0.24

MPH = Midparental height; IGF-1 = insulin-like growth factor 1; BMI = body mass index.

Patient Characteristics before GH Treatment

The background data and auxological characteristics of the total cohort of 429 patients with NS are shown in table 1. As in other Noonan studies, the number of male patients was twice that of the females. Birth weight and birth length in both boys and girls were significantly reduced with respect to the normal population. The median age at the start of GH treatment was the same for boys and girls (9.7 years), with a range for the whole group of 4.3–14.4 years. The height at the start of GH therapy was comparable for boys and girls: −3.6 SD for Prader standards and −1.1 SD for Noonan-specific standards. Bone age was delayed (7.2 vs. 9.7 years).

GH stimulatory tests were reported in 321 patients, with peak GH levels of 10.1 μg/l and a 10th percentile value of 4.8 μg/l. The median dose of GH at the commencement of therapy was 0.25 mg/kg/week, with a range of 0.16–0.36. The majority of patients received 6 or 7 injections of GH per week.

Figures 1 and 2 represent the heights of females and males at the start of treatment. With only a few exceptions, all patients had a height well below −2 standard deviation (SD).

Results of Growth Hormone Therapy

The results of the 3-year longitudinal cohort, for both females and males, together with the median cross-sectional data are presented in table 2.

Background data of the longitudinal cohort did not differ essentially from those of the total patient group, except for a somewhat higher midparental height. At GH start, the median age was 7.5 years, i.e. 2 years younger in the longitudinal cohort than in the total group, but the height SD score (SDS) and bone age delay were the same.

Over the 3-year period, the height velocity increased from 4.8 cm/year before treatment to 7.3 cm/year during the first year and to 5.9 cm/year during the second and third year. The height SDS according to Prader increased over the subsequent years from −3.6 to −3.1, −2.8 and −2.4, and according to Noonan standards, from −1.2 to −0.6, −0.3 and −0.2, respectively.

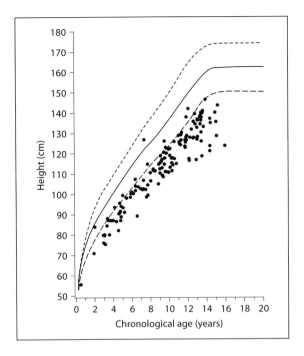
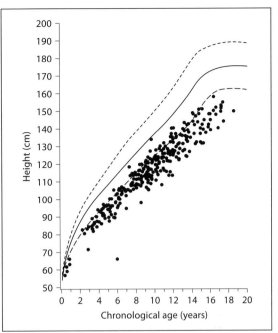

Fig. 1. Correlation of height and age at treatment start for female NS patients. Dashed lines = ± 2 SD; solid line = 0 SD.

Fig. 2. Correlation of height and age at treatment start for male NS patients. Dashed lines = ± 2 SD; solid line = 0 SD.

The data on the cohort of 38 patients who reached NAH are summarized in table 3 and figure 3. The mean total duration of GH treatment was 7.1 years, with a range of 4.4–11.3.

The mean age at the start of GH treatment was 9.1 years, which is equal to that of the total group, but 2 years older than that of the longitudinal cohort. They started GH therapy at a mean height of –3.5 SD according to Prader and –1.1 SD according to the Noonan standards; thus, they are comparable with the data of the whole group as well as with the longitudinal cohort. There were no significant differences between boys and girls.

In the first year, the height SDS increased to –3.0 and –0.8 for Prader and Noonan references, respectively. At the start of puberty, at a mean age of 13.8 years, the mean height SDS was –2.3 and –0.7 for Prader and Noonan references, i.e. a gain of 1.3 (Prader) and 0.4 SD (Noonan), respectively.

Figure 3 visualizes the progress of the height SDS in the NAH cohort according to Noonan standards and shows a gradual increase in the height SDS. NAH was –2.4 SD according to Prader and 0.0 SD according to Noonan standards, whereas the same data at the start of treatment were –3.5 and –1.1 SD. In figure 4, these data are combined in a graph, showing that about half of the boys reached an adult height above the –2 SD Prader limit, whereas for the girls, this percentage is lower.

Effect of Gender

In the longitudinal cohort, at the start of GH treatment, females were shorter than males (–4.3 vs. –3.5 SD, according to Prader references). This remained during the first and second year of

Table 2. Prepubertal longitudinal growth and cross-sectional data of NS patients

	Prepubertal longitudinal growth								Cross-sectional data	
	all				females		males			
	n	median	10th percentile	90th percentile	n	median	n	median	n	median
Background										
Birth weight SDS	81	−0.3	−2.1	1.0	23	−0.4	58	−0.3	393	−0.4
Birth length SDS	62	−0.7	−2.0	1.4	19	−1.2	43	−0.6	269	−0.7
MPH SDS (Prader)	77	−0.5	−2.3	1.1	22	−0.3	55	−0.6	394	−1.0
Maximum GH, μg/l	67	9.8	4.5	25.0	21	9.8	46	9.7	321	10.1
IGF-1 SDS	14	−2.0	−2.5	−0.6	3	−2.1	11	−2.0	121	−2.0
At start of GH treatment										
Age, years	85	7.5	3.3	11.0	24	6.8	61	7.9	429	9.7
Bone age, years	23	5.8	2.3	8.5	4	6.9	19	5.5	120	7.2
Height, cm					24	101.0	61	109.4		
Height SDS (Prader)	85	−3.6	−5.0	−2.4	24	−4.3	61	−3.5	429	−3.6
Height SDS (Noonan)	80	−1.2	−2.5	0.0	23	−1.4	57	−1.2	423	−1.1
Height velocity, cm/year	40	4.8	3.5	7.1	10	4.8	30	4.7	193	4.4
BMI SDS	85	−0.6	−1.9	0.8	24	−0.6	61	−0.6	429	−0.6
GH dose, mg/kg/week	85	0.24	0.16	0.36	24	0.28	61	0.23	429	0.25
1 year of GH therapy										
Age, years	85	8.6	4.3	12.0	24	7.7	61	9.1	348	10.9
Height, cm					24	107.7	61	117.1		
Height SDS (Prader)	85	−3.1	−4.3	−1.8	24	−3.4	61	−2.9	348	−3.1
Height SDS (Noonan)	85	−0.6	−2.3	0.7	24	−0.7	61	−0.5	348	−0.6
Height velocity, cm/year	85	7.3	5.5	11.3	24	7.1	61	7.5	348	7.2
BMI SDS	83	−0.7	−1.8	0.7	23	−0.7	60	−0.6	344	−0.7
2 years of GH therapy										
Age, years	85	9.5	5.3	12.9	24	8.8	61	9.9	289	12.0
Height, cm					24	113.6	61	123.0		
Height SDS (Prader)	85	−2.8	−4.1	−1.3	24	−3.1	61	−2.6	289	−2.8
Height SDS (Noonan)	85	−0.3	−2.1	1.0	24	−0.5	61	−0.2	289	−0.3
Height velocity, cm/year	84	5.9	4.6	8.4	23	6.5	61	5.7	272	6.0
BMI SDS	85	−0.6	−1.9	0.8	24	−0.6	61	−0.6	289	−0.5
3 years of GH therapy										
Age, years	85	10.6	6.4	13.9	24	9.8	61	10.8	204	12.6
Height, cm					24	119.0	61	127.0		
Height SDS (Prader)	85	−2.4	−3.6	−1.0	24	−2.7	61	−2.4	204	−2.5
Height SDS (Noonan)	85	−0.2	−1.9	1.3	24	−0.3	61	0.0	204	0.0
Height velocity, cm/year	82	5.9	3.8	7.4	23	6.3	59	5.7	193	5.7
BMI SDS	85	−0.7	−2.1	0.7	24	−0.5	61	−0.8	204	−0.4

MPH = Midparental height; IGF-1 = insulin-like growth factor 1; BMI = body mass index.

Table 3. NAH of NS patients

	NAH n	all median	10th percentile	90th percentile	females n	median	males n	median
Background								
Birth weight SDS	36	−0.3	−2.2	1.0	17	−0.3	19	−0.3
Birth length SDS	20	−0.5	−1.9	0.9	12	−0.7	8	−0.2
MPH SDS (Prader)	35	−0.9	−2.6	0.1	16	−1.1	19	−0.6
Maximum GH, μg/l	37	11.5	3.2	24.2	19	11.2	18	12.3
IGF-1 SDS	3	−1.8	−2.9	−1.7	3	−1.8	–	–
At start of GH treatment								
Age, years	38	9.1	4.8	13.0	19	8.9	19	9.5
Bone age, years	8	7.4	5.0	11.9	4	8.1	4	5.8
Height, cm					19	110.7	19	116.9
Height SDS (Prader)	38	−3.5	−5.0	−2.5	19	−3.9	19	−3.4
Height SDS (Noonan)	37	−1.1	−2.5	−0.1	19	−1.2	18	−1.1
Height velocity, cm/year	16	4.4	2.6	5.6	9	4.7	7	4.4
BMI SDS	38	−0.5	−1.9	1.3	19	−0.3	19	−0.6
GH dose, mg/kg/week	38	0.23	0.13	0.33	19	0.23	19	0.23
1 year of GH therapy								
Age, years	38	10.0	5.9	14.0	19	9.9	19	10.5
Height, cm					19	115.7	19	123.7
Height SDS (Prader)	38	−3.0	−4.5	−2.0	19	−3.1	19	−2.9
Height SDS (Noonan)	38	−0.8	−2.2	0.4	19	−0.7	19	−0.8
Height velocity, cm/year	38	6.9	4.5	9.2	19	7.0	19	6.8
BMI SDS	36	−9.5	−2.1	0.5	19	−0.4	19	−0.7
At start of puberty								
Age, years	15	13.8	11.1	15.6	9	13.7	6	13.9
Height, cm					9	135.0	6	140.2
Height SDS (Prader)	15	−2.3	−3.7	−0.6	9	−1.9	6	−2.5
Height SDS (Noonan)	15	−0.7	−2.1	1.7	9	0.1	6	−0.8
BMI SDS	15	−0.5	−1.9	0.5	9	−0.8	6	−0.1
NAH								
Age, years	38	18.0	16.3	19.8	19	16.6	19	18.5
Height, cm					19	149.5	19	161.0
Height SDS (Prader)	38	−2.4	−4.7	−1.5	19	−2.5	19	−2.4
Height SDS (Noonan)	38	0.0	−1.8	1.1	19	0.0	19	0.0
Height – MPH SDS (Prader)	35	−1.5	−3.1	−0.3	16	−1.5	19	−1.5
Δ height SDS (latest – puberty, Prader)	16	−0.4	−1.6	0.3	9	−0.7	6	0.0
Δ height SDS (latest – puberty, Noonan)	15	0.3	−0.5	1.0	9	0.2	6	0.5
Δ height SDS (latest – start, Prader)	38	1.0	0.2	2.0	19	1.0	19	0.9
Δ height SDS (latest – start, Noonan)	37	1.1	0.5	1.9	19	0.9	18	1.3
BMI SDS	38	−0.2	−2.5	1.4	19	0.1	19	−0.4

MPH = Midparental height; IGF-1 = insulin-like growth factor 1; BMI = body mass index.

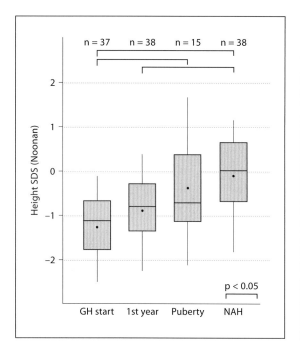

Fig. 3. Height SDS (Noonan-specific standard) at GH start, after 1 year of treatment, at puberty and at NAH.

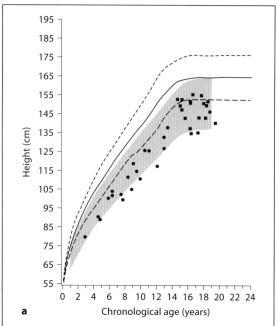

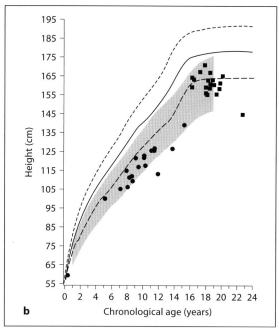

Fig. 4. Correlation of height and age at treatment start (●) and at NAH (■) for female (**a**) and male (**b**) NS patients. Dashed lines = ± 2 SD; solid line = 0 SD; shaded area = Noonan references.

therapy, but the difference had disappeared at 3 years of follow-up. However, according to Noonan standards, there was no significant difference, neither at GH start, nor at any follow-up period.

In the NAH cohort, neither at the start of therapy, at 1 year of therapy, at the start of puberty nor at NAH, any significant difference between males and females was found.

Effects of GH Dosage

Figure 5 shows the relation between the Δ height SDS during the first year of treatment and the dose of GH used at the start of therapy, as analyzed in a cohort of 63 patients <12 years of age. A slight positive correlation is suggested (Δ height SDS = 0.954 × GH dose + 0.248) ($p = 0.054$); however, after correction for extreme values, the significance disappeared ($p = 0.17$).

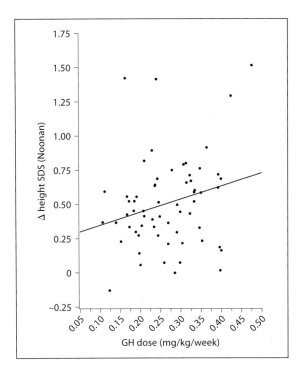

Fig. 5. Correlation between the Δ height SDS during the first year of treatment and the GH dose used at the start of therapy.

Table 4. Discontinuation of GH therapy

Main reason	n	%
Normal height reached	10	7.87
Growth plate fusion	13	10.24
Height velocity	37	29.13
Patient/parent decision	22	17.32
Treatment trial	4	3.15
Noncompliance	9	7.09
No funds for GH	4	3.15
Adverse event	1	0.79
Other reason	27	21.26

Discontinuation

One hundred and twenty-seven patients with reasons for discontinuation reported to KIGS are shown in table 4. The main reasons were low height velocity and patient/parent decision, which may, at least in part, represent insufficient response. Satisfaction with the height attained was the reason for discontinuation in 10 cases (8%). Only in 1 case an adverse event was mentioned as the reason for discontinuation.

At the start of treatment, these patients did not significantly differ from the total group or the longitudinal cohort with respect to height according to Prader or Noonan standards, height velocity or the GH dose instituted. Only the body mass index was somewhat lower (–0.7 vs. 0.4; p = 0.03) than that of the total group, but equal to that of the longitudinal group.

Comparison with the longitudinal group during the first 3 years of treatment learned that the group that discontinued GH treatment got a significantly lower GH dose, declining over the years, with a mean over 3 years of 0.20 versus 0.29 mg/kg/week ($p < 0.01$), which may account for the somewhat smaller although not significant response in the second and third year of therapy.

Cardiac Adverse Events

In 7 patients, cardiac adverse events were reported. Cyanotic periods (after 2.3 years of GH treatment) were reported in 1 patient, cardiac arrhythmias (after 2.9, 4.5 and 5.1 years) in 3 patients and angina pectoris in 1 patient (after 4.1 years). Of the 4 arrhythmia patients, 1 needed a pacemaker implantation. The most severe adverse events reported were left ventricular hypertrophy (after 2.0 years) and cardiomyopathy requiring cardiac transplantation (after 10.7 years), where the pre-existing situation was not clear.

Discussion

This database on NS surely represents the largest cohort of NS patients in the literature.

Since the publication of the 10-year KIGS data [11], the total number of NS patients in the database has increased from 143 to 429. However, the main characteristics of this population, such as age and low height SDS at GH start (even for Noonan-specific references), as well as the GH dose used and the response to GH treatment, have essentially remained the same.

Subsets of 3-year longitudinal and NAH cohorts were studied. The positive response during the first years of treatment of about 1 SD was sustained during the following years and even up to adult height. Thus, the main gain in the height SDS appears to be in the first years of treatment.

However, this response is less than that reported by Swedish investigators [12] who found an improvement in final height of 1.7 SD (= 10.4 cm). A possible explanation for this difference may be the selection of the patients: in the Swedish database, all diagnoses were made by 1 experienced investigator, whereas in the KIGS database, there are a large number of doctors making the diagnoses, which may have led to the inclusion of other Noonan-like patient groups as well. Also, a selection with regard to height may have contributed to this difference, as the KIGS patients had a lower height SDS according to Noonan standards at the start of treatment than the Swedish cohort (–1.1 SD vs. –0.1 to –0.7 SD).

An important point of consideration is the GH dose used. In the Swedish study, in which 25 prepubertal NS children were treated with GH in 2 different doses of 0.23 and 0.46 mg/kg/week, no difference was found between the 2 GH doses used. In the KIGS database, the median GH dose at the start of treatment was 0.25 mg/kg/week, with a range of 0.16–0.36. In linear regression analysis, the contribution of the dosage to the response was only minimally significant. Still, the GH dosage seems important, as evidenced from older studies [13], and certainly, there is a threshold in achieving a good response. This is in line with the growing evidence that PTPN11 and thus SHP-2 mutations cause mild GH resistance by a postreceptor signaling defect [14]. Therefore, it can be argued that NS patients should be treated by a higher dosage than substitution dosages, e.g., 0.35 mg/kg/week, or more, as in the Swedish study.

Of course, the evaluation of such a large and unselected database has its limitations. The lack of analysis of genetic data, the selection on shortness and the wide range of GH dosages used are characteristics of such a retrospective sampled database.

Furthermore, although the total cohort may be rather large (n = 429), the number of patients eligible for the 3-year longitudinal follow-up (n = 85) or for adult height analysis (n = 38) is more limited, although still higher than that in other reports.

An important matter of concern is the possible bias by the high number (108/429) of dropouts. While the first-year response of this dropout group was not significantly lower than that of the longitudinal group, in the second and third year of therapy, the response was lower, most probably due to a lower GH dose used.

Despite all these restrictions and biases, there seems to be no doubt that there is a positive effect of GH treatment on height velocity and adult height. The total gain may be about 1 SD and is already reached in the first years of therapy.

References

1. Noonan J, Ehmke DA: Associated noncardiac malformations in children with congenital heart disease. J Pediatr 1963;63:468–470.
2. Allanson JE: Noonan syndrome. J Med Genet 1987;24:9–13.
3. Sharland M, Burch M, McKenna WJ, Patton MA: A clinical study of Noonan syndrome. Arch Dis Child 1992;67:178–183.
4. Tartaglia M, Mehler EL, Goldberg R, Zampino G, Brunner HG, Kremer H, van der Burgt I, Crosby AH, Ion A, Jeffery S, Kalidas K, Patton MA, Kucherlapati RS, Gelb BD: Mutations in PTPN11, encoding the protein tyrosine phosphatase SHP-2, cause Noonan syndrome. Nat Genet 2001;29:465–468.
5. Schubbert S, Zenker M, Rowe SL, Boll S, Klein C, Bollag G, van der Burgt I, Musante L, Kalscheuer V, Wehner LE, Nguyen H, West B, Zhang KY, Sistermans E, Rauch A, Niemeyer CM, Shannon K, Kratz CP: Germline KRAS mutations cause Noonan syndrome. Nat Genet 2006;38:331.
6. Tartaglia M, Kamini K, Shaw A: PTPN11 mutations in Noonan syndrome: molecular spectrum, genotype-phenotype correlation, and phenotypic heterogeneity. Am J Hum Genet 2002;70:1555–1563.
7. Allanson JE, Hall JG, Hughes HE, Prens M, Wilt RD: Noonan syndrome: the changing phenotype. Am J Med Genet 1985;21:507–514.
8. Van der Burgt I, Berends E, Lommen E, van Beersum S, Hamel B, Mariman E: Clinical and molecular studies in a large Dutch family with Noonan syndrome. Am J Med Genet 1994;53:187–191.
9. Witt D R, Keena B A, Hall J G, Allanson JE: Growth curves for height in Noonan syndrome. Clin Genet 1986;30:150–153.
10. Ranke M, Heidemann P, Knupfer C, Enders H, Schmaltz AA, Bierich JR: Noonan syndrome: growth and clinical manifestations in 144 cases. Eur J Pediatr 1988;148:220–227.
11. Otten BJ, Noordam K: Short stature in Noonan syndrome demography and response to growth hormone treatment in KIGS; in Ranke MB, Wilton P (eds): Growth Hormone Therapy in KIGS – 10 Years Experience. Heidelberg, Johan Ambrosius Barth Verlag, 1999.
12. Osio D, Dahlgren J, Wikland KA, Westphal O: Improved final height with long-term growth hormone treatment in Noonan syndrome. Acta Paediatr 2005;94:1232–1237.
13. Cianfarani S, Spadoni GL, Finocchi G: Trattamento con ormonne della crescita (GH) in tre casi di sindrome di Noonan. Minerva Pediatr 1987;39:281–284.
14. Binder G, Neuer K, Ranke MB, Wittekindt NE: PTPN11 mutations are associated with mild growth hormone resistance in individuals with Noonan syndrome. J Clin Endocrinol Metab 2005;90:5377–5381.

Growth Hormone Treatment in Skeletal Dysplasias: The KIGS Experience

Thomas Hertel

Skeletal dysplasia is a heterogeneous group of diseases affecting the skeleton, and almost all types cause moderate to severe disproportionate short stature. The group comprises more than 200 different disorders with genetic defects ranging from collagen defects to defects in growth factor receptors. The final height differs substantially between the various disorders, but is often in the range of 110–130 cm [1]. The most prevalent type is probably achondroplasia, with an estimated incidence of 1 in 25,000 births [2]. Other skeletal dysplasias include hypochondroplasia, dyschondrosteosis (Leri-Weill syndrome), congenital spondyloepiphyseal dysplasia, pseudoachondroplasia, multiple epiphyseal dysplasia, metaphyseal dysplasias like Jansen, McKusick and Schmid type, pycnodysostosis, diastrophic dwarfism, and many others. Some mucopolysaccharidoses also exhibit bone dysplasia like Morquio syndrome. All in all, the estimated incidence is in the order of 3–5 per 10,000 births.

The KIGS registry comprises data from approximately 58,000 individuals treated with growth hormone (GH); of these, 601 patients have been reported as having a skeletal dysplasia (table 1). This review will focus in more detail on the results in individuals with achondroplasia, hypochondroplasia, spondyloepiphyseal dysplasia, Leri-Weill syndrome (dyschondrosteosis) and pseudoachondroplasia. The KIGS registry lists several other skeletal dysplasias; however, there are too few cases in each group to make a meaningful analysis in disorders like metaphyseal dysplasia or trichorhinophalangeal syndrome.

KIGS Patients and Results

Birth length and weight were moderately reduced in all of the five groups. The maximal GH value during a stimulation test was normal in most individuals (tables 2, 3).

Achondroplasia (OMIM No. 100800)
In the KIGS registry, 73 patients were registered as having achondroplasia. Data are given in table 2. The median age at the start of therapy was 5.4 years, and the median height standard devia-

Department of Paediatrics
Odense University Hospital
Sdr. Boulevard 29
DK–5000 Odense C (Denmark)

Table 1. Number of patients with skeletal dysplasia included in the KIGS registry

Condition	N
Hypochondroplasia	177
Achondroplasia	73
Leri-Weill dyschondrosteosis (dyschondrosteosis)	46
Osteogenesis imperfecta	39
Spondyloepiphyseal dysplasia	23
Cornelia de Lange syndrome (Brachmann-de Lange syndrome)	23
Metaphyseal chondrodysplasia	23
Pseudoachondroplastic dysplasia (pseudoachondroplasia)	14
Langer-Giedion syndrome (trichorhinophalangeal syndrome)	15
Seckel syndrome (bird-headed dwarfism, Seckel-type dwarfism, nanocephalic dwarfism, microcephalic primordial dwarfism)	13
Cleidocranial dysplasia (cleidocranial dysostosis)	10
Multiple epiphyseal dysplasia (epiphyseal dysplasia)	10
Cartilage hair hypoplasia (metaphyseal chondrodysplasia, McKusick type)	9
Spondylometaphyseal dysplasia	9
Ellis van Creveld syndrome (chondroectodermal dysplasia, mesoectodermal dysplasia)	8
Hypophosphatasia	6
Mucopolysaccharidosis type I (Hurler syndrome, Hurler-Scheie syndrome, Scheie syndrome)	6
Metaphyseal chondrodysplasia, Schmid type	5
Chondrodysplasia punctata (chondrodystrophia calcificans punctata)	4
Acromesomelic dysplasia (St. Helena dysplasia, Grebe dysplasia, Grebe chondrodysplasia)	3
Asphyxiating thoracic dystrophy (Jeune syndrome, thoracic-pelvic-phalangeal dystrophy)	3
Kniest dysplasia (metatropic dwarfism, metatropic dysplasia)	3
Shwachman-Diamond syndrome (Shwachman-Bodian syndrome)	3
Diastrophic dysplasia	2
Hallermann-Streiff syndrome (Francois dyscephalic syndrome)	2
Immunoosseous dysplasia, Schimke type (Schimke immunoosseous dysplasia)	2
Larsen syndrome	2
Mesomelic dysplasia	2
Mucopolysaccharidosis type IV (Morquio syndrome)	2
Conradi-Hunermann syndrome	1
Metatropic dwarfism (metatropic dysplasia)	1
Microcephalic osteodysplastic primordial dwarfism (brachymelic primordial dwarfism, Taybi-Linder syndrome)	1
Mucopolysaccharidosis type II (Hunter syndrome)	1
Mucopolysaccharidosis type VI (Maroteaux-Lamy syndrome)	1
Spondylocostal dysostosis (Jarcho-Levin syndrome, spondylothoracic dysplasia)	1
Spondyloepimetaphyseal dysplasia	1

tion score (SDS) was –5.6. Body proportions reported as sitting height ratio (sitting height/total height) were clearly abnormal, with a median sitting height ratio SDS of 9.1. Midparental height was also affected and below average. The parental height data, with the 10th percentile at –3.8 SD, indicate that some of the parents may have suffered from achondroplasia themselves.

Table 2. Auxological characteristics of patients with achondroplasia and hypochondroplasia

	Achondroplasia				Hypochondroplasia			
	n	median	10th percentile	90th percentile	n	median	10th percentile	90th percentile
Background								
Birth weight SDS	62	−0.5	−1.8	0.5	150	−0.5	−2.4	0.7
Birth length SDS	29	−1.3	−3.1	0.5	100	−0.9	−3.0	0.9
MPH SDS (Prader)	59	−1.0	−3.8	0.7	162	−1.3	−3.2	0.5
Maximum GH, µg/l	39	9.5	3.3	19.8	122	11.1	4.7	28.5
Start of GH treatment								
Age, years	73	5.4	1.7	11.8	177	10.1	4.8	13.7
Bone age, years	21	7.0	3.3	12.0	52	8.6	3.3	12.5
Height SDS (Prader)	73	−5.6	−7.3	−4.2	177	−3.5	−4.7	−2.3
Sitting height ratio SDS	33	9.1	4.4	10.3	71	3.0	0.5	5.7
Height − MPH SDS (Prader)	59	−4.8	−6.8	−2.5	162	−2.0	−4.2	−0.2
Height velocity, cm/year	27	4.5	3.0	7.6	93	4.3	3.1	6.4
BMI SDS	73	2.0	0.8	3.3	177	0.6	−0.7	2.5
GH dose, mg/kg/week	73	0.32	0.17	0.50	177	0.25	0.16	0.38

MPH = Midparental height; BMI = body mass index.

Table 3. Auxological characteristics of patients with dyschondrosteosis and spondyloepiphyseal dysplasia

	Dyschondrosteosis				Spondyloepiphyseal dysplasia			
	n	median	10th percentile	90th percentile	n	median	10th percentile	90th percentile
Background								
Birth weight SDS	44	−0.9	−2.2	0.3	19	−0.6	−1.5	1.0
Birth length SDS	34	−1.1	−2.2	0.1	15	−0.9	−2.8	1.2
MPH SDS (Prader)	46	−2.0	−3.1	−0.4	21	−1.4	−2.4	0.9
Maximum GH, µg/l	37	9.0	2.9	25.0	13	10.0	2.0	20.0
Start of GH treatment								
Age, years	46	10.3	6.3	13.7	23	7.0	3.5	12.7
Bone age, years	16	10.4	6.4	13.0	8	8.3	4.5	10.0
Height SDS (Prader)	46	−3.0	−4.7	−1.9	23	−4.3	−6.4	−3.0
Sitting height ratio SDS	22	2.7	1.9	4.8	8	2.3	−0.9	3.7
Height − MPH SDS (Prader)	46	−1.1	−2.9	0.4	21	−4.0	−6.0	−1.5
Height velocity, cm/year	22	4.5	3.6	5.7	9	5.5	1.9	6.2
BMI SDS	46	0.4	−0.7	1.8	23	1.1	−0.6	2.6
GH dose, mg/kg/week	46	0.25	0.16	0.36	23	0.28	0.17	0.41

MPH = Midparental height; BMI = body mass index.

Table 4. Prepubertal longitudinal growth – achondroplasia

	All				Females		Males	
	n	median	10th percentile	90th percentile	n	median	n	median
Start of GH treatment								
Age, years	51	4.8	1.6	9.9	20	4.4	31	5.3
Bone age, years	13	4.0	1.5	10.5	5	5.8	8	3.9
Height, cm					20	83.7	31	88.4
Height SDS (Prader)	51	–5.6	–7.3	–4.4	20	–6.5	31	–5.2
Sitting height ratio SDS	26	9.2	7.6	10.3	9	9.6	17	8.7
Height – MPH SDS (Prader)	44	–4.8	–6.8	–2.6	16	–5.5	28	–4.3
Height velocity, cm/year	23	4.9	3.1	7.6	8	4.1	15	5.0
BMI SDS	51	2.1	0.8	3.4	20	2.1	31	2.1
GH dose, mg/kg/week	51	0.33	0.17	0.50	20	0.32	31	0.33
One year of GH therapy								
Age, years	51	5.8	2.5	10.9	20	5.5	31	6.1
Height, cm					20	93.4	31	93.5
Height SDS (Prader)	51	–5.0	–6.2	–3.6	20	–5.8	31	–4.8
Sitting height ratio SDS	34	8.7	7.5	11.0	13	9.6	21	8.4
Height – MPH SDS (Prader)	44	–4.2	–6.3	–2.2	16	–4.6	28	–3.5
Height velocity, cm/year	51	6.5	4.1	10.1	20	6.5	31	6.4
BMI SDS	51	2.1	0.9	3.4	20	1.7	31	2.4
Mean GH dose, mg/kg/week	51	0.33	0.16	0.46	20	0.33	31	0.33

MPH = Midparental height; BMI = body mass index.

Fifty-one patients could be followed for 1 year, and the gain in the height SDS was marginally statistically significant at 0.4 (table 4, fig. 1). However, in 44 of these patients, the height SDS – the midparental height SDS only showed a nonsignificant gain from –4.8 to –4.2 (fig. 2). The median age at the start of GH therapy in this group was 4.8 years, and the median height SDS at the start of therapy was –5.6. The GH dose was moderately high at 0.33 mg/kg/week, with a median of 7 injections per week. The sitting height percentage of total height (sitting height ratio) SDS changed from 9.2 (n = 26) to 8.7 (n = 34) during 1 year of therapy, indicating that GH treatment did not worsen body proportions. The body mass index SDS did not change during treatment. Data on near adult height are not yet available.

Hypochondroplasia (OMIM No. 146000)
The KIGS registry lists 177 patients with a diagnosis of hypochondroplasia. Detailed data from these patients (77 females/100 males) could be evaluated for this analysis (table 2). It should be noted that some parents may have had hypochondroplasia themselves, as the lower limit for height SDS (10th percentile) is –3.2 SD. The median height SDS in the 177 individuals was –3.5, and the age at the start of therapy was 10.1 years. In hypochondroplasia, there are also abnormal body proportions, although not as severe as in achondroplasia. The median sitting height ratio SDS was 3.0 ranging from 0.5 to 5.7, leaving some doubt as to the certainty of the diagnosis in some of the patients diagnosed as having hypochondroplasia.

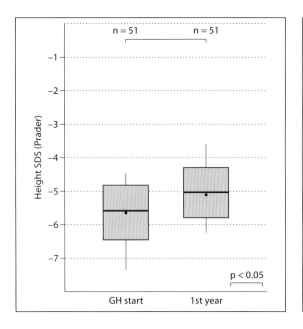 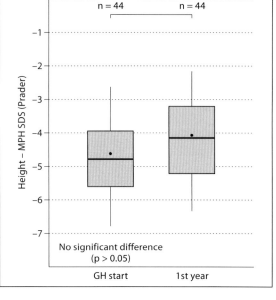

Fig. 1. Height SDS prior to and after 1 year of GH treatment in patients with achondroplasia.

Fig. 2. Height – midparental height (MPH) SDS prior to and after 1 year of GH treatment in patients with achondroplasia.

The prepubertal height gain during the first year of GH therapy was evaluated in 97 patients (41 females/56 males) (table 5). The age at the start of therapy in these patients was 8.6 years at a dose of 0.24 mg/kg/week. The median injection frequency was 7/week. The height SDS at the start of therapy was –3.6 in the 97 prepubertal individuals, and after 1 year of prepubertal longitudinal treatment, the gain in the height SDS was 0.4 ($p < 0.05$; fig. 3). Body proportions measured as sitting height ratio SDS changed from 3.0 (n = 37) to 3.4 (n = 41) during 1 year of GH therapy.

Near adult height was available from 19 patients, started on GH at a median age of 9.6 years. The gain in the height SDS was significant, with a median gain of 0.9 SD ($p < 0.05$) during a median 6.4 years of therapy (fig. 4, table 6); some patients had a marked benefit of treatment, as the 90th percentile in the Δ height SDS was 3.2. The median total GH dose was 0.25 mg/kg/week. The dose did change during puberty. The injection frequency per week in this cohort was less than optimal, with a median frequency of 6.

Dyschondrosteosis (OMIM No. 127300)
The KIGS registry lists 46 patients with a diagnosis of dyschondrosteosis (Leri-Weill syndrome) (table 3). The age at the start of GH therapy was rather late at 10.3 years, and the height SDS at the start was –3.0. In 20 patients (10 females/10 males), prepubertal GH therapy for 1 year could be evaluated (table 7). The median age at the start of treatment was 9.5 years. The GH dose was 0.26 mg/kg/week, given at 7 injections per week in most patients. The gain in the height SDS during the first year of GH therapy showed an increase of 0.7 SD (fig. 5). The sitting height ratio SDS did not change during 1 year of treatment. The body mass index SDS was likewise not affected during treatment, from 0.2 to 0.3 (n = 20). Data on near adult height are not yet available.

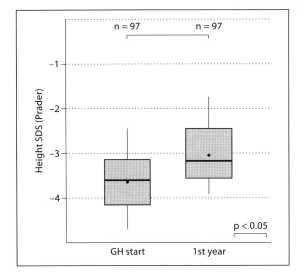
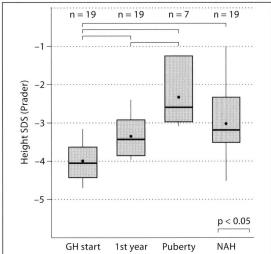

Fig. 3. Height SDS prior to and after 1 year of GH treatment in prepubertal patients with hypochondroplasia.

Fig. 4. Height – midparental height (MPH) SDS at GH start, after 1 year, at puberty onset and at near adult height (NAH) in patients with hypochondroplasia.

Table 5. Prepubertal longitudinal growth – hypochondroplasia

	All				Females		Males	
	n	median	10th percentile	90th percentile	n	median	n	median
Start of GH treatment								
Age, years	97	8.6	4.6	11.7	41	8.5	56	8.8
Bone age, years	31	7.1	3.3	10.1	18	6.5	13	7.1
Height, cm					41	109.2	56	112.5
Height SDS (Prader)	97	–3.6	–4.7	–2.4	41	–3.6	56	–3.6
Sitting height ratio SDS	37	3.0	0.3	5.8	9	9.6	20	2.1
Height – MPH SDS (Prader)	90	–2.1	–4.2	–0.3	38	–3.1	52	–1.4
Height velocity, cm/year	49	4.2	3.2	7.0	22	4.5	27	3.8
BMI SDS	97	0.6	–0.8	2.1	41	0.6	56	0.7
GH dose, mg/kg/week	97	0.24	0.16	0.33	41	0.27	56	0.23
One year of GH therapy								
Age, years	97	9.7	5.7	12.7	41	9.5	56	9.9
Height, cm					41	116.6	56	120.4
Height SDS (Prader)	97	–3.2	–3.9	–1.7	41	–3.2	56	–3.1
Sitting height ratio SDS	41	3.4	0.8	5.8	20	3.7	21	2.5
Height – MPH SDS (Prader)	90	–1.5	–3.6	0.2	38	–2.3	52	–1.0
Height velocity, cm/year	97	7.4	5.2	9.3	41	7.7	56	7.2
BMI SDS	96	0.6	–0.8	2.3	40	0.6	56	0.6
Mean GH dose, mg/kg/week	97	0.24	0.16	0.35	41	0.3	56	0.23

MPH = Midparental height; BMI = body mass index.

Table 6. Near adult height – hypochondroplasia

	All			
	n	median	10th percentile	90th percentile
Start of GH treatment				
Age, years	19	9.6	7.3	12.2
Bone age, years	8	6.4	4.5	12.0
Height SDS (Prader)	19	–4.1	–4.7	–3.2
Sitting height ratio SDS	5	2.5	2.3	3.2
Height – MPH SDS (Prader)	18	–1.6	–4.0	–0.9
Height velocity, cm/year	14	3.9	3.2	4.8
BMI SDS	19	0.2	–1.8	1.3
GH dose, mg/kg/week	12	0.22	0.16	0.32
One year of GH therapy				
Age, years	19	10.6	8.4	13.2
Height SDS (Prader)	19	–3.4	–4.0	–2.4
Sitting height ratio SDS	7	2.5	1.2	3.6
Height – MPH SDS (Prader)	18	–1.1	–3.3	–0.3
Height velocity, cm/year	19	7.6	4.1	9.0
BMI SDS	19	0.2	–1.3	1.3
GH dose, mg/kg/week	19	0.23	0.15	0.30
At start of puberty				
Age, years	7	12.0	11.4	14.7
Height SDS (Prader)	7	–2.6	–3.1	–1.3
Sitting height ratio SDS	5	2.1	0.9	2.8
Height – MPH SDS (Prader)	6	0.0	–1.7	0.5
Δ height SDS between GH start and puberty (Prader)	7	1.1	0.6	2.9
BMI SDS	7	–0.3	–2.1	1.4
Near adult height				
Age, years	19	16.6	15.7	18.4
Height SDS (Prader)	19	–3.2	–4.5	–1.0
Sitting height ratio SDS	13	2.1	0.6	5.9
Height – MPH SDS (Prader)	18	–0.9	–4.0	0.4
Δ height SDS between puberty and latest visit (Prader)	7	–0.2	–0.7	0.4
Δ height SDS between GH start and latest visit (Prader)	19	0.9	0.1	3.2
BMI SDS	18	0.5	–0.2	1.8

MPH = Midparental height; BMI = body mass index.

Spondyloepiphyseal Dysplasia (OMIM No. 183900)

The KIGS registry lists 23 patients with spondyloepiphyseal dysplasia (10 females/13 males) (table 3). The age at the start of therapy was 7.0 years with a GH dose of 0.28 mg/kg/week at 7 injections per week. GH therapy in 17 prepubertal patients did not result in a significant increase in the height SDS during the first year of therapy, although some patients did seem to benefit

Table 7. Prepubertal longitudinal growth – dyschondrosteosis

	All			
	n	median	10th percentile	90th percentile
Start of GH treatment				
Age, years	20	9.5	5.0	12.2
Bone age, years	5	10.0	6.4	13.0
Height SDS (Prader)	20	–3.2	–5.0	–2.1
Sitting height ratio SDS	10	2.7	2.3	6.9
Height – MPH SDS (Prader)	20	–1.0	–3.4	0.0
Height velocity, cm/year	13	4.5	3.2	5.4
BMI SDS	20	0.2	–0.4	1.2
GH dose, mg/kg/week	20	0.26	0.17	0.38
One year of GH therapy				
Age, years	20	10.6	5.9	13.3
Height SDS (Prader)	20	–2.5	–4.0	–1.6
Sitting height ratio SDS	11	2.7	1.7	3.4
Height – MPH SDS (Prader)	20	–0.3	–2.4	0.6
Height velocity, cm/year	20	7.8	6.2	9.5
BMI SDS	20	0.3	–0.5	1.3
Mean GH dose, mg/kg/week	20	0.26	0.16	0.37

MPH = Midparental height; BMI = body mass index.

Table 8. Prepubertal longitudinal growth – spondyloepiphyseal dysplasia

	All			
	n	median	10th percentile	90th percentile
Start of GH treatment				
Age, years	17	7.0	3.3	10.9
Bone age, years	7	7.7	4.5	10.0
Height SDS (Prader)	17	–4.5	–7.4	–2.5
Sitting height ratio SDS	7	2.7	–0.9	3.7
Height – MPH SDS (Prader)	16	–3.8	–6.2	–1.5
Height velocity, cm/year	7	5.5	2.7	6.2
BMI SDS	17	1.5	–1.4	2.7
GH dose, mg/kg/week	17	0.29	0.17	0.42
One year of GH therapy				
Age, years	17	8.0	4.3	11.9
Height SDS (Prader)	17	–3.9	–7.2	–1.4
Sitting height ratio SDS	10	1.8	–2.3	4.3
Height – MPH SDS (Prader)	16	–3.3	–6.0	–0.7
Height velocity, cm/year	17	6.7	5.3	9.1
BMI SDS	17	1.4	–0.9	2.6
Mean GH dose, mg/kg/week	17	0.29	0.20	0.41

MPH = Midparental height; BMI = body mass index.

Table 9. Auxological characteristics of patients with pseudoachondroplasia

	All			
	n	median	10th percentile	90th percentile
Background				
Birth weight SDS	10	–0.7	–3.8	0.8
Birth length SDS	5	–0.2	–4.7	1.9
MPH SDS (Prader)	14	–0.5	–1.8	0.8
Maximum GH, μg/l	8	11.1	2.8	23.5
Start of GH treatment				
Age, years	14	7.4	2.5	11.8
Bone age, years	4	3.3	1.0	4.5
Height SDS (Prader)	14	–4.8	–6.2	–3.5
Sitting height ratio SDS	8	5.8	2.4	11.9
Height – MPH SDS (Prader)	14	–4.2	–6.0	–2.5
Height velocity, cm/year	5	2.8	0.8	5.2
BMI SDS	14	1.6	–0.1	3.5
GH dose, mg/kg/week	14	0.26	0.19	0.49

MPH = Midparental height; BMI = body mass index.

(table 8, fig. 6). Body proportions could be followed in a few individuals with a change in the sitting height SDS from 2.7 (n = 7) to 1.8 (n = 10). No near adult heights were available.

Pseudoachondroplasia

The KIGS registry lists 14 patients with pseudoachondroplasia. All provide sufficient data for analysis (table 9). The median age at the start of therapy was 7.4 years, with a GH dose of 0.26 mg/kg/week at 7 injections per week. The height SDS at the start of treatment was –4.8, and the sitting height ratio SDS was 5.8. In 8 patients that could be followed through 1 year of prepubertal GH therapy the median age at the start of treatment was 5.6 years. The increase in height was not significant, with a median gain of 0.2 SD. The sitting height ratio changed from 5.8 to 7.8 SD, indicating a worsening of body propor-

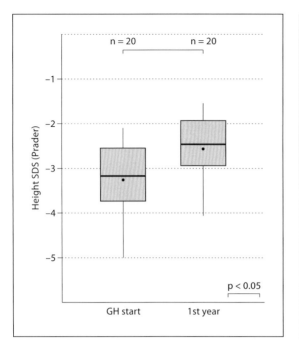

Fig. 5. Height SDS prior to and after 1 year of GH treatment in patients with dyschondrosteosis.

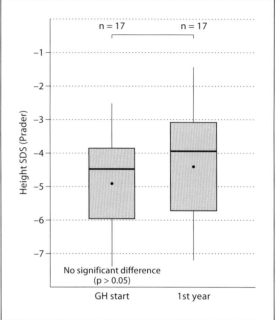

Fig. 6. Height SDS prior to and after 1 year of GH treatment in patients with spondyloepiphyseal dysplasia.

tions. Near adult height was not available in any patient.

Metaphyseal Chondrodysplasia
(McKusick, Schmid, Undescribed)
In the KIGS registry, 23 patients are reported as having a metaphyseal dysplasia, but the precise subtype is not given. A further 9 patients are reported to have the McKusick type and 5 patients the Schmid subtype of metaphyseal dysplasia. Thus, it is not possible to give further data on the effect of GH therapy in this patient group.

Discussion

The severe growth deficiency in these disorders has led to many attempts to alleviate this setback, and the first report on GH treatment in a patient with achondroplasia was published in 1964 [3]. The majority of investigations of the effect of GH therapy relate to children with achondroplasia and hypochondroplasia. No randomized, placebo-controlled studies have been published in this area. There are only a few studies of children with other skeletal dysplasias treated with GH, and most of these include few patients [4–6]. There is also a lack of information on the development of body proportions during GH therapy [7].

The grouping in the KIGS registry is based on the diagnosis made by the treating physician. This diagnosis is primarily obtained by a radiological diagnosis, which in several cases may present some difficulty. There are no records of molecular diagnosis in the KIGS registry. Consequently, there is an amount of uncertainty surrounding the reported diagnoses. One exception may be achondroplasia, which is quite recognizable both clinically and radiologically. On the other hand, there are few studies of these patients where larger numbers of patients with skeletal dysplasia have been reported. Therefore, a review of the KIGS experience is warranted.

This review of the KIGS data reveals a moderate, but significant gain in the height SDS after 1 year in 3 of the 5 diagnoses described; however, a long-term effect can only be partly assessed in hypochondroplasia and remains to be demonstrated in achondroplasia and Leri-Weill syndrome.

Achondroplasia

This disease is caused by an almost uniform mutation in the FGFR3 gene in all patients [8, 9]. The mutation in the transmembrane region of the FGFR3 protein leads to a gain in function of FGFR3, and thus, to premature growth cessation of the chondrocytes, especially in the long bones [10]. The mean final height in untreated patients with achondroplasia is around 124 cm in girls and 132 cm in boys, with a range of approximately 106–142 cm [1, 11]. Several papers have described GH treatment in this condition [12–15]. The effect varies, with a gain of 1–1.5 SD over 3–5 years. No final height data have been presented so far.

Only a minor gain in the height SDS was found in the results from the KIGS registry, and the result was lower than that found in the studies mentioned above. This could be due to a somewhat lower dose of GH during therapy. However, the dose is larger than the one used in the hypochondroplasia group and also comparable with the doses used in some of the other studies. Nonetheless, a high dose may be preferable [12].

In the group of patients that had records of body proportions, no deterioration in the sitting height ratio was seen, indicating that GH therapy does not influence body proportions adversely in accordance with previous studies [12].

The growth impairment in patients with achondroplasia is probably of such magnitude that GH therapy is unlikely to benefit the patients, if not a very high dose is used.

Hypochondroplasia

Hypochondroplasia is the most frequent skeletal dysplasia in the KIGS registry. In about 60% of the patients, the mutation causing hypochondroplasia is found in the FGFR3 gene, whereas in up to 40% of patients with a radiologically and clinically confirmed diagnosis of hypochondroplasia, no mutation could be found in the FGFR3 gene or other genes. The most prevalent FGFR3 mutation is the Asn540Lys (N540K). Other mutations in the FGFR3 gene have also been found to cause hypochondroplasia [16–20]. The mutation is often situated in the tyrosine kinase part of the protein leading to a gain in function, although at a milder level than in achondroplasia or thanatophoric dysplasia [21]. One early study has suggested a link to the insulin-like growth factor 1 gene [22], although this has not since been confirmed. In most cases, the final height in hypochondroplasia is compromised and in the range of 132–147 cm [1, 23]. However, a few cases have been reported to have normal height, although with abnormal body proportions [17, 24]. Several investigators have studied the effect of GH in children with hypochondroplasia [15, 22, 25, 26]. The gain in the height SDS was found to be in the order of approximately 1 SD after 2–3 years of treatment, but with some variation. The results in the KIGS registry are in line with the published results. The final height gain in hypochondroplasia of about 1 SD is in the same order as that obtained in the KIGS registry for Turner syndrome. A previous analysis from the KIGS registry of 3 years of GH therapy in 33 prepubertal patients with hypochondroplasia also revealed a gain of approximately 1 SD [27]. The dose used in the KIGS patients is lower than that used in for example Turner studies, and a better effect using a higher dose might be expected [28]. The range in the effect of treatment certainly supports this view, although some patients had no improvement by the therapy. On the other hand, some patients actually experienced a marked effect of the treatment with a gain of more than 3 SD. Of special note is also the age at the start of therapy, as most studies have shown better results if treatment is started at an early age. There was a slight increase in the body disproportion parameter (sitting height ratio). However, this is also seen in normal patients at this stage of childhood growth, and therefore, it is not an indication of worsening in the body disproportion during GH therapy. One caveat in interpreting the data is the missing DNA confirmation of the diagnosis, and thus, the possible heterogeneity in this group of patients. The large range in the response to GH treatment in the patients who had reached near adult height may imply that a subgroup of patients with hypochondroplasia benefits significantly from GH therapy. A clinical study of GH treatment, including thorough investigations of the genetic background, in these patients seems warranted.

Dyschondrosteosis

Dyschondrosteosis or Leri-Weill syndrome is a mesomelic skeletal disorder caused by a deletion or mutation in the SHOX gene. Several mutations and deletions have been described [29–34]. A genotype-phenotype correlation has also been described, especially when considering the wrist X-ray [30]. There are abnormal body proportions due to short legs (increased sitting height ratio), and the adult height in individuals with dyschondrosteosis is variable but in most patients reduced, whereas the height reduction seems to be gender specific with a greater loss of height in females compared with males [35, 36].

The effect in the KIGS registry patients was moderate, but statistically significant. As in the previous 2 disorders, the dose was reasonable but lower than the recommended dose in Turner syndrome. GH therapy has been investigated in a number of studies, and the effect has been comparable with that observed in other skeletal dysplasias [5, 6, 30].

Spondyloepiphyseal Dysplasia

This is the fourth most common skeletal dysplasia in the KIGS registry (excluding osteogenesis imperfecta). The cause of spondyloepiphyseal dysplasia is a deletion or mutation in the gene coding for collagen type II (COL2A1). Mutations in the COL2A1 gene can cause a variety of phenotypes ranging from lethal hypochondrogenesis to almost no symptoms, except for mild arthrosis [37]. The phenotype of congenital spondyloepiphyseal dysplasia comprises severe short stature (although variable in some), with final heights in most individuals of 100–125 cm. Other symptoms include a markedly short trunk, short limbs, myopia, platyspondyly and a risk of luxation of the dens axis when hyperextending the cervical columna. Hands and feet often have normal size and proportions. Despite the severe growth impairment seen in this disorder, very few papers have reported on GH treatment in these individuals, and mostly, the results have been disappointing. The effect reported from the KIGS registry is also poor, as no effect could be demonstrated during 1 year of therapy with a reasonable dose. The reason for the poor response in congenital spondyloepiphyseal dysplasia, in contrast to the effect seen in for example achondroplasia and hypochondroplasia, might originate in the cause of the disease. The mutation in the collagen type II molecule leads to defective 'building blocks' of the bone, and therefore, to shortened growth. In the other disorders, the growth impairment is due to a defective growth process, which can be enhanced and enlarged by GH treatment.

Pseudoachondroplasia

This disorder is caused by mutations in the COMP gene leading to a defect in the cartilage oligomeric matrix protein [38]. The mutations interfere with the normal folding of the protein leading to an accumulation of the proteins in the endoplasmatic reticulum of this and other proteins (including collagen type IX and chondroitin sulfate), thus leading to death of the cell. The result is a decrease in viable cells in the bone matrix and reduced bone size. The final height is severely affected, with final heights of around 80–130 cm. The growth pattern differs somewhat from most skeletal dysplasias, showing almost normal growth during the first year or so. The phenotype of pseudoachondroplasia also involves a waddling gait, deformity of the legs, short fingers, loose joint and ligamentous laxity [39]. The effect of GH therapy has only been reported in one earlier study including 4 children, but no effect of GH therapy was found [4]. The result from the KIGS registry supports this finding, as well as raising the question of an aggravation of the body disproportion; therefore, treatment of this disorder with GH is inadvisable. The reason for the poor response in this disorder and the aforementioned spondyloepiphyseal dysplasia is likely due to the disordered bone structure.

Conclusion

A moderate effect of GH therapy was seen during the first year of therapy in 3 of the 5 disorders described. This modest effect of GH was possibly due to doses below the optimal dose for severe growth impairment in these disorders. The abnormal body proportions of the patients were not affected. Only for a group of patients with hypochondroplasia could the final height be reported, and in this group, there was a small but significant gain in height equivalent to approximately 5–6 cm.

References

1 Scott CI Jr: Dwarfism. Summit, Ciba-Geigy, 1988.
2 Oberklaid F, Danks DM, Jensen F, Stace L, Rosshandler S: Achondroplasia and hypochondroplasia. J Med Genet 1979; 16:140–146.
3 Gershberg H, Mari S, Hulse M, St Paul H: Long-term treatment of hypopituitary and of achondroplastic dwarfism with human growth hormone. Metabolism 1964;13:152–160.
4 Kanazawa H, Tanaka H, Inoue M, Yamanaka Y, Namba N, Seino Y: Efficacy of growth hormone therapy for patients with skeletal dysplasia. J Bone Miner Res 2003;21:307–310.
5 Munns CF, Berry M, Vickers D, Rappold GA, Hyland VJ, Glass IA, Batch JA: Effect of 24 months of recombinant growth hormone on height and body proportions in SHOX haploinsufficiency. J Pediatr Endocrinol Metab 2003;16: 997–1004.
6 Thuestad IJ, Ivarsson SA, Nilsson KO, Wattsgård C: Growth hormone treatment in Leri-Weill syndrome. J Pediatr Endocrinol Metab 1996;9:201–204.
7 Hagenäs L, Hertel T: Skeletal dysplasia, growth hormone treatment and body proportions: comparison with other syndromic and non-syndromic short children. Horm Res 2003;60:65–70.
8 Horton WA, Lunstrum GP: Fibroblast growth factor receptor 3 mutations in achondroplasia and related forms of dwarfism. Rev Endocr Metab Disord 2002;3:381–385.
9 Shiang R, Thompson LM, Zhu YZ, Church DM, Fielder TJ, Bocian M, Winokur ST, Wasmuth JJ: Mutations in the transmembrane domain of FGFR3 cause the most common genetic form of dwarfism, achondroplasia. Cell 1994; 78:335–342.
10 Ornitz DM, Marie PJ: FGF signaling pathways in endochondral and intramembranous bone development and human genetic disease. Genes Dev 2002;16:1446–1465.
11 Horton WA, Rotter JI, Rimoin DL, Scott CI Jr, Hall JG: Standard growth curves for achondroplasia. J Pediatr 1978;93:435–438.
12 Hertel NT, Eklof O, Ivarsson S, Aronson S, Westphal O, Sipila I, Kaitila I, Bland J, Veimo D, Muller J, Mohnike K, Neumeyer L, Ritzen M, Hagenas L: Growth hormone treatment in 35 prepubertal children with achondroplasia: a five-year dose-response trial. Acta Paediatr 2005;94:1402–1410.
13 Horton WA, Hecht JT, Hood OJ, Marshall RN, Moore WV, Hollowell JG: Growth hormone therapy in achondroplasia. Am J Med Genet 1992;42:667–670.
14 Ramaswami U, Rumsby G, Spoudeas HA, Hindmarsh PC, Brook CGD: Treatment of achondroplasia with growth hormone: six years of experience. Pediatr Res 1999;46:435–439.
15 Tanaka N, Katsumata N, Horikawa R, Tanaka T: The comparison of the effects of short-term growth hormone treatment in patients with achondroplasia and with hypochondroplasia. Endocr J 2003;50:69–75.

16 Bellus GA, Spector EB, Speiser PW, Weaver CA, Garber AT, Bryke CR, Israel J, Rosengren SS, Webster MK, Donoghue DJ, Francomano CA: Distinct missense mutations of the FGFR3 lys650 codon modulate receptor kinase activation and the severity of the skeletal dysplasia phenotype. Am J Hum Genet 2000;67:1411–1421.

17 Grigelioniené G, Hagenäs L, Eklöf O, Neumeyer L, Haereid PE, Anvret M: A novel missense mutation Ile538Val in the fibroblast growth factor 3 in hypochondroplasia. Hum Mutat 1998;11:333.

18 Heuertz S, Le Merrer M, Zabel B, Wright M, Legeai-Mallet L, Cormier-Daire V, Gibbs L, Bonaventure J: Novel FGFR3 mutations creating cysteine residues in the extracellular domain of the receptor cause achondroplasia or severe forms of hypochondroplasia. Eur J Hum Genet 2006;14:1240–1247.

19 Thauvin-Robinet C, Faivre L, Lewin P, De Monleon JV, Francois C, Huet F, Couailler JF, Campos-Xavier AB, Bonaventure J, Le Merrer M: Hypochondroplasia and stature within normal limits: another family with an Asn540Ser mutation in the fibroblast growth factor receptor 3 gene. Am J Med Genet 2003;119A:81–84.

20 Winterpacht A, Hilbert K, Stelzer C, Schweikardt T, Decker H, Segerer H, Spranger J, Zabel B: A novel mutation in FGFR-3 disrupts a putative N-glycosylation site and results in hypochondroplasia. Physiol Genomics 2000;2:9.

21 Bellus GA, McIntosh I, Smith EA, Aylsworth AS, Kaitila I, Horton WA, Greenhaw GA, Hecht JT, Francomano CA: A recurrent mutation in the tyrosine kinase domain of fibroblast growth factor 3 causes hypochondroplasia. Nat Genet 1995;10:357–359.

22 Mullis PE, Patel MS, Brickell PM, Hindmarsh PC, Brook CGD: Growth characteristics and response to growth hormone therapy in patients with hypochondroplasia: genetic linkage of the insulin-like growth factor I gene at chromosome 12q23 to the disease in a subgroup of these patients. Clin Endocrinol 1991;34:265–274.

23 Appan S, Laurent S, Chapman M, Hindmarsh PC, Brook CGD: Growth and growth hormone therapy in hypochondroplasia. Acta Paediatr Scand 1990;79:796–803.

24 Riepe FG, Krone N, Sippell WG: Disproportionate stature but normal height in hypochondroplasia. Eur J Pediatr 2005;164:397–399.

25 Bridges NA, Hindmarsh P, Brook CGD: Growth of children with hypochondroplasia treated with growth hormone for up to three years. Horm Res 1991;36(suppl 1):56–60.

26 Ramaswami U, Hindmarsh PC, Brook CGD: Growth hormone therapy in hypochondroplasia. Acta Paediatr Suppl 1999;428:116–117.

27 Hertel NT, Hagenäs L, Otten BJ, De Schepper J, Gregory JW, Sipilä I: Three years of growth hormone treatment in 33 prepubertal children with hypochondroplasia. The KIGS experience. Horm Res 2005;64(suppl 1):51.

28 van Pareren YK, de Muinck Keizer-Schrama S, Stijnen T, Sas TCJ, Jansen M, Otten BJ, Hoorweg-Nijman JJG, Vulsma T, Stokvis-Brantsma WH, Rouwe CW, Reeser HM, Gerver WJ, Gosen JJ, Rongen-Westerlaken C, Drop SLS: Final height in girls with Turner syndrome after long-term growth hormone treatment in three dosages and low dose estrogens. J Clin Endocrinol Metab 2003;88:1119–1125.

29 Belin V, Cusin V, Viot G, Girlich D, Toutain A, Moncla A, Vekemans M, Le Merrer M, Munnich A, Cormier-Daire V: SHOX mutations in dyschondrosteosis (Leri-Weill syndrome). Nat Genet 1998;19:67–69.

30 Binder G, Renz A, Martinez A, Keselman A, Hesse V, Riedl SW, Hausler G, Fricke-Otto S, Frisch H, Heinrich JJ, Ranke MB: SHOX haploinsufficiency and Leri-Weill dyschondrosteosis: prevalence and growth failure in relation to mutation, sex, and degree of wrist deformity. J Clin Endocrinol Metab 2004;89:4403–4408.

31 Cormier-Daire V, Belin V, Cusin V, Viot G, Girlich D, Toutain A, Moncla A, Vekemans M, Le MM, Munnich A: SHOX gene mutations and deletions in dyschondrosteosis or Leri-Weill syndrome. Acta Paediatr Suppl 1999;88:55–59.

32 Grigelioniené G, Schoumans J, Neumeyer L, Ivarsson SA, Eklöf O, Enkvist O, Tordai P, Fosdal I, Myhre AG, Westphal O, Nilsson NÖ, Elfving M, Ellis I, Anderlid BM, Fransson I, Tapia-Paez I, Nordenskjöld M, Hagenäs L, Dumanski JP: Analysis of short stature homeobox-containing gene (SHOX) and auxological phenotype in dyschondrosteosis and isolated Madelung deformity. Hum Genet 2001;109:551–558.

33 Ogata T: SHOX: pseudoautosomal homeobox containing gene for short stature and dyschondrosteosis. Growth Horm IGF Res 1999;9(suppl B):53–57.

34 Ogata T: SHOX haploinsufficiency and its modifying factors. J Pediatr Endocrinol Metab 2002;15(suppl 5):1289–1294.

35 Munns CF, Glass IA, Flanagan S, Hayes M, Williams B, Berry M, Vickers D, O'Rourke P, Rao E, Rappold GA, Hyland VJ, Batch JA: Familial growth and skeletal features associated with SHOX haploinsufficiency. J Pediatr Endocrinol Metab 2003;16:987–996.

36 Ross JL, Scott C Jr, Marttila P, Kowal K, Nass A, Papenhausen P, Abboudi J, Osterman L, Kushner H, Carter P, Ezaki M, Elder F, Wei F, Chen H, Zinn AR: Phenotypes associated with SHOX deficiency. J Clin Endocrinol Metab 2001;86:5674–5680.

37 Nishimura G, Haga N, Kitoh H, Tanaka Y, Sonoda T, Kitamura M, Shirahama S, Itoh T, Nakashima E, Ohashi H, Ikegawa S: The phenotypic spectrum of COL2A1 mutations. Hum Mutat 2005;26:36–43.

38 Briggs MD, Hoffmann SMG, King LM, Olsen AS, Mohrenweiser H, Leroy JG, Mortier GR, Rimoin DL, Lachman RS, Gaines ES, Cekleniak JA, Knowlton RG, Cohn DH: Pseudoachondroplasia and multiple epiphyseal dysplasia due to mutations in the cartilage oligomeric matrix protein gene. Nat Genet 1995;10:330–336.

39 McKeand J, Rotta J, Hecht JT: Natural history study of pseudoachondroplasia. Am J Med Genet 1996;63:406–410.

Prader-Willi Syndrome and Growth Hormone Treatment

Ann Christin Lindgren

Prader-Willi syndrome (PWS) is a neurogenetic disorder characterized by both mental and physical abnormalities. It is considered the most common genetic syndrome leading to life-threatening obesity. The main characteristics are muscular hypotonia, present at birth as 'floppy infant' resulting in a failure to thrive during the first months of life, and after 1–2 years of life, developing excessive appetite with progressive obesity if the caloric intake is not restricted, hypogonadism present as cryptorchidism in boys and small labia and clitoris in girls, mental retardation, behaviour abnormalities such as temper tantrums, autistic traits [1] and psychological disturbances. Respiratory and sleep disturbances (including sleep apnoea), short final stature and typical dysmorphic facial features with small hands and feet are also typical signs of PWS.

Diagnosis of PWS is made according to a set of consensus clinical criteria that were published in 1993 [2]. Recently, these clinical criteria have been revised to be able to identify the appropriate patients for DNA testing for PWS [3] (table 1). DNA testing is mandatory for the diagnosis of PWS.

Table 1. Suggested new criteria to prompt DNA testing for PWS

Age at assessment	Features sufficient to prompt DNA testing
Birth to 2 years	– hypotonia with poor suck
2–6 years	– hypotonia with a history of poor suck – global developmental delay
6–12 years	– history of hypotonia with poor suck (hypotonia often persists) – global developmental delay – excessive eating (hyperphagia, obsession with food) with central obesity if uncontrolled
13 years through adulthood	– cognitive impairment, usually mild mental retardation – excessive eating (hyperphagia, obsession with food) with central obesity if uncontrolled – hypothalamic hypogonadism and/or typical behaviour problems (including temper tantrums and obsessive-compulsive features)

Adapted from Gunay-Aygun et al. [3].

Pediatric Endocrinology Unit
Department of Woman and Child Health
Astrid Lindgren Children's Hospital, Karolinska Hospital
SE–171 76 Stockholm (Sweden)

The PWS disorder arises from a lack of expression of a paternally inherited gene or genes known to be imprinted and located in the region of chromosome 15q11-q13 [4]. Occurring in 70–75% of affected individuals, the principal genetic mutation associated with PWS is deletion of a segment of the paternally derived chromosome 15q11-q13. Several other abnormalities have been linked with the syndrome: 20–25% of patients with PWS exhibit maternal disomy of the same region of chromosome 15q, 2–5% have imprinting centre mutations, and approximately 1% of affected individuals have a balanced translocation [5–7]. The individual gene or genes from within 15q11-q13 that cause the condition have yet to be identified, but two genes involved in the development of central nervous system functioning have been demonstrated not to be expressed in PWS, namely the small nuclear ribonucleoprotein polypeptide N gene and the necdin gene [8–10].

Growth and Body Composition in Prader-Willi Syndrome

Restriction of growth is a frequently observed sequel of PWS [11]. Specific growth charts for PWS are available. In an American chart based on a study of the weight and height of 71 Caucasian Americans with PWS, aged 4–24 years, compared with healthy subjects, the 50th percentile for height in the patient group fell below the normal 5th percentile by the age of 12–14 years, whereas the 50th percentile for weight in the affected individuals approximated the 95th percentile in the healthy population [12]. As a result of their feeding difficulties, affected infants often fail to thrive and, during the first year, this may result in growth below the 3rd percentile. Thereafter, linear growth is only slightly compromised, remaining at the 10th percentile or below until the age of 10 years for females and 12 years for males, after which height velocity often declines relative to the norm at these ages, due to a lack of growth spurt [11, 12]. This growth pattern may vary in the individual child, partly as a consequence of evolving overweight or dietary interventions. Thus, it is not uncommon to see temporary growth arrest when caloric restrictions take effect after late diagnosis, or, conversely, an improvement in growth rate may be seen when overweight develops (personal observations). Cassidy [6] reports that the mean adult height achieved by men and women with PWS is 155 and 148 cm, respectively. In the German study by Wollmann et al. [13], the mean height was slightly higher, i.e. 162 and 150 cm for men and women, respectively, and similar results were found by Hauffa et al. [14] who noticed a near final mean height of 159 cm in boys and 149 cm in girls (fig. 1).

Evaluation of body composition in PWS has shown that the syndrome is associated with high body fat mass and low muscle mass independent of body weight when compared with healthy controls. Studies have shown that the mean percent body fat in PWS was 42–51% [15–17], while in healthy children and young adults, the mean percent body fat was only 11% in males, 15.5% in girls <15 years old, and 24% in females >15 years old [18, 19].

The study by Brambilla et al. [15] shows that patients with PWS have a low lean body mass (LBM) as well as a higher ratio of fat mass to LBM compared with both healthy individuals of normal weight and, importantly, those with simple obesity. The study also shows that LBM declines further with age. Young children with PWS (<12 years old) have an LBM that is 81–93% of that found in children of normal weight, whereas in older patients, LBM is only 63–83% of the normative values. Limb areas appear to be most compromised. In addition, the bone mineral content is found to be lower than in the healthy obese and normal weight populations. Notably, Eiholzer et al. [20] have shown that even in the first years of life, children with PWS have an abnormally low LBM.

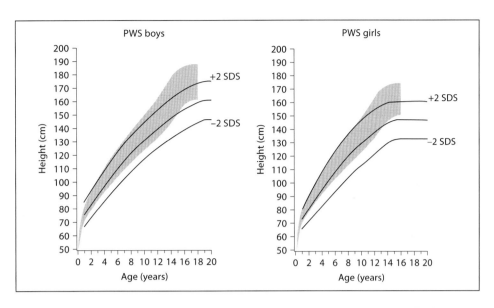

Fig. 1. Growth charts for children with PWS, ±2 standard deviation score (SDS). Shaded area = Growth chart for the normal healthy population. Adapted from the publication by Hauffa et al. [14].

The low LBM associated with PWS is likely to reflect a reduced muscle mass, and thus, it may contribute to the observed moderate clinical hypotonia and poor physical performance of these individuals [15, 21]. Muscle is a metabolically active tissue, and a small mass of this tissue, in conjunction with reduced physical activity [16], may explain the low energy expenditure found in patients with the syndrome [21–25]. In one study, patients with the condition expended approximately 50% less energy than healthy obese controls [26].

PWS is associated with increased morbidity and premature mortality, the main cause of which is thought to be overweight [27, 28]. Many of the medical complications of overweight including type II diabetes mellitus, hypertension, atherosclerosis, hyperlipidemia, compromised cardiopulmonary function, respiratory and sleep disturbances, and psychological problems such as depression and lack of self-esteem [29–32] have also been described in young patients with PWS [33, 34]. Affected individuals are at risk of developing scoliosis due to the muscular hypotonia, and this may be of concern when considering treatment with growth hormone (GH) to improve growth rate. Up to 80% of patients are reported to have a scoliosis exceeding 10°, and 15–20% have clinically significant scoliosis [35]. Similarly, there are indications that the incidence of osteoporosis is higher among patients with PWS, to which reduced GH secretion and hypogonadism could contribute [36].

The respiratory function in subjects with PWS is impaired and of multi-factorial origin including disturbed respiratory control with low response to high pCO_2 and/or to low pO_2 [36–39]. In some cases, this is present already at birth. Sleep apnoea is frequently found in children with PWS resulting in alveolar hypoventilation. The insufficiency of respiratory muscles and the pharyngeal narrowness may be important in the pathogenesis of respiratory abnormalities seen in PWS [40]. These respiratory abnormalities and the anatomical pharyngeal deviation are thought to play an important role in the cases of death reported in children with PWS treated with GH as well as in those untreated [41].

Insulin-Like Growth Factor 1/Growth Hormone Axis in Prader-Willi Syndrome

There are many data indicating a reduced GH secretion in patients with PWS. Low peak GH response to stimulation tests, decreased spontaneous GH secretion and low serum insulin-like growth factor 1 (IGF-1) levels have been documented in at least 14 studies involving about 300 affected children [42–56]. Depending on the stimulation test used, 40–100% of children with this condition fulfilled the criteria for GH deficiency (GHD), which is generally defined as 'peak GH levels of <10 μg/l in response to one or two stimulation tests'. The majority of affected children also have low GH secretion when measured by frequent blood sampling over 24 h. Low IGF-1 and GH levels are not limited to those who are severely overweight but have also been found in patients who are of normal weight [42, 53]. In addition, they have depressed levels of IGF binding protein 3 [43]. Clinical features of the condition also support the presence of GHD in PWS. Both PWS and GHD are characterized by short stature, overweight with extra fat deposits over the abdomen, abnormal body composition with reduced muscle mass, low bone density and, in some patients, retarded bone age [2, 15, 57, 58]. In summary, as a group, patients with PWS are GH deficient, though the degree of GHD may vary from mild to severe insufficiency.

Effects of Growth Hormone Treatment in Prader-Willi Syndrome

The GH-deficient state commonly associated with PWS, as evidenced by reduced GH secretion, low serum IGF-1 levels and clinical features typical of GHD, has provided a rationale for trials assessing the efficacy of GH treatment. Recently, treatment with GH has become an approved indication in Europe, the US and Japan based on the experience of three controlled randomized studies [44, 53, 59, 60]. However, up to now, the duration of treatment is limited. Longitudinal growth has been shown to increase by GH therapy [44, 50, 53, 59–66]. The initial positive effects on height velocity appear to be sustained throughout treatment. Furthermore, a report involving children treated with GH over a period of 7.5 years and other reports of shorter duration show that growth continues to improve, with the result that the target height standard deviation score can be reached [62–66].

The effect of GH therapy on body composition in PWS has been assessed in several studies [52, 60, 61], including two controlled studies [58, 65]. In these, a controlled diet was initiated before the start of therapy and maintained throughout the trial. The results show that GH treatment leads to an overall improvement in body composition by reducing fat mass and increasing muscle mass. Follow-up of long-term GH treatment has shown a reduction in fat mass and a sustained increase in LBM. However, LBM did not reach values observed in healthy children [62–66]. Improved motor performance and agility have also been documented in children with PWS who received GH therapy [58, 60, 61, 65]. Furthermore, some reports suggest that such treatment has beneficial effects on physical appearance, energy and endurance, thus improving the psychosocial functioning of affected children [44, 58, 63, 64, 67]. Adding a note of caution, it is recognized that many of these observations are based on spontaneous reports by parents and attending physicians; therefore, further studies are required to confirm these particular benefits. The patients participating in the reported studies are in most cases above the age of 3 years. However, recently controlled studies on younger children with PWS, <3 years of age, treated with GH have shown beneficial effects on body composition and mobility [20, 68]. These results suggest that early institution of GH therapy may normalize LBM, delay fat accumulation and improve motor development.

There are studies that have shown a favourable effect of GH treatment on respiratory functions in children with PWS [69] by improving respiratory muscle strength [44, 65] in connection with an improved body composition and growth. Treatment with GH has also been shown to have a direct or indirect effect on the central respiratory regulatory system resulting in increased ventilation and sensitivity of peripheral chemoreceptors to carbon dioxide [38].

Side Effects of Growth Hormone Treatment in Prader-Willi Syndrome

The reported adverse events during GH therapy of patients with PWS are generally similar to those observed during treatment of children with classic GHD, Turner syndrome or chronic renal insufficiency. Recent studies have shown that insulin levels in children with PWS are lower than in obese controls at baseline [43, 69, 70], but increase during GH treatment [69, 71]. Glucose levels tend to remain unchanged or increase within the normal reference range [69, 71]. However, considering the limited experience of prolonged GH treatment in these patients and the increased incidence of diabetes mellitus associated with the disorder, carbohydrate metabolism (glucose, haemoglobin A_{1C}) should be closely monitored in patients receiving GH therapy.

Attributed to a combination of overweight and muscular hypotonia, scoliosis is common in both children and adolescents with PWS. The rapid growth associated with GH treatment may aggravate this spinal deformity, and therefore, the occurrence and development of scoliosis should be monitored by clinical examination at every check-up of the patient during therapy. If clinical quantification of scoliosis is difficult, in extreme overweight for example, X-ray monitoring should be used. In the controlled randomized studies performed, the majority of the patients had a mild scoliosis (<20°) occurring equally among the control and treatment groups [44, 53]. Furthermore, there was no significant worsening of the condition in either group during the studies and during the follow-ups [62–66, 72].

GH treatment has not been shown to increase the rate of mortality in this condition, which is increased due to respiratory failure, although there have been some cases of mortality during therapy [41]. On the contrary, in the few studies that have been performed, GH therapy has been shown to improve respiratory function [38, 44, 73].

Conclusion

The care of children with PWS should be in close collaboration with a comprehensive team, including a paediatrician trained in endocrinology and neurology, a dietician, a physiotherapist and a psychologist. The main medical focus is to avoid development of overweight and its complications by keeping an appropriate diet with an adjusted caloric intake and physical activity. GH therapy is a complement to be able to maintain an appropriate body composition by decreased fat mass and increased muscle mass, and to improve the compromised final height. It seems as if this treatment also has a favourable effect on glucose homeostasis and blood lipids, as well as improving the respiratory function compromised in PWS. The side effects of GH treatment in PWS are few and similar to those seen in other conditions treated with GH. However, as the long-term experience of GH therapy is limited, further long-term follow-up studies and studies on infants with PWS are needed.

The present recommendations before initiating GH therapy are to avoid development of overweight by a vigorous diet and weight control, to perform polysomnography and otorhinolaryngologic examination, and to have the patient undergo tonsil/adenoidectomy if necessary. If the child snores and the snoring increases during therapy, the child must be further evaluated regarding respiratory functions. During GH treatment in subjects with PWS, carbohydrate metabolism as well as the development of scoliosis must be closely monitored.

References

1 Greaves N, Prince E, Evans DW, Charman T: Repetitive and ritualistic behaviour in children with Prader-Willi syndrome and children with autism. J Intellect Disabil Res 2006;50:92–100.
2 Holm VA, Cassidy SB, Butler MG, Hanchett JM, Greenswag LR, Whitman BY, Greenberg F: Prader-Willi syndrome. Consensus diagnostic criteria. Pediatrics 1993;91:398–402.
3 Gunay-Aygun M, Schwartz S, Heeger S, O'Riordan MA, Cassidy SB: The changing purpose of Prader-Willi syndrome clinical diagnostic criteria and proposed revised criteria. Pediatrics 2001; 108:e92.
4 Horsthemke B, Buiting K: Imprinting defects on human chromosome 15. Cytogenet Genome Res 2006;113:292–299.
5 Wharton RH, Loechner KJ: Genetic and clinical advances in Prader-Willi syndrome. Curr Opin Pediatr 1996;8: 618–624.
6 Cassidy SB: Prader-Willi syndrome. J Med Genet 1997;34:917–923.
7 Nicholls RD, Ohta T, Gray TA: Genetic abnormalities in Prader-Willi syndrome and lessons from mouse models. Acta Paediatr Suppl 1999;88:99–104.
8 MacDonald HR, Wevrick R: The necdin gene is deleted in Prader-Willi syndrome and is imprinted in human and mouse. Hum Mol Genet 1997;6:1873–1878.
9 Muscatelli F, Abrous DN, Massacrier A, Boccaccio I, Le Moal M, Cau P, Cremer H: Disruption of the mouse necdin gene results in hypothalamic and behavioral alterations reminiscent of the human Prader-Willi syndrome. Hum Mol Genet 2000;9:3101–3110.
10 Bittel DC, Butler MG: Prader-Willi syndrome: clinical genetics, cytogenetics and molecular biology. Expert Rev Mol Med 2005;7:1–20.

11 Bray GA, Dahms WT, Swerdloff RS, Fiser RH, Atkinson RL, Carrel RE: The Prader-Willi syndrome. A study of 40 patients and a review of the literature. Medicine 1983;62:59–80.
12 Butler MG, Meaney FJ: Standards for selected anthropometric measurements in Prader-Willi syndrome. Pediatrics 1991;88:853–860.
13 Wollmann HA, Schultz U, Grauer ML, Ranke MB: Reference values for height and weight in Prader-Willi syndrome based on 315 patients. Eur J Pediatr 1998;157:634–642.
14 Hauffa BP, Schlippe G, Roos M, Gillessen-Kaesbach G, Gasser T: Spontaneous growth in German children and adolescents with genetically confirmed Prader-Willi syndrome. Acta Paediatr 2000;89:1302–1311.
15 Brambilla P, Bosio L, Manzoni P, Pietrobelli A, Beccaria L, Chiumello G: Peculiar body composition in patients with Prader-Labhart-Willi syndrome. Am J Clin Nutr 1997;65:1369–1374.
16 Davies PSW, Joughlin C: Using stable isotopes to assess reduced physical activity of individuals with Prader-Willi syndrome. Am J Ment Retard 1993;3: 349–353.
17 Lee PD, Hwu K, Henson H, Brown BT, Bricker JT, LeBlanc AD, Fiorotto ML, Greenberg F, Klish WJ: Body composition studies in Prader-Willi syndrome: effects of growth hormone therapy. Basic Life Sci 1993;60:201–205.
18 Boot AM, Bouquet J, de Ridder MAJ, Krenning EP, de Muinck Keizer-Schrama SMPF: Determinants of body composition measured by dual-energy X-ray absorptiometry in Dutch children and adolescents. Am J Clin Nutr 1997;66:232–238.

19 Ogle GD, Allen JR, Humphries IR, Lu PW, Briody JN, Morley K, Howman-Giles R, Cowell CT: Body composition assessment by dual-energy X-ray absorptiometry in subjects aged 4–26. Am J Clin Nutr 1995;61:746–753.
20 Eiholzer U, l'Allemand D, Schlumpf M, Rousson V, Gasser T, Fusch T: Growth hormone and body composition in children younger than 2 years with Prader-Willi syndrome. J Pediatr 2004;144: 753–758.
21 Davies PSW, Joughin C, Cole TJ, Livingstone MBE, Barnes ND: Total energy expenditure in the Prader-Willi syndrome. Am J Clin Genet 1992;44: 75–78.
22 Coplin SS, Hine J, Gormican A: Outpatient dietary management in the Prader-Willi syndrome. J Am Diet Assoc 1976;68:330–334.
23 Nelson RA, Anderson LF, Gastineau CF, Hayles AB, Stamnes CL: Physiology and natural history of obesity. JAMA 1973;223:627–630.
24 van Mil EG, Westerterp KR, Kester AD, Curfs LM, Gerver WJ, Schrander-Stumpel CT, Saris WH: Activity related energy expenditure in children and adolescents with Prader-Willi syndrome. Int J Obes Relat Metab Disord 2000;24:429–434.
25 van Mil EG, Westerterp KR, Gerver WJ, Curfs LM, Schrander-Stumpel CT, Kester AD, Saris WH: Energy expenditure at rest and during sleep in children with Prader-Willi syndrome is explained by body composition. Am J Clin Nutr 2000;71:752–756.
26 Schoeller DA, Levitsky LL, Bandini LG, Dietz WW, Walczak A: Energy expenditure and body composition in Prader-Willi syndrome. Metabolism 1988;37: 115–120.
27 Greenswag L: Adults with Prader-Willi syndrome. A survey of 232 cases. Dev Med Child Neurol 1987;29:145–152.

28 Laurance BM, Brito A, Wilkinson J: Prader-Willi syndrome after the age of 15 years. Arch Dis Child 1981;56:181–186.
29 Klish WJ: Childhood obesity: pathophysiology and treatment. Acta Paediatr Jpn 1995;37:1–5.
30 Rosengren A, Wedel H, Wilhelmsen L: Body weight and weight gain during adult life in men in relation to coronary heart disease and mortality. A prospective population study. Eur Heart J 1999; 20:269–277.
31 Csabi G, Torok K, Jeges S, Molnar D: Presence of metabolic cardiovascular syndrome in obese children. Eur J Pediatr 2000;159:91–94.
32 Karason K, Lindroos AK, Stenlof K, Sjostrom L: Relief of cardiorespiratory symptoms and increased physical activity after surgically induced weight loss: results from the Swedish Obese Subjects Study. Arch Intern Med 2000; 160:1797–1802.
33 Burman P, Ritzén EM, Lindgren AC: Endocrine dysfunction in Prader-Willi syndrome: a review with special reference to GH. Endocr Rev 2001;22:787–799.
34 Höybye C, Hilding A, Jacobsson H, Thorén M: Metabolic profile and body composition in adults with Prader-Willi syndrome and severe obesity. J Clin Endocrinol Metab 2002;8:3590–3597.
35 Holm VA, Laurnen EL: Prader-Willi syndrome and scoliosis. Dev Med Child Neurol 1981;23:192–201.
36 Arens R, Gozal D, Burrell BC, Bailey SL, Bautista DB, Keens TG, Ward SL: Arousal and cardiorespiratory responses to hypoxia in Prader-Willi syndrome. Am J Respir Crit Care Med 1996;153:283–287.
37 Schluter B, Buschatz D, Trowitzsch E, Aksu F, Andler W: Respiratory control in children with Prader-Willi syndrome. Eur J Pediatr 1997;156:65–68.
38 Lindgren AC, Hellström LG, Ritzén EM, Milerad J: Growth hormone treatment increases CO(2)-response, ventilation and central respiratory drive in children with Prader-Willi syndrome. Eur J Pediatr 1999;158:936–940.
39 Nixon GM, Brouillette RT: Sleep and breathing in Prader-Willi syndrome. Pediatr Pulmonol 2002;34:209–217.

40 Richards A, Quaghebeur G, Clift S, Holland A, Dahlitz M, Parkes D: The upper airway and sleep apnoea in the Prader-Willi syndrome. Clin Otolaryngol Allied Sci 1994;19:193–197.
41 Eiholzer U: Deaths in children with Prader-Willi syndrome. Horm Res 2005;63:33–39.
42 Lee PDK: Endocrine and metabolic aspects of Prader-Willi syndrome; in Greenswag LR, Alexander RC (eds): Management of Prader-Willi Syndrome. New York, Springer, 1995, pp 32–57.
43 Eiholzer U, Stutz K, Weinmann C, Torresani T, Molinari L, Prader A: Low insulin, IGF-I and IGFBP-3 levels in children with Prader-Labhart-Willi syndrome. Eur J Pediatr 1998;157:890–893.
44 Carrel AL, Myers SE, Whitman BY, Allen DB: Growth hormone improves body composition, fat utilization, physical strength and agility, and growth in Prader-Willi syndrome: a controlled study. J Pediatr 1999;134:215–221.
45 Fesseler WH, Bierich JR: Untersuchungen beim Prader-Labhart-Willi-Syndrome. Monatsschr Kinderheilkd 1983; 131:844–847.
46 Costeff H, Holm VA, Ruvalcaba R, Shaver J: Growth hormone secretion in Prader-Willi syndrome. Acta Paediatr Scand 1990;79:1059–1062.
47 Calisti L, Giannessi N, Cesaretti G, Saggese G: Studio endocrino nella sindrome di Prader-Willi. A proposito di 5 casi. Minerva Pediatr 1991;43:587–593.
48 Huw K, Klish WJ, Henson H, Brown BT, Bricker JT, LeBlanc AD, Fiorotto ML, Greenberg F, Lee PDK: Endocrine status, growth hormone therapy and body composition in Prader-Willi syndrome (abstract 710). Abstr 74th Annu Meet Endocr Soc, San Antonio, Texas, 1992, p 229.
49 Cappa M, Grossi A, Borrelli P, Ghigo E, Bellone J, Benedetti S, Carta D, Loche S: Growth hormone (GH) response to combined pyridostigmine and GH-releasing hormone administration in patients with Prader-Labhardt-Willi syndrome. Horm Res 1993;39:51–55.

50 Angulo M, Castro-Magana M, Mazur B, Canas JA, Vitollo PM, Sarrantonio M: Growth hormone secretion and effects of growth hormone therapy on growth velocity and weight gain in children with Prader-Willi syndrome. J Pediatr Endocrinol Metab 1996;3:393–399.
51 Grosso S, Cioni M, Buoni S, Peruzzi L, Pucci L, Berardi R: Growth hormone secretion in Prader-Willi syndrome. J Endocrinol Invest 1998;21:418–422.
52 Grugni G, Guzzaloni G, Moro D, Bettio D, De Medici C, Morabito F: Reduced growth hormone (GH) responsiveness to combined GH-releasing hormone and pyridostigmine administration in the Prader-Willi syndrome. Clin Endocrinol (Oxf) 1998;48:769–775.
53 Lindgren AC, Hagenäs L, Müller J, Blichfeldt S, Rosenborg M, Brismar T, Ritzén EM: Growth hormone treatment of children with Prader-Willi syndrome affects linear growth and body composition favourably. Acta Paediatr 1998;87:28–31.
54 Sipilä I, Alanne S, Apajasalo M, Hietanen H: Growth hormone therapy in children with Prader-Willi syndrome. A preliminary report of one year treatment in 19 children (abstract). Horm Res 1998;50(suppl 3):1–150.
55 Thacker MJ, Hainline B, St Dennis-Feezle L, Johnson NB, Pescovitz OH: Growth failure in Prader-Willi syndrome is secondary to growth hormone deficiency. Horm Res 1998;49:216–220.
56 Corrias A, Bellone J, Beccaria L, Bosio L, Trifiro G, Livieri C, Ragusa L, Salvatoni A, Andreo M, Ciampalini P, Tonini G, Crino A: GH/IGF-I axis in Prader-Willi syndrome: evaluation of IGF-I levels and of the somatotroph responsiveness to various provocative stimuli. Genetic Obesity Study Group of Italian Society of Pediatric Endocrinology and Diabetology. J Endocrinol Invest 2000; 23:84–89.
57 Rosenbaum M, Gerner J, Leibel R: Effects of systemic (GH) administration on regional adipose tissue distribution in GH-deficient children. J Clin Endocrinol Metab 1989;69:1274–1281.
58 Lindgren AC, Hagenäs L, Müller J, Blichfeldt S, Rosenborg M, Brismar T, Ritzén EM: Effects of growth hormone treatment on growth and body composition in Prader-Willi syndrome: a preliminary report. Acta Paediatr Suppl 1997;423:60–62.

59 Hauffa BP: One-year results of growth hormone treatment of short stature in Prader-Willi syndrome. Acta Paediatr Suppl 1997;423:63–65.
60 Davies PSW, Evens S, Broomhead S, Clough H, Day JME, Laidlaw A, Barnes ND: Effect of growth hormone on height, weight, and body composition in Prader-Willi syndrome. Arch Dis Child 1998;78:474–476.
61 Eiholzer U, Gisin R, Weinmann C, Kriemler S, Steinert H, Torresani T, Zachmann M, Prader A: Treatment with human growth hormone in patients with Prader-Labhart-Willi syndrome reduces body fat and increases muscle mass and physical performance. Eur J Pediatr 1997;157:368–377.
62 Lindgren AC, Ritzén EM: Five years of growth hormone treatment in children with Prader-Willi syndrome. Acta Paediatr Suppl 1999;433:109–111.
63 Eiholzer U, l'Allemand D: Growth hormone normalizes height, prediction of final height and hand length in children with Prader-Willi syndrome after 4 years of therapy. Horm Res 2000;53:185–192.
64 Lindgren AC: Long-term growth hormone therapy in children with Prader-Willi syndrome. Proc 36th Int Symp Growth Horm Growth Factors Endocrinol Metab, Geneva, 2004.
65 Myers SE, Carrel AL, Whitman BY, Allen DB: Sustained benefit after 2 years of growth hormone on body composition, fat utilization, physical strength and agility, and growth in Prader-Willi syndrome. J Pediatr 2000;137:42–49.
66 Carrel AL, Myers SE, Whitman BY, Allen DB: Benefits of long-term GH therapy in Prader-Willi syndrome: a 4-year study. J Clin Endocrinol Metab 2002;87:1581–1585.
67 Whitman BY, Myers S, Carrel A, Allen D: The behavioral impact of growth hormone treatment for children and adolescents with Prader-Willi syndrome: a 2-year controlled study. Pediatrics 2002;109:E35.
68 Carrel AL, Moerchen V, Myers SE, Bekx T, Whitman BY, Allen DB: Growth hormone improves mobility and body composition in infants and toddlers with Prader-Willi syndrome. J Pediatr 2004;145:744–749.
69 Lindgren AC, Hagenas L, Ritzen EM: Growth hormone treatment of children with Prader-Willi syndrome: effects on glucose and insulin hemostasis. Swedish National Growth Hormone Advisory Group. Horm Res 1999;51:157–161.
70 Zipf WB: Glucose homeostasis in Prader-Willi syndrome and potential implications of growth hormone therapy. Acta Paediatr Suppl 1999;433:115–117.
71 L'Allemand D, Eiholzer U, Schlumpf M, Torresani T, Girard J: Carbohydrate metabolism is not impaired after 3 years of growth hormone therapy in children with Prader-Willi syndrome. Horm Res 2003;59:239–248.
72 Nagai T, Obata K, Ogata T, Murakami N, Katada Y, Yoshino A, Sakazume S, Tomita Y, Sakuta R, Niikawa N: Growth hormone therapy and scoliosis in patients with Prader-Willi syndrome. Am J Med Genet A 2006;140:1623–1627.
73 Haqq AM, Stadler DD, Jackson RH, Rosenfeld RG, Purnell JQ, LaFranchi SH: Effects of growth hormone on pulmonary function, sleep quality, behavior, cognition, growth velocity, body composition and resting energy expenditure in Prader-Willi syndrome. J Clin Endocrinol Metab 2003;88:2206–2212.

Effects of Growth Hormone Treatment in Children Presenting with Prader-Willi Syndrome: The KIGS Experience

Maïthé Tauber

Growth hormone (GH) treatment was approved very recently in 2000 in the USA and Europe, based on few studies, and a review on the effects of GH treatment has been published in 2002 [1–7]. The indications were different in the USA and Europe, i.e. for growth in the USA and for growth and/or body composition effects in Europe. KIGS represents a unique opportunity to evaluate the effect of GH in a large number of patients with Prader-Willi syndrome (PWS). Side effects have recently been reported using the KIGS database in 675 children with PWS [8].

Patients and Methods

One thousand and one hundred and thirty-five children, 603 boys (53.1%) and 532 girls, presenting with PWS [9] were entered into the KIGS database as of January 2006. The duration of GH treatment was 1.9 years (range 0.2–5.3). Six hundred and fifty-two children, 368 boys (57.4%) and 284 girls, were treated for at least 1 year and were prepubertal at the start of treatment. Ten percent of these children were treated for more than 5 years, and near final height was achieved in 33 patients (21 boys and 12 girls).

Data Collected
We chose Prader charts for the standard deviation score (SDS) [10], as it was a multinational cohort. We also used a syndrome-specific chart of PWS [11]. Midparental height (MPH) was calculated as defined previously [12]. Data are presented as medians with 10th and 90th percentiles.

Overall Group
Baseline characteristics of the 1,135 children are shown in table 1. Briefly, at the start of GH treatment, chronological age was 6.4 years with a bone age of 6.0 years; the height SDS (Prader chart) was –2.2 and the height – MPH SDS –2.0. The height SDS using the syndrome-specific chart was –0.3, height velocity was 5.1 cm/year, and the body mass index (BMI) SDS was 2.0. The birth weight SDS was –1.4 and the birth length SDS –0.5. Among 1,062 children with data on pubertal status, 10% were pubertal.

Figure 1 shows the height of the patients plotted in a combined general population and syndrome-specific charts for girls and boys.

Four hundred and twenty-four GH tests were performed (in 37% of the patients) with a maximum GH peak of 5.9 µg/l. Three hundred and ninety-three insu-

Department of Endocrinology, Hôpital des Enfants
330 avenue de Grande-Bretagne, TSA 70034
FR–31059 Toulouse Cedex 9 (France)

Table 1. Auxological and biological data at the start of GH treatment in the whole population and in boys and girls separately

	All			Boys			Girls		
	n	median	10–90th percentile	n	median	10th–90th percentile	n	median	10–90th percentile
Chronological age, years	1,135	6.4	1.3–12.9	603	6.5	1.4–12.9	532	6.3	1.3–12.8
Bone age, years	308	6.0	1.5–13.0	151	6.0	1.5–13.0	157	6.8	1.5–12.8
MPH SDS	932	−0.2	−1.8 to 1.2	495	−0.3	−1.7 to 1.2	437	−0.2	−1.8 to 1.2
Height SDS	1,135	−2.2	−4.1 to −0.3	603	−1.9	−3.8 to −0.3	532	−2.5	−4.4 to −0.7
Height − MPH SDS	932	−2.0	−4.0 to 0	495	−1.7	−3.6 to 0.1	437	−2.2	−4.3 to −0.2
Height SDS (syndrome specific)	1,058	−0.3	−1.7 to 0.9	558	−0.2	−1.8 to 1.1	500	−0.4	−1.7 to 0.7
Height velocity, cm/year	352	5.1	2.6–8.6	176	5.2	2.6–8.9	176	4.9	2.7–8.4
BMI SDS	1,135	2.0	−1.0 to 3.8	603	2.2	−0.8 to 4.0	532	1.7	−1.1 to 3.6
Birth weight SDS	1,026	−1.4	−2.8 to 0.2	538	−1.5	−3.0 to 0.1	488	−1.3	−2.7 to 0.2
Birth length SDS	783	−0.5	−2.1 to 1.4	416	−0.5	−2.2 to 1.3	367	−0.5	−2.0 to 1.6
GH dose, mg/kg/week	1,135	0.23	0.15–0.31	603	0.23	0.15–0.31	532	0.23	0.15–0.30
Maximum GH peak, μg/l	424	5.9	1.3–16.7	229	5.8	1.0–15.7	195	6.1	1.4–20.3
IGF-1 SDS	393	−1.6	−2.9 to 0.1	205	−1.55	−2.8 to −0.3	188	−1.7	−3.1 to 0.2
Years on GH treatment at latest visit	1,135	1.9	0.2–5.3	603	1.92	0.1–5.5	532	1.9	0.3–4.6

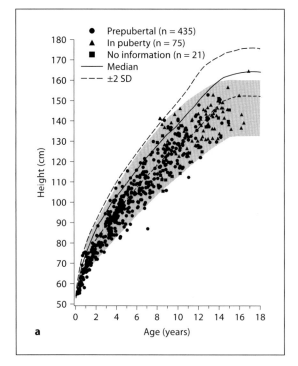 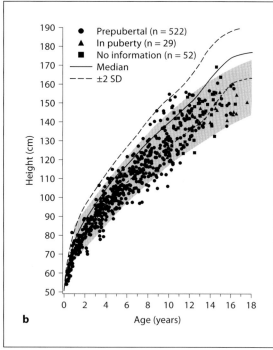

Fig. 1. Heights of girls (**a**) and boys (**b**) at the start of GH treatment plotted both in the Prader chart (white area, from −2 to +2 SD) and the Prader-Willi chart (grey area, from −2 to +2 SD).

Table 2. Auxological data at the start and after 1 year of GH treatment in the whole group and in boys and girls separately

	All			Boys			Girls		
	n	median	10–90th percentile	n	median	10–90th percentile	n	median	10–90th percentile
At start of GH treatment									
Chronological age, years	652	5.5	1.3–10.9	368	6.1	1.4–11.9	284	5.1	1.2–10.2
MPH SDS (Prader)	548	–0.2	–1.8 to 1.2	310	–0.2	–1.7 to 1.2	238	–0.2	–1.9 to 1.1
Height SDS (Prader)	652	–2.2	–4.1 to 0.4	368	–1.0	–2.7 to 0.8	284	–1.6	–3.6 to 0.3
Height – MPH SDS (Prader)	548	–2.0	–3.9 to 0.1	310	–1.8	–3.6 to 0.2	238	–2.4	–4.3 to –0.1
Height SDS (syndrome specific)	652	0.3	–1.3 to 1.8	368	0.5	–1.3 to 1.8	284	0.1	–1.3 to 1.2
Height velocity, cm/year	229	5.1	2.7–8.7	128	5.2	2.6–8.9	101	4.9	3.0–7.5
Height velocity SDS (Prader)	229	–1.4	–4.1 to 0.9	128	–1.4	–4.2 to 1.1	101	–1.5	–4.0 to 0.6
BMI SDS	652	1.7	–1.2 to 3.7	368	2.0	–1.1 to 3.9	284	1.4	–1.3 to 3.5
After 1 year on GH									
Height SDS (Prader)	652	–1.2	–3.2 to 0.6	368	–1.0	–2.7 to 0.8	284	–1.6	–3.6 to 0.3
Height velocity, cm/year	652	10.4	6.7–14.7	368	10.5	6.6–14.9	284	10.3	6.9–14.7
Height velocity SDS (Prader)	651	4.0	–0.2 to 9.0	367	4.8	–0.1 to 9.8	284	3.2	–0.2 to 7.6
Height – MPH SDS (Prader)	548	–1.0	–2.9 to 0.9	310	–0.8	–2.5 to 1.0	238	–1.2	–3.2 to 0.7
Δ height SDS (Prader)	652	0.9	0.9–0.0	368	0.9	0.0–1.8	284	0.9	0.0–1.9
BMI SDS	651	1.3	–0.9 to 3.4	368	1.6	–0.9 to 3.6	283	1.1	–0.9 to 3.1
Studentized residual	375	0.1	–1.6 to 2.0	215	0.4	–1.2 to 2.3	160	–0.2	–1.9 to 1.6

lin-like growth factor 1 (IGF-1) values were reported with a value of –1.6 SDS.

Girls were significantly shorter (p < 0.05), with a height SDS of –2.5 versus –1.9, and lighter, with a BMI SDS of 1.7 versus 2.2, compared with boys. The height – MPH SDS was higher in girls than in boys (–2.2 vs. –1.7; p < 0.05).

The median GH dose was 0.23 mg/kg/week at the start of treatment, with a duration of 1.9 years.

Subgroups of Patients
Data from 652 children (368 boys and 284 girls) regarding growth (height, growth velocity, height – MPH and gain in height, all expressed in SDS) and BMI were analyzed after 1 year of GH treatment. We divided this group according to their age at the start of GH treatment (before or after 6 years), their BMI (those with a BMI SDS >2, classified as obese, vs. those with a BMI SDS <2) and their height: short stature (SS) children with a height – MPH SDS below –2 versus non-short (NS) children with a height – MPH SDS above –2. We chose these definitions of obese/nonobese and SS/NS to limit discrepancies between countries. Data on the 33 patients who reached near final height were also analyzed.

Prediction Model
The idiopathic GH deficiency prediction model [12] without maximum GH peak was applied to these children after 1 year. Differences between observed and predicted height velocities were expressed in terms of studentized residuals. The residual is calculated as the observed height velocity – the predicted height velocity for each observation, and the studentized residual is the residual divided by its standard error. A studentized residual of 0 means that the prediction was completely fulfilled. Positive values indicate growth exceeding the prediction, negative values are the expression of growth slower than predicted.

Statistical Analysis
We used Student's t test for the comparison of data before and after treatment regarding height, BMI, gain in height and gain in BMI, as well as between boys and girls. The Wilcoxon rank sum test was used for the other variables which were not normally distributed.

Results

Effect on Growth after 1 Year of GH Treatment
Growth Effect in the Whole Group
After 1 year of GH treatment, the height SDS rose from –2.2 to –1.2 (p < 0.05) (table 2). The gain in

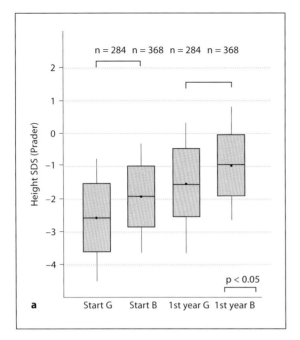
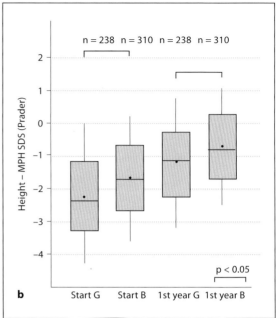
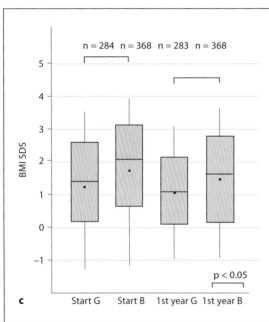

Fig. 2. Height SDS (**a**), height – MPH SDS (**b**) and BMI SDS (**c**) for girls (G) and boys (B) at the start and after 1 year of GH treatment. All data are presented as median and interquartile range (grey box) with the mean indicated as a black dot and the 10th and 90th percentiles as vertical lines.

height was 0.9 SDS. Growth velocity increased from 5.1 to 10.4 cm/year, and when expressed as SDS, increased from –1.4 to 4.0 ($p < 0.05$). The height – MPH SDS rose from –2.0 to –1.0 ($p < 0.05$) (fig. 2).

Analysis of studentized residuals with the idiopathic GH deficiency prediction model in 375 children showed that these children grew significantly better than predicted (fig. 3).

The height SDS remained lower in girls than in boys, i.e. –1.6 versus –1.0 ($p < 0.05$), and the gain in the height SDS was not significantly different (0.9).

Effect of GH in SS versus NS children

Two hundred and seventy-four children (134 boys, 140 girls) were included in the SS group and 274 (176 boys and 98 girls) in the NS group. The SS children were significantly younger than the NS children (5.0 vs. 6.9 years), and at the start of GH treatment, showed a height SDS of –2.9 versus –1.5, a height – MPH SDS of –3.0 versus –1.0 ($p < 0.05$), and a height velocity SDS of –1.6 versus –1.2 (not significant), respectively (table 3). There was no significant difference in maximum GH peak (6.4 vs. 5.9 µg/l), but SS children had significantly lower IGF-1 values (–1.9 vs. –1.4 SDS) than NS children.

The gain in the height SDS was significantly greater in SS children, i.e. 1.1 (0.4–2.0) versus 0.8 (–0.2 to 1.7; p < 0.05), but the height velocity SDS was not significantly different (4.1 vs. 4.3). Studentized residuals were significantly lower in the SS versus the NS group, i.e. –0.2 (–1.9 to 1.7) versus 0.4 (–1.2 to 2.3), indicating that SS children grew less while NS grew more than predicted by the model (fig. 4).

Growth Effect in Obese versus Nonobese Children

Two hundred and ninety-five children (194 boys and 101 girls) were classified as obese, compared with 357 (174 boys and 183 girls) who were nonobese. Obese children were significantly taller and had a lower MPH. IGF-1 levels were significantly lower in nonobese children compared with obese children, i.e. –1.7 SDS (–2.9 to –0.5) versus –1.4 SDS (2.7–0.4), while GH peak levels were nonsignificantly different.

The gain in the height SDS was not significantly different between these groups, 0.9 (0.0 to –1.8) versus 0.9 (0.0 to –1.8). Obese children had a greater decrease in BMI SDS compared with nonobese children, i.e. –0.4 (–1.3 to –0.2) versus –0.2 (–1.2 to –1.8). Growth velocity studentized residuals were significantly higher in obese children, 0.4 (–1.5 to 2.3) versus –0.2 (–1.7 to 1.6), suggesting that nonobese children grew less while obese children grew better than predicted (table 3).

Growth Effect in Children Younger and Older than 6 Years

Three hundred and forty-six children started GH treatment before 6 years of age (181 boys and 165 girls) and 306 (187 boys and 119 girls) after 6 years of age. At baseline, the younger children were significantly shorter, –2.4 SDS (–4.3 to –0.7) versus –2.1 SDS (–3.9 to –0.7), and had a lower

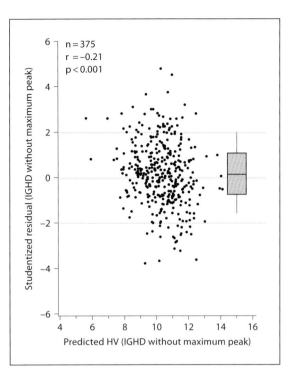

Fig. 3. Predicted height velocity (HV) during the first year on GH presented as studentized residuals (0 ± 2 SD). IGHD = Idiopathic GH deficiency.

BMI SDS, 1.1 (–2.0 to 3.8) versus 2.2 (0.5–3.7). The height – MPH SDS was –2.3 (–4.2 to 0.2) in the younger and –1.7 SDS (–3.5 to 0.2) in the older children, whereas the IGF-1 levels were lower in the older children, –1.9 SDS (–3.0 to 0.5), than in the younger children, –1.4 SDS (–2.6 to 0.2).

The height gain was significantly higher in the younger children than in the older children, i.e. 1.2 (0.3–2.0) versus 0.8 SDS (–0.2 to 1.4). Studentized residuals were significantly lower, –0.1 (–1.9 to 2.0), in the younger than in the older children, 0.3 (–1.2 to 2.1), suggesting that older children grew better than predicted by the model (table 3).

Effect on BMI after 1 Year of GH Treatment
In the whole group, the BMI SDS significantly decreased from 1.7 to 1.3 (table 2). The BMI SDS

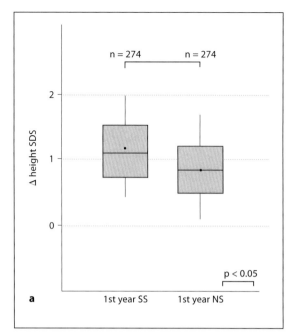
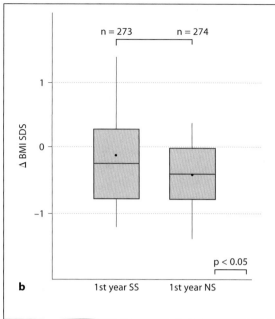
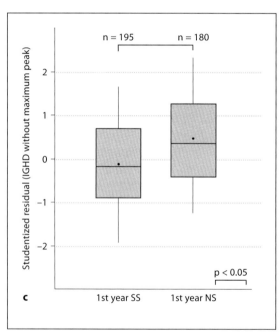

Fig. 4. Gain in height SDS (**a**), Δ BMI SDS (**b**) and studentized residuals (**c**) in SS and NS children. All data are presented as median and interquartile range (grey box) with the mean indicated as a black dot and the 10th and 90th percentiles as vertical lines. IGHD = Idiopathic GH deficiency.

remained lower ($p < 0.05$) in girls than in boys after 1 year of GH treatment (1.1 vs. 1.6). The decrease in the BMI SDS was significantly different in the 6 subgroups: –0.3 (–1.5 to 0.4) in SS children versus –0.4 (–1.4 to 1.1) in NS children, –0.4 (–1.3 to 0.2) in obese versus –0.2 (–1.2 to 1.1) in nonobese children, and –0.2 (–1.5 to 1.8) in children younger than 6 years versus –0.4 (–1.1 to 0.1) in children older than 6 years.

Effect on Near Adult Height
The characteristics of the 33 patients are given in table 4. The height SDS rose from –2.5 to –1.3 at 1 year of treatment, to –0.5 at the start of puberty, and decreased to –1.0 at near final height. There was no significant difference between boys and girls. Six among 21 boys and 4 among 12 girls remained below –2 SDS of the Prader chart. Loss in the height SDS during puberty was 0.8. The BMI SDS at the start of treatment was 1.7, 1.1 at 1 year of treatment, 1.3 at the start of puberty and 1.6 at near final height. The height at treatment start and the near final height were plotted in growth charts (fig. 5).

Table 3. Auxological and biological data at baseline and after 1 year on GH in the 3 groups (SS vs. NS, obese vs. nonobese, and children <6 years vs. >6 years at the start of GH treatment)

	Short		NS		p	Obese		Nonobese		p	<6 years		>6 years		p
	n	median	n	median		n	median	n	median		n	median	n	median	
At start of GH treatment															
Sex ratio (boys/girls)	134/140		176/98			194/101		174/183			181/165		187/119		
Chronological age, years	274	5.0	274	6.9	<0.05	295	6.7	357	4.4	<0.05	346	3.3	306	8.9	<0.05
MPH SDS	274	0.3	274	−0.7	<0.05	256	−0.5	292	0.1	<0.05	278	0.1	270	−0.4	<0.05
Height SDS	274	−2.9	274	−1.5	<0.05	295	−1.6	357	−2.6	<0.05	346	−2.4	306	−2.1	<0.05
Height − MPH SDS	274	−3.0	274	−1.0	<0.05	256	−1.3	292	−2.6	<0.05	278	−2.3	270	−1.7	<0.05
Height SDS (syndrome specific)	260	−0.7	256	0.1	<0.05	294	0	317	−0.6	<0.05	305	−0.2	306	−0.5	<0.05
Height velocity SDS	107	−1.6	94	−1.2	n.s.	103	−1.1	126	−1.5	n.s.	113	−1.2	116	−1.5	n.s.
BMI SDS	274	1.1	274	2.5	<0.05	295	2.9	357	0.6	<0.05	346	1.1	306	2.2	<0.05
Birth weight SDS	262	−1.4	253	−1.4	n.s.	269	−1.4	340	−1.4	n.s.	328	−1.3	281	−1.5	n.s.
Birth length SDS	217	−0.3	190	−0.5	n.s.	198	−0.5	272	−0.4	n.s.	262	−0.4	208	−0.5	n.s.
Maximum GH peak, μg/l	114	6.4	99	5.9	n.s.	117	5.5	133	6.8	n.s.	102	6.1	148	5.9	n.s.
IGF-1 SDS	117	−1.9	97	−1.4	<0.05	109	−1.4	132	−1.7	<0.05	123	−1.4	118	−1.9	<0.05
After 1 year on GH															
Height SDS	274	−1.7	274	−0.6	<0.05	295	−0.7	357	−1.7	<0.05	346	−1.2	306	−1.2	n.s.
Δ height SDS	274	1.1	274	0.8	<0.05	295	0.9	357	0.9	n.s.	346	1.2	306	0.8	<0.05
Height − MPH SDS	274	−1.9	274	0.1	<0.05	256	−0.2	292	−1.6	<0.05	278	−1.1	270	−0.9	<0.05
Height SDS (syndrome specific)	274	−0.0	274	0.7	<0.05	295	0.6	357	0.0	<0.05	346	0.5	306	0.0	<0.05
Height velocity SDS	274	4.1	273	4.3	n.s.	295	5.4	356	2.6	<0.05	345	2.4	306	5.4	<0.05
BMI SDS	273	0.8	274	2.1	<0.05	295	2.6	356	0.3	<0.05	346	0.8	305	1.7	<0.05
Δ BMI SDS	273	−0.3	274	−0.4	<0.05	295	−0.4	356	−0.2	<0.05	346	−0.27	305	−0.4	<0.05
Studentized residual	195	−0.2	180	0.4	<0.05	197	0.4	178	−0.2	<0.05	190	−0.1	185	0.3	<0.05

n.s. = Not significant.

Table 4. Near adult height in PWS patients

	All				Females		Males		SS		NS	
	n	median	10th percentile	90th percentile	n	median	n	median	n	median	n	median
Background												
Birth weight SDS	28	-1.7	-3.1	-0.3	9	-1.8	19	-1.6	15	-1.5	10	-2.2
Birth length SDS	19	-0.19	-2.0	1.2	7	-0.5	12	0.1	11	0.3	8	-1.1
MPH SDS (Prader)	28	0.0	-1.6	1.4	11	0.3	17	-0.3	16	0.4	12	-0.5
Maximum GH, µg/l	18	5.8	1.9	11.8	7	8.0	11	5.5	9	4.3	4	5.0
IGF-1 SDS	11	-1.7	-2.7	-1.2	4	-2.6	7	-1.4	5	-2.1	5	-1.4
At start of GH treatment												
Age, years	33	8.9	5.4	12.2	12	9.1	21	8.9	16	8.9	12	8.9
Bone age, years	21	6.3	3.9	11.4	6	7.7	15	6.3	10	6.0	9	7.5
Height, cm					12	112.8	21	115.5				
Height SDS (Prader)	33	-2.5	-4.5	-0.5	12	-2.8	21	-2.3	16	-3.1	12	-1.9
Height SDS (syndrome specific)	33	-0.6	-2.7	0.6	12	-1.1	21	-0.5	16	-1.1	12	-0.4
Height velocity, cm/year	25	4.1	2.6	6.6	8	4.2	17	4.0	13	4.4	10	3.7
BMI SDS	33	1.7	0.6	3.0	12	1.3	21	2.0	16	1.5	12	2.0
GH dose, mg/kg/week	33	0.21	0.13	0.33	12	0.19	21	0.24	16	0.21	12	0.24
After 1 year on GH												
Age, years	33	9.9	6.4	13.2	12	10.0	21	9.9	16	9.8	12	9.9
Height, cm					12	122.4	21	127.8				
Height SDS (Prader)	33	-1.3	-3.4	0.1	12	-2.2	21	-0.8	16	-2.3	12	-0.6
Height SDS (syndrome specific)	33	0.1	-1.9	1.2	12	-0.3	21	0.2	16	-0.6	12	0.6
Height velocity, cm/year	33	9.7	7.0	15.1	12	9.3	21	9.8	16	9.4	12	10.8
BMI SDS	33	1.1	-0.6	2.4	12	0.9	21	1.3	16	0.9	12	1.5
At start of puberty												
Age, years	10	11.7	9.9	17.6	3	10.7	7	13.5	5	11.7	3	13.5
Height, cm					3	137.5	7	145.7				
Height SDS (Prader)	10	-0.5	-3.6	2.2	3	-0.2	7	-1.7	5	-1.7	3	1.5
Height SDS (syndrome specific)	10	0.8	-3.4	2.9	3	1.0	7	1.0	5	-1.0	3	2.3
BMI SDS	10	1.3	-0.2	2.4	3	0.9	7	1.6	5	1.0	3	1.6
Near adult height												
Age, years	33	17.5	15.7	20.4	12	16.3	21	18.0	16	17.1	12	18.3
Height, cm					12	157.0	21	171.2				
Height SDS (Prader)	33	-1.0	-3.7	0.7	12	-1.0	21	-1.0	16	-1.2	12	-1.0
Height SDS (syndrome specific)	33	1.7	-0.9	3.7	12	1.4	21	2.2	16	1.4	12	2.2
Height – MPH SDS (Prader)	28	-1.1	-2.4	0.0	11	-1.2	17	-1.1	16	-1.4	12	-0.5
Δ height SDS (latest – puberty, Prader)	10	-0.8	-1.2	0.5	3	-0.4	7	-0.9	5	-0.8	3	-1.0
Δ height SDS (latest – puberty, syndrome specific)	10	0.9	0.5	2.6	3	0.5	7	1.5	5	0.8	3	1.5
Δ height SDS (latest – start, Prader)	33	1.3	0.1	2.7	12	1.3	21	1.3	16	1.9	12	1.0
Δ height SDS (latest – start, syndrome specific)	33	2.4	1.1	4.0	12	2.3	21	2.9	16	2.4	12	2.4
BMI SDS	33	1.6	0.3	2.9	12	1.6	21	1.6	16	1.5	12	1.7

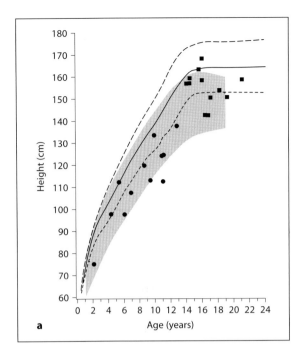
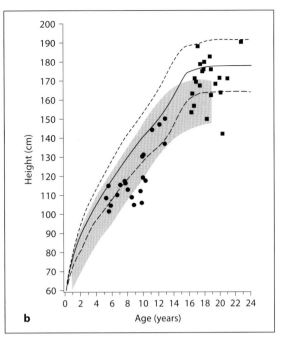
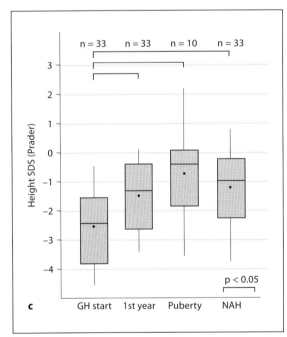

Fig. 5. Heights before (●) and after (■) GH treatment in boys (**a**) and girls (**b**) are plotted in the Prader chart (white area, mean 0 ± 2 SD) and the syndrome-specific chart (grey area, from –2 to +2 SD). **c** The heights at GH start, at 1 year of treatment, at the start of puberty and at near final height are given as median and interquartile range (grey box), with the mean indicated as a black dot and the 10th and 90th percentiles as vertical lines. NAH = Near adult height.

In this group, separating SS and NS children, again, we found that SS patients grew during the first year, as did GH-deficient patients, when the prediction model was applied, but that NS patients grew better, as studentized residuals were 0.1 (–0.8 to 2.3) versus 1.8 (0.1–3). During puberty, the loss of growth was similar in both groups, i.e. –0.8 SDS (–1.4 to 1.2) in the SS group versus –1.0 SDS (–1.0 to –0.8) in the NS group. There was no significant difference in near final height, i.e.–1.2 SDS (–3.1 to 0.4) for the SS group versus –1.0 SDS (–2.3 to 0.8) for the NS group. Interestingly, the height – MPH SDS was 0.4 (–1.6 to 2.0) at treatment start and decreased to –1.4 (–2.7 to

–0.6) at final height in the SS group, while it was –0.5 at treatment start (–1.3 to 1.1) and –0.5 at final height (–1.2 to 0.7) in the NS group. At the start of treatment, the girls were shorter, i.e. –2.8 SDS (–4.5 to –0.8) versus –2.3 SDS (–4.3 to –0.5), and had a lower BMI SDS of 1.3 (0.6–2.7) versus 2.0 (0.8–3.1) compared with the boys. Nevertheless, the near adult height SDS and the BMI SDS were not significantly different, i.e. –1.0 in girls (–3.7 to 0.0) versus –1.0 (–3.1 to 0.8) in boys, whereas the BMI SDS was 1.6 (0.6–2.0) in girls versus 1.6 (0.3–3.2) in boys. Loss in height during puberty was significantly less in girls, –0.4 SDS (–0.8 to –0.2), compared with boys, –0.9 SDS (–1.4 to 1.2).

The mean pubertal GH dose was 0.17 mg/kg/week. The mean duration of treatment was 8.4 ± 2.3 years, with 4.2 ± 1.4 years during puberty. Boys started puberty at 14.0 ± 2.7 years and girls at 10.2 ± 1.0 years. We did not have bone age records during puberty to analyze bone maturation or data on whether or not puberty was induced in some patients.

Discussion

This cohort is unique, as it is an international and large cohort of children with PWS. In this respect, baseline characteristics are interesting to analyze in order to describe the natural history of this rare disorder. A gender difference was reported for the first time, with girls being shorter and lighter than boys at a mean age of 6.8 years. Forty-five percent of these children are obese, with a BMI SDS >2, and 50% of them are short. Interestingly, obese children at a median age of 6.7 years were in the normal range of height for specific growth charts, while the nonobese children showed a SDS of –0.6, suggesting that the growth chart had been done with a majority of obese children.

The 53% of boys versus the 47% of girls could represent a bias, as parents could be more concerned with SS or obesity in boys, but it could also be specific for the syndrome.

Birth weight is significantly more impaired (–1.3 ± 1.2 SDS) than birth length (–0.4 ± 1.4 SDS). We could not analyze if there is an effect of the genetic mechanism (deletion or disomy) in auxological differences at birth as it has been reported in some studies that patients with deletion were shorter at birth [13]. In 424 tests, maximum GH peak was 5.9 µg/l, showing the high frequency of low GH peak in these patients [3, 14–17]. IGF-1 values were also low at –1.5 SDS, confirming the GH-deficient status of the majority of these patients and particularly the low IGF-1 values contrasting with rather high BMIs.

We analyzed the first-year response to GH treatment in 652 children and showed that they respond as well or slightly better than GH-deficient patients, without gender difference. Interestingly, the patients who are not growth retarded responded better than the short children both in terms of height and BMI, suggesting that PWS per se is a very GH-sensitive condition.

The decrease in the BMI is statistically significant for the first year, with a very wide individual variation, as previously reported [3]. We do not have data on whether or not a comprehensive care of these children was set up, nor on their dietetic habits and physical activities.

The lack of a consistent decrease in the BMI could not be analyzed as a failure of GH treatment. In these patients, we know that the BMI does greatly increase with time, and therefore, the stabilization of the BMI may be considered efficacious. Interestingly, obese children responded better both in terms of BMI and height velocity. For the first time, it was possible to report near final height in a cohort of 33 patients.

While the overall growth effect in the prepubertal period is clearly as good as that obtained in GH-deficient patients, pubertal growth of PWS patients is not satisfactory, with a median loss of height of –0.8 SDS, being worse in boys than in girls, while the BMI did not significantly change during puberty. We could not precisely analyze pubertal growth, as we do not have data on bone age before and during puberty to evaluate bone maturation. We also lack data on pubertal management given the fact that most of these patients have hypogonadism, mainly partial hypogonadism both of central and peripheral origins [18, 19]. This condition requires treatment to induce a complete puberty for which we do not have any data in this cohort. We could hypothesize that some of the results in terms of growth are due to the impaired treatment of hypogonadism, particularly in boys, as it is well known that some physicians are reluctant to prescribe testosterone therapy, particularly in patients with behavioral problems, thinking that they could become more aggressive. The GH dose decreased during puberty. Therefore, optimizing pubertal growth is a challenge in this population. Ten patients among 33 (30% in both boys and girls) did not reach normal height, and the median height SDS at NAH for the whole group was –1.0.

In conclusion, this analysis based on a large cohort allows us to describe the history of the syndrome and the effect of GH treatment. A major effect on body weight is reported for the first time, as well as a sex ratio in height and BMI, with girls being shorter and lighter.

These patients are more sensitive to GH treatment than GH-deficient patients, and NS children even respond better both in terms of height and BMI. Near final height was obtained in 33 patients and showed a consistent positive effect of GH treatment with a Δ height SDS at 2.4 for the specific growth chart for the syndrome, most of them reaching normal near adult height.

References

1 Carrel AL, Myers SE, Whitman BY, Allen DB: Benefits of long-term GH therapy in Prader-Willi syndrome: a 4-year study. J Clin Endocrinol Metab 2002;87:1581–1585.
2 Lindgren AC, Ritzen EM: Five years of growth hormone treatment in children with Prader-Willi syndrome. Swedish National Growth Hormone Advisory Group. Acta Paediatr Suppl 1999;88:109–111.
3 Burman P, Ritzen EM, Lindgren AC: Endocrine dysfunction in Prader-Willi syndrome: a review with special reference to GH. Endocr Rev 2001;22:787–799.
4 Haqq AM, Stadler DD, Jackson RH, Rosenfeld RG, Purnell JQ, LaFranchi SH: Effects of growth hormone on pulmonary function, sleep quality, behavior, cognition, growth velocity, body composition, and resting energy expenditure in Prader-Willi syndrome. J Clin Endocrinol Metab 2003;88:2206–2212.
5 Lindgren AC, Hagenas L, Muller J, Blichfeldt S, Rosenborg M, Brismar T, Ritzen EM: Growth hormone treatment of children with Prader-Willi syndrome affects linear growth and body composition favourably. Acta Paediatr 1998;87:28–31.
6 Tauber M, Barbeau C, Jouret B, Pienkowski C, Malzac P, Moncla A, Rochiccioli P: Auxological and endocrine evolution of 28 children with Prader-Willi syndrome: effect of GH therapy in 14 children. Horm Res 2000;53:279–287.
7 Eiholzer U, Schlumpf M, Nordmann Y, l'Allemand D: Early manifestations of Prader-Willi syndrome: influence of growth hormone. J Pediatr Endocrinol Metab 2001;14:1441–1444.
8 Craig ME, Cowell CT, Larsson P, Zipf WB, Reiter EO, Albertsson-Wikland K, Ranke MB, Price DA, KIGS International Board: Growth hormone treatment and adverse events in Prader-Willi syndrome: data from KIGS (the Pfizer International Growth Database). Clin Endocrinol (Oxf) 2006;65:178–185.
9 Prader A, Labhart A, Willi H: Ein Syndrom von Adipositas, Kleinwuchs, Kryptorchidismus und Oligophrenie nach myotonieartigem Zustand im Neugeborenenalter. Schweiz Med Wochenschr 1956;6:1260–1261.
10 Prader A, Largo RH, Molinari L, Issler C: Physical growth from birth to 20 years of age. First Zürich longitudinal study of growth and development. Helv Paediatr Acta Suppl 1988;52:1–125.
11 Butler MG, Meaney FJ: Standards for selected anthropometric measurements in Prader-Willi syndrome. Pediatrics 1991;88:853–860.
12 Ranke MB, Lindberg A, Albertsson-Wikland K, Wilton P, Price DA, Reiter EO: Increased response, but lower responsiveness, to growth hormone (GH) in very young children (aged 0–3 years) with idiopathic GH deficiency: analysis of data from KIGS. J Clin Endocrinol Metab 2005;90:1966–1971.

13 Gillessen-Kaesbach G, Robinson W, Lohmann D, Kaya-Westerloh S, Passarge E, Horsthemke B: Genotype-phenotype correlation in a series of 167 deletion and non-deletion patients with Prader-Willi syndrome. Hum Genet 1995;96:638–643.

14 Grugni G, Guzzaloni G, Moro D, Bettio D, De Medici C, Morabito F: Reduced growth hormone (GH) responsiveness to combined GH-releasing hormone and pyridostigmine administration in the Prader-Willi syndrome. Clin Endocrinol (Oxf) 1998;48:769–775.

15 Cappa M, Raguso G, Palmiotto T, Faedda A, Gurreri F, Neri G, Deghenghi R, Loche S: The growth hormone response to hexarelin in patients with Prader-Willi syndrome. J Endocrinol Invest 1998;21:501–505.

16 Angulo M, Castro-Magana M, Mazur B, Canas JA, Vitollo PM, Sarrantonio M: Growth hormone secretion and effects of growth hormone therapy on growth velocity and weight gain in children with Prader-Willi syndrome. J Pediatr Endocrinol Metab 1996;9:393–400.

17 Beccaria L, Bosio L, Sanzari A, Aimaretti G, Ghigo E, Chiumello G: GH secretion in Prader-Labhart-Willi syndrome: somatotrope responsiveness to GHRH is enhanced by arginine but not by pyridostigmine. J Pediatr Endocrinol Metab 1996;9:577–583.

18 Eiholzer U, l'Allemand D, Rousson V, Schlumpf M, Gasser T, Girard J, Gruters A, Simoni M: Hypothalamic and gonadal components of hypogonadism in boys with Prader-Labhart-Willi syndrome. J Clin Endocrinol Metab 2006; 91:892–898.

19 Crino A, Schiaffini R, Ciampalini P, Spera S, Beccaria L, Benzi F, Bosio L, Corrias A, Gargantini L, Salvatoni A, Tonini G, Trifiro G, Livieri C, Genetic Obesity Study Group of the Italian Society of Pediatric Endocrinology and Diabetology (SIEDP): Hypogonadism and pubertal development in Prader-Willi syndrome. Eur J Pediatr 2003; 162:327–333.

Growth and Growth Hormone Treatment in Children Born Small for Gestational Age and with Silver-Russell Syndrome

Wayne S. Cutfield[a] Edward O. Reiter[b]
on behalf of the KIGS International Board

[a]Liggins Institute, University of Auckland
2–6 Park Avenue, Grafton, Auckland (New Zealand)
[b]Baystate Children's Hospital, Tufts University School of Medicine
759 Chestnut Street, Springfield, MA 01199 (USA)

Definitions

Small for gestational age (SGA) is a term used to describe an infant's birth size based upon appropriate auxological standards for healthy infants. Until 10 years ago, intrauterine growth retardation (IUGR) and SGA were used interchangeably to describe newborn infants born small when compared with population standards. However, these terms are not always synonymous and the conditions may occur independently. IUGR more accurately refers to poor fetal growth, usually in the last trimester, that leads to reduced birth size. However, IUGR may be associated with either normal or reduced birth size when based upon population rather than individualized growth standards [1]. Approximately 20% of SGA infants are thought to have suffered from IUGR [2, 3]. An arbitrary range of anthropometric criteria has been used to define SGA that extends from a birth weight <10th percentile for gestational age to a birth weight standard deviation score (SDS) of less than –2 [4–7]. Unfortunately, comparison between SGA childhood studies using different definitions is difficult as the greater the reduction in birth weight the greater the likelihood of short stature and metabolic abnormalities [4, 8]. In an attempt to standardize the definition of SGA, the International SGA Advisory Board recently recommended that SGA be defined as a birth weight (SGA_W) or length (SGA_L) or both weight and length (SGA_{WL}) ≤2 SD below the mean for gestational age [9]. Although SGA_L occurs 1.5 times more commonly in developed countries than SGA_W or SGA_{WL}, birth length is seldom accurately measured at birth [10]. Whichever definition is employed to define SGA, it is important to recognize that it has been arbitrarily set and there will be some infants born with a birth weight or length above the SGA cut-off who have suffered appreciable nutritional constraint in utero. Conversely, 22% of SGA children are 'constitutionally small' when maternal factors are considered [11].

Children with Silver-Russell syndrome (SRS) are usually very SGA and exhibit a variable number of other clinical features that include limb asymmetry, triangular face with small pointed chin, frontal prominence, very slim phenotype, generalized camptodactyly, hypospadias, sweating and pallor in the early weeks of life and reduced intellectual function [12]. Price et al. [12] proposed the following diagnostic criteria for SRS: (1) birth weight below or equal to –2 SD from the mean, (2) poor postnatal growth below or equal to –2 SD from the mean at diagnosis, (3) preservation of occipitofrontal head circumference, (4) classic facial phenotype, and (5) asymmetry. There is no single radiographic feature that is pathognomonic of SRS; however, during childhood, delayed bone age, clinodactyly, fifth middle or distal phalangeal hypoplasia, ivory epiphyses and a second metacarpal pseudoepiphysis are suggestive [13].

Aetiology

SGA is a descriptive rather than a diagnostic term for a very heterogeneous group with influences from maternal, placental, fetal, environmental and genetic factors on birth size. Whilst there are a multitude of causes of SGA, the majority of SGA infants are assumed to have suffered placental dysfunction without another obvious diagnosis. Although severe mutations in genes involved in the metabolism, growth and skeletal development lead to a SGA infant, these are rare causes of SGA and are usually associated with a range of dysmorphic features. Although no association has been found between insulin-like growth factor 1 (IGF-1) gene polymorphism and SGA, lower IGF-1 levels have been found in an IGF-1 gene polymorphism in short SGA children [14, 15].

Future studies will determine whether IGF-1, IGF-1 receptor or IGF-2 polymorphisms play a meaningful role in the incidence of SGA infants.

Recently, genetic mutations have been identified that are common causes of SRS and include chromosome 11p15 (epi)genetic mutations (35% of cases) and maternal uniparental disomy of chromosome 7 (10% of cases) [16–18]. Interestingly, SRS and Beckwith-Wiedemann syndrome may be regarded as two disorders caused by opposite (epi)genetic disturbances of the same chromosomal region displaying opposite clinical pictures. It appears that 11p15 epigenetic mutations are rare in SGA children without the clinical features of SRS [19].

Auxology

One of the most commonly studied long-term sequelae of SGA infants is poor postnatal growth and short stature with an adult height that is approximately 1 SD below the mean [2, 3, 6, 7]. Typically, SGA infants display marked growth acceleration in early infancy. Approximately 80% of SGA children achieve a length within the normal range by 6 months of age which is further increased to 86% by 12 months [2, 7]. Catch-up growth into the normal height range is virtually always complete by 2 years of age [2, 20]. Overall, 8–14% of SGA infants become short adults [2, 4]. There is a greater risk of short adult stature in those with a birth length of –2 SDS or less compared with those with a birth weight of –2 SDS or less [2, 4]. Amongst short adults, SGA is a common finding, with SGA_L found in 22% and SGA_W found in 14% of all short adults [2, 6].

Genetic height potential as reflected in midparental height is one of the most important factors influencing the growth pattern and adult height achieved in an SGA child. When adjustment is made for parents' heights, SGA subjects of both sexes achieve an adult height that is approximately 4 cm below their midparental height

[6]. In the first 2 years of life, shorter birth length is the major influence on SGA catch-up growth, whereas throughout the rest of childhood, genetic height potential had the greatest influence, with SGA children who had tall parents showing the most impressive catch-up growth [21].

A major portion of SGA children are born prematurely. These children often display a delayed pattern in catch-up growth into the normal range that may extend to the age of 4 years [20, 22]. Greater prematurity (lower gestational age at birth) may exacerbate delayed catch-up growth and further increase the risk of short adult height [23, 24]. Infants born of very low birth weight and SGA have delayed catch-up growth that may extend to 6 years of age [24]. In addition, up to 54% of very-low-birth-weight SGA infants fail to show a progressive improvement in height SDS during infancy and/or childhood [24].

Children with SRS are a very small subgroup of SGA children; thus, less is known about growth and the endocrine axes than in SGA children without a diagnosed syndrome. Birth weight is very low in SRS infants and is typically only 1.9–2.0 kg at term [25, 26]. Growth during infancy and early childhood is poor without any catch-up growth in infancy. By the age of 4 years, these children have a height SDS of −3.5 to −4.4 [25–27]. During the remainder of childhood, growth is constant and parallel to the 3rd percentile; thus, final adult height is poor with males achieving a height of 151.2 cm and females a height of 139.9 cm [26].

Growth Hormone and Insulin-Like Growth Factor 1 Axis

SGA children exhibit alterations in the growth hormone (GH) and insulin axes. In late gestation and at birth, changes to the insulin substrate and GH-IGF axes can be largely attributed to poor nutrition, with the majority of studies demonstrating elevated serum GH, low IGF-1, IGF-2 and IGF-binding protein 3 (IGFBP-3) together with low insulin and increased IGFBP-1 levels [28–30]. These changes are in sharp contrast to changes seen in these axes when nutritional constraint is removed. Spontaneous pulsatile GH hypersecretion occurs in the first few days of life [31], and exogenous GH-releasing hormone has been shown to elicit an exaggerated GH response in SGA neonates during the early phase of catch-up growth [32]. Three days after birth, exaggerated GH secretion in SGA neonates has been associated with increased levels of circulating IGF-1, suggesting that nutritional inhibition of IGF-1 secretion is removed before GH hypersecretion is inhibited [32]. This transient GH hypersecretion may drive the early growth acceleration that occurs to some degree in most SGA infants.

There have been conflicting reports regarding the characteristics of the GH-IGF axis in children born SGA. Both diminished and elevated spontaneous GH secretions in short SGA children have been reported [33–35]. Diminished GH secretion rates reported could simply be due to the younger ages of SGA compared with appropriate for gestational age control children [33, 35]. Stanhope et al. [36] found a reduction in the number of overnight GH pulses in short SGA children; however, these occurred almost exclusively in children with SRS. Reduced stimulated GH levels have not been found in short SGA children [34, 35]. Cross-sectional analysis shows that growth responses to a range of GH doses are lower in SGA children than in either GH-deficient children or Turner syndrome girls, indirectly suggesting that short SGA children may have mild partial GH resistance [37].

There have also been conflicting reports in serum IGF-1, IGF-2 and IGFBP-3 in short SGA children. Investigators have reported both lower and similar levels of serum IGF-1 and IGF-2 and comparable IGFBP-3 levels in SGA when compared with normal children of normal height. Low IGF-1 values have been interpreted to be due to either GH deficiency or GH resistance [30, 33,

34]. Unfortunately, height and weight were not matched between the SGA and control groups in these studies. Unlike normal stature children, short SGA children are usually thin. Age, height and nutritional status (as measured by body mass index) have all been shown to positively influence IGFBP-3 and IGF-1 levels in normal and SGA children [33, 36]. However, when short prepubertal SGA children are matched to normal prepubertal children for age, height and weight, SGA children display higher serum IGF-1, IGF-2 and IGFBP-3 values [38]. However, when short SGA children are compared with normal height controls, the SGA children have lower serum IGF-1 and IGFBP-3 levels [38]. In addition, fasting hyperinsulinaemia was correlated with fasting plasma IGF-1 levels in SGA children, suggesting that insulin may be regulating IGF-1 levels [38].

Children with SRS appear to have impaired spontaneous GH secretion; however, the contribution of these subtle abnormalities to the extreme short stature and poor early childhood growth has not been determined. Chromosome 11p15 mutations involving growth-regulating genes IGF2 and CDKN1C are more likely to have constrained fetal and early childhood growth. Limited data suggest that these children secrete diminished amounts of GH with reduced pulse frequency overnight [5]. Although the IGF-1 receptor gene was considered to be a good candidate to explain the small size and poor growth of SRS children, IGF-1 receptor mutations were not found in a small childhood SRS cohort [39].

Puberty and Gonadal Function

The age of onset of puberty in SGA children occurs within the age range of normal puberty [40]. However, within the age range of normal puberty, there are conflicting reports as to whether puberty occurs slightly earlier, on time or is delayed in SGA children [6, 41–44]. Collectively, evidence suggests slightly earlier or normal onset of puberty rather than delayed puberty, with menarche reported 4–6 months earlier [40, 42, 43]. A similar pattern of normal or slightly earlier than normal puberty has been found in children with SRS [25, 26, 45]. Earlier onset of puberty in SGA females and not males was found in one large study, raising the possibility of sexual dimorphism [42]. Precocious puberty occurs more commonly in females, and thus, it is conceivable that SGA females are more vulnerable to the effects of SGA on pubertal timing. The duration of puberty, the magnitude of the pubertal growth spurt and peak height velocity all suggest a normal pubertal tempo in SGA children [40]. However, the timing of the peak height velocity occurred earlier in SGA males and females [40].

There are a number of studies across ethnicities that have found an association between low birth weight and premature pubarche or exaggerated pubarche (characterized by higher androgen levels and more abundant pubic and axillary hair) [46–48]. Premature adrenarche characterized by elevated serum dehydroepiandrosterone sulphate and/or androstenedione levels has been reported in SGA children without premature pubarche, suggesting that altered adrenal function in SGA children occurs more commonly than is clinically evident [49, 50]. There is a group of SGA girls who appear to manifest the sequence of rapid weight gain in childhood, premature adrenarche and pubarche with early onset of puberty and early menarche with an increased risk of polycystic ovarian syndrome [50–52]. Biochemical features of polycystic ovarian syndrome in SGA adolescent girls have been reported as common in the absence of overt evidence. Ibanez et al. [53] found a 10-fold increased incidence of anovulation, hyperandrogenism and hyperinsulinaemia in lean SGA girls.

Zhang et al. [54] have proposed an explanation for the association between hyperandrogenism and insulin resistance in SGA girls. SGA could lead to programmed enhanced serine phosphorylation of cytochrome P450c17 (manifest as enhanced 17,20-lyase activity) and the insulin receptor (reflected in reduced insulin signalling).

There is evidence of alterations in the hypothalamic gonadal axis in those born SGA. Structural and functional gonadal abnormalities are suggested by reduction in ovarian and testicular size, reduced uterine volume in females and hypersecretion of follicle-stimulating hormone in infancy (suggesting a diminished production of inhibin B and oestrogen by gonads) [54–56]. These detailed studies in Spanish children have been extended in other countries to show a lower percentage of primordial follicles in ovaries of IUGR female fetuses and unexplained male subfertility (assessed by semen analysis) associated with a low birth weight [57, 58].

Metabolism

Barker et al. [59–64] proposed the 'fetal origins of adult disease' hypothesis as explanation for the association between a reduction in birth weight and a range of metabolic and cardiovascular diseases that included type 2 diabetes mellitus, syndrome X, hypertension, cerebrovascular and coronary heart disease. Other groups have confirmed these observations across ethnicities and countries [65–67]. Short SGA children have been found to be insulin resistant with normal insulin secretory capacity [8, 68, 69]. Subsequently, indirect evidence of insulin resistance has been reported in SGA children as young as 12 months of age, adding weight to the view that the defect in insulin sensitivity occurs prior to birth [70].

SGA children at risk of insulin resistance and type 2 diabetes mellitus in later adult life are more likely to have had rapid childhood weight gain, with increased fat mass that continues into adult life. In early childhood, SGA children already display altered body composition that is not evident using standard anthropometric indices. By 4 years of age, SGA children with the same height, weight and body mass index as normal birth weight children had an increase in fat mass and a reduction in lean mass [71]. Predictably, SGA children are at greater risk of insulin resistance if they experience accelerated weight gain during childhood compared with those who do not experience accelerated weight gain [68]. Interestingly, childhood weight acceleration has a greater impact on insulin sensitivity in SGA than in normal birth weight children [68]. Retrospective adult studies of type 2 diabetes mellitus have found that those in the lowest birth weight tertile are more likely to display a pattern of accelerated weight gain during childhood and early adulthood than those in the middle or upper birth weight tertile [72].

Adiponectin is secreted from adipose tissue and has important roles in enhancing insulin sensitivity and preventing atherosclerosis and inflammation. Plasma adiponectin levels are lower in SGA neonates [73]. In addition, plasma adiponectin levels are lower in SGA children that exhibit catch-up growth compared with normal or obese children [74]. It is conceivable that the low adiponectin levels seen in SGA children will enhance the risk of future atherosclerosis given the potent anti-atherosclerotic and anti-inflammatory role that adiponectin displays [75].

Other metabolic changes seen in short SGA children include elevated free fatty acids and cholesterol levels in the upper quartile, increased daytime systolic blood pressure and diminished nighttime blood pressure dipping [69, 76, 77]. In a large cohort of normal children, multivariate analysis revealed that with every kilogram reduction in birth weight there was an increase in systolic blood pressure of 1.3 mm Hg and diastolic blood pressure of 0.6 mm Hg [78]. Lipoprotein(a), an independent risk factor for coronary artery disease, was found to be higher in SGA adolescents than in controls [79]. Despite the range of metabolic changes reported in SGA children, it is important to recognize that overt clinical metabolic diseases such as impaired glucose tolerance, type 2 diabetes mellitus, dyslipidaemia and hypertension have not been reported to occur more commonly is SGA children.

Growth Hormone Treatment

In the early 1970s, GH treatment did not appear to appreciably improve growth rates of SGA children. However, these initial studies used treatment regimens now considered suboptimal of low-dose cadaveric GH administered 3 times per week [80, 81]. Following the introduction of recombinant GH, larger GH doses administered to a range of SGA study groups became possible. The impressive impact of high-dose GH therapy administered for up to 6 years on growth was shown in a collection of European randomized multi-centred studies [82]. Over 6 years, GH treatment at 67 μg/kg/day led to an increase in height SDS of +2.7, which was greater than that achieved with GH at 33 μg/kg/day with an increase in height SDS of +2.0 [82]. Furthermore, GH administered at the very high dose of 100 μg/kg/day for 2 years and then stopped for 4 years achieved the same height gain as seen in patients treated for 6 years with the more conventional dose of 33 μg/kg/day. These authors showed that high-dose GH therapy can accelerate height into the normal range and they suggested that individualized dosing strategies could be used that may include discontinuous regimens. However, premature discontinuation of higher-dose therapy leads to considerable catch-down growth, limiting the benefit of earlier treatment. GH doses of 68–100 μg/kg/day resulted in a reduction of 1 SDS in height 4–5 years after treatment was stopped [82, 83]. In the first study of GH treatment to final height in SGA children, 85% of those randomized to treatment achieved a height within the normal height range after 7.8 years of treatment [84]. Surprisingly, unlike other final height studies in GH-treated growth disorders, there was no difference in the final height achieved in those treated with GH at 33 compared with 67 μg/kg/day [84]. If GH treatment is delayed until adolescence, there is still an improvement in final height although it is far less impressive than when treatment is started in mid-childhood. GH therapy at 67 μg/kg/day from approximately the start of puberty (12.5 years in boys and 10.5 years in girls) achieved an increase in final height of 0.6 SDS compared with an improvement of 2.1 SDS from mid-childhood at the same dose [85].

The concept of polymorphisms in growth-related genes regulating growth response to GH treatment was recently introduced by Dos Santos et al. [86]. These authors found that a common polymorphism of the GH receptor (GHR; an exon 3 deletion) expressed in either the homozygous (*d3/d3* GHR) or heterozygous states (*d3/fl* GHR) was associated with a greater response to GH therapy than the homozygous full length state (*fl/fl* GHR). However, two subsequent studies have not found that the GHR exon 3 deletion is associated with initial growth response to GH therapy [87, 88]. Conversely, it appears that the biologically less active *fl/fl* GHR form occurs twice as commonly in short SGA children than in the normal adult population [89]. Although the GHR exon 3 deletion does not characterize responsiveness to GH across populations, the search for other polymorphisms of growth-regulating genes in SGA children is likely to continue.

GH therapy was approved to treat short SGA children in the USA in 2001 and in Europe in 2003. Despite the growing evidence that GH improves final height in these children, there remain discrepancies in GH funding for SGA in developed and developing countries. In late 2006, GH has been approved to treat short children with SGA as part of either a specific SGA indication or a broader indication for short non-GH-deficient children in countries that include the USA, UK, Europe, New Zealand and Australia. GH is neither government nor insurance funded in Canada, Japan, China, Hong Kong, Thailand, Singapore, the Philippines, Indonesia and India.

The effects of GH extend beyond linear growth and include potentially important effects on body composition, muscle mass and function, bone mass, metabolism, behaviour and cognitive function. To date, almost all GH treatment studies in these children have focused exclusively on linear growth. Almost all assessment beyond linear growth has been conducted in a single centre in a single population. In a large cohort of adolescents, those born SGA were more likely to suffer from learning and attention problems, which were more pronounced with more severe SGA [90]. GH therapy was associated with improvement in aspects of quality of life from a disorder-specific questionnaire that included improved physical abilities, contact with adults and body image [91]. In the same centre, GH therapy was associated with a small improvement in IQ compared with historical reference data [84]. Diminished lean mass evident before GH therapy was increased within 3 years of treatment, without a sustained change in fat mass [92]. Bone mineral content was also increased within 3 years of GH treatment [92].

Remarkably few adverse events have been reported during GH therapy in SGA children. GH therapy is associated with a 60% reduction in insulin sensitivity in prepubertal children that improves after treatment is stopped [93, 94].

Data regarding long-term GH therapy in children with SRS are scarce. Low-dose GH therapy (≥25 μg/kg/day) led to an improvement in the height SDS of 1.8 in a group of 33 children [95]. There have been few recent treatment studies published in these children and no final height studies aside from collected case reports. This initial gain in height with GH treatment appears at least comparable with SGA children; however, the full impact of treatment cannot be gauged until final height studies are published. Little information about possible adverse events during GH treatment in SRS is reported. Limited data suggest that GH treatment does not exaggerate limb asymmetry [96].

Conclusions

SGA children do not usually have a clearly defined aetiology for their small size at birth, unlike SRS children. Generally, SGA children do not achieve their genetic height potential and some become short adults. The endocrine changes that occur in SGA children include subtle changes in the GH-IGF-1 axis and a range of metabolic changes of which many could be attributed to an underlying reduction in insulin sensitivity. Acceleration in weight gain through childhood characterizes those most at risk of later type 2 diabetes mellitus. GH therapy started in mid-childhood will lead to an adult height in the normal range in the vast majority of SGA children. Added benefits of therapy include increased muscle mass, bone mineral content and improved quality of life and cognitive function. Although we have learnt much about the endocrine and body composition alterations in SGA children over the past 10 years, there are still some fundamental unanswered issues that include identification of the trigger(s) and mechanism(s) that lead to the endocrine changes that can be associated with significant metabolic disease later in adult life.

References

1 McCowan L, Stewart AW, Francis A, Gardosi J: A customised birthweight centile calculator developed for a New Zealand population. Aust N Z J Obstet Gynaecol 2004;44:428–431.
2 Karlberg J, Albertsson-Wikland K: Growth in full-term small-for-gestational-age infants: from birth to final height. Pediatr Res 1995;38:733–739.
3 Fitzhardinge PM, Steven EM: The small-for-date infant. 1. Later growth patterns. Pediatrics 1972;49:671–681.
4 Albertsson-Wikland K, Karlberg J: Natural growth in children born small for gestational age with and without catch-up growth. Acta Paediatr Suppl 1994: 399:64–70.
5 Ackland EM, Stanhope R, Eyre C, Hamill G, Jones J, Preece MA: Physiological growth hormone secretion in children with short stature and intra-uterine growth retardation. Horm Res 1988;30:241–245.
6 Leger J, Levy-Marchal C, Bloch J, Pinet A, Chevenne D, Porquet D, et al: Reduced final height and indications for insulin resistance in 20 year olds born small for gestational age: regional cohort study. BMJ 1997;315:341–347.
7 Tenovuo A, Kero P, Piekkala P, Korvenranta H, Sillanpaa M, Erkkola R: Growth of 519 small for gestational age infants during the first two years of life. Acta Paediatr Scand 1987;76:636–646.
8 Hofman PL, Cutfield WS, Robinson EM, Bergman RN, Menon RK, Sperling MA, et al: Insulin resistance in short children with intrauterine growth retardation. J Clin Endocrinol Metab 1997;82:402–406.
9 Lee P, Chernausek S, Hokken-Koelega A, Czernichow P: International Small for Gestational Age Advisory Board consensus development conference statement: management of short children born small for gestational age. Pediatrics 2003;111:1253–1261.
10 Albertsson-Wikland K, Wennergren G, Wennergren M, Vilbergsson G, Rosberg S: Longitudinal follow-up of growth in children born small for gestational age. Acta Paediatr 1993;82: 438–443.

11 Mamelle N, Cochet V, Claris O: Definition of fetal growth restriction according to constitutional growth potential. Biol Neonate 2001;80:277–285.
12 Price SM, Stanhope R, Garrett C, Preece MA, Trembath RC: The spectrum of Silver-Russell syndrome: a clinical and molecular genetic study and new diagnostic criteria. J Med Genet 1999; 36:837–842.
13 Herman TE, Crawford JD, Cleveland RH, Kushner DC: Hand radiographs in Russell-Silver syndrome. Pediatrics 1987;79:743–744.
14 Johnston LB, Leger J, Savage MO, Clark AJ, Czernichow P: The insulin-like growth factor-I (IGF-I) gene in individuals born small for gestational age (SGA). Clin Endocrinol 1999;51:423–427.
15 Johnston LB, Dahlgren J, Leger J, Gelander L, Savage MO, Czernichow P, et al: Association between insulin-like growth factor I (IGF-I) polymorphisms, circulating IGF-I, and pre- and postnatal growth in two European small for gestational age populations. J Clin Endocrinol Metab 2003;88:4805–4810.
16 Gicquel C, Rossignol S, Cabrol S, Houang M, Steunou V, Barbu V, et al: Epimutation of the telomeric imprinting center region on chromosome 11p15 in Silver-Russell syndrome. Nat Genet 1003;37:1003–1007.
17 Eggermann T, Schonherr N, Meyer E, Obermann C, Mavany M, Eggermann K, et al: Epigenetic mutations in 11p15 in Silver-Russell syndrome are restricted to the telomeric imprinting domain. J Med Genet 2006;43:615–616.
18 Monk D, Bentley L, Hitchins M, Myler RA, Clayton-Smith J, Ismail S, et al: Chromosome 7p disruptions in Silver Russell syndrome: delineating an imprinted candidate gene region. Hum Genet 2002;111:376–387.
19 Schonherr N, Meyer E, Eggermann K, Ranke MB, Wollmann HA, Eggermann T: (Epi)mutations in 11p15 significantly contribute to Silver-Russell syndrome: but are they generally involved in growth retardation? Eur J Med Genet 2006;49:414–418.
20 Hokken-Koelega AC, De Ridder MA, Lemmen RJ, Den Hartog H, De Muinck Keizer-Schrama SM, Drop SL: Children born small for gestational age: do they catch up? Pediatr Res 1995;38:267–271.

21 Luo ZC, Albertsson-Wikland K, Karlberg J: Length and body mass index at birth and target height influences on patterns of postnatal growth in children born small for gestational age. Pediatrics 1998;102:E72.
22 Gibson AT, Carney S, Cavazzoni E, Wales JK: Neonatal and post-natal growth. Horm Res 2000;1:42–49.
23 Sung IK, Vohr B, Oh W: Growth and neurodevelopmental outcome of very low birth weight infants with intrauterine growth retardation: comparison with control subjects matched by birth weight and gestational age. J Pediatr 1993;123:618–624.
24 Brandt I, Sticker EJ, Gausche R, Lentze MJ: Catch-up growth of supine length/height of very low birth weight, small for gestational age preterm infants to adulthood. J Pediatr 2005;147:662–668.
25 Angehrn V, Zachmann M, Prader A: Silver-Russell syndrome. Observations in 20 patients. Helv Paediatr Acta 1979; 34:297–308.
26 Wollmann HA, Kirchner T, Enders H, Preece MA, Ranke MB: Growth and symptoms in Silver-Russell syndrome: review on the basis of 386 patients. Eur J Pediatr 1995;154:958–968.
27 Tanner JM, Lejarraga H, Cameron N: The natural history of the Silver-Russell syndrome: a longitudinal study of thirty-nine cases. Pediatr Res 1975;9: 611–623.
28 Giudice LC, de Zegher F, Gargosky SE, Dsupin BA, de las Fuentes L, Crystal RA, et al: Insulin-like growth factors and their binding proteins in the term and preterm human fetus and neonate with normal and extremes of intrauterine growth. J Clin Endocrinol Metab 1995;80:1548–1555.
29 Lassarre C, Hardouin S, Daffos F, Forestier F, Frankenne F, Binoux M: Serum insulin-like growth factors and insulin-like growth factor binding proteins in the human fetus. Relationships with growth in normal subjects and in subjects with intrauterine growth retardation. Pediatr Res 1991;29:219–225.

30 Leger J, Oury JF, Noel M, Baron S, Benali K, Blot P, et al: Growth factors and intrauterine growth retardation. 1. Serum growth hormone, insulin-like growth factor (IGF)-I, IGF-II, and IGF binding protein 3 levels in normally grown and growth-retarded human fetuses during the second half of gestation. Pediatr Res 1996;40:94–100.

31 de Zegher F, Devlieger H, Veldhuis JD: Properties of growth hormone and prolactin hypersecretion by the human infant on the day of birth. J Clin Endocrinol Metab 1993;76:1177–1181.

32 Deiber M, Chatelain P, Naville D, Putet G, Salle B: Functional hypersomatotropism in small for gestational age (SGA) newborn infants. J Clin Endocrinol Metab 1989;68:232–234.

33 Boguszewski M, Rosberg S, Albertsson-Wikland K: Spontaneous 24-hour growth hormone profiles in prepubertal small for gestational age children. J Clin Endocrinol Metab 1995;80:2599–2606.

34 de Waal WJ, Hokken-Koelega AC, Stijnen T, de Muinck Keizer-Schrama SM, Drop SL: Endogenous and stimulated GH secretion, urinary GH excretion, and plasma IGF-I and IGF-II levels in prepubertal children with short stature after intrauterine growth retardation. The Dutch Working Group on Growth Hormone. Clin Endocrinol (Oxf) 1994;41:621–630.

35 Woods KA, van Helvoirt M, Ong KK, Mohn A, Levy J, de Zegher F, et al: The somatotropic axis in short children born small for gestational age: relation to insulin resistance. Pediatr Res 2002;51:76–80.

36 Stanhope R, Ackland F, Hamill G, Clayton J, Jones J, Preece MA: Physiological growth hormone secretion and response to growth hormone treatment in children with short stature and intrauterine growth retardation. Acta Paediatr Scand Suppl 1989;349:47–52.

37 Ranke MB, Lindberg A, Cowell CT, Albertsson-Wikland K, Reiter EO, Wilton P, et al: A growth prediction model for short children born small for gestational age. J Pediatr Endocrinol Metab 2002;87:235–239.

38 Cutfield WS, Hofman PL, Vickers M, Breier B, Blum WF, Robinson EM: IGFs and binding proteins in short children with intrauterine growth retardation. J Clin Endocrinol Metab 2002;87:235–239.

39 Binder G, Mavridou K, Wollmann HA, Eggermann T, Ranke MB: Screening for insulin-like growth factor-I receptor mutations in patients with Silver-Russell syndrome. J Pediatr Endocrinol Metab 2002;15:1167–1171.

40 Lazar L, Pollak U, Kalter-Leibovici O, Pertzelan A, Phillip M: Pubertal course of persistently short children born small for gestational age (SGA) compared with idiopathic short children born appropriate for gestational age (AGA). Eur J Endocrinol 2003;149:425–432.

41 Vicens-Calvet E, Espadero RM, Carrascosa A: Longitudinal study of the pubertal growth spurt in children born small for gestational age without postnatal catch-up growth. J Pediatr Endocrinol Metab 2002;15:381–388.

42 Persson I, Ahlsson F, Ewald U, Tuvemo T, Qingyuan M, von Rosen D, et al: Influence of perinatal factors on the onset of puberty in boys and girls: implications for interpretation of link with risk of long term diseases. Am J Epidemiol 1999;150:747–755.

43 Koziel S, Jankowska EA: Effect of low versus normal birthweight on menarche in 14-year-old Polish girls. J Paediatr Child Health 2002;38:268–271.

44 Boonstra V, van Pareren Y, Mulder P, Hokken-Koelega A: Puberty in growth hormone-treated children born small for gestational age (SGA). J Clin Endocrinol Metab 2003;88:5753–5758.

45 Davies PS, Valley R, Preece MA: Adolescent growth and pubertal progression in the Silver-Russell syndrome. Arch Dis Child 1988;63:130–135.

46 Auchus RJ, Rainey WE: Adrenarche – physiology, biochemistry and human disease. Clin Endocrinol (Oxf) 2004;60:288–296.

47 Ibanez L, Potau N, Francois I, de Zegher F: Precocious pubarche, hyperinsulinism, and ovarian hyperandrogenism in girls: relation to reduced fetal growth. J Clin Endocrinol Metab 1998;83:3558–3562.

48 Neville KA, Walker JL: Precocious pubarche is associated with SGA, prematurity, weight gain, and obesity. Arch Dis Child 2005;90:258–261.

49 Ghirri P, Bernardini M, Vuerich M, Cuttano AM, Coccoli L, Merusi I, et al: Adrenarche, pubertal development, age at menarche and final height of full-term, born small for gestational age (SGA) girls. Gynecol Endocrinol 2001;15:91–97.

50 Ong KK, Potau N, Petry CJ, Jones R, Ness AR, Honour JW, et al: Opposing influences of prenatal and postnatal weight gain on adrenarche in normal boys and girls. J Clin Endocrinol Metab 2004;89:2647–2651.

51 Ibanez L, Jimenez R, de Zegher F: Early puberty-menarche after precocious pubarche: relation to prenatal growth. Pediatrics 2006;117:117–121.

52 Ibanez L, Ferrer A, Ong K, Amin R, Dunger D, de Zegher F: Insulin sensitization early after menarche prevents progression from precocious pubarche to polycystic ovary syndrome. J Pediatr 2004;144:23–29.

53 Ibanez L, Potau N, Ferrer A, Rodriguez-Hierro F, Marcos MV, de Zegher F: Reduced ovulation rate in adolescent girls born small for gestational age. J Clin Endocrinol Metab 2002;87:3391–3393.

54 Zhang LH, Rodriguez H, Ohno S, Miller WL: Serine phosphorylation of human P450c17 increases 17,20-lyase activity: implications for adrenarche and the polycystic ovary syndrome. Proc Natl Acad Sci USA 1995;92:10619–10623.

55 Ibanez L, Potau N, Enriquez G, de Zegher F: Reduced uterine and ovarian size in adolescent girls born small for gestational age. Pediatr Res 2000;47:575–577.

56 Ibanez L, Valls C, Cols M, Ferrer A, Marcos MV, de Zegher F: Hypersecretion of FSH in infant boys and girls born small for gestational age. J Clin Endocrinol Metab 2002;87:1986–1988.

57 de Bruin JP, Dorland M, Bruinse HW, Spliet W, Nikkels PG, Te Velde ER: Fetal growth retardation as a cause of impaired ovarian development. Early Hum Dev 1998;51:39–46.

58 Francois I, de Zegher F, Spiessens C, D'Hooghe T, Vanderschueren D: Low birth weight and subsequent male subfertility. Pediatr Res 1997;42:899–901.

59 Barker DJ, Osmond C, Golding J, Kuh D, Wadsworth ME: Growth in utero, blood pressure in childhood and adult life, and mortality from cardiovascular disease. BMJ 1989;298:564–567.

60 Barker DJ, Winter PD, Osmond C, Margetts B, Simmonds SJ: Weight in infancy and death from ischaemic heart disease. Lancet 1989;ii:577–580.

61 Barker DJ, Hales CN, Fall CH, Osmond C, Phipps K, Clark PM: Type 2 (non-insulin-dependent) diabetes mellitus, hypertension and hyperlipidaemia (syndrome X): relation to reduced fetal growth. Diabetologia 1993;36:62–67.

62 Hales CN, Barker DJ, Clark PM, Cox LJ, Fall C, Osmond C, et al: Fetal and infant growth and impaired glucose tolerance at age 64. BMJ 1991;303:1019–1022.

63 Barker DJ, Osmond C, Law CM: The intrauterine and early postnatal origins of cardiovascular disease and chronic bronchitis. J Epidemiol Community Health 1989;43:237–240.

64 Hales CN, Barker DJ: Type 2 (non-insulin-dependent) diabetes mellitus: the thrifty phenotype hypothesis. Diabetologia 1992;35:595–601.

65 Lithell HO, McKeigue PM, Berglund L, Mohsen R, Lithell UB, Leon DA: Relation of size at birth to non-insulin dependent diabetes and insulin concentrations in men aged 50–60 years. BMJ 1996;312:406–410.

66 Curhan GC, Willett WC, Rimm EB, Spiegelman D, Ascherio AL, Stampfer MJ: Birth weight and adult hypertension, diabetes mellitus, and obesity in US men. Circulation 1996;94:3246–3250.

67 Ravelli AC, van der Meulen JH, Michels RP, Osmond C, Barker DJ, Hales CN, et al: Glucose tolerance in adults after prenatal exposure to famine. Lancet 1998;351:173–177.

68 Veening MA, van Weissenbruch MM, Heine RJ, Delemarre-van de Waal HA: β-Cell capacity and insulin sensitivity in prepubertal children born small for gestational age: influence of body size during childhood. Diabetes 2003;52:1756–1760.

69 Arends NJT, Boonstra VH, Duivenvoorden HJ, Hofman PL, Cutfield WS, Hokken-Koelega ACS: Reduced insulin sensitivity and the presence of cardiovascular risk factors in short prepubertal children born small for gestational age (SGA). Clin Endocrinol (Oxf) 2005;62:44–50.

70 Soto N, Bazaes RA, Pena V, Salazar T, Avila A, Iniguez G, et al: Insulin sensitivity and secretion are related to catch-up growth in small-for-gestational-age infants at age 1 year: results from a prospective cohort. J Clin Endocrinol Metab 2003;88:3645–3650.

71 Ibanez L, Ong K, Dunger DB, de Zegher F: Early development of adiposity and insulin resistance after catch-up weight gain in small-for-gestational-age children. J Clin Endocrinol Metab 2006;91:2153–2158.

72 Hypponen E, Power C, Smith GD: Prenatal growth, BMI, and risk of type 2 diabetes by early midlife. Diabetes Care 2003;26:2512–2517.

73 Kamoda T, Saitoh H, Saito M, Sugiura M, Matsui A: Serum adiponectin concentrations in newborn infants in early postnatal life. Pediatr Res 2004;56:690–693.

74 Cianfarani S, Martinez C, Maiorana A, Scire G, Spadoni GL, Boemi S: Adiponectin levels are reduced in children born small for gestational age and are inversely related to postnatal catch-up growth. J Clin Endocrinol Metab 2004;89:1346–1351.

75 Goldstein BJ, Scalia R: Adiponectin: a novel adipokine linking adipocytes and vascular function. J Clin Endocrinol Metab 2004;89:2563–2568.

76 Primatesta P, Falaschetti E, Poulter NR: Birth weight and blood pressure in childhood: results from the Health Survey for England. Hypertension 2005;45:75–79.

77 Bazaes RA, Salazar TE, Pittaluga E, Pena V, Alegria A, Iniguez G, et al: Glucose and lipid metabolism in small for gestational age infants at 48 hours of age. Pediatrics 2003;111:804–809.

78 Yiu V, Buka S, Zurakowski D, McCormick M, Brenner B, Jabs K: Relationship between birth weight and blood pressure in childhood. Am J Kidney Dis 1999;33:253–260.

79 Pulzer F, Haase U, Kratzsch J, Richter V, Rassoul F, Kiess W, et al: Lipoprotein(a) levels in formerly small-for-gestational age children. Horm Res 1999;52:241–246.

80 Tanner JM, Whitehouse RH, Hughes PCR, Vince FP: Effect of human growth hormone for one to seven years on growth of 100 children, with growth hormone deficiency, low birth weight, inherited smallness, Turner's syndrome and other complaints. Arch Dis Child 1971;46:745–782.

81 Grunt JA, Enriquez AR, Daughaday WH, Budd S: Acute and long-term responses to hGH in children with idiopathic small-for-dates dwarfism. J Clin Endocrinol Metab 1972;35:157–168.

82 de Zegher F, Albertsson-Wikland K, Wollmann HA, Chatelain P, Chaussain JL, Lofstrom A, et al: Growth hormone treatment of short children born small for gestational age: growth responses with continuous and discontinuous regimens over 6 years. J Clin Endocrinol Metab 2000;85:2816–2821.

83 Fjellestad-Paulsen A, Simon D, Czernichow P: Short children born small for gestational age and treated with growth hormone for three years have an important catch-down five years after discontinuation of treatment. J Clin Endocrinol Metab 2004;89:1234–1239.

84 Van Pareren Y, Mulder P, Houdijk M, Jansen M, Reeser M, Hokken-Koelega A: Adult height after long-term, continuous growth hormone (GH) treatment in short children born small for gestational age: results of a randomized, double-blind, dose-response GH trial. J Clin Endocrinol Metab 2003;88:3584–3590.

85 Carel JC, Chatelain P, Rochiccioli P, Chaussain JL: Improvement in adult height after growth hormone treatment in adolescents with short stature born small for gestational age: results of a randomized controlled study. J Clin Endocrinol Metab 2003;88:1587–1593.

86 Dos Santos C, Essioux L, Teinturier C, Tauber M, Goffin V, Bougneres P: A common polymorphism of the growth hormone receptor is associated with increased responsiveness to growth hormone. Nat Genet 2004;36:720–724.

87 Carrascosa A, Esteban C, Espadero R, Fernandez-Cancio M, Andaluz P, Clemente M, et al: The $d3/fl$-growth hormone receptor polymorphism does not influence the effect of growth hormone treatment (66 μg/kg/day) or the spontaneous growth in short non-growth hormone deficient small for gestational-age children: results form a two-year controlled prospective study in 170 Spanish patients. J Clin Endocrinol Metab 2006;91:3281–3286.

88 Binder G, Baur F, Schweizer R, Ranke MB: The d3-growth hormone receptor polymorphism is associated with increased responsiveness to GH in Turner syndrome and short SGA children. J Clin Endocrinol Metab 2006;91:659–664.

89 Audi L, Esteban C, Carrascosa A, Espadero R, Perez-Arroyo A, Arjona R, et al: Exon 3-deleted/full-length growth hormone receptor polymorphism genotype frequencies in Spanish short small-for-gestational age (SGA) children and adloescents (n = 247) and in an adult control population (n = 289) show increased *fl/fl* in short SGA. J Clin Endocrinol Metab 2006;91:5038–5043.

90 O'Keeffe MJ, O'Callaghan M, Williams GM, Najman JM, Bor W: Learning, cognitive, and attentional problems in adolescents born small for gestational age. Pediatrics 2003;112:301–307.

91 Bannink EMN, van Pareren Y, Theunissen NCM, Raat H, Mulder PGM, Hokken-Koelega ACS: Quality of life in adolescents born small for gestational age: does growth hormone make a difference. Horm Res 2005;64:166–174.

92 Hokken-Koelega ACS, van Pareren Y, Sas T, Arends N: Final height data, body composition and glucose metabolism in growth hormone-treated short children born small for gestational age. Horm Res 2003;60(suppl 3):113–114.

93 Cutfield WS, Jackson WE, Jefferies C, Robinson EM, Breier BH, Richards GE, et al: Reduced insulin sensitivity during growth hormone therapy for short children born small for gestational age. J Pediatr 2003;142:113–116.

94 de Zegher F, Ong K, Helviort M, Woods K, Dunger D: High-dose growth hormone (GH) treatment in non-GH-deficient children born small for gestational age induces growth responses related to pretreatment GH secretion and associated with a reversible decrease in insulin sensitivity. J Clin Endocrinol Metab 2002;87:148–151.

95 Rakover Y, Dietsch S, Ambler GR, Chock C, Thomsett M, Cowell CT: Growth hormone therapy in Silver Russell syndrome: 5 years experience of the Australian and New Zealand Growth database. Eur J Pediatr 1996;155:851–857.

96 Rizzo V, Traggiai C, Stanhope R: Growth hormone treatment does not alter lower limb asymmetry in children with Russell-Silver syndrome. Horm Res 2001;56:114–116.

KIGS 20 Years: Children Born Small for Gestational Age

David B. Dunger

Children born small for gestational age (SGA) generally catch up in the first 12 months of life, but in around 10% of cases, this may not be the case, and particularly where there are recognisable syndromes, such as the Silver-Russell syndrome, adult height will be compromised. The use of growth hormone in short children born SGA has been explored for over 30 years, but the indication was not approved by the Food and Drug Administration and the European Agency for the Evaluation of Medicinal Products until 2001 and 2003, respectively. Approval of the growth hormone indication was based on gains in final height in two pivotal trials, but there remain some concerns about the safety of long-term treatment, as SGA infants may be predisposed to the development of insulin resistance and type 2 diabetes.

SGA children starting on growth hormone therapy have been registered in the KIGS database since its conception 20 years ago. The purpose of this article is to review the data in the KIGS database and to reflect on the contribution made by KIGS to our overall understanding of the effects of growth hormone in this condition.

The KIGS Database

More than 2,000 children have been entered into the KIGS database over the last 20 years with a diagnosis relating to being born SGA. The KIGS classifications are summarised in table 1. To

Table 1. Classification of SGA in the KIGS database

3.4	SGA/IUGR with persisting short stature
	3.4.1 Cause known
	3.4.2 Cause unknown
3.5	SGA/IUGR with persisting short stature with minor dysmorphic stigma
	3.5.1 IUGR due to prenatal infection
	3.5.2 IUGR due to drugs (including smoking and alcohol)
	3.5.9 Others
3.3.1	Silver-Russell syndrome

IUGR = Intrauterine growth retardation.

Department of Paediatrics
Addenbrooke's Hospital, University of Cambridge
Hills Road, Level 8, Box 116
Cambridge CB2 2QQ (UK)

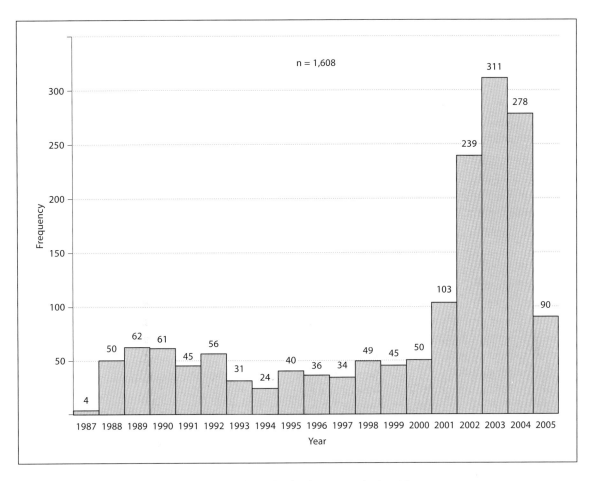

Fig. 1. Number of SGA children registered yearly in the database over the last 20 years.

date, 472 children with Silver-Russell syndrome and 2,097 children with SGA/intrauterine growth retardation have been registered in the database. The number of children registered over the last 20 years has gradually increased and accelerated over the last 4 years, and more than 900 children have now completed 1 year of growth hormone therapy (fig. 1). Around 65 children born SGA and 43 with Silver-Russell syndrome have reached near adult height. Over the years, the study of the database has led to a large number of publications relating either to Silver-Russell syndrome or children born SGA [see chap. by Cutfield, this vol., pp. 389–399]. As a post-marketing surveillance study, KIGS can always be criticised, as the ascertainment figures are unknown and the data may not always be reliable. However, the shear size of the database means that a lot of the 'flaws' in the system become less important and KIGS has made a valuable contribution to the development of prediction models, the study of gains in final height and long-term surveillance of the safety of growth hormone treatment.

Table 2. Regression equation variables for predicting the first-year growth response to growth hormone therapy in 613 children born SGA

	Parameter estimate	Rank	Partial r^2
Intercept (constant)	9.4		
Age at treatment start	–0.3	2	0.1
Weight SDS at treatment start	0.3	3	0.1
Growth hormone dose	56.5	1	0.4
Midparental height SDS	0.1	4	0.01
r^2	0.5		
Error SD	1.3		

Prediction Models

Michael Ranke and other colleagues from the KIGS International Board have been at the forefront of the development of prediction models that allow physicians to individualise growth hormone treatment in many conditions, including children born SGA. In 2003, they reported on first-year growth hormone treatment in 613 children from the KIGS database [1]. In the first year of treatment, the growth response correlated positively with the growth hormone dose, the weight at the start of growth hormone treatment and the midparental height standard deviation score (SDS), and negatively with the age at treatment start. Using this model, 52% of the variability of the growth hormone response could be explained with the mean error SD of 1.3 cm (table 2). The growth hormone dose was the most important response predictor (35% of variability) followed by age at treatment start (fig. 2). The second-year growth response was best predicted by height velocity at 1 year of treatment, age at the start of treatment and growth hormone dose, which together accounted for 34% of the variability with an error SD of 1.1 cm. However, the first-year response to growth hormone was by far the most important predictor of the second-year response, accounting for 29% of the variability.

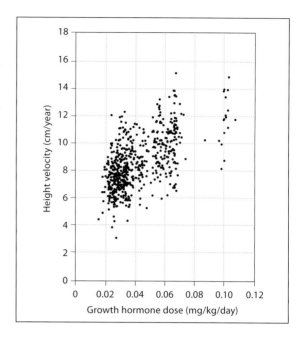

Fig. 2. Linear correlation between height velocity during the first year of growth hormone treatment and the growth hormone dose in 613 children born SGA (r = 0.57, p < 0.001).

Growth hormone doses over the first year of treatment have been the source of some debate, as the dose range recommended by the Food and Drug Administration is 70 μg/kg/day in the first year and that approved by the European Agency for the Evaluation of Medicinal Products is 35 μg/kg/day. At the recent SGA consensus meeting organised by the European Society for Paediatric Endocrinology, the Growth Hormone Research Society and the Lawson Wilkins Paediatric Endocrine Society, there was general agreement that the higher dose of growth hormone should be available for children who showed the most marked growth retardation at the beginning of treatment [2]. Prediction models developed through the study of KIGS provide a further opportunity to optimise treatment and to identify children who are not compliant with therapy. It is likely that such models can be refined in the future with the study of treatment outcome in

Table 3. Characteristics of all patients with SGA and Silver-Russell syndrome at treatment start and after 1 year of treatment

	SGA				Silver-Russell syndrome			
	n	median	10th percentile	90th percentile	n	median	10th percentile	90th percentile
Background								
Birth weight SDS	891	−2.7	−4.1	−1.7	342	−3.0	−4.8	−0.9
Birth length SDS	712	−2.7	−4.5	−1.6	241	−3.1	−5.4	−0.6
MPH SDS (Prader)	828	−1.2	−2.7	0.3	328	−0.6	−2.0	0.7
Maximum GH, µg/l	640	15.0	6.4	34.0	260	12.1	4.4	32.1
IGF-1 SDS	329	−1.2	−2.4	−0.4	104	−0.9	−2.8	0.9
At start of GH treatment								
Age, years	891	7.1	3.4	11.2	357	5.0	2.2	9.9
Bone age, years	314	4.7	2.2	9.0	120	3.2	1.0	8.0
Height SDS (Prader)	891	−3.4	−4.9	−2.4	357	−4.1	−6.0	−2.8
Height velocity, cm/year	353	5.1	3.4	7.5	170	5.8	3.5	9.0
BMI SDS	891	−1.1	−2.9	0.5	357	−2.4	−4.9	−0.2
GH dose, mg/kg/week	891	0.28	0.17	0.47	357	0.30	0.17	0.46
After 1 year of GH therapy								
Age, years	891	8.1	4.4	12.2	357	6.0	3.1	11.0
Height SDS (Prader)	891	−2.7	−4.1	−1.7	357	−3.3	−5.0	−2.0
Height velocity, cm/year	891	8.4	6.1	11.1	357	8.6	6.1	11.9
BMI SDS	887	−1.1	−2.6	0.5	357	−2.2	−4.8	−0.4
GH dose, mg/kg/week	891	0.33	0.17	0.47	357	0.30	0.18	0.46
Studentised residual of height velocity	632	−0.4	−1.8	0.7	251	−0.8	−1.9	0.6

MPH = Midparental height; GH = growth hormone; IGF-1 = insulin-like growth factor 1; BMI = body mass index.

relation to genes effecting growth response to growth hormone. Such studies involving the KIGS database are currently under consideration. The KIGS database also provides an opportunity to explore the influence of identified methylation defects affecting imprinted genes on chromosome 11 in cases of Silver-Russell syndrome in response to growth hormone therapy.

Comparison of Children Born Small for Gestational Age for Unknown Reasons and Those with Silver-Russel Syndrome

Children with Silver-Russell syndrome and those born SGA are often grouped together, although it has long been recognised that the prognosis for final height is probably worse in the former. Such decisions largely relate to the number of children available for study and it is only through the KIGS database that enough data have been accumulated to make some comparisons between the two groups. Currently, there are data from around 900 children born SGA and 400 born with Silver-Russell syndrome available for comparison. The baseline characteristics of these two prepubertal cohorts are summarised in table 3. Although the size at birth is comparable between the two groups, the Silver-Russell syndrome subjects are shorter at birth and at the start of growth hormone treatment even though they tend to be started on treatment at around 5 years of age, in contrast to SGA children who are started on treatment around the age of 7 years. Interestingly, there were no differences in maximum growth hormone response to stimulation, and if anything, the insulin-like growth factor 1 levels were marginally higher in the Silver-Russell syndrome group. Finally, the body mass index difference at diagnosis is quite striking, being –2.4 SD in the Silver-Russell syndrome group compared with –1 SD in the SGA group.

Response to treatment in the first year was comparable between the two groups, as was the growth hormone dose (table 3). The response to growth hormone therapy in the subgroup with near final height data is summarised in table 4. The growth hormone dose in both groups was comparable, being on average around 0.23 mg/kg/week (30 μg/kg/day). Final height in the SGA group was around –2 SDS (–1 SDS for height adjusted for midparental height). The Silver-Russell syndrome subjects fared less well, with a median final height SDS of –2.9, which was –2 SDS when adjusted for midparental height. The median Δ change in the height SDS in the SGA children was 1.3, which was identical to that observed in the subjects with Silver-Russell syndrome. Thus, the height gain and the response to therapy were comparable between the two groups, the major difference being the height SDS at the start of treatment which was lower in the Silver-Russell syndrome group and never regained during treatment.

The mean height SDS gain in the pivotal registration studies was around 1.8 (0.7 SD) in contrast to the 1.4 SD gain in the KIGS data. This could relate to the differences in doses, as the mean dose used in the KIGS database in patients reaching near final height was 30 μg/kg/day; in the registration studies, two doses were explored, one group receiving 33 and the other 67 μg/kg/day. The other major difference is that the registration trials were carefully controlled and randomised, whereas the KIGS database reflects wide variation in treatment regimens and growth hormone doses used in an unselected population. Nevertheless, comparison between the KIGS database and the registration studies provides reassurance that growth hormone treatment outside of the restricted confines of a controlled trial will still bring the expected benefits in terms of final height.

Adverse Events

Wayne Cutfield [3] recently reviewed adverse events in the KIGS database relating to children born SGA. At the time, a total of 1,909 children born SGA were identified. Comparisons were made with children treated with growth hormone diagnosed as having idiopathic short stature, also derived from the KIGS database. The total number of adverse events (187 vs. 183 per 1,000 patients) and the total number of serious adverse events (14 vs. 10 per 1,000 patients) were no different between the children with SGA and those with idiopathic short stature. There were no differences in the incidence of adverse events in comparison of data from the USA, where a higher dose of growth hormone tends to be used during the first year of treatment, with data from Europe, where the lower dose is used. There was no increased incidence of neoplasia, or perhaps more importantly, diabetes in the SGA group. These data are reassuring, but further surveillance of the long-term effects of growth hormone therapy in SGA children is required, perhaps into adult life, and the KIGS database provides a unique opportunity to establish such long-term studies as part of a successful academic pharmaceutical partnership.

Conclusions

The KIGS database has made a valuable contribution to our understanding of the variability in response to growth hormone therapy in children born SGA. It provides an opportunity to identify variation related to underlying genetic

Table 4. Near adult height in patients with SGA and Silver-Russell syndrome

	SGA				Silver-Russell syndrome			
	n	median	10th percentile	90th percentile	n	median	10th percentile	90th percentile
Background								
Birth weight SDS	65	−2.6	−3.9	−2.0	39	−3.2	−5.9	−1.4
Birth length SDS	50	−2.9	−4.5	−1.9	25	−2.9	−5.7	−0.2
MPH SDS (Prader)	65	−1.1	−2.6	0.0	41	−0.6	−2.7	0.5
Maximum GH, μg/l	60	12.8	3.9	33.0	39	11.9	3.4	35.0
IGF-1 SDS	5	−1.7	−2.9	−0.6	3	−1.4	−2.6	0.4
At start of GH treatment								
Age, years	65	7.9	3.6	11.9	43	7.9	4.0	11.7
Bone age, years	39	5.0	2.5	9.5	23	4.5	2.0	11.0
Height SDS (Prader)	65	−3.6	−5.0	−2.6	43	−4.0	−5.5	−2.3
Height velocity, cm/year	37	4.8	2.4	7.9	26	4.6	2.5	7.7
BMI SDS	65	−1.1	−3.3	0.2	43	−2.0	−4.4	−0.1
GH dose, mg/kg/week	65	0.24	0.16	0.43	43	0.25	0.17	0.46
After 1 year of GH therapy								
Age, years	65	8.9	4.6	12.9	43	9.0	5.0	12.7
Height SDS (Prader)	65	−3.0	−4.6	−2.0	43	−3.3	−4.7	−1.9
Height velocity, cm/year	65	7.5	5.6	10.0	43	8.5	5.8	10.8
BMI SDS	64	−1.2	−3.1	−0.1	43	−2.3	−4.1	0.3
GH dose, mg/kg/week	65	0.23	0.16	0.42	43	0.25	0.18	0.48
At start of puberty								
Age, years	27	12.4	10.4	14.3	16	12.3	10.8	14.7
Height SDS (Prader)	27	−1.7	−2.9	−0.7	16	−2.1	−2.9	−0.2
BMI SDS	26	−0.9	−2.7	0.7	15	−1.7	−4.0	0.2
GH dose, mg/kg/week	26	0.23	0.16	0.40	15	0.25	0.16	0.37
Near adult height								
Age, years	65	16.8	14.7	18.3	43	16.8	15.2	18.9
Height SDS (Prader)	65	−2.1	−3.5	−1.3	43	−2.9	−4.2	−1.0
Height − MPH SDS (Prader)	65	−1.0	−2.4	0.0	41	−2.0	−3.3	−0.3
Δ height SDS (latest − puberty, Prader)	27	−0.2	−1.1	0.3	16	−0.7	−1.7	0.2
Δ height SDS (latest − start, Prader)	65	1.3	0.2	2.6	43	1.3	0.1	2.8
BMI SDS	64	−0.5	−2.3	1.2	42	−1.3	−2.9	0.4
Mean pubertal GH dose, mg/kg/week	27	0.23	0.17	0.36	16	0.23	0.16	0.35
Mean total GH dose, mg/kg/week	65	0.24	0.16	0.37	43	0.26	0.17	0.35
Years on GH treatment	65	7.7	5.1	11.7	43	7.9	5.0	11.5

MPH = Midparental height; GH = growth hormone; IGF-1 = insulin-like growth factor 1; BMI = body mass index.

defects, and when these are identified, to develop robust prediction models based on both baseline phenotypic data and future genetic data. The KIGS database also provides insight into national prescribing and the effects of dose variation on final height data. Finally, the KIGS database provides an opportunity to build on the existing database to provide long-term data on the safety of growth hormone for the SGA indication into adult life.

References

1 Ranke MB, Lindberg A, Cowell CT, Albertsson Wikland K, Reiter EO, Wilton P, Price DA: Prediction of response to growth hormone treatment in short children born small for gestational age: analysis of data from KIGS (Pharmacia International Growth Database). J Clin Endocrinol Metab 2003;88:125–131.

2 Clayton PE, Cianferani S, Czernichov P, Johannsson G, Rapaport R, Rogol A: The child born small for gestational age (SGA): a consensus statement on management through to adulthood. J Clin Endocrinol Metab, in press.

3 Cutfield WS, Lindberg A: Adverse events during growth hormone treatment of children born small for gestational age and children with idiopathic short stature enrolled in the Pfizer International Growth Database (KIGS). KIGS Annual Report 2006;23:19–24.

Growth Hormone Treatment in Short Children with Chronic Kidney Disease

Otto Mehls[a] Anders Lindberg[b] Richard Nissel[c] Elke Wühl[a]
Franz Schaefer[a] Burkhard Tönshoff[a] Dieter Haffner[c]

[a]University Hospital of Pediatric and Adolescent Medicine
Im Neuenheimer Feld 151, DE–69120 Heidelberg (Germany)
[b]Pfizer Endocrine Care
KIGS/KIMS/ACROSTUDY Medical Outcomes
Vetenskapsvägen 10, SE–191 90 Sollentuna (Sweden)
[c]University Hospital of Pediatric and Adolescent Medicine
Rembrandtstrasse 17–18, DE–18075 Rostock (Germany)

Recombinant human growth hormone (rhGH) as a new treatment modality for short stature in chronic kidney disease (CKD) became available about 17 years ago. Since then, many studies have shown that this treatment is able to reverse progressive growth failure in CKD. GH treatment for short stature following CKD has become approved as an indication for GH treatment in 1994 in the US and in 1995 in Europe. This chapter summarizes the pathogenesis of growth failure in CKD patients and the therapeutic efficacy of GH including its effects on final height. The review of clinical data is based on a recent analysis of data from KIGS and data from important prospective clinical trials.

Growth Disturbance in Chronic Renal Failure

Since the early 1970s, the survival of children with end-stage renal disease (ESRD) has been made possible by renal replacement therapy, e.g., long-term dialysis and renal transplantation. The incidence of ESRD in children is about 1.5–2.0 per million population or 6–10 per million children. Whereas these numbers are representative of the patients who newly enter programs for renal replacement therapy, the number of patients with CKD seen by physicians for conservative treatment is about 8–10 times higher, because the mean time from the start of CKD to the start of renal replacement therapy amounts to about 10 years.

The majority of children with CKD suffer from congenital renal disorders, whereas less children present with acquired renal diseases such as glomerulonephritis or acute renal failure like hemolytic uremic syndrome. In the ESCAPE trial, a representative number of 400 children with all stages of CKD are followed [1]. About 70% of these children have chronic renal failure (CRF) due to renal hypodysplasia with or without vesicoureteral reflux or obstructive uropathy [1]. Another 15% of the patients have congenital hereditary disorders and only 15% glomerulonephritis or hemolytic uremic syndrome. The progression rate of CKD is higher in patients with glomerulonephritis than in patients with congenital renal disorders [2]. In a representative European multicenter study, the mean loss of glomerular filtration rate (GFR) was 6 ml/min × 1.73 m^2 per year for children with glomerulonephritis and 2.5 ml/min × 1.73 m^2 per year for children with hypodysplasia [2].

Growth failure is still a major obstacle to successful rehabilitation of children with CKD. The mean height standard deviation score (SDS) at the start of renal replacement therapy is about –2, indicating that half of the patients have short stature [3–5]. Likewise, the mean final height SDS is reported to be significantly reduced and varied between –1.4 in girls and –2.2 in boys in various reports [6–8]. In the study of Hokken-Koelega et al. [7], 77% of male and 71% of female transplanted patients were below the third percentile of normal adult height.

The pathogenesis of impaired growth in CKD is complex. Several factors like the patient's age, the type, duration and severity of renal disease, the treatment modality and the patient's social environment all play important roles [9]. Malnutrition [10–13] and complex disturbances of the somatotropic hormone axis seem to be the most frequent and most important factors contributing to the degree of growth disturbance.

Optimizing nutrition during the nutrition-sensitive phase of growth, e.g., during infancy and early childhood [14], might improve growth, whereas this treatment strategy is less efficient at later age. However, optimized clinical management (without GH treatment) is not able to prevent stunting in a significant percentage of children. In the recent annual report of the NAPRTCS (North American Pediatric Renal Cooperative Study) in the United States, growth data of CKD patients were analyzed over a period of 5 years. The results showed that improvement in growth without GH treatment was only observed in young patients below the age of 5 years [5]. The younger the patients at the start of observation, the higher the increase in height SDS during the observation period. The age- and height-related same pattern was seen after successful renal transplantation [5].

Growth Hormone Resistance in Chronic Renal Failure

In experimental uremia, GH was able to improve growth and conversion of food into lean body mass [15]. However, the growth response was relatively better in sham-operated pair-fed control animals. In children with CRF, normal or elevated circulating GH levels were noted despite a reduced growth rate [16, 17]. Both seminal observations led to the concept that uremia induces a state of insensitivity to GH. Today, this concept is substantiated and it became clear that many factors contribute to the resistance to GH in CKD (table 1).

Whereas the GH secretion rate in CKD is variable between patients and studies [18, 19], a prolonged half-life of GH as a result of the reduced renal metabolic clearance rate is a consistent finding [17]. The hepatic and local insensitivity to the action of GH is partly the consequence of reduced GH receptor expression [20, 21]. Independent of the GH receptor expression, GH receptor signaling is disturbed [22]. Similar to the recently described genetic defect of the JAK2-STAT5 pathway [23], the phosphorylation and dimerization of STAT5 and its translation into the nucleus as well as its binding to GH-dependent genes are functionally impaired in uremic rats. The consequence is a low insulin-like growth factor 1 (IGF-1) production evidenced by both clinical and experimental studies [24, 25]. Nevertheless, serum levels of IGF-1 and IGF-2 are normal in preterminal CKD, while in ESRD, IGF-1 levels are slightly decreased and IGF-2 levels slightly increased [26]. The discrepancy between

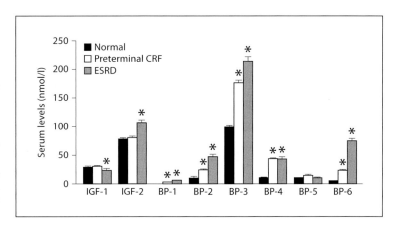

Fig. 1. Comparison of the molar serum concentrations of IGFs and IGFBPs (BP-1 to BP-6) in children with preterminal CRF and children with ESRD. The mean molar concentrations in normal age-matched children are given for comparison. Data are means + SEM. * p < 0.05, significant versus control. With permission from Ulinski et al. [26].

Table 1. Factors contributing to insensitivity to GH/IGF in CKD

Disturbed GH secretion	pulsatile secretion disturbed
	circulating levels not decreased because of impaired (renal) metabolic clearance
Reduced IGF bioactivity	IGF production low
	IGF binding to binding proteins increased
Endorgan resistance to GH and IGF	GH receptor expression decreased
	GH receptor signaling disturbed
	IGF type 1 receptor expression decreased
	IGF postreceptor defect

the decreased production of IGF-1 and near-normal IGF serum concentration is explained by the increased concentration of IGF-binding proteins (IGFBPs) [26–28] (fig. 1). CRF serum has an IGF-binding capacity that is increased by 7- to 10-fold, leading to decreased IGF bioactivity of CRF serum despite normal total IGF levels. Serum levels of intact IGFBP-1, IGFBP-2, IGFBP-4, IGFBP-6 and low-molecular-weight fragments of IGFBP-3 are elevated in CRF serum in relation to the degree of renal dysfunction, whereas serum levels of intact IGFBP-3 are normal [29]. Levels of immunoreactive IGFBP-5 are not altered in CRF serum, but the majority of IGFBP-5 is fragmented. Decreased renal filtration and increased hepatic production of IGFBP-1 and IGFBP-2 both contribute to high levels of serum IGFBP. Experimental and clinical evidence suggests that these excessive high-affinity IGFBPs in CRF serum inhibit IGF action in growth plate chondrocytes by competition with the type 1 IGF receptor for IGF binding [30]. These data indicate that growth failure in CRF is mainly due to functional IGF deficiency. In addition to the reduced IGF activity, there is an end-organ resistance to IGF-1 as to GH [31].

GH exerts its stimulatory effect mainly on longitudinal growth, not by normalizing increased serum levels of inhibitory IGFBPs [32, 33], but by increasing serum IGF levels [34]. Some of the GH-induced IGF is bound in new serum ternary complexes, but the majority of stimulated IGF circulates in the 35-kDa serum fractions bound to previously unsaturated excess IGFBPs [32]. This GH-induced rise in levels of IGFs relative to IGFBPs in the 35-kDa fractions of CRF serum presumably leads to an increase in IGFs in extravascular fluids, from where circulating IGFs

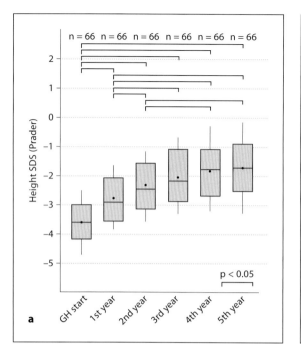
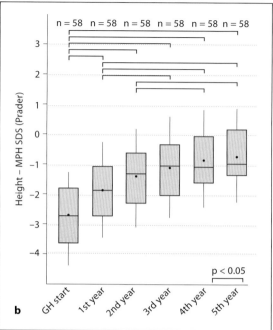

Fig. 2. Improvement in height SDS (**a**) and height SDS corrected for MPH (**b**) within 5-year GH treatment in prepubertal children with CRF under conservative treatment. Longitudinal data are shown as box plots representing ranges (whiskers), quartiles (shaded boxes), means (dots) and medians (horizontal lines).

have access to their target tissues (the growth plate), to interact with the type 1 IGF receptor for stimulation of longitudinal growth.

Data from KIGS

In the KIGS database, more than 1,700 patients in all stages of CKD including renal transplantation were recorded by January 1, 2006. Sixty-nine percent of patients were boys. The mean chronological age at the start of GH treatment was 9.1 ± 4.4 years, and the mean bone age was retarded by nearly 2 years. Of all patients, 19.8% were pubertal. The mean height SDS was –2.5 ± 1.2 according to Tanner [35] and –3.1 ± 1.3 according to Prader [36]. The mean height SDS corrected for midparental height (MPH) was –2.4 ± 1.5. The body mass index SDS was nearly normal (–0.3 ± 1.4). The patients were treated with a mean GH dose of 0.32 ± 0.12 mg/kg/week. Male patients were slightly more growth retarded than females. Their MPH corrected SDS (Prader) was –2.7 compared with –2.3 in girls.

The prepubertal longitudinal growth is shown in figure 2. There were complete data up to 5 years of treatment in 66 patients. These patients were prepubertal at the start of treatment and were conservatively treated. Some of them required dialysis treatment during the 5-year observation period.

Eighty-two percent of the patients were boys. The mean chronological age at the start of GH treatment was 5.5 ± 3.3 years (median age 4.8), and the mean height SDS was –3.6 ± 0.9 (Prader). The MPH corrected SDS was –2.7 ± 1.3.

The mean increase in height SDS (fig. 2a) over 5 years of GH therapy as well as the increase in

MPH corrected SDS (fig. 2b) was nearly 1.8. Height velocity was significantly higher during the first years of GH treatment compared with baseline height velocity (fig. 3). Thereafter, height velocity was not significantly different anymore. However, this has to be balanced to the decreasing height velocity with age and the prepubertal growth dipping seen in normal children. In addition, the therapeutic effect of GH treatment on the height SDS might even be higher than seen from the graphs, because a decrease in height SDS would be expected in untreated controls with CKD.

In an earlier analysis of the KIGS data [37], we have shown that the response of short children with CKD to GH treatment is lower than that expected for children with GH deficiency. It has also been shown that the response to GH treatment is lower in dialysis patients compared with patients on conservative treatment.

Figure 4 illustrates the respective data for the second treatment year. One hundred and sixty-one patients with conservative treatment and 23 patients with dialysis treatment presented with a complete data set and could be analyzed. The figures demonstrate that the growth response to GH did not significantly differ in patients on conservative treatment from the response in children with primary GH deficiency, whereas the growth in dialysis patients was less than predicted by the idiopathic GH deficiency model.

In 87 patients, near final height was reached. Near final height was defined as a growth <2 cm/year at age 17 years. At the start of GH therapy, the mean chronological age of these patients was 10.1 ± 2.2 years and the mean height was 118.2 ± 12.5 cm. The mean chronological age at near adult height was 17.7 ± 1.6 years and the mean height 155.9 ± 12.0 cm. The mean increase in height SDS was 0.9 (fig. 5).

In 65 patients, the MPH corrected SDS according to Prader could be calculated. These patients had a mean MPH corrected SDS of –2.5 ± 1.5 at the start of GH treatment and –1.6 ± 1.6 at the time of near final height. The body mass in-

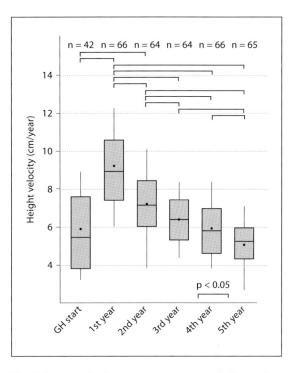

Fig. 3. Longitudinal analysis over 5 years of height velocity in a subgroup of 66 patients with CRF (same patients as in fig. 2). Box plots represent ranges (whiskers), 25th and 75th percentiles (shaded boxes), means (dots) and medians (horizontal lines).

dex SDS was –0.4 ± 1.3 at the start of treatment and –0.5 ± 1.3 at the time of near final height.

The mean treatment time until the start of puberty was 3.4 ± 1.6 years, and the mean time on GH treatment was 6.7 ± 1.7 years. It is of note that despite the longer treatment time compared with the 5-year treatment time in prepubertal children (fig. 2), the Δ height SDS was only 0.9 ± 1.9 within 6.7 years compared with 1.9 within 5 years. This difference is explained by the younger mean age at treatment start in the prepubertal children (5.5 vs. 10.1 years).

There was no significant difference between males and females regarding age at start, height SDS at start, duration of treatment, Δ height SDS and final height. Patients who reached near final height and in whom GH treatment was started

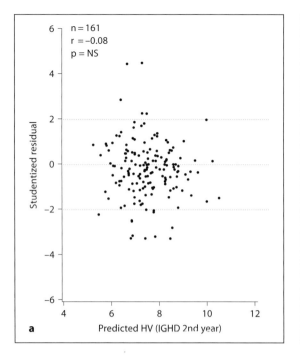 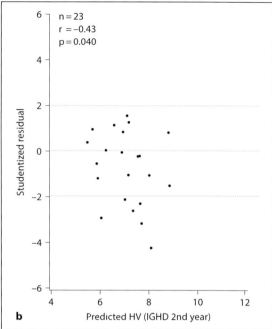

Fig. 4. Second-year response to GH treatment of patients with CRF on conservative treatment (**a**) and on dialysis (**b**) compared with the KIGS prediction model for children with idiopathic GH deficiency (IGHD). Growth response in dialyzed children was significantly reduced. NS = Not significant.

during conservative treatment (n = 20) had a slightly higher increase in height SDS than patients in whom GH treatment was started during dialysis (n = 35), despite identical duration of GH treatment (0.8 ± 0.8 vs. 0.7 ± 1.1 SD).

Factors Predictive of Short- and Long-Term Efficacy of Growth Hormone Treatment

The first proof that GH treatment with a dose of 0.045–0.05 mg/kg/day (25–30 mg/m^2/week) is effective to stimulate growth in uremia came from a placebo-controlled study [38] in children with CRF under conservative treatment. Shortly thereafter, it has been shown that GH treatment is also effective in dialyzed children [34]. Although there is no doubt on the efficacy of GH in short children with CKD [39], the response to GH therapy in the individual patients varies widely, and the reason for this variability remains to be elucidated.

Several studies on factors predictive of the growth response to rhGH in short children before and after renal transplantation have been performed [40–42]. Those studies do not always present identical results. This might be explained by the small number of patients in most of the studies, the different age groups and the different baseline treatment modalities like conservative treatment, dialysis and renal transplantation.

The largest study is from Haffner et al. [41]. The authors evaluated the growth-stimulating effect of GH in 103 prepubertal children with CKD on conservative treatment (n = 74) or dialysis (n = 29) with a treatment time of up to 5 years. The height SDS increased persistently, and the mean predicted adult height increased by 7.7 cm during

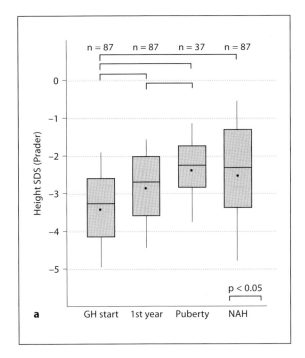
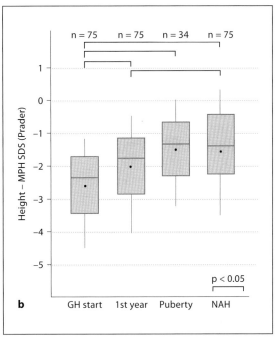

Fig. 5. The height SDS after Prader (**a**) and the height SDS corrected for MPH (**b**) at the start of GH treatment and at the time of near final height. Box plots represent ranges (whiskers), 25th and 75th percentiles (shaded boxes), means (dots) and medians (horizontal lines). NAH = Near adult height.

the first 3 treatment years. Both standardized height and predicted height were significantly more increased in conservatively treated than in dialyzed children. Age, GFR, target height and pre-GH treatment growth rate were identified as independent predictors of the response to rhGH treatment during the first and second treatment year. GFR and target height were positively correlated with the change in height SDS and the change in absolute or age-standardized height velocity. Age affected growth response depending on which outcome measure was used (fig. 6). Although the first-year change in height SDS was inversely correlated with age, the change in absolute height velocity was independent of age, and the change in standardized height velocity was positively correlated with age. These findings may demonstrate that the replication of cells within the growth zone can be stimulated by GH only to a certain extent which is independent of age. This results in a slightly better improvement in the height velocity SDS in older children in whom the physiologic growth velocity prior to puberty is low. However, the best therapeutic effect (change of the height SDS) is seen in young children because the SD values physiologically increase over time and the absolute height deficit indicated by SDS values is inversely related to the patient's age. The growth response during the first treatment year positively predicted the long-term response.

If uremia induces a state of GH resistance, it is expected that the resistance is increasing with decreasing renal function. In contrast to the study by Haffner et al. [41], a correlation between renal function and growth response was mostly not found [43], but this is due to the small number of patients studied, the wide age range and the great variability in absolute response. However, there

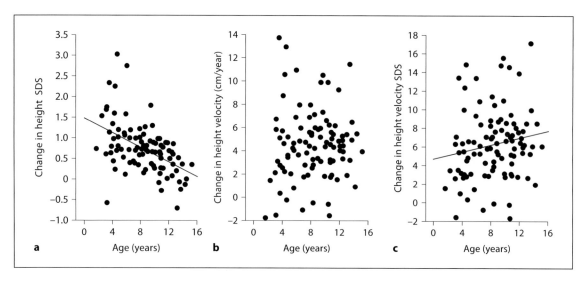

Fig. 6. Change in height SDS (**a**), height velocity (**b**) and height velocity SDS (**c**) during the first year of rhGH treatment as a function of age. While absolute height increment induced by treatment is independent of age, a positive correlation with age appears when the change in height velocity is standardized, and there is a negative correlation when the change in height SDS is related to age. With permission from Haffner et al. [41].

are several studies clearly demonstrating that patients with end-stage renal failure, e.g., on dialysis treatment, respond significantly less to GH than children on conservative treatment [30, 41, 44–46]. Dialysis treatment, e.g., three times 5-hour hemodialysis per week or daily peritoneal dialysis, does not completely reverse the uremic state. However, this can be obtained by daily hemodialysis, e.g., 12 h during the night. Recently, it has been demonstrated that daily dialysis not only reversed uremia but also induced catch-up growth in children on GH treatment (fig. 7). Obviously, daily hemodialysis reversed the insensitivity to GH in these patients [47].

Patients after renal transplantation responded to GH treatment as well as children on conservative treatment [41, 48]. The height velocity was positively correlated with GFR and negatively with age and prednisolone dose.

In multivariate analysis, age is the strongest predictor of an increase in height SDS and growth velocity. This was noted in patients on conservative treatment [41, 42] and in patients on renal replacement therapy [49]. There is no doubt that the dose of GH is an important factor for the treatment response, as shown in many studies in short children with different primary diseases including idiopathic GH deficiency and Turner syndrome [50]. A correlation between the GH dose and the degree of growth response has also been noted for renal patients [37, 51, 52]. However, in most of the studies, the same GH dose of 0.045–0.050 mg/kg/day was used during the last 15 years. Therefore, the influence of the GH dose on the growth response could not be systematically analyzed. But, there are two randomized studies from Hokken-Koelega et al. [51, 52] using two different doses of GH. These studies clearly demonstrated that 2 IU rhGH/m²/day (0.022 mg/kg/day) is less effective than 4 IU rhGH/m²/day (0.045 mg/kg/day) [51]. In contrast, a doubling of the dose to 8 IU/m²/day (0.09 mg/kg/day) did not further increase growth velocity and a change in height SDS [52].

Age at the start of GH treatment and the duration of GH treatment are the strongest positive

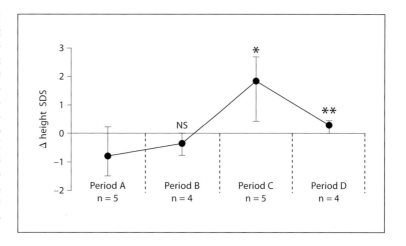

Fig. 7. Median (range) normalized height standard changes (Δ height SDS per year) between the considered periods of treatment. Period A: conventional dialysis without rhGH; period B: conventional dialysis under rhGH therapy; period C: intensified daily dialysis; period D: transplantation up to last follow-up, no GH treatment. * $p < 0.01$, period C versus period A, and period C versus period B. ** $p < 0.05$, period D versus period C, period D versus period A, and period D versus period B. With permission from Fischbach et al. [47].

predictors of the improvement of final height (see below), whereas the time spent on dialysis is a negative predictor.

In conclusion, the optimal treatment strategy out of all above considerations is to start GH treatment at an early age and at an early state of CKD prior to renal replacement therapy. A GH dose of 0.050 mg/kg/day seems to be optimal.

Final Height

In 2001, Haffner and Schaefer [53] reviewed 11 studies on GH treatment in children with CKD in which final height was reached. They concluded that the eventual height benefit of extended GH treatment appears to be on average 1.0–1.5 SD. Since then, only 2 further studies on final height in GH-treated children with CKD have been published [8, 54, 55]. The reason for this might be that most of the short children with CKD and GH treatment receive transplantation before they have reached final height. However, after renal transplantation, GH treatment is withheld for at least 1 year, because a significant number of children with a well-functioning renal graft grow normally. Therefore, in most of the centers, GH treatment is not reintroduced after successful renal transplantation in the majority of the patients. Restart of GH therapy might be initiated in the slowest growing children only, who present at the same time with a significant impairment of renal allograft function. The analysis of those patients is not representative.

Hokken-Koelega et al. [56] followed 45 children with CKD, who were prepubertal at start, for up to 8 years of GH treatment. The treatment resulted in a sustained and significant improvement in height SDS compared with baseline values. The mean height SDS reached the lower end (–1.9) of the normal growth chart after 3 years and even approached genetic target height after 6 years of therapy [56]. Hokken-Koelega et al. [56] also documented that a sufficient pubertal growth spurt occurred if GH treatment was continued during puberty. In the study of Haffner et al. [49], the increase in height SDS during puberty was not significantly better than in untreated control patients, although the growth response during prepuberty was striking. The discrepancy might be explained by the fact that GH treatment was not continued in all pubertal children because of renal transplantation. On the other hand, Haffner et al. [49] documented that puberty was not advanced, and no exaggerated loss in growth potential occurred during puberty.

In transplanted children, in whom GH treatment was started either in early or late puberty, a significant total height gain of 19 cm as a mean was observed [52]. The height gain was greater in children with a start of GH treatment in early puberty than in those with a start in late puberty.

The only study with an untreated matched cohort group for control was published by Haffner et al. [49], who followed 38 initially prepubertal children with CKD treated with GH until they reached their final height. Patients were treated with GH during only 70% of the 8-year observation period, mainly due to renal transplantation when GH treatment was stopped. Fifty children with CKD who did not receive GH because their height was above the third percentile served as controls. These children were matched for age, the degree of CKD, time spent on dialysis and time after renal transplantation. The children treated with GH showed sustained catch-up growth, whereas the control children developed progressive growth failure. The mean adult final height of GH-treated children was 1.5 SD (boys) and 1.2 SD (girls) above their standardized height at baseline. In contrast, the final height of untreated children decreased from baseline by a mean of 0.6 SD. Thus, the growth benefit was 15 cm in boys and 10.5 cm in girls.

The patients in the study of Haffner et al. [49] have not been treated with GH during 30% of the observation time because of renal transplantation which is mostly performed at pubertal age. Therefore, it is not surprising that the main increase in height SDS was observed during the prepubertal time and that the final increase in height SDS was correlated with the duration of GH treatment prior to puberty.

The greatest number of CKD patients with a final height following GH treatment comes from the KIGS registry (see above). The mean observed increase in height SDS was 0.9. Like in the study of Haffner et al. [49], the increase in height SDS was slightly better in boys than in girls. Whereas the start of GH treatment was initiated at a mean age of 8 years in the study of Haffner et al. [49], the mean age at the start of GH treatment in the KIGS cohort was 10 years. Apart from differences in patient selections, the different age at start is certainly a major factor which might explain the slightly different results.

Adverse Events

It has been expected in the past that the frequency of adverse events of GH treatment in children with CRF would be higher than in other treatment groups. This was based on the fact that patients with CKD, independently of GH treatment, present with clinical signs and symptoms which are also known as adverse events of treatment with GH. Benign intracranial hypertension is rarely observed in children on conservative treatment, on dialysis and after renal transplantation [57], also without GH treatment. Patients with CKD develop glucose intolerance and insulin resistance [58]. In transplanted children, corticosteroid treatment might further contribute [59]. Slipped epiphyses and femoral head necrosis might be observed in CKD independent of GH treatment [60, 61].

Given its remarkable efficacy, GH treatment causes surprisingly few side effects in children with CKD which has recently been summarized in the Cochrane review [39]. Despite a decreased metabolic clearance for GH, regular treatment with 0.05 mg rhGH/kg/day does not result in accumulation [62]. In the chapter by Patrick Wilton [this vol., pp. 432–441], the latest information on serious adverse events during GH treatment including patients with CKD is given. It is of note that between all patient groups treated with GH, the frequency of benign intracranial hypertension is highest in patients with CKD. However, Fine et al. [63] have pointed out the need for an untreated control group of patients with CKD. According to the investigations of Fine in children on conservative treatment and dialysis and also in children with renal allografts, no increased incidence of adverse events was noted in

GH-treated patients when compared with untreated patients. Not only was there no difference between treated and untreated patients, but also the incidence of intracranial hypertension was much less than that calculated earlier by Koller et al. [57].

This group reported on symptoms or signs of intracranial hypertension with papilledema during GH treatment in 15 cases of approximately 1,670 patients (0.9%) with renal disease. All of the 15 patients were using medications which could predispose them to intracranial hypertension; in addition, fluid retention due to chronic renal disease was noted as another predisposing factor. The median duration of GH treatment before the onset of signs and symptoms was 13 weeks. Temporal relation suggests that GH treatment was the precipitating factor. All but 2 patients were symptomatic, the symptoms generally abating when GH therapy was discontinued, but 2 patients had persistent blindness. At least 4 of these patients had a recurrence of intracranial hypertension after reinitiation of GH treatment.

Although the frequency of intracranial hypertension in renal patients is debatable, the occurrence might be a serious event in the patients. Therefore, it might be prudent to perform routine funduscopy examinations before and during initiation of GH therapy and whenever signs or symptoms of intracranial hypertension develop. In addition, one might start GH therapy with half of the maintenance dose during the first weeks. Furthermore, GH should be discontinued when intracranial hypertension is verified by papilledema and should not be resumed after relief of symptoms because of the risk of recurrence.

It is further remarkable that an irreversible diabetes mellitus has not been reported in patients with CKD including renal transplantation so far, although an increase in insulin resistance with a rise in circulating insulin levels is regularly seen [64]. Diabetes mellitus was only reported in patients with nephropathic cystinosis in whom the development of diabetes regularly occurs during adolescence, when patients are not treated with cysteamine [65, 66].

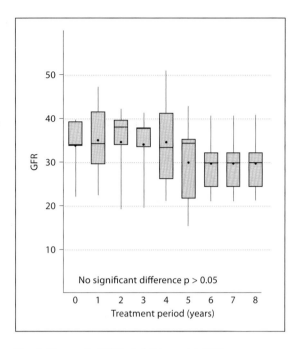

Fig. 8. Change in GFR in 5 children with CRF on conservative treatment and GH treatment for a period of 8 years. Box plots represent ranges (whiskers), 25th and 75th percentiles (shaded boxes), means (dots) and medians (horizontal lines). The mean cumulative loss of GFR was <5 ml/min/1.73 m^2.

Another concern was the deterioration in renal function following GH treatment. This concern was based on observations in mice transgenic for GH. The animals die by progressive damage of the kidney. However, in transgenic animals, GH is not only produced by the pituitary gland but also from renal cells. Furthermore, the circulating GH levels in transgenic mice were about 100 times higher than those in patients treated with rhGH.

The acute effect of GH on GFR is obliterated in CRF [67]. So far, there is no evidence that renal function is deteriorated by GH in doses used for treatment in CKD. Neither in the study of Fine et al. [68] nor in the study of Wühl et al. [65], an accelerated decline in renal function was observed for a treatment time of 5 years. The KIGS database observations up to 8 years did not give evidence for a rapid decline in renal function either (fig. 8).

GH is an immune modulatory substance [69], which might trigger rejection episodes in patients with renal allografts. Several uncontrolled studies have not disclosed an effect on rejection activity [70–72], whereas a randomized prospective study provided some evidence for an increased incidence of acute rejection episodes [73]. Whereas the number of patients with acute rejection episodes did not differ significantly, patients who had experienced more than one rejection episode prior to the start of GH treatment were at risk of developing one and more rejection episodes [73]. In a placebo-controlled randomized study, there was no evidence that GH induced rejection episodes [74]. In fact, the number of patients with rejection episodes was higher in the placebo group. However, the number of patients was limited to 37 patients followed for 1 year in a placebo-controlled fashion.

Slipped epiphyses [75] and femoral head necrosis [76] have been reported as rare events during treatment with GH. It is unlikely that these complications were caused by GH because both complications are noted in children with CRF without GH treatment [60, 61]. The number of events is too small to allow to calculate any incidence rates.

An aggravation of secondary hyperparathyroidism has also been reported [77]. A direct stimulation of parathyroid hormone by GH is not known. Therefore, the increase in parathyroid hormone serum concentration might be due to small decreases in ionized calcium as a consequence of GH-stimulated bone apposition or due to an increase in serum phosphate concentration secondary to a higher protein and phosphate intake.

References

1 Wühl E, Mehls O, Schaefer F, ESCAPE Trial Group: Antihypertensive and antiproteinuric efficacy of ramipril in children with chronic renal failure. Kidney Int 2004;66:768–776.
2 Wingen AM, Fabian-Bach C, Schaefer F, Mehls O: Randomised multicentre study of a low-protein diet on the progression of chronic renal failure in children. European Study Group of Nutritional Treatment of Chronic Renal Failure in Childhood. Lancet 1997;349:1117–1123.
3 Gorman G, Fivush B, Frankenfield D, Warady B, Watkins S, Brem A, Neu A: Short stature and growth hormone use in pediatric hemodialysis patients. Pediatr Nephrol 2005;20:1794–1800.
4 North American Pediatric Renal Transplant Cooperative Study: Annual report. Renal transplantation, dialysis, chronic renal insufficiency. 2006. http://web.emmes.com/study/ped/annlrept/annlrept2006.pdf.
5 Shroff R, Rees L, Trompeter R, Hutchinson C, Ledermann S: Long-term outcome of chronic dialysis children. Pediatr Nephrol 2006;21:257–264.
6 Schaefer F, Gilli G, Schärer K: Pubertal growth and final height in chronic renal failure; in Schärer K (ed): Growth and Endocrine Changes in Children and Adolescents with Chronic Renal Failure. Pediatr Adolesc Endocrinol. Basel, Karger, 1989, vol 22, pp 59–69.
7 Hokken-Koelega AC, Van Zaal MA, van Bergen W, de Ridder MA, Stijnen T, Wolff ED, de Jong RC, Donckerwolcke RA, De Muinck Keizer-Schrama SM, Drop SL: Final height and its predictive factors after renal transplantation in childhood. Pediatr Res 1994;36:323–328.
8 André JL, Bourquard R, Guillemin F, Krier MJ, Briancon S: Final height in children with chronic renal failure who have not received growth hormone. Pediatr Nephrol 2003;18:685–689.
9 Mehls O, Schaefer F, Tönshoff B: Growth Disorders in Chronic Renal Failure. Oxford, Oxford Pharma Genesis Ltd, 2003.
10 Arnold WC, Danford D, Holliday MA: Effects of calorie supplementation on growth in uremia. Kidney Int 1983;24:205–209.
11 Wingen AM, Mehls O: Nutrition in children with preterminal chronic renal failure. Myth or important therapeutic aid? Pediatr Nephrol 2002;17:111–120.
12 Norman LJ, Macdonald IA, Watson AR: Optimising nutrition in chronic renal insufficiency – growth. Pediatr Nephrol 2004;19:1245–1252.
13 Rees L, Shaw V: Nutrition in children with CRF and on dialysis. Pediatr Nephrol DOI: 10.1007/s00467-006-0279-z.

14 Karlberg J, Schaefer F, Hennicke M, Wingen AM, Rigden S, Mehls O: Early age-dependent growth impairment in chronic renal failure. European Study Group for Nutritional Treatment of Chronic Renal Failure in Childhood. Pediatr Nephrol 1996;10:283–287.
15 Mehls O, Ritz E, Hunziker EB, Eggli P, Heinrich U, Zapf J: Improvement of growth and food utilization by human recombinant growth hormone in uremia. Kidney Int 1988;33:45–52.
16 Samaan NA, Freeman RM: Growth hormone levels in severe renal failure. Metabolism 1970;19:102–113.
17 Haffner D, Schaefer F, Girard J, Ritz E, Mehls O: Metabolic clearance of recombinant human growth hormone in health and chronic renal failure. J Clin Invest 1994;93:1163–1171.
18 Schaefer F, Veldhuis JD, Jones J, Schärer K: Alterations in growth hormone secretion and clearance in peripubertal boys with chronic renal failure and after renal transplantation. J Clin Endocrinol Metab 1994;78:1298–1306.
19 Tönshoff B, Veldhuis JD, Heinrich U, Mehls O: Deconvolution analysis of spontaneous nocturnal growth hormone secretion in prepubertal children with chronic renal failure. Pediatr Res 1995;37:86–93.
20 Tönshoff B, Eden S, Weiser E, Carlsson B, Robinson IC, Blum WF, Mehls O: Reduced hepatic growth hormone (GH) receptor gene expression and increased plasma GH binding protein in experimental uremia. Kidney Int 1994;45:1085–1092.
21 Tönshoff B, Cronin MJ, Reichert M, Haffner D, Wingen AM, Blum WF, Mehls O: Reduced concentration of serum growth hormone (GH)-binding protein in children with chronic renal failure: correlation with GH insensitivity. J Clin Endocrinol Metab 1997;82:1007–1013.
22 Schaefer F, Chen Y, Tsao T, Nouri P, Rabkin R: Impaired JAK-STAT signal transduction contributes to growth hormone resistance in chronic uremia. J Clin Invest 2001;108:467–475.
23 Kofoed EM, Hwa V, Little B, Woods KA, Buckway CK, Tsubaki J, Pratt KL, Bezrodnik L, Jasper H, Tepper A, Heinrich JJ, Rosenfeld RG: Growth hormone insensitivity associated with a STAT5b mutation. N Engl J Med 2003;349:1139–1147.
24 Tönshoff B, Powell DR, Zhao D, Durham SK, Coleman ME, Domene HM, Blum WF, Baxter RC, Moore LC, Kaskel FJ: Decreased hepatic insulin-like growth factor (IGF)-I and increased IGF binding protein-1 and -2 gene expression in experimental uremia. Endocrinology 1997;138:938–946.
25 Blum WF: Insulin-like growth factors (IGFs) and IGF binding proteins in chronic renal failure: evidence for reduced secretion of IGFs. Acta Paediatr Scand Suppl 1991;379:24–31.
26 Ulinski T, Mohan S, Kiepe D, Blum WF, Wingen AM, Mehls O, Tönshoff B: Serum insulin-like growth factor binding protein (IGFBP)-4 and IGFBP-5 in children with chronic renal failure: relationship to growth and glomerular filtration rate. Pediatr Nephrol 2000;14:589–597.
27 Tönshoff B, Blum WF, Wingen AM, Mehls O: Serum insulin-like growth factors (IGFs) and IGF binding proteins 1, 2, and 3 in children with chronic renal failure: relationship to height and glomerular filtration rate. J Clin Endocrinol Metab 1995;80:2684–2691.
28 Tönshoff B, Blum WF, Mehls O: Serum insulin-like growth factors and their binding proteins in children with end-stage renal disease. Pediatr Nephrol 1996;10:269–274.
29 Powell DR, Liu F, Baker B, et al: Characterization of insulin-like growth factor binding protein-3 in chronic renal failure serum. Pediatr Res 1993;33:136–143.
30 Blum WF, Ranke MB, Kietzmann K, Tönshoff B, Mehls O: Growth hormone resistance and inhibition of somatomedin activity by excess of insulin-like growth factor binding protein in uraemia. Pediatr Nephrol 1991;5:539–544.
31 Mak RH, Pak Y: End-organ resistance to growth hormone and IGF-I in epiphyseal chondrocytes of rats with chronic renal failure. Kidney Int 1996;50:400–406.
32 Powell DR, Liu F, Baker BK, et al: Modulation of growth factors by growth hormone in children with chronic renal failure. The Southwest Pediatric Nephrology Study Group. Kidney Int 1997;51:1970–1979.
33 Powell DR, Durham SK, Liu F, Baker BK, Lee PD, Watkins SL, Campbell PG, Brewer ED, Hintz RL, Hogg RJ: The insulin-like growth factor axis and growth in children with chronic renal failure: a report of the Southwest Pediatric Nephrology Study Group. J Clin Endocrinol Metab 1998;83:1654–1661.
34 Tönshoff B, Mehls O, Heinrich U, Blum WF, Ranke MB, Schauer A: Growth-stimulating effects of recombinant human growth hormone in children with end-stage renal disease. J Pediatr 1990;4:561–566.
35 Tanner JM, Whitehouse RH: Clinical longitudinal standards for height, weight, height velocity, weight velocity, and stages of puberty. Arch Dis Child 1976;51:170–179.
36 Prader A, Largo RH, Molinari L, Issler C: Physical growth of Swiss children from birth to 20 years of age. First Zürich longitudinal study of growth and development. Helv Paediatr Acta Suppl 1989;52:1–125.
37 Mehls O, Berg U, Broyer M, Rizzoni G: Chronic renal failure and growth hormone treatment: review of the literature and experience in KIGS; in Ranke MB, Wilton P (eds): Growth Hormone Therapy in KIGS – 10 Years Experience, ed 1. Heidelberg, Barth, 1999, pp 327–340.
38 Fine RN, Kohaut EC, Brown D, Perlman AJ: Growth after recombinant human growth hormone treatment in children with chronic renal failure: report of a multicenter randomized double-blind placebo-controlled study. Genentech Cooperative Study Group. J Pediatr 1994;124:374–382.
39 Vimalachandra D, Hodson EM, Willis NS, Craig JC, Cowell C, Knight JF: Growth hormone for children with chronic kidney disease. Cochrane Database Syst Rev 2006;3:1–41.
40 Wühl E, Haffner D, Tönshoff B, Mehls O: Predictors of growth response to rhGH in short children before and after renal transplantation. German Study Group for Growth Hormone Treatment in Chronic Renal Failure. Kidney Int Suppl 1993;43:S76–S82.

41 Haffner D, Wühl E, Schaefer F, Nissel R, Tönshoff B, Mehls O: Factors predictive of the short- and long-term efficacy of growth hormone treatment in prepubertal children with chronic renal failure. German Study Group for Growth Hormone Treatment in Children with Chronic Renal Failure. J Am Soc Nephrol 1998;9:1899–1907.

42 Tönshoff B, Haffner D, Albers N, Offner G, Mehls O: Predictors of the response to growth hormone in short prepubertal children post-renal transplant. German Study Group for Growth Hormone Treatment in Children Post Renal Transplantation Study Group Members. Br J Clin Pract Suppl 1996;85:34–37.

43 Rees L, Maxwell H: Factors influencing the response to growth hormone in children with renal disease. Pediatr Nephrol 1996;10:337–339.

44 Mehls O, Broyer M: Growth response to recombinant human growth hormone in short prepubertal children with chronic renal failure with or without dialysis. The European/Australian Study Group. Acta Paediatr Suppl 1994;399:81.

45 Wühl E, Haffner D, Nissel R, Schaefer F, Mehls O: Short dialyzed children respond less to growth hormone than patients prior to dialysis. German Study Group for Growth Hormone Treatment in Chronic Renal Failure. Pediatr Nephrol 1996;10:294–298.

46 Perfumo F, Verrina E, Edefonti A, Trivelli A, Canepa A, Gusmano R: Is the response to rhGH in peritoneal dialysis patients less effective than in patients with chronic renal insufficiency. Br J Clin Pract Suppl 1996;85:18–20.

47 Fischbach M, Terzic J, Menouer S, Dhcu C, Soskin S, Helmstetter A, Burger MC: Intensified and daily hemodialysis in children might improve statural growth. Pediatr Nephrol 2006;21:1746–1752.

48 Van Es A: Growth hormone treatment in short children with chronic renal failure and after renal transplantation: combined data from European clinical trials. The European Study Group. Acta Paediatr Scand Suppl 1991;379:42–48.

49 Haffner D, Schaefer F, Nissel R, Wühl E, Tönshoff B, Mehls O, German Study Group for Growth Hormone Treatment in Chronic Renal Failure: Effect of growth hormone treatment on adult height of children with chronic renal failure. N Engl J Med 2000;343:923–930.

50 Ranke MB, Lindberg A: Growth hormone treatment of idiopathic short stature: analysis of the database from KIGS, the Kabi Pharmacia International Growth Study. Acta Paediatr Suppl 1994;406:18–23.

51 Hokken-Koelega AC, Stijnen T, de Muinck Keizer-Schrama SM, Wit JM, Wolff ED, de Jong MC, Donckerwolcke RA, Abbad NC, Bot A, Blum WF, et al: Placebo-controlled, double-blind, cross-over trial of growth hormone treatment in prepubertal children with chronic renal failure. Lancet 1991;338:585–590.

52 Hokken-Koelega A, Stijnen T, de Ridder MA, de Muinck Keizer-Schrama SM, Wolff ED, de Jong MC, Donckerwolcke RA, Groothoff JW, Blum WF, Drop SL, et al: Growth hormone treatment in growth-retarded adolescents after renal transplant. Lancet 1994;343:1313–1317.

53 Haffner D, Schaefer F: Does recombinant growth hormone improve adult height in children with chronic renal failure? Semin Nephrol 2001;21:490–497.

54 Fine RN, Stablein D: Long-term use of recombinant human growth hormone in pediatric allograft recipients: a report of the NAPRTCS Transplant Registry. Pediatr Nephrol 2005;20:404–408.

55 Crompton CH, Australian and New Zealand Paediatric Nephrology Association: Long-term recombinant human growth hormone use in Australian children with renal disease. Nephrology (Carlton) 2004;9:325–330.

56 Hokken-Koelega A, Mulder P, De Jong R, Lilien M, Donckerwolcke R, Groothof J: Long-term effects of growth hormone treatment on growth and puberty in patients with chronic renal insufficiency. Pediatr Nephrol 2000;14:701–706.

57 Koller EA, Stadel BV, Malozowski SN: Papilledema in 15 renally compromised patients treated with growth hormone. Pediatr Nephrol 1997;11:451–454.

58 Mak RH, Haycock GB, Chantler C: Glucose intolerance in children with chronic renal failure. Kidney Int 1983;24:S22.

59 Shishido S, Sato H, Asanuma H, Shindo M, Hataya H, Ishikura K, Hamasaki Y, Goto M, Ikeda M, Honda M: Unexpectedly high prevalence of pretransplant abnormal glucose tolerance in pediatric kidney transplant recipients. Pediatr Transplant 2006;10:67–73.

60 Mehls O, Ritz E, Krempien B, Gilli G, Link K, Willich W, Schärer K: Slipped epiphyses in renal osteodystrophy. Arch Dis Child 1975;50:545–554.

61 Mehls O, Ritz E, Oppermann HC, Guignard JP: Femoral head necrosis in uremic children without steroid treatment or transplantation. J Pediatr 1981;6:926–929.

62 Tönshoff B, Heinrich U, Mehls O: How safe is the treatment of uraemic children with recombinant human growth hormone? Pediatr Nephrol 1991;5:454–460.

63 Fine RN, Ho M, Tejani A, Blethen S: Adverse events with rhGH treatment of patients with chronic renal insufficiency and end-stage renal disease. J Pediatr 2003;142:539–545.

64 Haffner D, Nissel R, Wühl E, Schaefer F, Bettendorf M, Tönshoff B, Mehls O: Metabolic effects of long-term growth hormone treatment in prepubertal children with chronic renal failure and after kidney transplantation. Pediatr Res 1997;43:209–215.

65 Wühl E, Haffner D, Offner G, Broyer M, van't Hoff WG, Mehls O, European Study Group on Growth Hormone Treatment in Children with Nephropathic Cystinosis: Long-term treatment with growth hormone in short children with nephropathic cystinosis. J Pediatr 2001;138:880–887.

66 Wühl E, Haffner D, Gretz N, Offner G, van't Hoff WG, Broyer M, Mehls O, The European Study Group on Growth Hormone Treatment in Short Children with Nephropathic Cystinosis: Treatment with recombinant human growth hormone in short children with nephropathic cystinosis: no evidence for increased deterioration rate of renal function. Pediatr Res 1998;43:484–488.

67 Haffner D, Zacharewicz S, Mehls O, Heinrich U, Ritz E: The acute effect of growth hormone on GFR is obliterated in chronic renal failure. Clin Nephrol 1989;32:266–269.

68 Fine RN, Kohaut E, Brown D, Kuntze J, Attie KM: Long-term treatment of growth retarded children with chronic renal insufficiency, with recombinant human growth hormone. Kidney Int 1996;49:781–785.

69 Melk A, Daniel V, Mehls O, Opelz G, Tönshoff B: Longitudinal analysis of T-helper cell phenotypes in renal-transplant recipients undergoing growth hormone therapy. Transplantation 2004;78:1792–1801.

70 Fine RN, Yadin O, Nelson PA, Pyke-Grimm K, Boechat MI, Lippe BH, Sherman BM, Ettenger RB, Kamil E: Recombinant human growth hormone treatment of children following renal transplantation. Pediatr Nephrol 1991; 5:147–151.

71 van Dop C, Jabs KL, Donohue PA, Bock GH, Fivush BA, Harmon WE: Accelerated growth rates in children treated with growth hormone after renal transplantation. J Pediatr 1992;120:244–250.

72 Hokken-Koelega AC, Stijnen T, de Jong RC, Donckerwolcke RA, Groothoff JW, Wolff ED, Blum WF, de Munick Keizer-Schrama SM: A placebo-controlled, double-blind trial of growth hormone treatment in prepubertal children after renal transplant. Kidney Int Suppl 1996;53:S128–S134.

73 Guest G, Berard E, Crosnier H, Chevallier T, Rappaport R, Broyer M: Effects of growth hormone in short children after renal transplantation. Pediatr Nephrol 1998;12:437–446.

74 Fine RN, Stablein D, Cohen AH, Tejani A, Kohaut E: Recombinant human growth hormone post-renal transplantation in children: a randomized controlled study of the NAPRTCS. Kidney Int 2002;62:688–696.

75 Watkins SL: Is severe renal osteodystrophy a contraindication for recombinant human growth hormone treatment? Pediatr Nephrol 1996;10:351.

76 Boechat M, Winters W, Hogg R, Fine RN, Watkins S: Avascular necrosis of the femoral head in children with chronic renal disease. Radiology 2001; 218:411–413.

77 Picca S, Cappa M, Martinez C, Moges SI, Osborn J, Perfumo F, Ardissino G, Bonaudo R, Montini G, Rizzoni G: Parathyroid hormone levels in pubertal uremic adolescents treated with growth hormone. Pediatr Nephrol 2004;19:71–76.

Predicting Growth in Response to Growth Hormone Treatment – The KIGS Approach

Michael B. Ranke[a]   Anders Lindberg[b]

Treatment of short children with growth hormone (GH) should be guided by the following goals: (1) normal height should be reached as soon as possible; (2) adult height attained should be within the normal range; (3) the risk of therapy should be minimised, and (4) the aims of treatment should be obtained with the least possible costs. It is obvious to every clinician that even in GH deficiency (GHD), we will not reach all of these goals in every individual. We assume that this is probably due to the fact that our current modalities of treatment are too simple and too inflexible for patients of great individual variability – including age, sex, weight and target height – even within the same diagnostic category. The development and application of growth prediction models is the attempt to consider the definable variability of an individual during GH treatment. Accurate prediction models will allow for GH treatment to be tailored to individual needs from the beginning and allow for adjustments during the whole growth process in order to achieve optimal growth, safety and cost outcomes. In addition, the models will provide physicians and patients with realistic expectations of the treatment. Discrepancies between predicted and observed growth will allow for an early detection of causes and, possibly, corrective measures.

Growth prediction models are based on identifying those variables that correlate with growth. Many such variables were originally identified from small-scale prospective studies [1–4], and their significance was often first assessed by simple univariate linear regression analyses. In order to develop prediction models, data from the variables that may be of predictive value are required from large well-defined cohorts of patients in which there has been sufficient variation in the growth response over a defined period [5–11]. Computer programs are then used to identify predictive algorithms (mathematical descriptions of variables that correlate with growth) using complex multiple regression analyses [12–14]. These algorithms retrospectively describe the growth of the cohort, e.g., in centimetres (mean ± standard deviation, SD), as a function of the variables investigated. Prediction of growth in

[a] Paediatric Endocrinology Section
University Children's Hospital, University of Tübingen
Hoppe-Seyler-Strasse 1, DE–72076 Tübingen (Germany)
[b] Pfizer Endocrine Care
KIGS/KIMS/ACROSTUDY Medical Outcomes
Vetenskapsvägen 10, SE–191 90 Sollentuna (Sweden)

Table 1. Predicted height velocity during GH treatment in children with IGHD and early onset IGHD, including prepubertal years and total pubertal growth

	1st year		2nd year	3rd year	4th year	5–8th year	TPG	1st year early-onset GHD	
	with max. peak	without max. peak						with max. peak	without max. peak
Patients	592	592	572	333	179	179	303	260	260
R^2	0.6	0.5	0.4	0.4	0.3	0.3	0.7	0.5	0.5
Error SD	1.5	1.7	1.2	1.1	1.0	1.0	4.2	2.1	2.3
Predictor									
Intercept	14.6	12.4	5.7	5.6	6.0	6.0	48.3	19.3	17.8
Age	−0.3	−0.4	−0.1	−0.1	−0.1	−0.1	−3.0	−2.3	−2.3
Birth weight SDS	0.3	0.5						0.1	0.4
ln GH dose	1.6	1.5	0.6	0.7	0.9	0.9		2.3	2.1
Weekly GH dose							6.5		
ln maximum GH	−1.4							−1.0	
Height – MPH SDS	−0.4	−0.6					−1.3	−0.3	−0.4
Weight SDS	0.3	0.3	0.2	0.3	0.4	0.4		0.2	0.2
Height velocity – previous year			0.3	0.3	0.2	0.2			
Gender (boys = 1)							11.3		

Predictors and parameter estimates are shown.
Max. peak = Maximum GH level to tests; TPG = total pubertal growth; MPH = midparental height.

response to GH treatment in an individual patient is generated by prospectively entering the patient's data into the selected algorithm. Algorithms are useful for predictive purposes when the combination of predictors describes a high percentage of the variation in response (high R^2) with a low margin of error (low error SD).

Based on data from KIGS, a number of prediction models have been developed and published for a variety of groups of children treated with GH: (1) GHD: 1st to 8th prepubertal year [15], total pubertal growth [16], early onset [17]; (2) Turner syndrome (TS): 1st to 8th prepubertal year [18]; (3) small for gestational age (SGA): 1st and 2nd prepubertal year [19], and (4) idiopathic short stature (ISS): 1st prepubertal year [20; also see chap. by Ranke et al., this vol., pp. 319–325]. The components of the respective algorithms to predict height velocity are listed in tables 1 and 2. The predictors and the parameter estimates can be used to calculate the mean predicted height velocity, such as idiopathic GHD (IGHD), first prepubertal year, model without maximum GH to tests: velocity (cm/year) = 12.41 + [age (years) × −0.36] + [birth weight SD score (SDS) × 0.47] + [ln GH dose (IU/kg/week) × 1.54] + (height – midparental height SDS × −0.60) + (weight SDS × 0.28).

To date, there is a growing number of articles investigating the utility of KIGS prediction models when applied to other cohorts. Moreover, other prediction models have been published [8, 11, 21–23], giving further support to the concept which was first put forward by Sherman et al. [5]. However, the development of prediction models is an ongoing process. The aim of this article is not only to document the KIGS development but also to discuss the aspects which have been discussed critically within and outside the KIGS environment.

Table 2. Predicted height velocity during GH treatment in children with TS, SGA and ISS, including prepubertal years

	TS, year					SGA 1st year	SGA 2nd year		ISS 1st year
	1st	2nd	3rd	4th	5–8thr		with HV	without HV	
Patients	686	681	293	291	291	607	385	379	657
R^2	0.5	0.3	0.3	0.3	0.3	0.5	0.3	0.3	0.4
Error SD	1.3	1.1	1.0	1.0	1.0	1.4	1.1	1.1	1.2
Predictor									
Intercept	8.1	6.0	5.6	4.8	4.8	9.4	4.7	8.0	9.1
Age	–0.3	–0.1	–0.1	–0.1	–0.1	–0.3	–0.1	–0.2	–0.3
Injections	0.4								
ln GH dose	2.2	1.1	0.9	0.6	0.6				
Weekly GH dose									7.3
Daily GH dose						56.5	13.5	27.5	
Oxandrolone (yes = 1)	1.6	1.0	0.7	0.6	0.6				
Height – MPH SDS	–0.2								–0.3
MPH SDS						0.1		0.2	
Weight SDS	0.4	0.1	0.2	0.2	0.2	0.3		0.2	0.3
Previous HV		0.2	0.2	0.3	0.3		0.3		

Predictors and parameter estimates are shown. HV = Height velocity; MPH = midparental height.

Response and Responsiveness

The response to treatment is defined by the quantitative change measured during treatment (e.g., height) in causal relationship to the modality of treatment (e.g., dose, frequency of injection, mode of application). In principle, it can be investigated by systematically studying the dose-response relationship in a group of defined patients. For example, it has been documented that in children with GHD, there is a positive relationship between the GH dose and the observed annual height velocity [2]. Other studies have proven that in other diagnoses such as TS and SGA, higher doses of GH are required in order to induce a growth response comparable with GHD. Thus, girls with TS – as a group – are relatively less responsive to GH. This observation shows that the responsiveness which is determined by the diagnosis influences the mode of treatment (e.g., dose). At the same time, there is heterogeneity of the response to a given GH dose between individuals of the same diagnostic category. Consequently, the mode of treatment required to achieve a certain response varies between individuals. Ideally, the responsiveness should be determined by establishing a dose-response relationship in each individual which could then be taken as a measure of responsiveness. Prediction models describe the most likely mean response considering the qualitative and quantitative variability of the predictors (sex, age, height, weight, GH dose) of the diagnostic group investigated with a certain degree of error. This algorithm is then applied to an individual. The difference between the predicted response and the observed response can be expressed in terms of a 'studentised residual' [(observed – predicted)/error SD of predicted]. This is a calculation equivalent to the calculation of a SDS. If the height response observed is greater or lower than the predicted average of the reference group, it can be deduced that the individual is more or less responsive to GH. Thus, the studentised residual is an 'index of

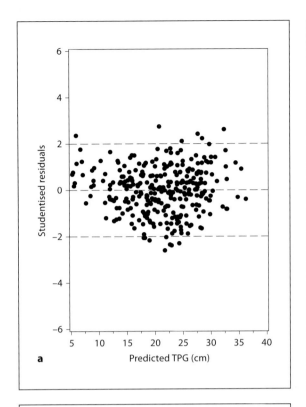
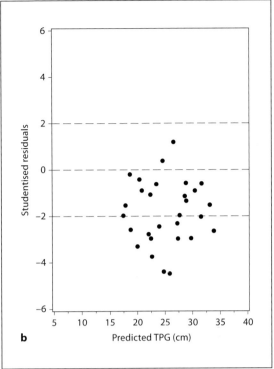
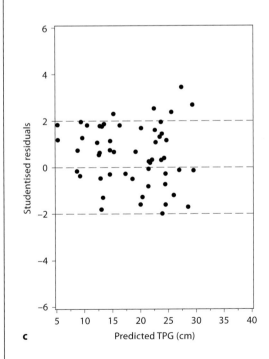

Fig. 1. a Studentised residuals versus predicted height for total pubertal growth (TPG) during GH treatment in children with IGHD used for model development [19]. **b, c** Studentised residuals versus predicted height velocity for total pubertal growth (TPG) during GH treatment in children with medulloblastoma (**b**) or craniopharyngioma (**c**) at near adult height, based on the prediction model for IGHD by Ranke et al. [19].

responsiveness'. This calculation takes into consideration the variability of the GH dose and can therefore be determined at any dose level used in the reference population. We have used the 'studentised plot' in order to illustrate the variability in the responsiveness of groups and individuals. The plots of the studentised residuals of total pubertal growth in patients from KIGS with IGHD (model group), medulloblastoma and craniopharyngioma are illustrated in figure 1. The graphs show lesser responsiveness in medulloblastoma but equal responsiveness in craniopharyngioma compared with IGHD. Treatment according to the responsiveness of an individual is the key to the optimal (also in terms of costs) and individual use of GH.

KIGS Cohorts

Patient data are voluntarily submitted to KIGS by the investigators. After a plausibility check and a possible dialogue with the investigators, they are then documented within the KIGS database [24]. Diagnoses are given according to the KIGS Aetiology Classification System [25] and can only be modified by the investigator. One of the ongoing debates relates to the issue whether or not patients documented within KIGS are representative. For example, it can be asked whether patients designated to have TS within KIGS are likely to be identical to such patients collected within studies which were conducted to prove the long-term efficacy of recombinant human GH. If one accepts that chromosomal analysis is sufficiently standardised worldwide, the question must be answered positively. However, the degree of standardisation is less developed in other areas such as GH determination for defining GHD. In addition, there are no control patients within KIGS. And, not least, it is not easy to collect information about drop-outs in order to conduct the data in an 'intention-to-treat' manner. However, when comparing the KIGS cohorts which were used for the development of prediction models (or many other analyses) with cohorts from other similar pharmacoepidemiological surveys [8, 26] and within case control studies, the level of concordance is remarkably high. Thus, even though the formal level of evidence deducible from KIGS data is not the highest possible, it is substantial since it mirrors the real life situation of treatment and not the 'artificial' setting of studies conducted in study centres, which are not without bias either [27].

Model Validation

The validation of the developed KIGS models was mainly based on analytical processes which are part of the statistical analysis [14] and on the application of cohorts from KIGS and other sources which were not part of the primary analytical process. Recently, several investigators have applied KIGS models to their own cohorts in order to support or falsify the models. As an example, Vasahlo et al. [28] have compared predicted and observed height velocity in 38 prepubertal children with IGHD over 6 years. They came to the conclusion that the KIGS models underpredicted the response (0.1–1.1 cm/year depending on the year of treatment). Such studies pose the question whether the observed differences are the consequence of the large (n ≥600) but not truly representative KIGS cohort used for model development, or the inherent biases of small groups from single centres. Next to this approach, other authors are discussing our analytical approach. De Ridder et al. [29] applied the first-year GHD KIGS model to 136 Dutch children and observed 'overfitting' of the KIGS model in the extremes. When applying their corrected (calibrated) model and the original KIGS model to 226 cases from Genesis database, they observed a significantly smaller margin or error compared with the original [30]. However, the absolute error of the modified model was so small (mean ± SD: –0.11 ± 2.05 vs. 0.28 ± 2.11 cm/year) that the practical relevance of the calibration must be questioned. Thus, the future will tell which model/modification will better serve the outlined goals of treatment in the long run.

Response Variables

It is extremely difficult to decide which of the potential response parameters of height is the most appropriate – in general and in view of the development of prediction models. For prepubertal children, height velocity in terms of centimetres/year with its characteristic decline with age appears to be a simple, straightforward parameter. On the other hand, it can be argued that the gain in height velocity over basal pretreatment height velocity gives a more accurate description of a gain in growth. However, height velocity to GH is a composite of the underlying growth rate during treatment, which differs from pretreatment height velocity and induced height velocity. In KIGS, as in most studies, pretreatment height velocity is not documented, or not documented with the same degree of accuracy. In order to control for the effect of age, some investigators propose to choose the change in height SDS as the response parameter. However, change in height SDS is a complex parameter. Its calculation depends on the calculation of the height SDS at the beginning and the end of the observational period. At both time points, the value is dependent on the patient's height measurement, the mean reference value for age and the respective SD of the mean. Mean height tends to increase with age, and the SD tends to increase with the magnitude of height. Thus, depending on age, the same change in height in terms of centimetres leads to different results in calculations of Δ height SDS. Attempts to correct for differences in the 'maturity' of short children by substituting chronological age with bone age have no true empirical foundation and are subject to major calculation error since bone age readings have a high degree of error determination. This is probably one reason why bone age has not been a better predictor than age in any of the KIGS models. Bone age development may also depend on the underlying disorder, independent of GH treatment. Automated bone age reading is desperately needed to explore its role for the interpretation of growth and the response to GH.

The analysis of a height response during pubertal age and during puberty remains an unsolved problem. This is why we have restricted analyses of pubertal growth to total pubertal growth (from the apparent beginning of puberty to the nearing of adult height).

Predictors

The KIGS prediction models are based on information collected within the worldwide survey. These are parameters which are easily accessible to each clinician, are available before treatment and can be determined with a relatively high degree of accuracy. Most important, the models contain treatment modalities (dose, frequency of injections) as variables.

The KIGS models have been criticised since they can only explain 40–60% of the variability of the response. In order to value the magnitude of these figures, one needs to consider the low margin of error of the predictions and the fact that a degree of explained variability of more than 80% cannot be reached based on statistical grounds if very large cohorts are investigated. Nevertheless, the degree of explained variability needs to be increased with the incorporation of additional predictors. We believe that parameters potentially improving the prediction may be collected. These can be classified into various categories such as anthropometrical parameters, parameters of body composition, biochemical and genetic parameters.

Anthropometrical parameters in addition to those already documented within KIGS (e.g., height, weight) can be easily collected within a clinical setting. These are for example measures like head circumference, sitting height, leg length, limb length and fat folds. These parameters can probably be measured with a similar degree of accuracy, such as height and weight.

Components of body composition such as fat mass, muscle mass and characteristics of bone structure can be measured with the help of more sophisticated and more expensive equipment such as computed tomography, peripheral quantitative computed tomography, dual-energy X-ray absorptiometry or magnetic resonance tomography. Not all of these methods have reached a level of standardisation to allow pooling of data from various sources. In addition, they are expensive and time-consuming. However, deviations of components of body composition from the normal population may be part of the disorders treated (e.g., obesity in Prader-Willi syndrome), and changes during GH treatment may be important response parameters in their own right in addition to height.

Biochemical parameters can be related to the underlying growth disorders, e.g., insulin-like growth factor 1 (IGF-1) in GHD, or can be subject to change due to the growth process induced by GH, e.g., components of collagen, the bone matrix or products of cells of the growth plate, and may thus be predictors of the growth process. However, presently, it is still difficult to explain which role such biochemical parameters in the circulation play for the growth process. For example, blood levels of IGF-1 are correlated to the extent of GHD. When trying to use both maximum GH levels to tests and basal IGF-1 levels for the development of a first-year prediction model for GHD, we observed these two parameters to be exclusive. This suggests that in this disorder, the two parameters contain, to a certain degree, the same information. Nonetheless, in both GHD and in other growth disorders, they may independently contribute to the explained variability of the response to GH. However, the degree of measurement error of a biochemical parameter determined by means of immunoassay, even under the circumstance of standardisation, is in the order of 15–20%. Thus, any attempt to incorporate biochemical parameters must be accompanied by measures for standardisation, which pose problems of logistics and costs, which cannot be taken on by the KIGS organisation. Since IGF-1 is not only considered to be a surrogate parameter for the efficacy of GH treatment in adults with GHD but is also considered an important indicator of safety and efficacy of GH treatment in children [31], it can be assumed that standardisation and collection of IGF-1 levels will progress more rapidly.

The genetic make-up of an individual may be the most important component of its ability to respond to GH in terms of height growth. Recently, this concept was proven by showing that children with the abbreviated variable of the GH receptor show a greater response to GH than those with the full-length variant [32]. Further studies correlating the response to GH with the gene structure of the GH receptor in various cohorts of patients (GHD, SGA, TS) show conflicting results [33–35]. Possibly, these divergences are the result of differences in the cohorts, the doses of GH given, methodological aspects of data analysis and the fact that the contribution of this single genetic polymorphism to the overall growth response is not very large. However, in our opinion, there is no doubt that pharmacogenomics will play an important role in the attempt to explain the responsiveness – in terms of desired affects and side effects – of an individual to therapeutic agents. The practical advantage of this approach is that we are dealing with unchangeable qualities of an individual which with time is going to be increasingly less expensive to investigate.

Short-Term Response Variables

The ability to determine a change in height depends on the height velocity and the accuracy of the height determination. If the height velocity is large and the error of measurement is small, two height measurements can be distinguished from each other after a shorter period of time has elapsed between the readings (and vice versa). Thus, the accurate determination of a response to GH may not always require a full year. During the first year of treatment and in young children, sufficient information may be gained after 6 months or even earlier. Thus, prediction models for the first months of treatment may be devel-

Table 3. Adult height after GH treatment in children with IGHD, ISS and TS

	IGHD	ISS	TS
Patients, n	319	238	413
R^2	0.6	0.6	0.7
Error SD	0.8	0.6	3.6
Predictor			
Intercept	−0.8	1.3	142.9
Age		−0.1	−0.3
Age at puberty start			0.74
Injections	0.2		
GH dose			4.8
Duration of GH	0.1		
Birth weight SDS	0.1		
MPH SDS	0.3	0.4	1.4
Height SDS at GH start	0.6	0.7	
TS height SDS at GH start			4.1
ln maximum GH	−0.3		
First studentised residuals		0.2	2.0

Predictors and parameter estimates are shown. SDS is used for the IGHD and the ISS models, and cm for the TS model.

Table 4. Total gain in height during GH treatment in children with ISS and TS

	ISS	TS
Patients, n	238	389
R^2	0.4	0.9
Error SD	0.6	3.7
Predictor		
Intercept	1.1	64.0
Age	−0.05	−4.8
Age at puberty start		1.0
GH dose		6.7
Birth weight SDS		0.3
Height − MPH SDS	−0.4	
MPH SDS		1.4
TS height SDS at GH start		−0.7
First studentised residuals	0.2	2.1

Predictors and parameter estimates are shown. MPH = Midparental height. SDS is used for the ISS model, and cm for the TS model.

oped with a sufficient degree of accuracy. However, we doubt whether clinicians are likely to change therapeutic decisions on the results of short-term growth data.

Some investigators who have developed alternative prediction models have decided to include short-term changes in growth or biochemical parameters [23, 36–38] into models predicting a full year of growth. The model published by Schönau et al. [23] was based on 58 prepubertal children with GHD. First-year height velocity (centimetres/year) was explained by bone age retardation over chronological age at GH start, pre-treatment IGF-1 serum levels, urinary levels of deoxypyridinoline (a marker of bone resorption) after 1 month on GH, and height velocity during the first 3 months on GH. This model, derived from children on a fixed dose of GH, explained 89% of the variability of the response with a standard error of 0.9 cm/year. The high degree of explained variability is partly due to the small numbers of individuals and the fact that the biochemical parameters were determined centrally within a study. More important is the fact that height velocity during GH treatment is part of both sides of the equation. Thus, much of the 12-month height velocity is already explained by the first 3 months of growth. Adding to this principal methodological flaw in terms of 'prediction' is the fact that the GH dose is not included as a predictive variable. Thus, there is doubt that such a model, though giving information about potential predictors, has clinical utility in a process aimed at optimising and individualising GH treatment in a worldwide setting.

Description of Long-Term Growth

Many children from various diagnostic groups have been followed within KIGS to their adult height. These data can be analysed to describe in numerical terms the outcomes of long-term treatment in terms of height or gain in height. The parameters and the parameter estimates required for the calculations of adult height in IGHD, ISS and TS are listed in table 3. The parameters and the parameter estimates required for the calculations of the total gain in height are listed in table 4.

Outlook

It appears obvious that the response to a drug is dependent on specific features of the treated individual (e.g., sex, age, weight). Prediction models are an attempt to calculate the most likely response to the chosen treatment based on available information. The aim is to predict as much of the variability of the response with the lowest possible error. In the future, it must be our goal to collect further predictors (e.g., anthropometrical parameters, biochemical parameters, molecular genetic information – including short-term changes in response to GH) in order to improve these models. We are convinced that such models will guide us towards a rational approach in GH treatment in order to optimise and individualise outcomes in terms of efficacy, safety and costs.

References

1 Preece MA, Tanner JM, Whitehouse RM, Cameron N: Dose dependence of growth response to human growth hormone in growth hormone deficiency. J Clin Endocrinol Metab 1976;42:477–483.
2 Frasier SD, Costin G, Lippe BM, Aceto T Jr, Bunger PF: A dose-response curve for human growth hormone. J Clin Endocrinol Metab 1981;53:1213–1217.
3 Albertsson-Wikland K: The effect of human growth hormone injection frequency on linear growth rate. Acta Paediatr Scand 1987;337:110–116.
4 Wit JM, van't Hof MA, van den Brande JL: The effect of human growth hormone therapy on skinfold thickness in growth hormone-deficient children. Eur J Pediatr 1988;147:588–592.
5 Sherman B, Frane J, Johanson AJ, Kaplan SL: Predictors of response in treatment with methionyl human growth hormone; in Underwood LE (ed): Human Growth Hormone. Progress and Challenges. New York, Marcel Dekker, 1988, pp 131–142.
6 Ranke MB, Guilbaud O: Growth response in prepubertal children with idiopathic growth hormone deficiency during the first two years of treatment with growth hormone. Analysis of the Kabi Pharmacia International Growth Study. Acta Paediatr Scand Suppl 1991;379:109–115.
7 Ranke MB, Guilbaud O, Lindberg A, Cole T: Prediction of the growth response in children with various growth disorders treated with growth hormone: analysis of data from the Kabi Pharmacia International Growth Study. Acta Paediatr Scand Suppl 1993;391:82–88.
8 Blethen SL, Compton P, Lippe BM, Rosenfeld RG, August GP, Johanson A: Factors predicting the response to growth hormone (GH) therapy in prepubertal children with GH deficiency. J Clin Endocrinol Metab 1993;76:574–579.
9 Ranke MB, Lindberg A, Guilbaud O: Prediction of growth response to treatment with growth hormone; in Ranke MB, Gunnarsson R (eds): Progress in Growth Hormone Therapy – 5 Years of KIGS. Mannheim, J&J Verlag, 1994, pp 97–111.
10 Ranke MB, Lindberg A, Chatelain P, Wilton P, Cutfield, Albertsson-Wikland K, Price DA: Development of the KIGS model for predicting growth response to growth hormone replacement therapy in children with idiopathic growth hormone deficiency from start of treatment until final height; in Ranke MB, Wilton P (eds): Growth Hormone Therapy in KIGS – 10 Years' Experience. Heidelberg, Johann Ambrosius Barth, 1997, pp 371–384.
11 Albertsson-Wikland K, Kriström B, Rosberg S, Svensson B, Nierop AFM: Validated multivariate models predicting the growth response to GH treatment in individual short children with a broad range in GH secretion capacities. Pediatr Res 2000;48:475–484.
12 Cook RD, Weisberg S: Residuals and Influence in Regression. New York, Chapman and Hall, 1982.
13 Weisberg S: Applied Linear Regression, ed 2. Chichester, Wiley and Sons, 1985.
14 Harrell FEJ, Lee KL, Mark DB: Multivariable prognostic models: issues in developing models, evaluating assumptions and adequacy, and measuring and reducing errors. Stat Med 1996;15:361–387.
15 Ranke MB, Lindberg A, Chatelain P, Wilton P, Cutfield WS, Albertsson-Wikland K, Price DA: Derivation and validation of a mathematical model for predicting the response to exogenous recombinant human growth hormone (GH) in prepubertal children with idiopathic GH deficiency. J Clin Endocrinol Metab 1999;84:1174–1183.
16 Ranke MB, Lindberg A, Cowell CT, Wikland KA, Reiter EO, Wilton P, Price DA, KIGS International Board: Prediction of response to growth hormone treatment in short children born small for gestational age: analysis of data from KIGS. J Clin Endocrinol Metab 2003;88:125–131.

17 Ranke MB, Lindberg A, Albertsson-Wikland K, Wilton P, Price DA, Reiter EO: Increased response, but lower responsiveness to growth hormone (GH) in very young children (aged 0–3 years) with idiopathic GH deficiency: analysis of data from KIGS. J Clin Endocrinol Metab 2005;90:1966–1971.

18 Ranke MB, Lindberg A, Chatelain P, Wilton P, Cutfield W, Albertsson-Wikland K, Price DA, KIGS International Board: Prediction of long-term response to recombinant human growth hormone in Turner syndrome: development and validation of mathematical models. J Clin Endocrinol Metab 2000; 85:4212–4218.

19 Ranke MB, Lindberg A, Martin DD, Bakker B, Wilton P, Albertsson-Wikland K, Cowell CT, Price DA, Reiter EO: The mathematical model for total pubertal growth in idiopathic growth hormone deficiency suggests a moderate role of GH dose. J Clin Endocrinol Metab 2003;88:4748–4753.

20 Ranke MB, Guilbaud O: Growth hormone levels in response to stimulation tests and responsiveness to growth hormone in children with growth hormone deficiency and idiopathic short stature. Kabi Pharmacia International Growth Study, Report 8, Biannual Report 1992;1:34–41.

21 Spagnioli A, Spadoni GL, Boscherini B: Prediction of the outcome of growth hormone therapy in children with idiopathic short stature. A multivariate discriminant analysis. J Pediatr 1995; 126:905–909.

22 Südfeld H, Kiese K, Heinecke A, Brämswig JH: Prediction of growth response in prepubertal children treated with growth hormone for idiopathic growth hormone deficiency. Acta Paediatr 2000;89:34–37.

23 Schönau E, Westermann F, Rauch F, Stabrey A, Wassmer G, Keller E, Brämswig J, Blum WF: A new and accurate prediction model for growth response to growth hormone treatment in children with growth hormone deficiency. Eur J Endocrinol 2001;144:13–20.

24 Wallström A, Trulsson L: The Kabi International Growth Study: rationale, organisation and development; in Ranke MB, Gunnarsson R (eds): Progress in Growth Hormone Therapy – 5 Years of KIGS. Mannheim, J&J Verlag, 1994, pp 1–9.

25 Ranke MB: The Kabi Pharmacia International Growth Study: aetiology classification list with comments. Acta Paediatr Scand 1991;379:87–92.

26 Blethen SA, Baptista J, Kuntze J, Foley T, LaFranchi S, Johanson A, on behalf of the Genentech Study Group: Adult height in growth hormone (GH)-deficient children treated with biosynthetic GH. J Clin Endocrinol Metab 1997;82: 418–420.

27 Dowie J: What decision analysis can offer the clinical decision maker. Horm Res 1999;51(suppl):73–82.

28 Vasahlo J, Zidek T, Lebl J, Riedl S, Frisch H: Validation of a mathematical model predicting the response to growth hormone treatment in prepubertal children with idiopathic growth hormone deficiency. Horm Res 2004; 61:143–147.

29 De Ridder MAJ, Stijnen T, Hokken-Koelega AC: Validation and calibration of the Kabi Pharmacia International Growth Study prediction model for children with idiopathic growth hormone deficiency. J Clin Endocrinol Metab 2003;88:1223–1227.

30 De Ridder MAJ, Stijnen T, Drop SLS, Blum WF, Hokken-Koelega ACS: Validation of a calibrated prediction model for response to growth hormone treatment in an independent cohort. Horm Res 2006;66:13–16.

31 Lee KW, Cohen P: Individualized growth hormone therapy in children: advances beyond weight-based dosing. J Pediatr Endocrinol Metab 2003;16: 625–630.

32 Dos Santos C, Essioux L, Teinturier C, Tauber M, Goffin V, Bougneres P: A common polymorphism of the growth hormone receptor is associated with increased responsiveness to growth hormone. Nat Genet 2004;36:720–724.

33 Binder G, Baur R, Schweizer R, Ranke MB: The d3-growth hormone (GH) receptor polymorphism is associated with increased responsiveness to GH in Turner syndrome and short small-for-gestational-age children. J Clin Endocrinol Metab 2006;91:659–664.

34 Pilotta A, Mella P, Filisetti M, Felappi B, Prandi E, Parrinello G, Notarangelo LD, Buzi F: Common polymorphisms of the growth hormone (GH) receptor do not correlate with the growth response to exogenous recombinant human GH in GH-deficient children. J Clin Endocrinol Metab 2006;91:1178–1180.

35 Jorge AA, Marchisotti FG, Montenegro LR, Carvalho LR, Mendonca BB, Arnhold JJ: Growth hormone (GH) pharmacogenomics: influence of GH receptor exon 3 retention or deletion on first year growth response and final height in patients with severe GH deficiency. J Clin Endocrinol Metab 2006;91:1076–1080.

36 Kriström B, Jansson C, Rosberg S, Albertsson-Wikland K: Growth response to growth hormone (GH) treatment relates to insulin-like growth factor I (IGF-I) and IGF-binding protein-3 in short children with various GH secretion capacities: Swedish Study Group for Growth Hormone Treatment. J Clin Endocrinol Metab 1997;82:2889–2898.

37 Rauch F, Georg M, Stabrey A, Neu C, Blum WF, Remer T, Manz, Schönau E: Collagen markers deoxypyridinoline and hydroxylysine glucoside: pediatric reference data and use for growth prediction in growth hormone-deficient children. Clin Chem 2002;48:315–322.

38 Tobiume H, Kanzaki S, Hida S, Ono T, Moriwake, T, Yameuchi S, Tanka H, Seino Y: Serum bone alkaline phosphatase isoenzyme levels in normal children with growth hormone (GH) deficiency: a potential marker for bone formation and response to GH therapy. J Clin Endocrinol Metab 1997;82:2056–2061.

Adverse Events Reported in KIGS

Patrick Wilton

After more than 20 years of use in children with growth hormone deficiency (GHD), recombinant GH can be considered to have an excellent safety profile with few adverse drug reactions (ADRs) or, to use an older term, side effects [1, 2]. However, as the use of GH has been expanded to include other indications such as syndromes associated with short stature (e.g., Turner syndrome and Prader-Willi syndrome) and other patient groups such as adults with disorders associated with GHD, it is still important to monitor the safety of GH treatment. One of the main aims of KIGS is to study the safety of recombinant GH (Genotropin®, Pfizer Inc.) in children and adolescents. It is mandatory to report all adverse events (AEs) occurring in children enrolled in KIGS, regardless of whether or not the AE is suspected to be related to GH treatment. The definition of an AE in KIGS is broad and includes all unfavorable changes in signs, symptoms or laboratory tests occurring during treatment. With all AEs reported, an assessment of whether a particular AE is merely coincidental or is an ADR can be made. This article reports safety data from KIGS included in the database in January 2006.

Methods

Data from patients enrolled in KIGS are collected by means of a specifically designed case report form (CRF). One of the sections on the CRF requires investigators to describe any AEs that have occurred since the last visit of the patient. The description should include details of the duration and outcome of the AE. The information on the CRF is stored in the database as free text, and AEs are coded according to a list of 'preferred terms' for ADRs developed by the World Health Organization (WHO) Collaborating Centre for International Drug Monitoring [3]. In KIGS, the preferred terms are automatically grouped into 1 of 30 different organ system classes by means of specialized software. Implementing this system in KIGS sometimes poses problems because many of the AEs reported are concomitant diseases that cannot be coded according to the WHO system. In such cases, AEs are coded according to the criteria of the International Statistical Classification of Diseases, Injuries and Causes of Death [4] and are added manually to the appropriate organ system class in the WHO International Drug Monitoring List. The information is stored in the main database of KIGS and is available for further statistical evaluation. The diagnosis as given by the individual investigator is used in the analysis of AEs.

Pfizer Inc., 235 East 42nd Street, New York, NY 10017-15755 (USA)

Table 1. AEs reported in KIGS categorized according to the major diagnostic subgroups of patients

	Patients	AEs	Treatment years	AEs/100,000 treatment years
IGHD	28,620	6,661	84,329	79
Congenital GHD	2,448	1,227	8,758	140
Craniopharyngioma	1,145	814	4,044	201
Cranial tumors	2,163	1,016	6,819	149
Other tumors	168	41	527	78
Leukemia	625	247	1,929	128
Other causes of GHD	598	316	2,042	155
Idiopathic short stature	4,929	1,008	12,940	78
Turner syndrome	5,970	2,445	20,714	118
Prader-Willi syndrome	1,242	466	2,538	184
SGA/IUGR	2,536	435	4,722	92
Chronic renal failure	1,687	668	3,855	173
Other causes of short stature	3,451	1,551	10,475	148
Total	56,123	16,971	164,558	103

SGA = Small for gestational age; IUGR = intrauterine growth retardation.

Results

As of January 2006, 56,123 patients were included in the reported data set, representing 164,558 GH treatment years in KIGS. At this time, a total of 16,971 AEs have been reported. The number of patients and the total number of GH treatment years for the major diagnostic subgroups of patients in KIGS are listed in table 1. The numbers of AEs reported in KIGS, categorized by the organ system, are shown in table 2. The 10 most frequently reported AEs are listed in table 3. Clearly, the majority of AEs are coincidental illnesses. The incidence of AEs in patients with GHD of different etiologies is shown in table 4 and for other etiologies in table 5.

Idiopathic GHD
The incidence of ADRs of GH, edema, intracranial hypertension, arthralgia and myalgia was quite low in patients with idiopathic GHD (IGHD) compared with most other subgroups in KIGS. This was also true for AEs such as slipped capital femoral epiphysis (SCFE), diabetes mellitus and scoliosis. Eleven cases of benign intracranial hypertension corresponding to an incidence of 13/100,000 treatment years on GH were reported after 2 weeks to 8 years on a GH dose of 0.08–0.33 mg/kg/week. Thirteen cases of potential malignant de novo neoplasms were reported, 2 of them after GH therapy had been discontinued. Six patients had cranial tumors (2 germinomas and 4 other types), reported after 0.2–3.1 years on GH at a dose of 0.22–0.46 mg/kg/week. There were 2 cases of lymphoma reported after 0.3 and 3.8 years on a GH dose of 0.12 and 0.16 mg/kg/week, respectively, and 2 cases of acute myeloid leukemia (AML) after 0.5–1.5 years on a GH dose of 0.18 and 0.19 mg/kg/week, respectively. The latter patients were diagnosed as having Fanconi pancytopenia, a known risk factor associated with AML.

Congenital GHD
In the group of almost 2,500 congenital GHD patients, the incidence of idiopathic intracranial

Table 2. AEs reported in KIGS categorized by organ system according to the WHO International Drug Monitoring List

	AEs	Patients with AEs
Resistance mechanism disorders (e.g., infections)	2,514	2,082
Respiratory system disorders	2,442	1,713
Central and peripheral nervous system disorders	1,644	1,378
Gastrointestinal disorders	1,273	1,120
Musculoskeletal system disorders	1,448	1,347
Body as a whole/general disorders	1,169	1,075
Skin and appendage disorders	919	756
Urinary disorders	730	580
Metabolic and nutritional disorders	699	583
Endocrine disorders	513	465
Psychiatric disorders	436	399
Neoplasm	426	382
White cell and reticuloendothelial disorders	240	187
Application site disorder (injection reactions)	195	186
Liver and biliary disorders	183	159
Hearing and vestibular disorders	174	156
Vision disorders	199	189
Reproductive disorders	235	198
Red blood cell disorders	127	96
Cardiovascular disorders	160	145
Platelet, bleeding and clotting disorders	113	104
Vascular (extracardiac) disorders	102	97
Myo- and endopericardial disorders	31	31
Heart rate and rhythm disorders	42	38
Collagen disorders	26	19
Special sense disorders	3	3
Autonomic nervous system disorders	3	3

hypertension was 4 times higher than in IGHD patients. The incidence of seizures was also high (411/100,000), compared with 97/100,000 in patients with IGHD. There was only 1 neoplasm reported, a Hodgkin's disease in a 10-year-old boy after 3.2 years of GH treatment at a dose of 0.17 mg/kg/week.

Craniopharyngioma

There was a higher incidence of most AEs in patients treated for craniopharyngioma. Thirteen percent of the 1,145 patients reported a recurrence of craniopharyngioma after a median of 1.9 years on GH. The median time on GH was 4.1 years. There was no difference in the GH dose administered (0.17 mg/kg/week) between pa-

Table 3. The 10 most commonly reported AEs in KIGS

Upper respiratory tract infection	1,391
Headache	793
Otitis media	611
Pharyngitis	439
Viral infection	389
Influenza-like symptoms	344
Fracture	326
Convulsions/epilepsy	311
Fever	303
Gastroenteritis	293

Table 4. AEs in five subgroups of patients with GHD in KIGS

	IGHD		Craniopharyngioma		Cranial tumors		Leukemia		Congenital GHD	
	patients with AEs	AEs/100,000 treatment years	patients with AEs	AEs/100,000 treatment years	patients	AEs/100,000 treatment years	patients	AEs/100,000 treatment years	patients	AEs/100,000 treatment years
Arthralgia	66	78	6	148	5	73	1	52	8	91
Convulsions	82	97	15	371	41	601	2	104	36	411
Diabetes mellitus	14	17	6	148	5	73	2	104	1	11
IIH	11	13	2	49	3	44	2	104	5	58
Myalgia	15	18	2	49	2	29	0	–	1	11
SCFE	16	19	5	124	5	73	2	104	5	58
Scoliosis	82	97	5	124	10	147	4	207	11	126

Table 5. AEs in five subgroups of patients with other etiologies in KIGS

	Turner syndrome		SGA/IUGR		Idiopathic short stature		Chronic renal insufficiency		Prader-Willi syndrome		Other short stature	
	patients with AEs	AEs/100,000 treatment years	patients with AEs	AEs/100,000 treatment years	patients	AEs/100,000 treatment years	patients	AEs/100,000 treatment years	patients	AEs/100,000 treatment years	patients	AEs/100,000 treatment years
Arthralgia	21	101	3	64	16	118	2	52	2	79	18	172
Convulsions	17	82	8	169	17	125	7	182	8	315	18	172
Diabetes mellitus	8	39	0	–	2	14	1	26	8	315	4	38
IIH	12	58	1	21	0	–	5	130	2	79	3	29
Myalgia	4	19	0	–	1	7	0	–	1	40	5	48
SCFE	17	82	1	21	2	15	2	52	0	–	4	38
Scoliosis	48	232	7	148	9	70	6	157	66	2,600	31	296

SGA = Small for gestational age; IUGR = intrauterine growth retardation.

tients with or without recurrence. One patient was diagnosed with adrenal neuroblastoma after only 3 months on GH at a dose of 0.23 mg/kg/week. One unspecified brain tumor was reported after 3.1 years on GH at a dose of 0.18 mg/kg/week; however, there was no follow-up in this patient, and thus, the etiology of the 'brain tumor' could well be a recurrence of the craniopharyngioma.

Langerhans Cell Histiocytosis
Ten of the 175 patients diagnosed with Langerhans cell histiocytosis reported a detorioration in the disease. In addition, 4 patients were diagnosed with a neoplasm, including 2 cases with germinoma 0.6 and 0.7 years after GH start, 1 case with a primitive neuroectodermal tumor 1 year after GH start and 1 case with a parotis tumor after 3.5 years on GH. The GH dose administered in these cases was 0.19–0.21 mg/kg/week.

GHD after Treatment of Cranial Tumors
The group of patients treated for different types of cranial tumors had the highest incidence of seizures, but other AEs were not particular frequent. The largest subgroup included patients treated for medulloblastoma (n = 751) with a me-

Table 6. Recurrences in patients with different types of cranial tumors in KIGS

	Patients	Duration of GH treatment years	Treatment years	Patients with recurrence	Frequency of recurrence, %	Duration of GH treatment at recurrence, years
Craniopharyngioma	1,145	4.1 (0.7–9.6)	5,066	145	12.7	1.9 (0.4–6.1)
Astrocytoma/glioma	436	3.1 (0.8–8.0)	1,764	45	10.3	2.1 (0.4–5.4)
Ependymoma	128	2.8 (1.0–8.9)	523	8	6.3	0.8 (0.1–2.5)
Germinoma	336	2.4 (0.7–6.6)	1,136	14	4.2	0.8 (0.2–5.0)
Medulloblastoma	751	3.6 (0.8–8.0)	2,927	33	4.4	1.6 (0.3–3.7)
Other cranial tumors	490	3.6 (0.8–7.5)	2,141	26	5.3	1.5 (0.6–3.9)

Values are given as medians, with ranges in parentheses.

dian follow-up time in KIGS of 3.6 years; recurrence of medulloblastoma was reported in less than 5% after a median of 1.6 years on GH, with no difference in GH dose between those with or without recurrence, i.e. 0.20 and 0.21 mg/kg/week, respectively. The highest recurrence rate, 0.3%, was found in 436 patients treated for astrocytoma/glioma. Details regarding the recurrence of various cranial tumors are presented in table 6.

GHD after Treatment of Leukemia
In the group of 625 patients treated for leukemia and followed on GH in KIGS for a median of 3.1 years, 8 patients were diagnosed with a relapse between 3 and 13 years after the initial diagnosis and after 1 month to 5.2 years on GH at a dose of 0.16–0.34 mg/kg/week. One of the patients had discontinued GH treatment 0.4 years prior to the relapse. Six of the patients were bone marrow transplanted.

Second Neoplasms
In total, 38 patients with a potential malignant second neoplasm were reported during or up to 4.4 years after GH had been discontinued. Seven meningiomas and 11 other cranial tumors, 3 AML, 3 osteosarcomas, 2 lymphomas, 2 squamous cell carcinomas and 2 thyroid cancers were the most common neoplasms reported. The frequency of a second neoplasm was 9/751 (1.2%) in patients treated for medulloblastoma and 9/625 (1.4%) in patients treated for leukemia.

Turner Syndrome
Edema, but not arthralgia or myalgia, was more frequently reported in Turner syndrome compared with most other groups in KIGS. SCFE and scoliosis were also reported, with a higher incidence. There were 2 cases of benign tumors and 3 malignant tumors (lung carcinoma, thyroid papillary cancer, pilocytic astrocytoma) after 0.5–6.2 years on GH at a dose of 0.22–0.33 mg/kg/week. In addition, 1 case of malignant melanoma was reported after GH treatment had been discontinued.

Small for Gestational Age
There were very few reports of any ADRs (edema, intracranial hypertension or myalgia) associated with GH treatment in this group of about 2,500 patients. The incidence of seizures (169/100,000) and scoliosis (148/100,000) was higher than in IGHD patients. One neoplasm (AML) was reported after 4.7 years on GH treatment at a dose of 0.24 mg/kg/week.

Chronic Renal Failure

This group of 1,700 patients had a higher incidence of AEs than most other groups in KIGS. However, there was no report of myalgia and only 2 reports of arthralgia. The incidence of intracranial hypertension was the highest of any subgroup in KIGS, i.e. 130/100,000, and also scoliosis and seizures were among the highest. In 508 patients with a renal transplant, 3 developed adenocarcinoma in the graft. In addition, 1 transplanted patient developed a non-Hodgkin lymphoma after 0.4 years on GH at a dose of 0.30 mg/kg/week. This is one of the most common neoplasms in renal transplanted patients who are not on GH treatment, most likely because of the immunosuppressive therapy.

Prader-Willi Syndrome

In the group of 1,242 patients with Prader-Willi syndrome, the incidence of scoliosis was 27 times higher and that of diabetes mellitus 19 times higher than in IGHD patients. Both conditions are well-known comorbidities in this syndrome. There were only 8 reports of sleep apnea. Five patients died at the age between 2.1 and 15.8 years during GH treatment after 2–97 months on GH at a dose of 0.21 mg/kg/week. The cause of death was reported as respiratory insufficiency, pneumonia or dehydration, and 1 patient died in bed and another in the bath tub. A sixth patient died 12 months after GH had been discontinued when the patient developed diabetes. No neoplasm was reported.

Idiopathic Short Stature

This group of almost 5,000 patients had the lowest incidence of most AEs. Two pubertal patients developed teratocarcinoma of the testis after 3.3 and 3.9 years on GH at a dose of 0.19 mg/kg/week. None of them had cryptorchidism in their medical history, but 1 had a low birth weight which is another risk factor for testis neoplasm.

Discussion

KIGS is a large pharmacoepidemiological survey of children treated with GH which includes more than 56,000 patients receiving recombinant GH, corresponding to more than 164,000 treatment years. The definition of an AE in KIGS includes all concomitant diseases occurring during GH treatment, such as gastroenteritis and upper respiratory tract infections. Therefore, the finding of 0.1 AEs per patient per year shows that far from all AEs are reported. Although all AEs should be reported, it is understandable that illnesses that occur often in children are not always considered as AEs by investigators. However, events in which the influence of GH has been a subject of discussion (e.g., diabetes mellitus, SCFE and the recurrence of a neoplasm) are more likely to be reported. Safety data derived from clinical trials are often limited by the relatively small numbers of subjects. Therefore, KIGS provides a valuable resource for safety analysis, in which the incidence of AEs in a large group of patients with varied medical conditions can be compared with the incidence of these events in the general childhood population. If the incidence of a particular AE during GH treatment is significantly higher compared with published epidemiological data, then it is possible that GH is involved in the pathophysiology.

Leukemia

Since the first case of leukemia was reported in a child with GHD who was receiving GH replacement therapy [5], there have been many debates on whether GH increases the risk of leukemia [6]. Preclinical studies have proved contradictory results [for a review, see ref. 7]. The incidence of leukemia in untreated children with GHD is not known. There have been reports of a number of cases of leukemia in children with GHD who have never been treated with GH, supporting the hypothesis that there is an increased risk of leukemia associated with GHD regardless of GH treatment [8, 9]. The incidence of leukemia in normal children up to the age of 15 years is approximately 1 in 30,000, which is similar to the incidence in KIGS, supporting the hypothesis that there is no increased incidence of leukemia in children treated with GH. This is in accordance with a survey by Nishi et al. [10] of all GH-treated children in Japan. The incidence of 8 recurrences of leukemia in 625 (1.3%) children treated with GH (corresponding to 1,929 treatment years in KIGS) is less than the 7–8% recurrence rates reported in non-GH-treated leukemia cohorts [11, 12] and is most probably explained by a shorter follow-up time in KIGS. Eight of the 625 children with leukemia developed a secondary tumor. This equates to an incidence lower than the 2–3% reported in patients not treated with GH [13, 14]. Recently, Sklar et al. [15] showed that 3.3% (4/122) of GH-treated survivors of leukemia developed a secondary neoplasm, a higher percentage than expected, compared with 4,545 survivors not treated with GH. However, in a recent follow-up by this group, the risk was not significantly increased [16].

Craniopharyngioma

In the current analysis of KIGS data, 12.7% of patients experienced regrowth of a craniopharyngioma. The low frequency of relapse suggests that GH treatment does not increase the risk of regrowth of this type of tumor [11, 17, 18]. However, relapses have been reported to occur up to 20 years after treatment of craniopharyngioma [19]; thus, the median posttreatment follow-up of 4.1 years may be too short for an accurate assessment of relapse.

Malignant Cranial Tumors

Tumor histology and treatment influence the relapse rate of malignant cranial tumors. Unfortunately, the malignancy grade of brain tumors is seldom reported in KIGS. The relapse rate for medulloblastoma has been reported to be between 57 and 79% in a series of 122–287 children with a follow-up ranging from 5 to 15 years [20–23]. The majority of relapses occur within a few years of tumor treatment. However, few patients begin GH treatment during this period, and thus, the relapse rate in KIGS (4.7%) should be compared with that reported in the study by Ogilvy-Stuart et al. [11], in which 43 children without relapse were followed for 2 years after diagnosis of medulloblastoma. Of these patients, 15 (35%) experienced a relapse. In the same study, 26 children without a relapse 2 years after diagnosis were treated with GH and only 2 (8%) experienced a regrowth. In a later and more extensive survey, Swerdlow et al. [24] reported that 14% of 94 GH-treated patients experienced a recurrence compared with 53% of those not treated with GH. The fate of children with astrocytoma or glioma depends greatly on the histology of the tumor. The most malignant have a poor prognosis. Ilgren and Stiller [25] reported a 5-year survival rate of only 29% and a relapse rate of 31% in 112 children with astrocytoma observed for a mean of 1.9 years. The relapse rate in KIGS patients with astrocytoma or glioma (10.3%) with a median follow-up time since the initial diagnosis of 7 years compares favorably with the relapse rates for both astrocytoma of low (juvenile type) and high (adult type) malignancy (19 and 25%, respectively) reported by Ogilvy-Stuart et al. [11].

Diabetes Mellitus

It has been suggested that GH treatment could cause disturbances in carbohydrate metabolism. The high incidence of diabetes mellitus in patients with acromegaly and the knowledge that GH decreases insulin sensitivity, most probably via postreceptor mechanisms [26], support this view. A number of cases of type 2 diabetes mellitus developing during GH treatment have been reported [27–30]. In a review from Japan of all patients with GHD treated for at least 6 months between 1975 and 1982, 0.15% (3 of 1,959) of patients developed glucose intolerance [31]. The type of diabetes is not always reported in KIGS.

Some cases may be traditional type 1 or type 2 diabetes, but others could be mature-onset diabetes of the young or simply transient hyperglycemia, because a number of cases normalized when GH treatment was interrupted. It is known that the incidence of type 2 diabetes mellitus in the general childhood population has increased during the past 10–15 years. In Tokyo, between 1974 and 1990, the yearly incidence increased from 3.5 to around 8/100,000 in children under the age of 15 years [32]. The increase in the incidence of type 2 diabetes mellitus has been shown to be even higher in the Midwestern region of the USA, where it was reported to have reached 7.2/100,000 in 1996 [33].

Idiopathic Intracranial Hypertension
Treatment with tetracycline, vitamin A, insulin-like growth factor 1 and other drugs has been associated with an increased incidence of idiopathic intracranial hypertension (IIH, also known as pseudotumor cerebri), but otherwise, this condition is rare in childhood. The first cases occurring during GH treatment were reported by Otten et al. [34], and reports of IIH in children treated with GH for chronic renal failure, GHD, Turner syndrome and Prader-Willi syndrome have been published [35]. In KIGS, the highest incidence of IIH was found in patients with chronic renal failure in concordance with a survey of GH-treated children from the USA [36]. The percentage of KIGS patients who developed IIH during the first year of GH treatment is similar to that seen in a smaller survey of 3,332 GH-treated patients from Australia and New Zealand [37]. These results suggest that GH treatment increases the risk of IIH.

Slipped Capital Femoral Epiphysis
The incidence of SCFE in the general population aged between 7 and 17 years has been reported to be 10–13/100,000 [38, 39]. Suggested risk factors include rapid growth, obesity and hypothyroidism [40–42]. A number of cases have been reported in children with GHD before, during and after GH treatment [43–47]. The estimated yearly incidence of SCFE in KIGS patients with IGHD and idiopathic short stature has been estimated to be 19 and 15/100,000 treatment years of GH, respectively (tables 5, 6), rates similar to those in the general population. In a report from the USA, the incidence of SCFE during GH treatment in patients with IGHD was 7 times higher than that in KIGS, but a similar incidence was reported for children with organic GHD, and, in the US report, a lower incidence was seen in patients with idiopathic short stature [48]. The reason for these discrepancies is not obvious, but they are unlikely to be caused by different reporting strategies for different etiologies. Overall, the KIGS data suggest that SCFE is not an ADR to GH treatment. However, some patients treated with GH may have an increased risk of experiencing SCFE, for example, postleukemia and postcraniopharyngioma patients and those with Turner syndrome.

Seizures
The incidence of nonprovoked seizures in children has been reported to be 72–134/100,000 in different community-based studies [49–53]. The incidence of convulsions in KIGS varies considerably among the different patient subgroups. Patients with IGHD, Turner syndrome or idiopathic short stature did not show an increased incidence compared with the general population. However, a higher incidence than in the general population was found in patients in KIGS treated for cranial tumors. It is possible that surgery or irradiation in patients with tumors or leukemia can lead to a lower threshold for seizures, and, indeed, epilepsy has been reported in 7% of children treated for medulloblastoma who have survived for at least 2 years [54, 55].

Conclusions

KIGS is a pharmacoepidemiological survey of more than 56,000 children and adolescents treated with GH. The data in KIGS support the view that GH treatment does not increase the risk of recurrence of craniopharyngioma, malignant cranial tumors or leukemia, and neither that GH treatment increases the risk of de novo malignant neoplasms. The incidence of AEs among different diagnostic subgroups is of importance for the risk-benefit evaluation of GH treatment. The higher incidence of AEs among patients with organic GHD compared with IGHD is probably unrelated to GH treatment and merely reflects the higher morbidity in patients treated for craniopharyngioma or malignant neoplasms. The recent analysis of KIGS data has revealed no new ADR since the 10-year follow-up. In conclusion, treatment with GH seems to be a low-risk intervention in children and adolescents with various growth disorders.

References

1 Hintz LR: Untoward events in patients treated with growth hormone in the USA. Horm Res 1992;38:44–49.
2 Job JC, Maillard F, Goujard J: Epidemiologic survey of patients treated with growth hormone in France in the period 1959–1990: preliminary results. Horm Res 1992;38:35–43.
3 World Health Organization Collaborating Centre for International Drug Monitoring: International Monitoring of Adverse Reactions to Drugs: Adverse Reaction Terminology. Uppsala, World Health Organization, 1992.
4 World Health Organization: Manual of the International Statistical Classification of Diseases, Injuries and Causes of Death, ed 9. Geneva, World Health Organization, 1978.
5 Endo K, Kaneko Y, Shikano T, Minami H, Chino J: Possible association of human growth hormone treatment with an occurrence of acute myeloblastic leukaemia with an incision of chromosome in a child of pituitary dwarfism. Med Pediatr Oncol 1988;16:45–47.
6 Stahnke N: Leukaemia in growth hormone-treated patients: an update, 1992. Horm Res 1992;38:56–62.
7 Underwood L: The risks of growth hormone therapy: does growth hormone influence tumour formation or tumour growth?; in Frish H, Thomer M (eds): Hormonal Regulation of Growth (Serono Symposium). New York, Raven, 1998, p 58.
8 Rappaport R, Oberfield SE, Robison L, Salisbury S, David R, Rao J, Redmond GP: Relationship of growth hormone deficiency and leukaemia. J Pediatr 1995;126:759–761.
9 Watanabe S, Mizuno S, Tsunematsu Y, Komiyamu A, Fuji K, Kubota M: Leukaemia in GH-deficient children. Clin Pediatr Endocrinol 1994;3(suppl 5):53–60.
10 Nishi Y, Tanaka T, Takano K, Fujieda K, Igarashi Y, Hanew K, Hirano T, Yokoya S, Tachibana K, Saito T, Watanabe S: Recent status in the occurrence of leukaemia in growth hormone-treated patients in Japan. GH Treatment Study Committee of the Foundation for Growth Science, Japan. J Clin Endocrinol Metab 1999;84:1961–1965.
11 Ogilvy-Stuart AL, Ryder WDJ, Gattamaneni HR, Clayton PE, Shalet SM: Growth hormone and tumour recurrence. BMJ 1992;304:601–605.
12 Rivera G, Pui CH, Hancock M, Mahmoud H, Santana V, Sandbend J, Hurwitz C, Ribeiro R, Furman W, Crist W: Update of St Jude study XI for childhood acute lymphoblastic leukemia. Leukemia 1992;6(suppl 2):167–170.
13 Neglia JP, Meadows AT, Robison LL, Kim TH, Newton WA, Ruymann FB, Sather HN, Hammond GD: Second neoplasms after acute lymphoblastic leukemia in childhood. N Engl J Med 1991;325:1330–1336.
14 Nygaard R, Garwicz S, Haldorsen T, Hertz H, Johmundsson GK, Lanning M, Moe PJ: Second malignant neoplasms in patients treated for childhood leukemia. Acta Paediatr Scand 1991;80:1220–1228.
15 Sklar CA, Mertens AC, Mitby P, Occhiogrosso G, Qin J, Heller G, Yasui Y, Robinson LL: Risk of disease recurrence and second neoplasms in survivors of childhood cancer treated with growth hormone: a report from the childhood cancer survivor study. J Clin Endocrinol Metab 2002;87:3136–3141.
16 Ergun-Longmire B, Mertens A, Mitby P, Qin J, Heller G, Shi W, Yasui Y, Robinson L, Sklar C: Growth hormone treatment and risk of second neoplasms in the childhood cancer survivor. J Clin Endocrinol Metab 2006;91:3494–3498.
17 Arslanian S, Becker D, Lee P, Drash L, Foley T: Growth hormone and tumour recurrence: findings in children with brain neoplasms and hypopituitarism. Am J Dis Child 1995;139:347–350.
18 Darendeliler F, Karagiannis G, Wilton P, Ranke MB, Albertsson-Wikland K, Price DA, on behalf of the KIGS International Board: Recurrence of brain tumours in patients treated with growth hormone: analysis of KIGS (Pfizer International Growth Database). Acta Paediatr 2006;95:1284–1290.
19 Weiss M, Sutton L, Marcial V, Fowble B, Packer R, Zimmermann R, Schul L, Bruce D, D'Angio G: The role of radiation therapy in the management of childhood craniopharyngioma. Int J Radiat Oncol Biol Phys 1989;17:1313–1321.

20 Berry MP, Jenkin RDT, Keen CW, Nair BD, Simpson WJ: Radiation treatment for medulloblastoma: a 21-year review. J Neurosurg 1981;55:43–51.
21 Bloom HJG, Thornton H, Schweisguth O: SIOP medulloblastoma and high-grade ependymoma therapeutic clinical trial: preliminary results (1975–1981); in Raybaud C, Clement R, Lebrueil G, Bernard JL (eds): Pediatric Oncology: Proceedings of the 13th Annual Meeting of the International Society of Pediatric Oncology, Marseilles, September 1981. Amsterdam, Excerpta Medica, 1981, pp 309–322.
22 Stiller C, Lennox E: Childhood medulloblastoma in Britain 1971–1977: analyses of treatment and survival. Br J Cancer 1983;48:835–841.
23 Duffner PK, Cohen ME, Myers MH, Heise HW: Survival of children with brain tumours: SEER program, 1973–1980. Neurology 1986;36:597–601.
24 Swerdlow A, Reddingius R, Higgins C, Spoudeas H, Phipps K, Qiao Z, Ryder W, Brada M, Hayward R, Brook C, Hindmarsh P, Shalet S: Growth hormone treatment of children with brain tumours and risk of tumour recurrence. J Clin Endocrinol Metab 2000; 85:4444–4449.
25 Ilgren EB, Stiller CA: Cerebellar astrocytomas: therapeutic management. Acta Neurochir 1986;81:11–26.
26 Rosenfeld R, Wilson D, Dollar L, Bennett A, Hintz R: Both human pituitary growth hormone and recombinant DNA-derived human growth hormone cause insulin resistance at a post-receptor level. J Clin Endocrinol Metab 1982; 54:1033–1038.
27 Crawford BA, Cowell P, Greenacre NJ: Carbohydrate metabolism on high-dose growth hormone therapy in children treated for leukaemia. Aust Paediatr J 1989;25:236–240.
28 Czernichow P, Albertsson-Wikland K, Tuvemo T, Gunnarsson R, on behalf of the International Board of KIGS: Growth hormone treatment and diabetes: survey of the Kabi Pharmacia International Growth Study. Acta Paediatr Scand Suppl 1991;379:104–107.
29 Gard AA, Jones R: Growth hormone therapy and hyperglycaemia. Saudi Med J 1990;11:328–329.
30 Botero D, Danon M, Rosalind SB: Symptomatic non-insulin-dependent diabetes mellitus during therapy with recombinant human growth hormone. J Pediatr 1993;123:590–592.

31 Shizume K: Long-term effects of human growth hormone on 1,959 patients with pituitary dwarfism throughout Japan. Endocrinol Jpn 1984;31:201–206.
32 Kitagawa T, Owada M, Urakami T, Tajimu N: Epidemiology of type 1 (insulin-dependent) and type 2 (non-insulin-dependent) diabetes mellitus in Japanese children. Diabetes Res Clin Pract 1994;24:S7–S13.
33 Pinhas-Maniel O, Dolan LM, Daniels SR, Standiford D, Khoury PR, Zeiller P: Increased incidence of non-insulin-dependent diabetes mellitus among adolescents. J Pediatr 1996;128:608–615.
34 Otten BJ, Roittevel JJ, Cruysberg JRM: Pseudotumor cerebri following treatment with growth hormone (abstract). Horm Res 1992;37:16.
35 Malazowski S, Tanner L, Wysowski D, Fleming G: Growth hormone, insulin-like growth factor I and benign intracranial hypertension. N Engl J Med 1993;329:665–666.
36 Blethen SL, Allen DB, Graves D, August G, Moshang T, Rosenfeld R: Safety of recombinant deoxyribonucleic acid-derived growth hormone: the National Cooperative Growth Study experience. J Clin Endocrinol Metab 1996;81:1704–1710.
37 Crock PA, McKenzie JD, Nicoll AM, Howard NJ, Cutfield W, Shield LK, Byrne G: Benign intracranial hypertension and recombinant growth hormone therapy in Australia and New Zealand. Acta Paediatr 1998;87:381–386.
38 Henriksson B: The incidence of slipped capital femoral epiphysis. Acta Orthop Scand 1969;40:365–372.
39 Kelsey JL, Keggi KJ, Southwick WO: The incidence and distribution of slipped capital femoral epiphysis in Connecticut and Southwestern United States. J Bone Joint Surg 1970; 52A:1203–1216.
40 Crawford A, MacEwen G, Fonte D: Slipped capital femoral epiphysis coexistent with hypothyroidism. Clin Orthop 1977;122:135–139.
41 Kelsey J: The epidemiology of diseases of the hip: a review. Int J Epidemiol 1977;6:269–280.
42 Puri R, Smith C, Mathofra D, Williams A, Owen R, Harris F: Slipped capital femoral epiphysis and primary juvenile hypothyroidism. J Bone Joint Surg (Br) 1985;67:14–20.

43 Fidler MW, Brook CGD: Slipped upper femoral epiphysis following treatment with human growth hormone. J Bone Joint Surg 1974;56:1719–1722.
44 Heatley FW, Greenwood RH, Boase DL: Slipping of the upper femoral epiphyses in patients with intracranial tumours causing hypopituitarism and chiasmal compression. J Bone Joint Surg 1976; 58B:169–175.
45 Rennie W, Mitchell N: Slipped femoral capital epiphysis occurring during growth hormone therapy. J Bone Joint Surg 1974;56:703–705.
46 Prasad V, Greig F, Bastian W, Castells S, Juan C, AvRuskin TW: Slipped capital femoral epiphysis during treatment with recombinant growth hormone for isolated, partial growth hormone deficiency. J Pediatr 1990;116:397–399.
47 Rappaport EB, Fife D: Slipped capital femoral epiphysis in growth hormone-deficient patients. Am J Dis Child 1985; 139:396–399.
48 Blethen SL, Rundle AC: Slipped capital femoral epiphysis in children treated with growth hormone. Horm Res 1996; 46:113–116.
49 Van den Berg BJ, Yerushelmy J: Studies on convulsive disorders in young children. 1. Incidence of febrile and nonfebrile convulsions by age and other factors. Pediatr Res 1969;3:298–304.
50 Heijbel J, Blom S, Bergfors PG: Benign epilepsy of children with centro-temporal foci: a study of incidence rate in out-patient care. Epilepsia 1975;65: 657–664.
51 Shamansky SL, Glaser GH: Socioeconomic characteristics of childhood seizure disorders in the New Haven area: an epidemiological study. Epilepsia 1979;20:457–474.
52 Doose H, Sitepu B: Childhood epilepsy in a German city. Neuropediatrics 1983;14:220–224.
53 Sidenvall R, Forsgren L, Blomqvist HK, Heijbel J: A community-based prospective incidence study of epileptic seizures in children. Acta Paediatr Scand 1993;82:60–65.
54 Raimondi A, Tomita T: Medulloblastoma in childhood. Childs Brain 1979; 5:310–328.
55 Yssing M, Garwiezs S, Glomstein A, Jonmundsson G, Kruus S: Medulloblastoma in Nordic children. 2. Acta Paediatr Scand Suppl 1990;371:12–19.

Progress and Challenges in Understanding the Psychology of Growth Delay

Brian Stabler[a]   Louis E. Underwood[b]

In this chapter, we examine several questions focused on the psychological defects related to growth failure in children and short stature in adulthood. They include: (1) perceptions of society with regard to short stature; (2) opinions of pediatric endocrinologists with regard to the psychological problems and quality of life (QoL) of children with growth failure; (3) insights provided by prospective studies related to the psychological problems and QoL of short individuals, and (4) things that pediatric endocrinologists should do to improve the psychological adjustment and QoL of short children.

Perceptions of Society with Regard to Short-Statured Individuals

Societal perceptions of persons of short stature tend to be less positive than perceptions of persons of average or tall stature. Martel and Biller [1] adapted a test of semantic differential measures to assess how positively or negatively male university students felt about men who were short (157–166 cm), of average height (173–179 cm) or tall (183–193 cm). Students were asked to rate men of different heights on a 7-point scale ranging from extremely positive to extremely negative. Compared with tall men, short men were perceived as much more insecure, more submissive, less outgoing, less aggressive (more timid), less confident and less optimistic (more pessimistic). The same measures about men of different statures were collected from female university students. The results obtained from the females were similar to those of the male respondents. Females rated short males as much less confident, less positive, less optimistic and less 'complete' than tall males. When the men of different statures were questioned about the effects of their stature on their comfort in various social situations, i.e. first date, involved in contact sports, at a crowded party, or standing at a bar – short men indicated that they were significantly less comfortable than tall men (p < 0.05 for all categories).

Schumacher [2] observed that adult males in lower job ranks of several professions were shorter than those in the higher job ranks. These differences were significant even after educational

[a]Department of Psychiatry
CB 7160, School of Medicine
[b]Department of Pediatrics
CB 7039, 3341 Med Biomolecular Building
The University of North Carolina at Chapel Hill
Chapel Hill, NC 27599 (USA)

Table 1. Correlation between height and jobs of higher and lower rank

	n	Height, cm		p
		jobs of lower rank	jobs of higher rank	
Total group	489	178.2	182.2	<0.0001
Basic education	193	177.8	181.1	<0.001
Intermediate and higher education	296	178.8	182.3	<0.0001
Originally from lower social strata	329	177.8	181.4	<0.0001
Originally from higher social strata	160	179.5	183.1	<0.001

Data from Schumacher [2].

Table 2. Partial listing of the response of 100 mothers to items testing the perceived competence of male toddlers of different heights

Item	Mean scores		p
	tall	small	
Obeying rules or instructions	2.3	2.8	<0.05
Getting along with other children	2.3	3.2	<0.001
Understanding another person's point of view	2.9	3.7	<0.01
Being independent	3.0	3.8	<0.10
Not crying when frustrated	3.4	4.3	<0.01
Doing well in school	2.6	3.1	<0.05
Taking care of own needs	2.5	3.1	<0.01

A lower score implies more competency. Data from Eisenberg et al. [3].

attainment and social strata were taken into account (table 1). The same results were observed when the professional status of female nurses was correlated with their heights. Schumacher suggested that these findings indicate that taller people have a better opportunity to reach a higher level within a profession.

Adult perception of toddlers has also been shown to be based on height. Eisenberg et al. [3] conducted a study in which mothers (n = 100) of preschool children were asked to respond to a series of three photographs of two 19-month-old boys. Although the boys resembled one another in height and general appearance, they were photographed in such a way as to appear to be of different heights. The mothers completed a questionnaire to assess their perceptions of the various competencies of the two boys. A 6-point scale was used, with ratings ranging from 'extremely capable' to 'extremely incapable'. The questions assessed the mothers' expectations regarding social and cognitive skills and assignment of punishment for hypothetical wrongdoing. Of the 12 competency items tested, significant differences relating to height were observed in 10. Taller boys were consistently perceived as being more able (table 2).

Opinions of Pediatric Endocrinologists with Regard to Psychological Problems of Short Children

Cuttler et al. [4] reported on a detailed survey of the opinions of 434 North American pediatric endocrinologists with regard to the social and

Table 3. How often does height impair emotional well-being?

	If the height is between the 3rd and the 5th percentile	If the height is <3rd percentile
Always	0.3	6.2
Often	13.5	49.4
Sometimes	69.7	42.9
Seldom	16.5	
Never	0	
Seldom/never		2.1

Values are percentages. Opinions of 434 pediatric endocrinologists. Data from Cuttler et al. [4].

emotional effects of short stature. Two questions focused on the perceptions and beliefs related to the psychosocial effects of short stature. They asked how often height impairs the emotional well-being of children whose height is between the 3rd and 5th percentile? More than 83% of the pediatric endocrinologists expressed the opinion that there were adverse emotional consequences sometimes, often or always. When the question was rephrased to focus on children whose heights were below the 3rd percentile, adverse emotional effects were felt to be present in nearly 98% of the patients (table 3).

Insights Provided by Prospective Studies Related to Psychosocial Problems and the Quality of Life of Short Individuals

We assessed the psychological status of 195 short boys and girls, aged 5–16 years [5]. The children were recruited by pediatric endocrinologists at 28 centers in the US (National Cooperative Growth Study). For inclusion, the participants had to be below the 3rd percentile for height and have a diagnosis of growth hormone deficiency (GHD; n = 109; peak GH response to provocative stimuli <10 ng/ml) or idiopathic short stature (ISS; n = 86; peak GH >10 ng/ml). For comparison, 113 children of normal height (10th to 90th percentile) were recruited. The rate of grade failure in school among the short children was more than twice that of controls, and significantly more short children had received special education services. Using subscale scores from the Child Behavior Checklist (CBCL), short children exhibited significantly more behavior problems than controls. These included problems such as being socially withdrawn, being anxious/depressed, somatic complaints, having problems with attention and social interactions, and having aggression and/or delinquent behavior.

These short children were treated with GH and underwent repeat testing with CBCL each year for 3 years. Seventy-two children with GHD and 59 with ISS completed the study. After 3 years of GH therapy, the CBCL scores for total behavior problems were improved in the children with GHD ($p < 0.001$ vs. baseline scores) and in those with ISS ($p < 0.003$; fig. 1). Also, there was improvement among the children with GHD in the subscales measuring withdrawal ($p < 0.007$), somatic complaints ($p < 0.001$), anxiety/depression ($p < 0.001$), and attention, social and thought problems (each $p < 0.001$; fig. 1).

Findings and opinions of other health professionals are sometimes different from patients with slow growth who are referred to pediatric endocrine clinics. Voss and Mulligan [6] studied short children, identified by screening more than 14,000 children in two school districts in the UK. Compared with controls, these investigators found no significant deficits in intelligence, school performance, self-esteem or behavior, as rated by teachers. During follow-up, they reported on the emotional effects of GH therapy, showing that treatment produced no psychological benefit [7]. Sandberg et al. [8] compared short children (aged 6–10 years) referred to an endocrine clinic with children recruited from four elementary schools. They observed that the short

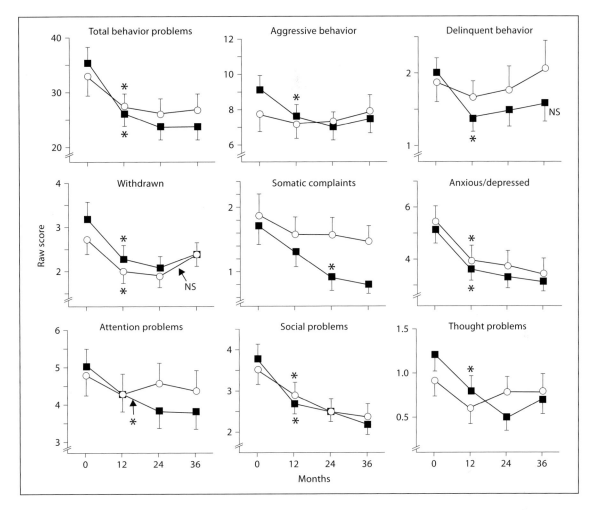

Fig. 1. Raw scores on CBCL at baseline (0 months) and during GH treatment (12, 24 and 36 months) of children with GHD (filled symbols and solid lines) and ISS (open symbols and dashed lines). Lower scores on each scale correspond to fewer behavior problems. Results for each group are displayed as means ± SEM. * p < 0.05, the point at which scores become different statistically from scores at baseline. From Stabler et al. [5].

boys had slightly lower scores, indicative of poorer adjustment on the CBCL for the scales dealing with activities, as well as with social and total competence. Short boys also exhibited higher social and thought problem scores. No differences were found between short and control girls. Vance et al. [9] compared data on short- and normal-statured children from a national health survey. They report that very tall males were better adjusted in school than very short males. Similar observations were made when comparing very tall females with short females.

We believe that the discrepancies between the studies cited above, showing problems among short children, and studies that show less compelling differences between short and normal children are the result of differences in the sources of the children studied (those referred to pediatric endocrinologists vs. population based) and/or differences in the tests used. Children referred to the pediatric endocrinologist most likely are children who are encountering difficulty with adjustment and coping, thus increasing the urgency to seek consultation.

Things that Pediatric Endocrinologists Should Do to Improve the Psychosocial Adjustment and Quality of Life of Short Children

Beyond doing the appropriate, diagnostic tests to determine why the child has growth failure and deciding whether to begin GH therapy (or whatever other medical therapy is appropriate), the physician should raise the following issues with the parents.
1. Is there a history of behavioral or psychological disturbance?
2. Has psychological testing occurred?
3. Is the patient functioning at grade level in school?
4. Does the patient relate well to age mates?
5. Does the patient behave in an age-appropriate fashion?

The answers to these questions will lead to further inquiry in many cases, focusing on specific areas of assessment. For example, it is frequently the case that short children are retained one grade in school and/or suffer from specific learning disability. Unless this information is actively sought it may never become apparent to the physician. The psychology of growth delay does not always evolve solely from the consequences of being short. Early studies suggested that short children had 'normal' intelligence and experienced few academic difficulties [10]. However, more recent findings raise the issue of discrepancy between academic potential, as represented by the intelligence quotient, and academic achievement as measured by standard educational tests [11].

Further assessment is better accomplished by a trained developmental specialist, such as a clinical psychologist. However, when this resource consultation is not available, there are screening techniques that can be employed in the pediat-ric clinic. The Child Health Questionnaire is a self-administered multifactorial questionnaire which elicits information related to general health, school achievement, problem behaviors and social relationships [12]. Scores are available with norms from both community- and health-impaired populations, balanced for gender, social class and age.

Maintaining Appropriate Expectations for Treatment Outcome

Issues which impact socially sensitive topics like height, strength or attractiveness are fraught with problems of subjectivity and bias. For short children and their parents, this can be particularly troublesome, because the obvious purpose of growth therapy is to improve height and appearance. When physicians and parents meet to discuss the implications of treatment, there may be misunderstandings, miscommunications and unexpressed hopes. These may give rise to unrealistic expectations for treatment outcome. We have shown that short patients (and also their parents) hold unrealistic beliefs about the amount and rate of growth change GH therapy may bring about [13]. Children may overestimate both their current height in relation to peers, but more importantly, may project final height to be in the 75th or 90th centile (fig. 2). These estimates are far beyond what might reasonably be expected based on growth projections. Without continued education and clarification, these hopes and expectations will be dashed by the reality that only minimal height effects are realized. Disappointment and dismay at this outcome could tarnish what is an otherwise excellent outcome from a purely medical standpoint.

The growth chart is a helpful tool for keeping the family and patient abreast of growth change

Each of us grows physically at our own pace: some of us grow fast, some of us grow slowly. This is why two children the same age may not be the same height. One may be a lot taller or a lot shorter than the other.
• These children are all your age. Choose the one who looks most like you.

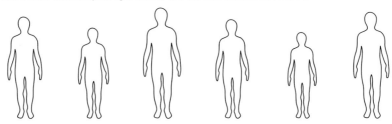

Each of us will grow until we become adults. Not all adults are the same size; some are bigger, some are smaller, even though they may be the same age.
• These people are all the same age. Which one will you look like when you are full grown?

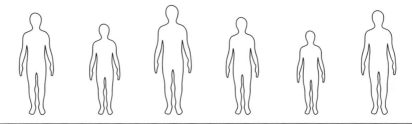

Fig. 2. The Silhouette Apperception Technique. From Grew et al. [13].

and can be the focus of clinical education during regular visits. However, what is sometimes overlooked is a means to inquire into what is expected or hoped for, and how this contrasts with what is actually happening. We have found that employing pictorial representations of the human figure, shown in ascending order from the 3rd to the 97th height percentile, is a more concrete and visually compelling means to elucidate the differences in height and expectations for change [13]. Using this approach, we are able to minimize the possibility of distortions or misunderstanding by both patients and parents.

Short children frequently experience delays in school achievement, often exhibited by test score results or by failure to be promoted academically [5]. Being retained a grade or more in school can have undesirable long-term effects on skill development, social relationships and self-concept.

The records of some short patients should contain information provided by the school on class or grade placement, intelligence testing, achievement test scores and history of behavioral or social problems. This information will likely indicate areas of special need such as learning disability, underachievement, or sensory deficiencies, such as hearing or vision problems.

Another area of useful inquiry is extracurricular activities such as hobby or sports groups, or religious and/or community associations. Involvement in these types of after-school activities may indicate positive social affiliations, which counter the potential for social isolation experienced by many growth-delayed children.

Other members of the care team should be actively involved at all stages of diagnosis and treatment. The optimal team should include a nurse, social worker, psychologist and/or educator. The role of the physician is a team leader and coordinator, responsible for directing the collection and integration of multiple forms of information and data about the patient and family.

A debate continues to wage over the question of what degree of pituitary deficiency is required to qualify for GH replacement therapy. From a purely biomedical standpoint, the answer seems straightforward; however, when the larger issues raised by growth failure, lack of development, social and emotional maturity are raised, simple answers do not suffice. When and until there is agreement on what constitutes the comprehensive assessment of growth delay, including any and all psychological issues, the question of whom to treat is likely to remain controversial. With a larger body of scientific evidence derived from controlled psychological investigations, clinicians might eventually become more comfortable making these decisions.

Thoughts about Final Outcomes of GH Therapy

By most biomedical criteria, the majority of child patients treated with GH show successful outcomes; growth rate accelerates and height begins to approach the normal range. However, there have been numerous follow-up studies which report that these same 'satisfactory' outcomes are not accompanied by good QoL and productivity in young and middle adulthood [14]. We initially believed that this might result from the stress and aversive social experience of being short in childhood. However, several reports implicating hypothalamic-pituitary functions in affective disorders such as anxiety and depression lead us to examine our adult patients more closely. We conducted a series of studies which compared the psychological and behavioral profiles of post-GHD short adults and non-GHD adults matched for age, sex and socioeconomic status. We found significantly more GHD-treated adults to carry lifetime diagnoses of social anxiety disorder and panic [15]. Non-GHD matched controls showed no evidence of these traits beyond that expected. We conclude that the lack of life satisfaction and low productivity among adults treated for GHD in childhood is more likely the result of hypothalamic-pituitary-related factors than the result of socialization. Further study is urgently needed to clarify why these outcomes continue to mar what is otherwise a triumph of endocrine therapy.

References

1 Martel LF, Biller HB: Stature and Stigma: The Biopsychosocial Development of Short Males. Lexington, DC Heath, 1987.
2 Schumacher A: On the significance of stature in human society. J Hum Evol 1982;11:697–701.
3 Eisenberg N, Roth K, Bryniarski KA, Murray E: Sex differences in the relationship of height to children's actual and attributed social and cognitive competencies. Sex Roles 1984;11:719–734.
4 Cuttler L, Silvers JB, Singh J, et al: Short stature and growth hormone therapy: a national study of physician recognition patterns. JAMA 1996;276:531.
5 Stabler B, Siegel PT, Clopper RR, et al: Behavior change after growth hormone treatment of children with short stature. J Pediatr 1998;133:366–373.
6 Voss LD, Mulligan J: The short normal child in school: self-esteem, behavior and attainment before puberty (The Wessex Growth Study); in Stabler B, Underwood LE (eds): Growth, Stature, and Adaptation. Chapel Hill, University of North Carolina, 1994.
7 Downey AB, Mulligan, J, McCaughery ES, Stratford RJ, Betts PR, Voss LD: Psychological response to growth hormone treatment in short normal children. Arch Dis Child 1996;75:32–35.
8 Sandberg DE, Brook AE, Campos SP: Short stature in middle childhood: a survey of psychological functioning in a clinically referred sample; in Stabler B, Underwood LE (eds): Growth, Stature, and Adaptation. Chapel Hill, University of North Carolina, 1994.
9 Vance MD, Ingersoll GM, Golden MP: Short stature in a nonclinical sample: not a big problem; in Stabler B, Underwood LE (eds): Growth, Stature, and Adaptation. Chapel Hill, University of North Carolina, 1994.
10 Money J, Pollitt E: Studies of the psychology of dwarfism: personality, maturation and response to growth hormone treatment in hypopituitary dwarfism. J Pediatr 1966;68:381–390.
11 Stabler B, Clopper RR, Siegel PT, Stoppani C, Compton PG, Underwood LE: Academic achievement and psychological adjustment in short children. J Dev Behav Pediatr 1994;15:1–6.
12 Eiser C, Morse R: Quality of life measures in chronic diseases of childhood. Health Technol Assess 2001;5:1–157.
13 Grew RS, Stabler B, Williams RW, Underwood LE: Facilitating patient understanding in the treatment of growth delay. Clin Pediatr 1983;22:685.
14 Stabler B, Tancer ME, Ranc J, Underwood LE: Evidence of social phobia and other psychiatric disorders in adults who were growth hormone deficient during childhood. Anxiety 1996;2:86–89.
15 Nicholas LM, Tancer ME, Silva SG, Underwood LE, Stabler B: Short stature, growth hormone deficiency and social anxiety. Psychosom Med 1997;59:372–375.

Growth Hormone and Brain Function

Fred Nyberg

Research on functions that growth hormone (GH) exerts on the central nervous system (CNS) has attracted many investigators during the past 2 decades. In various clinics, GH replacement therapy has been shown to improve several mental disabilities seen in adult GH deficiency (GHD) patients but also in individuals with childhood onset of GHD. Thus, in addition to normalizing growth and metabolism in adult GHD patients, the hormone has been seen to increase energy, motivation and wellbeing, as well as improving memory and cognition. Studies have also provided evidence that GH may cross the blood-brain barrier (BBB). Preclinical studies have revealed that specific receptors for GH are expressed in a variety of CNS regions including those that are believed to represent the functional anatomy of various behaviors, as mentioned above, associated with the hormone. Moreover, experimental animal models have been used to explore the mechanism at the molecular level by which GH may induce its effects on CNS-related behaviors.

Department of Pharmaceutical Biosciences
Uppsala University Biomedical Center
PO Box 591
Husargatan 6
SE–751 24 Uppsala (Sweden)

This article will review previous and current research on the significance of GH in relation to brain function. However, due to lack of space, it will be limited to certain functions that have reached particular attention in the clinical perspective.

Historical Aspects

Most of the biological actions that have been attributed to GH are related to its effects on peripheral organs and tissues. However, recent studies suggest that the hormone may induce profound effects on functions linked to the CNS. This appeared obvious from studies directed to the investigation of GH-induced effects on psychological functions that have been seen to be affected and improved during GH replacement therapy. Early work in this direction indicated that GH when systemically administered at physiological doses interacts with brain monoaminergic pathways. Thus, the rat hormone (rGH) given at physiological concentrations was shown to affect the catecholamine turnover in the rat hypothalamus [1]. From these studies, it was suggested that rGH inhibits its own secretion, partly via reduction of dopamine synthesis and release in the median eminence. This leads to increased release of somatostatin and attenuated synthesis and turnover of noradrenaline in the median eminence, which, in turn, causes a reduced secretion of a GH-releasing factor. Similar observations were made for prolactin [2]. At that time, reports providing evidence that both lactogenic and somatogenic binding sites are present in the brain appeared in the literature [3]. Thus, studies revealed that GH binding sites are present in brain areas such as the hypothalamus, pituitary and choroid plexus. Subsequent to these observations, specific binding sites for the hormone were identified not only in these brain regions but also in areas not directly connected to the hypothalamic-pituitary axis [4].

Furthermore, in parallel with these events, clinical researchers observed decreased ratings on psychological well-being and cognitive capabilities in individuals with deficient production of GH (GHD patients) and it was also found that GH replacement therapy improved these disabilities [5, 6]. Of special interest was the observation that GH may improve learning and memory performance. However, the mechanisms underlying these effects were not known. The identification and characterization of specific binding sites for the hormone in various areas of the human brain [4, 7] were reported. It was also found that the density of these sites was sex dependent and declined with age [7], and it was suggested that these sites are involved in the mediation of the GH effects on the brain [8, 9]. Furthermore, the GH receptor (GHR) in various tissues of the rat brain, including the choroid plexus, hippocampus, hypothalamus and spinal cord, has recently been cloned [10, 11]. The sequence of the gene transcript of the GHR in the human choroid plexus has also been determined [9]. From these studies, it became apparent that the nucleotide sequence of these receptor gene transcripts is almost identical to that determined for their liver congener.

In studies that followed, the identification of a brain variant of the GHR in the CNS and attempts to map the distribution of this protein and its message in various brain regions have been carried out. These studies revealed the presence of the GHR and its gene transcript in many tissues related to the functional anatomy of several behaviors known to be associated with the hormone [12, 13]. Functional studies in animals attempting to clarify the molecular mechanisms underlying these behaviors have also been carried out. Many of these studies are reviewed within this article. Our group has directed studies to the effects of the GH/insulin-like growth factor 1 (IGF-1) axis on the glutamate system including the N-methyl-D-aspartyl (NMDA) receptor and its subunits [14–16] in the rat hippocampus. As reviewed below, we observed that both GH and IGF-1 induce alterations in this system, which are compatible with the improvements in memory and learning processes as recorded from animal studies.

Many of the observations seen in animals are in agreement with the beneficial effect on memory and well-being seen during GH replacement therapy in human subjects [5, 6, 17]. E.g., an increased well-being observed in these patients may include the endogenous opioids, such as β-endorphin [18].

Evidence that Growth Hormone May Cross the Blood-Brain Barrier

The ability of GH to cross the BBB has been the subject of debate over the past 2 decades. The hormone represents a molecular size that is considered as too large for an easy penetration through the BBB. However, there are accumulating evidences speaking in favor of a possible pathway for GH to appear in the brain. First, immunoreactive GH has been detected in several brain areas, which suggests that the hormone may cross the BBB [19, 20]. Second, the presence of GH in the cerebrospinal fluid (CSF) is indicative of the ability of the hormone to penetrate this barrier [18, 21]. In addition, all beneficial effects seen for GH during replacement therapy suggest that the hormone may find its way from the circulatory system into the CNS [9]. There are several mechanisms suggested for the hormone to be transported across the BBB. For instance, GH may reach its responsive sites in the brain by circumventing the BBB through the median eminence of the hypothalamus. The median eminence serves as a circumventricular organ that permits hypothalamic polypeptides to leave the brain without disrupting the BBB and permits hormone compounds that do not cross the BBB to trigger changes in brain function [22]. Furthermore, like prolactin [23], GH has been suggested to cross the BBB through the choroid plexus via the CSF by a receptor-mediated mechanism and from this fluid is transported into the brain [24]. The hormone may also actively or passively cross the brain parenchyma capillaries through the BBB. A recent study suggests that GH may significantly diffuse into the CNS [25].

Extrapituitary Sources of Growth Hormone

Over the years, it has become evident that the source of GH is not restricted to the pituitary gland, and studies suggesting that the hormone may be produced in various areas in the brain have been reported [19, 26, 27]. Using radioimmunoassay, the distribution of GH immunoreactivity in the rodent and primate CNS was determined. High concentrations of extractable GH-like materials were detected in the rat amygdaloid nucleus, although other areas including the cortex, hippocampus and thalamus also contained immunoreactive GH [19]. Evidence that the gene transcript of GH is expressed in the brain has also been reported [28]. Additional reports indicating that the GH gene expression is not restricted to the pituitary gland and occurs in many extrapituitary tissues, including the CNS, are present in the literature [29, 30]. Studies have also shown that GH gene expression occurs in the brain prior to its ontogenic appearance in the pituitary gland,

suggesting that the hormone may have evolved phylogenetically as a neuropeptide, rather than an endocrine entity. Current and previous studies have shown that GH is produced within the hippocampal formation, a brain structure that has been associated with learning, memory, as well as aspects of emotional experience. It was demonstrated that GH production within the hippocampus is modulated by age and sex differences and the presence of estrogen [31]. Moreover, exposure to an acute stressful event increased both the expression of the GH gene transcript and the production of the hormone in both males and females. Thus, it appears that GH is produced in the hippocampal formation, where it is regulated by age, estrogen and exposure to environmental stimuli, such as stress [31]. However, it should be noted that evidence that GH may reach the hippocampal formation from the circulatory systems has also been presented [14–16].

Growth Hormone Receptors in the Central Nervous System

The presence of specific binding sites for GH in the CNS has been confirmed in many laboratories [for a review, see ref. 8, 9, 32, 33]. Binding studies have verified a high content of GH binding in the CNS, including the choroid plexus, pituitary, hypothalamus and hippocampus, but also in the spinal cord [4, 7, 34, 35]. In the human brain, the highest density of GH binding was detected in the choroid plexus [4]. In most areas in the human brain, an apparent decline in GH binding with increasing age was observed [7]. The distribution of GH binding sites in the rat CNS was found to be similar to that in humans [35]. Using rGH as radiolabel, it was confirmed that in the brain of this species, the highest content of GH binding is in the choroid plexus [20, 35, 36]. A sex-dependent GH binding in the rat was observed using the human variant of the hormone [36]. However, human GH is known to bind to lactogenic sites in the rat, and the binding of labeled rGH, which does not interact with lactogenic sites, did not show any sex differences [35, 36]. Therefore, it was suggested that the observed sex differences in the rat were due to a higher content of prolactin sites in the female animals.

Subsequent studies have shown that the identified binding sites for GH in the brain represent receptor proteins for the hormone [9, 35]. The expression of the gene transcripts of the GHR has been confirmed both in human and rat brain tissues. A study on the distribution of the GHR gene transcript in the rat brain has been reported by Burton et al. [12]. They used the in situ hybridization technique to probe the message in a variety of brain areas. Similar work has been carried out in other laboratories [37, 38]. Areas with a high expression of GHR mRNA-containing cells are the hypothalamus, the thalamus septal region, hippocampus, dentate gyrus and amygdala [12]. Moreover, the presence a 4.4-kb GHR transcript in an ovine choroid plexus cell line has been reported [39]. Also, the gene for the extracellular domain of the GHR in the human choroid plexus was cloned [9]. The predicted amino acid sequence of this part of the choroid plexus receptor was found to be homologous to the GHR in the human liver [40]. Using Northern blot analysis, no difference between sex and the expression of the GHR message in the choroid plexus was observed. The expression of the GHR in the human brain has also been studied in other laboratories [41]. The nucleotide sequence of the transcripts of the GHR in the rat hippocampus and spinal cord has been described [10], as well as those identified in the rat hypothalamus and choroid plexus [11].

Mechanisms of Action

At least three routes for the action of GH within the CNS have been discussed. First, the hormone has been proposed to undergo enzymatic degradation in the circulation to yield bioactive fragments that may gain access to the CNS and exert effects through interactions at peptide receptors [42]. A second possibility for GH to affect the brain is that it may elicit the release of mediators from peripheral tissue, such as IGF-1, that may cross the BBB and then exert central effects. A third route is that GH itself can penetrate the BBB and activate its receptors in the CNS. In this last case, stimulation of the GHR in the brain may lead to the release of brain-derived IGF-1, which in turn mediates the effect.

Clinical studies have shown that GH may cross the blood-CSF barrier, as the CSF levels of the hormone display a significant increase following GH replacement therapy [18, 21]. A concomitant enhancement of IGF-1 levels in the CSF of patients receiving GH was found [18], and a significant positive correlation between given doses of the levels of GH in the CSF was reported [21]. Also, it was shown in these studies that GH injections affected the levels of various transmitter substances in the CSF. For instance, GH elicited increased CSF concentrations of the opioid peptide β-endorphin [18], and the CSF levels of a dopamine metabolite and some amino acids were affected as well [21].

Our studies, using experimental animals, suggest that peripheral administration of GH may induce alterations in the glutamate transmission. Thus, the NMDA receptor subunit mRNAs in the hippocampus were affected in a fashion that is compatible with GH-promoting effects on memory and cognitive capabilities [14]. This effect of GH was mimicked by IGF-1, which induced a similar alteration in the expression of the NMDA subunit gene transcripts [15]. Thus, it seems that the effect of GH on the hippocampal formation may result from the release of IGF-1. In fact, we have observed that injection of rGH in the rat induces a significant increase in the CNS expression of the gene transcript of IGF-1 (unpublished observation). The involvement of a stimulatory effect on the brain GHR was suggested from the observation that peripherally administered GH elicited an effect on the NMDA receptor subunit NR2B that positively correlated with the expression of the GHR [14].

Knowledge about the mechanism of GH signaling at its target sites in the brain is still limited. However, it is anticipated that the hormone interacts with its brain receptors using a mechanism similar to that known for its action in peripheral cells [43]. Thus, it is hypothesized that when GH reaches its responsive sites in the brain, it binds to the extracellular component of the GHR and elicits receptor dimerization and/or a conformational change of predimerized receptor complexes. As a result of these events, the receptor-linked kinase, Janus kinase 2 (JAK2), is phosphorylated, leading to phosphorylation of the intracellular part of the GHR, which undergoes further tyrosine autophosphorylation. The formation of the JAK2 kinase-GHR complex results in a process that culminates in the activation of the signal transducer and activator of transcription (STAT) proteins, involved in the STAT pathway. The STAT proteins STAT1, STAT3 and STAT5 are cytoplasmic proteins that form homodimers and heterodimers. They are translocated to the nucleus, where they bind to response elements on DNA to stimulate transcription of genes. The interactions of the STAT proteins with their gene targets in the nucleus are believed to be essential for the actions of GH. In the brain, the JAK/STAT pathway has been suggested to be involved in the mediation of events that produce a calcium influx through NMDA receptors [44]. Chronic infusion of GH in male dwarf rats was shown to increased the expression of hypothalamic STAT5b, while a single injection of GH into similar rats induced the phosphorylation of STAT5 proteins [45]. The STAT5b protein has been directly implicated in the GH-induced production of IGF-1. This factor mediates many of the anabolic actions of GH. IGF-1 binds to a cell surface receptor (IGF1R), which mediates the action of IGF-1 on all types of cells.

Studies have suggested that GH may produce effects on cell proliferation and differentiation. GH has been shown to induce proliferation and differentiation that is blocked by IGF-1 antiserum [46]. The hormone increased IGF-binding protein 3, the IGF-1 receptor protein and its phosphorylation. It was demonstrated that GH promotes proliferation of neural precursors, neurogenesis and gliogenesis during brain development [46]. All these responses were suggested to be mediated by locally produced IGF-1.

The GH-induced activation of the JAK2/STAT system is also known to induce the expression of suppressors of cytokine signaling (SOCS) and/or cytokine-inducible SH2 protein (CIS). This effect leads to the attenuation of the GH signaling. Effects of GH in the brain also seem to involve an interaction with the SOCS/CIS system. Thus, studies directed to the rat hypothalamus have demonstrated that GH elicits an increase in the gene transcripts of SOCS3 and CIS in the arcuate nucleus and an enhancement of the SOCS3 message in the periventricular nucleus [47]. It was concluded that GH acts directly on hypothalamic neurons and enhances the gene expression of SOCS3 and CIS, which suggests that these regulators may be involved in the mechanism that regulates the GH action in these cells.

GH did not affect SOCS2 expression in the hypothalamus [47], but in studies using transgenic mice, SOCS2 is shown to block the effects of GH on neuronal differentiation [48]. It was suggested that GH, possibly regulated by SOCS2, is involved in several processes in the development and maturation of CNS regulating the number and size of multiple neurons and even glial cells [48, 49].

Functional Aspects of Growth Hormone Effects on Brain Function

GH has been suggested to be involved in several CNS-related behaviors. It is shown to produce a number of effects on CNS-related behaviors. Particular attention has been drawn to GH effects on appetite, cognitive and memory processes, as well as on neuroprotection. Many of these effects have been documented from in vitro studies using various types of cells, from in vivo studies in a variety of experimental animal models, and from clinical studies in humans [50–53]. An important issue in this regard is the well-known decline in the GH/IGF-1 axis that occurs with aging. The aging process is connected with losses in many functions related to the action of the somatotrophic axis in the brain.

Brain GH and Aging
Hypofunction in the somatotrophic axis in the brain during aging reflects a most important example of age-related changes that occur in man. It contributes a number of alterations in psychological capabilities seen during aging. Many of these are included in the spectrum of potential disabilities related to GHD, also in young subjects. Among these are decreased energy and motivation, disabilities in cognitive functions, and decreased mood and well-being, i.e. an overall impairment in quality of life [54].

The decline in GH secretion that occurs with increasing age is generally mirrored by a concomitant decrease in plasma levels of IGF-1, the best marker of GH status. Studies have also demonstrated that the decline in pituitary secretion of GH is paralleled with an age-related decreased in the density of GHR in the brain [7, 9]. The positive influence of GH replacement therapy seen in GHD patients has raised a discussion about the potential clinical implications of GH replacement at advanced age, as a treatment approach exerting anti-aging effects.

GH and Appetite
Clinical studies have shown that GHD patients increase their food intake when subjected to GH replacement therapy. These observations suggest that GH also has an appetite-stimulating effect. A recent study using transgenic mice with an overexpression of bovine GH in the CNS showed that it is possible to differentiate the effect of GH on body fat mass from that on appetite [55]. The transgenic mice were not deficient in GH, but they were obese and displayed an increased food intake, as well as increased hypothalamic expression of neuropeptide Y (NPY) and the agouti-related protein. Moreover, intracerebroventricular injections of the hormone in C57BL/6 mice induced an acute effect on food intake. It was concluded from this study that GH overexpression in the CNS causes hyperphagia-induced obesity, indicating a dual effect of GH, with a central stimulatory effect on appetite and a peripheral lipolytic effect. It is further shown that the GH releaser ghrelin increases food intake; however, it was also shown that the acute effect of ghrelin in this regard is dependent upon a functionally intact GHR signaling [56]. NPY has a well-documented role in the regulation of appetite, and a link between NPY and GH has been observed in several studies on food intake [57]. Also, the GH regulatory peptide GH secretagogue is coexpressed with NPY in the hypothalamic arcuate nucleus [58]. Finally, the distribution of GHR mRNA to visceral sensory and motor structures is consonant with a role of GH in the regulation of food intake and energy homeostasis [13].

GH in Cognition and Memory Function
The potential role of GH and IGF-1 in memory acquisition and cognitive functions has received attention during the past decade. GH replacement therapy in GHD patients has suggested that the hormone may induce improvements in both long-term and working memory [59–61]. From a very recent study, it was concluded that GH treatment for 6 months improved the long-term as well as the working memory in patients with GHD [61]. This improvement was associated with decreased brain activation in the ventrolateral prefrontal cortex, as visualized by means of functional magnetic resonance imaging. Thus, GH substitution in GHD patients results in ben-

eficial effects for the cognitive functioning, and the effects of this treatment can be visualized by means of neuroimaging [61]. Although many studies strongly suggest that GH is associated with cognitive function, there is still a need of studies on GH effects on cognitive functions in elderly healthy non-GHD individuals [62].

The mechanism by which GH exerts its beneficial effects on cognitive capabilities has attracted several researchers. It has been suggested that GH may produce these effects through the release of IGF-1. As mentioned above, this growth factor crosses the BBB, and in recent years, much attention has been focused on age-related decreases in serum GH and IGF-1 as potential mechanisms that may influence cognitive function in the elderly. However, according to the earlier discussion in this chapter, GH may pass the BBB or, alternatively, may be produced within the brain. In addition, following peripheral administration of GH in rats, the expression of the GHR message is altered in a mode that is compatible with a stimulatory effect on the GHR [14]. In behavioral animal experiments, it is shown that long-term GH/IGF-1 replacement improves learning and memory in aged rats. While the exact mechanism underlying these cognitive improvements is not yet clarified, GH and/or IGF-1 replacement to aged animals increases neurogenesis, vascular density and glucose utilization and alters NMDA receptor subunit composition in brain areas that are implicated in learning and memory [14, 16, 52, 53, 63].

In studies using experimental animals, GH is shown to influence the NMDA receptor system in the hippocampus, an essential component of long-term potentiation, which is highly involved in memory acquisition. It was observed that the hormone, in this case recombinant human GH (rhGH), affected the gene expression of the NMDA receptor subunits in a mode that would be compatible with enhanced memory and cognitive capabilities [14]. More recently, a similar effect was demonstrated for IGF-1 [15]. A very recent study, designed to examine the beneficial effects of rhGH on cognitive function in male rats with multiple hormone deficiencies resulting from hypophysectomy, indicated that the animals treated with the hormone performed much better than untreated controls using the Morris water maze to assess cognitive behavior [16]. The rhGH-treated animals performed significantly better in the spatial memory task than the control animals on the second and third days of trial. Assessment of the hippocampal expression of the gene transcripts of the NMDA receptor subunits NR1, NR2A and NR2B, the IGF-1 receptor and the postsynaptic density protein 95 indicated that there may exist a relationship between the message of the NMDA receptor subunits and learning ability, and that learning is improved by rhGH in the hypophysectomized rats. Moreover, a link between Morris water maze performance and the expression of postsynaptic density protein 95 was also suggested by this study [16].

GH and Neuroprotection

Quite recently, the concept of neuroprotection has appeared in the neuroscience literature. It includes a variety of processes and components that may be involved in preserving CNS functions. Evidence for neuroprotective effects of GH and IGF-1 is documented in the literature, and knowledge generated in this research area may have an impact on future treatment of brain or spinal cord trauma. Several review articles on this topic with particular focus directed to the GH/IGF-1 axis are present in the literature [53, 58, 64, 65].

A growing body of evidence suggests that the somatotrophic axis is integrally involved in the growth and development of the normal CNS. Some neuroprotective effects derive from locally produced IGF-1, whereas other effects originate from circulating IGF-1. Several of the neuroprotective effects seen for GH and IGF-1 emerged from their effects on adult cell genesis [53, 66]. For instance, in the hippocampus, IGF-1 is shown to increase oligodendrocyte recruitment and newborn cells with the endothelial phenotype. The increase in endothelial cell phenotype produced by IGF-1 may explain the increase in cerebral arteriole density observed following GH treatment [66]. All these findings seem to stress the role of IGF-1 being a putative regenerative agent in the CNS, whereas GH, which is less studied in this context, is believed to produce similar effects.

Experimental data have demonstrated [64] that as a consequence of brain injury, the IGF-1 gene transcript is induced, primarily within reactive microglia, and that the translation product, the IGF-1 protein, may act as neurotrophic and antiapoptotic substance that acts directly on the stressed cells. In a parallel phase, IGF-1 may act as a prohormone for the generation of the tripeptide glycine-proline-glutamate, released from the IGF-1 N terminus, and an additional N-terminal fragment of IGF-1, the des-N-(1–3) IGF-1. Both these IGF-1 fragments possess specific neuroprotective properties. Studies also revealed that centrally administered GH at 2 h subsequent to a hypoxic-ischemic brain injury in juvenile rats elicited a significant neuroprotection, which in a spatiotemporal pattern appeared distinct from the IGF-1-induced neuroprotective effect [64].

In some preliminary studies, it was previously shown that GH as well as IGF-1 may reduce the outcome of spinal cord trauma in the rat. Thus, topical application of the two hormones was shown to attenuate the trauma-induced edema and cell damages [9, 67]. It was further shown that GH has the capacity to improve spinal cord conduction and attenuate edema formation and cell injury in the cord indicating a potential therapeutic implication of this peptide in spinal cord injuries [68].

In human subjects, injury to the CNS is shown to attenuate the levels of circulating GH and IGF-1 [for a review, see for example ref. 9]. However, as both GH and IGF-1 display a wide array of neuroprotective activities, as demonstrated in both in vitro studies using various cell systems and in experimental animal studies, it is inviting to emphasize the potential therapeutic utility of both GH and IGF-1 in this context. As recent findings indicate that blood-born IGF-1 accounts for an important trophic source of brain cells [65], and as GH is known to use this factor as a mediator of its effects, the importance of the somatotrophic axis in therapeutic strategies for treatment of various types of CNS injury should be considered for further clinical research.

Concluding Remarks

It is evident from the above that GH as well its mediator IGF-1 may produce profound effects on brain function. The two hormones interact with the CNS on different levels. They have many effects in common, but available data also suggest that there are some differences. These differences may be of more importance in short-term treatments. There are target tissues containing receptors for both GH and IGF-1 in a variety of brain regions. They are both shown to represent important factors in the development and differentiation of the CNS and seem to induce beneficial effects on memory and cognitive disabilities. Also, both GH and IGF-1 are shown to produce protective effects in neurodegeneration and trauma to the CNS. The most important issue in this regard is to find routes for the implementation of GH and IGF-1 in therapeutic approaches to treat disorders related to impairments of the somatotrophic axis.

References

1 Andersson K, Fuxe K, Eneroth P, Isaksson O, Nyberg F, Roos P: Rat growth hormone and hypothalamic catecholamine nerve terminal systems. Evidence for rapid and discrete reductions in dopamine and noradrenaline levels and turnover in the median eminence of the hypophysectomized male rat. Eur J Pharmacol 1983;95:271–275.
2 Andersson K, Fuxe K, Eneroth P, Nyberg F, Roos P: Rat prolactin and hypothalamic catecholamine nerve terminal systems. Evidence for rapid and discrete increases in dopamine and noradrenaline turnover in the hypophysectomized male rat. Eur J Pharmacol 1981;76:261–265.
3 Posner BI, van Houten M, Patel B, Walsh RJ: Characterization of lactogen binding sites in choroid plexus. Exp Brain Res 1983;49:300–306.
4 Lai Z, Emtner M, Roos P, Nyberg F: Characterization of putative growth hormone receptors in human choroid plexus. Brain Res 1991;546:222–226.
5 Bengtsson BA, Eden S, Lonn L, Kvist H, Stokland A, Lindstedt G, Bosaeus I, Tolli J, Sjostrom L, Isaksson OG: Treatment of adults with growth hormone (GH) deficiency with recombinant human GH. J Clin Endocrinol Metab 1993;76:309–317.
6 McGauley GA, Cuneo RC, Salomon F, Sonksen PH: Psychological well-being before and after growth hormone treatment in adults with growth hormone deficiency. Horm Res 1990;33(suppl 4):52–54.
7 Lai Z, Roos P, Zhai O, Olsson Y, Fholenhag K, Larsson C, Nyberg F: Age-related reduction of human growth hormone-binding sites in the human brain. Brain Res 1993;621:260–266.
8 Nyberg F: Aging effects on growth hormone receptor binding in the brain. Exp Gerontol 1997;32:521–528.
9 Nyberg F: Growth hormone in the brain: characteristics of specific brain targets for the hormone and their functional significance. Front Neuroendocrinol 2000;21:330–348.
10 Thornwall-Le Greves M, Zhou Q, Lagerholm S, Huang W, Le Greves P, Nyberg F: Morphine decreases the levels of the gene transcripts of growth hormone receptor and growth hormone binding protein in the male rat hippocampus and spinal cord. Neurosci Lett 2001;304:69–72.

11 Le Grevés M: Growth hormone receptor message in the rat and human central nervous system; in Nyberg F (ed): The Somatotrophic Axis in Brain Function. San Diego, Elsevier Academic Press, 2006, pp 99–107.
12 Burton KA, Kabigting EB, Clifton DK, Steiner RA: Growth hormone receptor messenger ribonucleic acid distribution in the adult male rat brain and its colocalization in hypothalamic somatostatin neurons. Endocrinology 1992;131:958–963.
13 Kastrup Y, Le Greves M, Nyberg F, Blomqvist A: Distribution of growth hormone receptor mRNA in the brain stem and spinal cord of the rat. Neuroscience 2005;130:419–425.
14 Le Greves M, Steensland P, Le Greves P, Nyberg F: Growth hormone induces age-dependent alteration in the expression of hippocampal growth hormone receptor and N-methyl D aspartate receptor subunits gene transcripts in male rats. Proc Natl Acad Sci USA 2002;99:7119–7123.
15 Le Greves M, Le Greves P, Nyberg F: Age-related effects of IGF-1 on the NMDA-, GH- and IGF-1-receptor mRNA transcripts in the rat hippocampus. Brain Res Bull 2005;65:369–374.
16 Le Greves M, Zhou Q, Berg M, Le Greves P, Fholenhag K, Meyerson B, Nyberg F: Growth hormone replacement in hypophysectomized rats affects spatial performance and hippocampal levels of NMDA receptor subunit and PSD-95 gene transcript levels. Exp Brain Res 2006;173:267–273.
17 Deijen JB, de Boer H, van der Veen EA: Cognitive changes during growth hormone replacement in adult men. Psychoneuroendocrinology 1998;23:45–55.
18 Johansson JO, Larson G, Andersson M, Elmgren A, Hynsjo L, Lindahl A, Lundberg PA, Isaksson OG, Lindstedt S, Bengtsson BA: Treatment of growth hormone-deficient adults with recombinant human growth hormone increases the concentration of growth hormone in the cerebrospinal fluid and affects neurotransmitters. Neuroendocrinology 1995;61:57–66.

19 Hojvat S, Baker G, Kirsteins L, Lawrence AM: Growth hormone (GH) immunoreactivity in the rodent and primate CNS: distribution, characterization and presence posthypophysectomy. Brain Res 1982;239:543–557.
20 Mustafa A, Nyberg F, Bogdanovic N, Islam A, Roos P, Adem A: Somatogenic and lactogenic binding sites in rat brain and liver: quantitative autoradiographic localization. Neurosci Res 1994;20:257–263.
21 Burman P, Hetta J, Wide L, Mansson JE, Ekman R, Karlsson FA: Growth hormone treatment affects brain neurotransmitters and thyroxine. Clin Endocrinol (Oxf) 1996;44:319–324.
22 Ganong WF: Circumventricular organs: definition and role in the regulation of endocrine and autonomic function. Clin Exp Pharmacol Physiol 2000;27:422–427.
23 Walsh RJ, Slaby FJ, Posner BI: A receptor-mediated mechanism for the transport of prolactin from blood to cerebrospinal fluid. Endocrinology 1987;120:1846–1850.
24 Coculescu M: Blood-brain barrier for human growth hormone and insulin-like growth factor-I. J Pediatr Endocrinol Metab 1999;12:113–124.
25 Pan W, Yu Y, Cain CM, Nyberg F, Couraud PO, Kastin AJ: Permeation of growth hormone across the blood-brain barrier. Endocrinology 2005;146:4898–4904.
26 Pacold ST, Kirsteins L, Hojvat S, Lawrence AM: Biologically active pituitary hormones in the rat brain amygdaloid nucleus. Science 1978;199:804–806.
27 Lobie PE, Zhu T, Graichen R, Goh EL: Growth hormone, insulin-like growth factor I and the CNS: localization, function and mechanism of action. Growth Horm IGF Res 2000;10(suppl B):S51–S56.
28 Gossard F, Dihl F, Pelletier G, Dubois PM, Morel G: In situ hybridization to rat brain and pituitary gland of growth hormone cDNA. Neurosci Lett 1987;79:251–256.
29 Render CL, Hull KL, Harvey S: Neural expression of the pituitary GH gene. J Endocrinol 1995;147:413–422.

30 Harvey S, Kakebeeke M, Murphy AE, Sanders EJ: Growth hormone in the nervous system: autocrine or paracrine roles in retinal function? Can J Physiol Pharmacol 2003;81:371–384.
31 Donahue CP, Kosik KS, Shors TJ: Growth hormone is produced within the hippocampus where it responds to age, sex, and stress. Proc Natl Acad Sci USA 2006;103:6031–6036.
32 Han VK: Is the central nervous system a target for growth hormone and insulin-like growth factors? Acta Paediatr Suppl 1995;411:3–8.
33 Nyberg F, Burman P: Growth hormone and its receptors in the central nervous system – location and functional significance. Horm Res 1996;45:18–22.
34 Di Carlo R, Muccioli G, Papotti M, Bussolati G: Characterization of prolactin receptor in human brain and choroid plexus. Brain Res 1992;570:341–346.
35 Zhai Q, Lai Z, Roos P, Nyberg F: Characterization of growth hormone binding sites in rat brain. Acta Paediatr Suppl 1994;406:92–95.
36 Mustafa A, Adem A, Roos P, Nyberg F: Sex differences in binding of human growth hormone to rat brain. Neurosci Res 1994;19:93–99.
37 Hasegawa O, Minami S, Sugihara H, Wakabayashi I: Developmental expression of the growth hormone receptor gene in the rat hypothalamus. Brain Res Dev Brain Res 1993;74:287–290.
38 Lobie PE, Garcia-Aragon J, Lincoln DT, Barnard R, Wilcox JN, Waters MJ: Localization and ontogeny of growth hormone receptor gene expression in the central nervous system. Brain Res Dev Brain Res 1993;74:225–233.
39 Thornwall M, Chhajlani V, Le Greves P, Nyberg F: Detection of growth hormone receptor mRNA in an ovine choroid plexus epithelium cell line. Biochem Biophys Res Commun 1995;217:349–353.
40 Leung DW, Spencer SA, Cachianes G, Hammonds RG, Collins C, Henzel WJ, Barnard R, Waters MJ, Wood WI: Growth hormone receptor and serum binding protein: purification, cloning and expression. Nature 1987;330:537–543.
41 Castro JR, Costoya JA, Gallego R, Prieto A, Arce VM, Senaris R: Expression of growth hormone receptor in the human brain. Neurosci Lett 2000;281:147–150.
42 Nyberg F, Nalén B, Fhölenhag K, Fryklund L, Albertsson-Wikland K: Enzymatic release of peptide fragments from human growth hormone which displace (H)-dihydromorphine from rat brain opioid receptors. J Endocrinol Invest 1989;12(suppl 2):140.
43 Shafiei F, Herington AC, Lobie PE: Mechanism of signal transduction utilized by growth hormone; in Nyberg F (ed): The Somatotrophic Axis in Brain Function. San Diego, Elsevier Academic Press, 2006, pp 39–49.
44 Orellana DI, Quintanilla RA, Gonzalez-Billault C, Maccioni RB: Role of the JAKs/STATs pathway in the intracellular calcium changes induced by interleukin-6 in hippocampal neurons. Neurotox Res 2005;8:295–304.
45 Bennett E, McGuinness L, Gevers EF, Thomas GB, Robinson IC, Davey HW, Luckman SM: Hypothalamic STAT proteins: regulation of somatostatin neurones by growth hormone via STAT5b. J Neuroendocrinol 2005;17:186–194.
46 Ajo R, Cacicedo L, Navarro C, Sanchez-Franco F: Growth hormone action on proliferation and differentiation of cerebral cortical cells from fetal rat. Endocrinology 2003;144:1086–1097.
47 Kasagi Y, Tokita R, Nakata T, Imaki T, Minami S: Human growth hormone induces SOCS3 and CIS mRNA increase in the hypothalamic neurons of hypophysectomized rats. Endocr J 2004;51:145–154.
48 Ransome MI, Goldshmit Y, Bartlett PF, Waters MJ, Turnley AM: Comparative analysis of CNS populations in knockout mice with altered growth hormone responsiveness. Eur J Neurosci 2004;19:2069–2079.
49 Scott HJ, Stebbing MJ, Walters CE, McLenachan S, Ransome MI, Nichols NR, Turnley AM: Differential effects of SOCS2 on neuronal differentiation and morphology. Brain Res 2006;1067:138–145.
50 Savine R, Sonksen P: Growth hormone – hormone replacement for the somatopause? Horm Res 2000;53(suppl 3):37–41.
51 Svensson J, Johannsson G, Bengtsson BA: Body composition and quality of life as markers of the efficacy of growth hormone replacement therapy in adults. Horm Res 2001;55(suppl 2):55–60.
52 Sonntag WE, Ramsey M, Carter CS: Growth hormone and insulin-like growth factor-1 (IGF-1) and their influence on cognitive aging. Ageing Res Rev 2005;4:195–212.
53 Aberg ND, Brywe KG, Isgaard J: Aspects of growth hormone and insulin-like growth factor-I related to neuroprotection, regeneration, and functional plasticity in the adult brain. ScientificWorldJournal 2006;6:53–80.
54 Giordano R, Lanfranco F, Bo M, Pellegrino M, Picu A, Baldi M, Balbo M, Bonelli L, Grottoli S, Ghigo E, Arvat E: Somatopause reflects age-related changes in the neural control of GH/IGF-I axis. J Endocrinol Invest 2005;28(3 suppl):94–98.
55 Bohlooly-Y M, Olsson B, Bruder CE, Linden D, Sjogren K, Bjursell M, Egecioglu E, Svensson L, Brodin P, Waterton JC, Isaksson OG, Sundler F, Ahren B, Ohlsson C, Oscarsson J, Tornell J: Growth hormone overexpression in the central nervous system results in hyperphagia-induced obesity associated with insulin resistance and dyslipidemia. Diabetes 2005;54:51–62 (erratum published in Diabetes 2005;54:1249).
56 Egecioglu E, Bjursell M, Ljungberg A, Dickson SL, Kopchick JJ, Bergstrom G, Svensson L, Oscarsson J, Tornell J, Bohlooly-Y M: Growth hormone receptor deficiency results in blunted ghrelin feeding response, obesity, and hypolipidemia in mice. Am J Physiol Endocrinol Metab 2006;290:E317–E325.
57 Konturek SJ, Konturek JW, Pawlik T, Brzozowski T: Brain-gut axis and its role in the control of food intake. J Physiol Pharmacol 2004;55:137–154.
58 Willesen MG, Kristensen P, Romer J: Co-localization of growth hormone secretagogue receptor and NPY mRNA in the arcuate nucleus of the rat. Neuroendocrinology 1999;70:306–316.
59 Popovic V: GH Deficiency as the most common pituitary defect after TBI: clinical implications. Pituitary 2005;8:239–243.
60 Deijen JB, Arwert LI: Cognitive status of adult growth hormone (GH)-deficient patients and GH-induced neuropsychological changes; in Nyberg F (ed): The Somatotrophic Axis in Brain Function. San Diego, Elsevier Academic Press, 2006, pp 287–300.

61 Arwert LI, Veltman DJ, Deijen JB, van Dam PS, Drent ML: Effects of growth hormone substitution therapy on cognitive functioning in growth hormone deficient patients: a functional MRI study. Neuroendocrinology 2006;83:12–19.

62 van Dam PS: Neurocognitive function in adults with growth hormone deficiency. Horm Res 2005;64(suppl 3):109–114.

63 Sonntag WE, Lynch C, Thornton P, Khan A, Bennett S, Ingram R: The effects of growth hormone and IGF-1 deficiency on cerebrovascular and brain ageing. J Anat 2000;197:575–585.

64 Scheepens A, Williams CE, Breier BH, Guan J, Gluckman PD: A role for the somatotropic axis in neural development, injury and disease. J Pediatr Endocrinol Metab 2000;13(suppl 6):1483–1491.

65 Carro E, Trejo JL, Fernandez S, Fernandez AM, Torres-Aleman I: Insulin-like growth factor-1 and neuroprotection; in Nyberg F (ed): The Somatotrophic Axis in Brain Function. San Diego, Elsevier Academic Press, 2006, pp 209–215.

66 Anderson MF, Aberg MA, Nilsson M, Eriksson PS: Insulin-like growth factor-I and neurogenesis in the adult mammalian brain. Brain Res Dev Brain Res 2002;134:115–122.

67 Nyberg F, Sharma HS: Repeated topical application of growth hormone attenuates blood-spinal cord barrier permeability and edema formation following spinal cord injury: an experimental study in the rat using Evans blue, ^{125}I-sodium and lanthanum tracers. Amino Acids 2002;23:231–239.

68 Winkler T, Sharma HS, Stalberg E, Badgaiyan RD, Westman J, Nyberg F: Growth hormone attenuates alterations in spinal cord evoked potentials and cell injury following trauma to the rat spinal cord. An experimental study using topical application of rat growth hormone. Amino Acids 2000;19:363–371.

Review of Methods for Body Composition Assessment in Children

Jonathan C.K. Wells

Recent studies are increasingly emphasising the benefits of information about body composition in paediatric research and clinical practice. Almost all paediatric diseases adversely affect body composition, and treatments can influence and sometimes reverse such changes. Many such effects are too subtle to be inferred from changes in weight, leading to growing interest in the measurement of body composition itself. Whilst the recent emergence of an epidemic of childhood obesity has drawn attention to high levels of body fat, in many diseases, lean mass is also affected. Both fat mass and lean mass are important health outcomes. High levels of body fat adversely impact on health during childhood [1] and predispose to cardiovascular disease and diabetes in later life [2]. Low levels of lean mass tend to be associated with poorer physiological function and, through their association with bone deposition [3], may increase the risk of osteoporosis in later life.

Due to the ease with which weight and height can be measured in most contexts, weight for height and more recently body mass index (BMI; calculated as weight divided by the square of height) have long comprised the primary body composition outcome in paediatric clinical practice. With the growing interest in body composition has come increasing recognition that BMI is insufficient for this purpose. This review will first highlight the limitations of BMI as a measure of childhood body composition and then discuss other approaches with greater accuracy.

Body Mass Index and Body Composition

The statistical rationale of BMI is that it adjusts weight (WT) for variability in height (HT):

$$BMI = WT/HT^2 \qquad \text{(equation 1)}$$

Ideally, BMI should have zero correlation with stature, and hence, rank individuals in terms of their relative weight. Several studies have demonstrated its success in this context [4, 5], and even though at some ages (e.g., early infancy, puberty) a small residual correlation remains between weight and stature, this has a negligible effect on ranking. Thus, from a statistical point of view,

Childhood Nutrition Research Centre
Institute of Child Health
30 Guilford Street
London WC1N 1EH (UK)

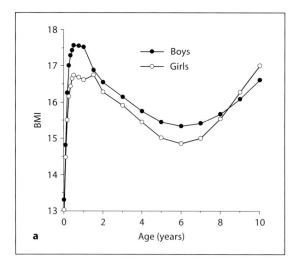
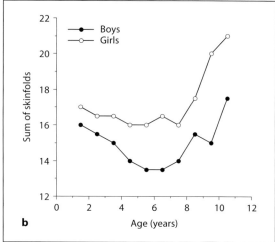
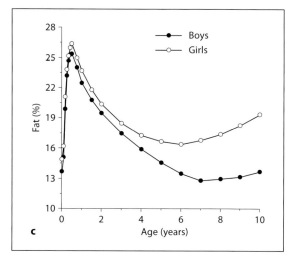

Fig. 1. Associations between indices of body composition and age. BMI (**a**); triceps skinfold (**b**); percentage of fat (**c**). Data are taken from Fomon et al. [7] and Ryan et al. [8].

BMI successfully adjusts weight for height. The critical question is, what information is actually conveyed by relative weight?

As demonstrated in numerous studies [6, 7], BMI has a characteristic relationship with age (fig. 1a). Values rise rapidly during infancy, decline to a nadir in mid-childhood and then increase again towards adult values. These patterns appear to have consistency with indices of adiposity, such as skinfold thicknesses [8] or percent fat [7] (although note that the sexual dimorphism for BMI is the reverse of that for the other two outcomes). Thus, figures 1b and c illustrate the age-related development of the sum of two skinfold thicknesses and the percentage of fat for comparison. The increase in BMI during mid-childhood has been referred to as the 'adiposity rebound' [9], and the time of its occurrence has been proposed to be an important factor in the risk of developing obesity. It is also clear that within any given age group, a group of individuals with very high BMI is likely to have high levels of body fat [10]. Collectively, this has led to a general perception that BMI is a useful index of adiposity in individuals, reflecting the approach adopted for adults.

In adults, BMI is used to categorise the nutritional status across the entire spectrum of body weight. The World Health Organisation categorises chronic energy deficiency as BMI <18.5 [11], while Garrow and Webster [12] proposed that normal weight be categorised as BMI 20–25, overweight as BMI 25–30, and obesity as BMI >30. This classification remains widely used despite evidence that central obesity (as indicated by waist circumference) varies widely for a given BMI value [13] and that waist circumference is a stronger predictor of cardiovascular risk factors [14]. Because in children BMI values change with age [6], the approach used in adults cannot be adopted directly. Instead, individual children are ranked in terms of BMI standard deviation scores, with centile cut-offs used to identify childhood overweight and obesity. Currently, these cut-offs are based on the back-extrapolation of adult values to equivalent values at earlier ages [15].

The hypothesis that individual variability in childhood BMI is proportional to variability in body fat is not well supported by evidence. Although some studies have reported relatively high correlations between BMI and percent fat [16, 17], this apparent level of agreement is an artefact of the wide range of body weights and percent fat studied. In the middle part of the range, where the majority of the population lie, the agreement between these variables is very poor. Furthermore, the use of percent fat as the reference index of adiposity in such analyses is also problematic. Percent fat refers to the proportion of fat in body weight. Since in all individuals percent fat and percent lean must add up to 100%, it can be seen that percent fat is not an independent index of adiposity, but is influenced by the relative amount of lean mass [18]. There are also statistical problems with the index, given that fat mass is present in both the numerator and the denominator (weight) [19].

These problems can be resolved by adopting a more sophisticated approach to the expression of body composition data. The simplest model of body composition divides weight (WT) into fat mass (FM) and lean mass (LM) components:

$$WT = LM + FM \qquad \text{(equation 2)}$$

Although a variety of more complex body composition models have been used, for example distinguishing the mineral, protein and water in lean mass, or the distribution of fat in different regional depots, the two-component model described in equation 2 is adequate for many purposes. Van Itallie et al. [20] proposed that equations 1 and 2 could be combined in order to divide BMI into its fat and lean components:

$$BMI = LM/HT^2 + FM/HT^2 \qquad \text{(equation 3)}$$

These two terms, known as the lean mass index (LMI) and the fat mass index (FMI), represent separate indices adjusting both lean mass and fat mass for height. Therefore, they are intended to be independent both of height and each other and allow investigation of two body composition outcomes. However, it is not inevitable that the power by which height should be raised, in order to adjust both lean and fat mass, will always be 2. An analysis of this issue in 8-year-old children found that whereas LM/HT^2 did adjust successfully for height, the optimal index for fat mass was FM/HT^6 [18]. This difference can be attributed to inconsistency in the degree of variability in the three terms HT, LM and FM, with FM having greater between-individual variability than the other two terms. Nevertheless, the index FM/HT^2 retains only a moderate correlation with height, such that <2% of the variability can be attributed to the effect of height [18]. Thus, the two indices derived from equation 3 are adequate for most purposes and will be problematic only when comparing 2 individuals or 2 groups differing markedly in height. The great advantage of LMI and FMI is that they are presented in the same units as BMI and hence facilitate analyses.

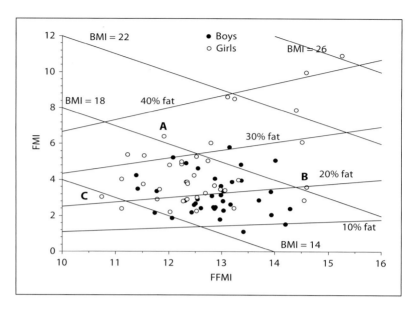

Fig. 2. Hattori chart plotting lean mass adjusted for height on the x-axis against fat mass adjusted for height on the y-axis. The data represent 75 children aged 8 years. The letters A and B identify 2 girls with almost identical BMI, but markedly different FMI and percent fat values, while the letters B and C identify 2 girls with almost identical FMI and percent fat values, but markedly different BMI. Reprinted with permission from Wells [83].

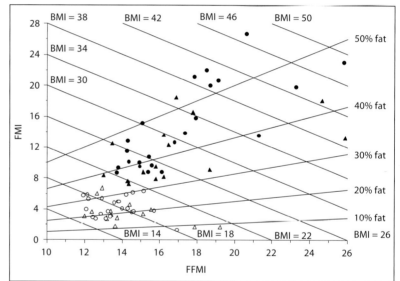

Fig. 3. Hattori chart illustrating the wide variety in proportions of lean and fat masses for a given BMI value in obese children. ○ = Non-obese girls; △ = non-obese boys; ● = obese girls; ▲ = obese boys. Reproduced with permission from Wells et al. [10].

For example, Hattori et al. [21] have devised a graph plotting FMI on the y-axis against LMI on the x-axis. Since in any individual, FMI and LMI must add up to BMI, the graph also shows diagonal lines of constant BMI value, and it is possible to add further nonparallel lines of constant percent fat value. These Hattori graphs elegantly illustrate the limitations of BMI as an index of adiposity in individuals. Figure 2 illustrates data from a sample of 75 normal healthy children aged 8 years. It can be seen that individual children of the same age and sex may vary up to 2-fold in percent fat for a given BMI value, which can be attributed to the fact that children vary substantially in their LMI as well as their FMI [22]. This variability is apparent from early

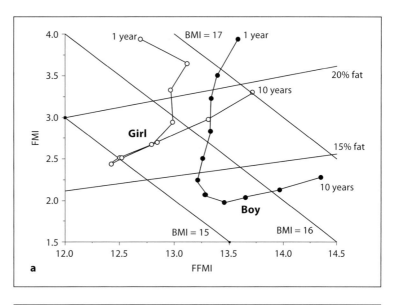

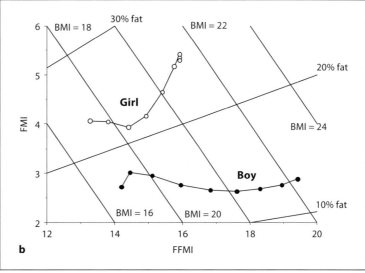

Fig. 4. Hattori charts illustrating the changing relationship between the fat and lean masses adjusted for height with age. **a** Data from the reference child of Fomon et al. [7], with sequential data points at 1 year, 18 months, and then annually from 2 to 10 years of age. **b** Data from the reference adolescent of Haschke [23], with sequential data points from 11.5 to 18.5 years. Both figures illustrate the significant contribution of increased lean mass to greater BMI with age, particularly in boys. Reproduced with permission from Wells et al. [10, 84].

infancy onwards [22] and remains present at the extremes of nutritional status. Figure 3 illustrates the same scenario for a population of obese children. Again, it can be seen that individuals, all with high BMI, vary substantially in the relative contributions of fat and lean to their weight [10].

The same graphs illustrate the limitations of BMI as an indicator of the developmental patterns of body composition. Figure 4 plots data from the reference child of Fomon et al. [7] and the reference adolescent of Haschke [23]. From 6 years of age, it can be seen that increases in BMI are substantially due to increasing LMI rather than FMI, particularly in boys [22]. In adolescence, the two sexes diverge markedly, with increasing BMI attributable almost entirely to LMI in the boy, but largely to FMI in the girl. Studies of individual children are consistent with these descriptions of average children, with the majority of increasing BMI attributable to lean mass [24]. Collectively, these data demonstrate the fallacy of the concept of a generic adiposity rebound expressed by increasing BMI. It has also been pointed out that the time of BMI rebound (the nadir in BMI value) is an artefact of BMI centile, such that heavier individuals, for statistical rather than biological reasons, tend to have an earlier increase in BMI centile [25].

In addition to the above limitations as an index of body fat in individuals, BMI is also confounded by population differences. In adults, for example, ethnic groups differ in the average body fat content for a given BMI value [26]. This has led to the derivation of ethnic-specific BMI cutoffs for defining overweight and obesity [27]. The same scenario is apparent in childhood [28, 29]. At any given BMI value, Asian children tend to have a higher level of body fat. These ethnic differences in body composition are of considerable importance given the central role of obesity, especially central obesity, in the aetiology of the metabolic syndrome, and ethnic variability in adiposity is believed to represent one of the mechanisms underlying the greater vulnerability to cardiovascular disease of some populations compared with others [30].

There is also some indication that the relationship between BMI and body fat alters over time. This issue remains difficult to reliably investigate due to the lack of high-quality data on children's body composition from prior decades. Nevertheless, several data sets indicate that secular increases in adiposity indices are greater than secular increases in BMI [31–33], an inconsistency that would imply a secular decrease in lean mass [31]. Such a decrease is highly plausible if children's activity levels have indeed declined, as is widely hypothesised. However, again, it is difficult to obtain reliable data on secular trends in childhood physical activity. Exercise is an established stimulant of lean mass during childhood [34]; hence, it remains plausible that changes in lifestyle have predisposed to both increasing levels of adiposity and lower levels of lean mass in contemporary children compared with those of previous decades. This hypothesis merits further attention, because it would indicate that the health consequences of high BMI could be worse in the current generation compared with previous generations of children [31].

BMI may be particularly misleading as an index of body fat in disease states where both fat mass and lean mass have been influenced. In some patients, growth of lean mass is constrained. Often dieticians feed up such patients on the assumption that the weight gain improves health; however, the weight gain may be entirely fat. In 2 patients with a rare condition called 'myofibromatosis', BMI Z scores were around –3, but measurements of body composition demonstrated 40% fat [35]. Thus, the low weight of these patients could be attributed to very low lean mass, and energy intake could not be assumed to be constraining growth. Similarly, a recent clinical trial evaluating provision of a gastrostomy to paediatric patients with cerebral palsy found that the additional weight gained by those receiving a gastrostomy was primarily fat [36].

A second area where BMI is particularly problematic as an outcome is the association between early growth and later body composition. Many studies have reported a positive correlation between birth weight and later BMI [37], which has often been interpreted as indicating that fat neonates have a higher risk of obesity in later life. A recent systematic review identified both high birth rate and rapid infant weight gain as risk factors for high childhood BMI [38]. However, more detailed studies have found that birth weight has little or no systematic association with later fat mass, and instead, predicts later lean mass [39–42]. Two studies undertaken in developing countries have extended these observations to weight gain in infancy, demonstrating that greater weight gain in the first few months of life is associated with greater lean mass but not fat mass in later childhood [42, 43]. However, similar studies in industrialised populations have suggested that infant weight gain may also predict later body fat [44]. This issue remains in need of further research, as the studies differ in the period of infancy investigated. Nevertheless, it is clear that there is a strong association between early weight gain and later lean mass, whereas high levels of weight gain in childhood tend to make a greater contribution to later adiposity [42, 43].

BMI is highly correlated with all the major components of body weight, including fat mass, lean mass and skeletal mineral mass. It is because it is correlated with each of these variables that it acts as a reliable proxy of none of them – for example, its capacity to express adiposity is confounded by its association with lean mass. There is no doubt that BMI remains an important tool for the paediatrician, enabling a simple, rapid and convenient evaluation of nutritional status. Rapid increases in BMI act as an index of excess weight gain in individuals, since any child rapidly increasing in BMI standard deviation score is likely to be gaining primarily fat and being at risk of obesity. For the epidemiologist, BMI may reveal broad trends within and between populations in relative weight and varying associations with variables such as socioeconomic status [45]. BMI also remains the current approach for categorising obesity, although its specificity for this task is better than its sensitivity, and waist circumference is increasingly used as a more sensitive index of central adiposity [46]. However, as an index of body composition in individuals, the limitations of BMI are unresolvable.

Body Composition in Different Contexts

Body composition itself is of interest in a number of different contexts. First, in order to guide clinical practice, clinicians require an evidence base derived from epidemiological studies and clinical trials. In such studies, the requirement is for a practical method capable of discerning the desired outcome with a relatively consistent level of error. Outcomes may range from global assessments of whole-body fat or lean masses to specific regional evaluations of muscle mass or visceral fat mass. Second, clinicians require methods capable of guiding the treatment of individual children in routine clinical practice. Once again, the optimal methods will depend on the outcome of interest.

A recent review of body composition techniques highlighted a wide variety of methods capable of contributing to these varied requirements [47]. The accuracy of any method requires evaluation against a reference method. The gold standard for body composition is cadaver dissection, and hence, all in vivo methods are imperfect and rely on assumptions. Currently, the most accurate in vivo techniques are multi-component models for the chemical composition of the body and magnetic resonance imaging (MRI) for regional tissue distributions. Where possible, other techniques should be evaluated against these references, and the literature increasingly reflects this ideal.

Simple Anthropometric Markers

Although BMI itself is a poor index of adiposity in individuals, other anthropometric measurements provide accurate and sensitive information about relative fat mass. Humans store fat largely in peripheral subcutaneous depots, which can be evaluated using skinfold calipers or girth measurements. Measurements of skinfold thicknesses have been used in paediatric clinical practice and research for decades. These measurements have a reputation for being unpopular with children and having poor precision particularly in relation to inter-observer error. In most cases, these concerns are unfounded. Infants and children from 4 years onwards tend to tolerate skinfold measurements very well. Toddlers are less accepting of the technique, but it can be used in research studies and in some patients in this age group. The imprecision of skinfold measurements derives from two factors: first, inconsistency in locating the site to be measured, and second, inconsistency in the style of measurement. In obese children, this error is significant, and it is often hard to identify an appropriate skinfold; hence, measurements are less useful in this disease state. However, in the vast majority of other scenarios, variability between individuals is substantially greater than inter-observer error, and the technique is worthwhile.

Skinfold thickness data are of greatest value if left in their raw state. In this form, they provide accurate evaluations of specific subcutaneous fat depots. The main difficulty lies in interpreting the data. Centile charts for children were published several decades ago [48] but are unlikely to be representative of contemporary children, given the recent obesity epidemic. Therefore, there is a need for updated reference data against which individual measurements can be evaluated. Such data have recently been published for UK infants [49] and are being collected for UK children. With such data, skinfold measurements represent a highly convenient and reliable assessment of subcutaneous adiposity, also suitable for longitudinal monitoring.

It is often assumed that skinfold data are of greatest benefit if incorporated into equations which predict whole-body fat mass, and hence, by difference in weight, lean mass [50, 51]. However, such equations suffer from a major limitation common to all predictive techniques in assuming that all individuals have the average relationship between the raw data and the predicted outcome. Figure 5 illustrates the generic scenario for a predictive method, showing the relationship between raw data on the x-axis (e.g., sum of four skinfolds) and outcome (e.g., body density) on the y-axis. Using the empirically determined regression line, all individuals are treated as if their

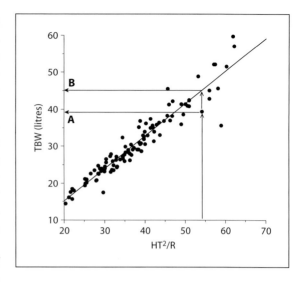

Fig. 5. Relationship between two variables in a predictive method, where the variable on the x-axis is used to predict the outcome on the y-axis. Here, impedance adjusted for height is used to predict TBW, while other examples include the sum of four skinfold thicknesses used to predict body density. The regression slope describes the best-fit relationship between the variables; however, the individual data points are scattered around this line. Therefore, use of the regression equation assumes that all individuals have the average y value for a given x value, resulting in a significant difference between the actual y value (A) and the predicted y value (B).

values lie along the line, whereas in reality, as shown in the plot, the individual data points are scattered around the line. The slope of the regression line also tends to differ between populations. Therefore, predictive equations introduce significant error to both individual and group data [52], and their values have substantially greater inaccuracy than the raw data. Finally, it is worth emphasising that regional data on adiposity may be much more informative than a single whole-body value.

The one limitation of skinfold thickness measurements is that they are unable to directly address intra-abdominal adipose tissue, the depot most strongly associated with adverse outcomes.

The gold standard for measuring internal adiposity is MRI, as discussed below. However, waist circumference has been shown to be a robust and valid index of abdominal adiposity in children [53], and a recent study found that waist circumference explained 65% of the variability in visceral adipose tissue [54]. These studies indicate an important role for waist circumference in monitoring abdominal adiposity, as increasingly advocated [46]. The availability of reference data [55] is also a major benefit for this outcome.

Arm anthropometry attempts to evaluate the relative contributions of fat mass and lean mass in the limb. Using a combination of mid upper arm girth and triceps skinfold thickness, the cross-sectional areas of lean and fat can be estimated [56]. Although this approach is widely used due to its convenience, a recent evaluation indicated that the derived index of arm fat was no better than the triceps skinfold itself at ranking body fat, and that after adjustment for body size, the derived index of arm lean explained only 30–40% of the variability in arm or whole-body lean mass [57].

Despite the profusion of more sophisticated techniques discussed below, anthropometry deserves to maintain a central role in the paediatrician's toolkit. Anthropometric techniques are convenient, cheap, portable, non-invasive and can be repeated at regular intervals. As with all techniques, they are of greatest value when used with high-quality reference data. The combination of raw skinfold thickness measurements and waist circumference standard deviation score offers a highly informative assessment of adiposity in individuals, arguably only bettered by MRI. Although other techniques are more accurate for determining total body fat mass, in many contexts, regional data are sufficient or even preferable for evaluating adiposity and monitoring progress. However, anthropometry cannot address lean mass satisfactorily.

Bioelectrical Impedance Analysis

Like anthropometric techniques, bioelectrical impedance analysis (BIA) appears to satisfy the requirements for a cheap, simple, portable and non-invasive method. Numerous studies have been undertaken in infants and children; however, the technique has so far failed to live up to its potential.

The generic theoretical basis of the technique is that the resistance or impedance of the body to a minor current passed between two anatomical locations is proportional to the water contained in the tissue in between. Using data from a sample of individuals, empirical equations can be developed relating an impedance index (typically height squared divided by impedance; HT^2/R) to total body water (TBW), allowing the prediction of TBW. In practice, a number of factors confound this association. First, as with skinfold equations, the slope of the regression line is dependent on the population studied, and hence, separate equations are required for different age groups, ethnic groups and patient groups [58, 59]. Second, individual variability in physique confounds the association between HT^2/R and TBW, leading to poor predictive accuracy in individuals [60]. Third, many diseases influence fluid distribution, and thus, distort the theoretical association. Even in healthy children, BIA has been shown to have poor accuracy in individuals, predicting percentage of fat with typical limits of agreement of ±8% [52]. This level of error indicates that BIA cannot be considered a robust approach for monitoring body composition in individuals at the current time. It is possible that future work may result in the development of more sophisticated equations with greater accuracy.

At present, the main role of conventional BIA is that of an epidemiological technique. In contrast to BMI, BIA expresses data in all age groups in the form of fat and lean masses and can therefore crudely identify trends within and between groups in both adiposity and lean masses. For example, BIA successfully illustrates the fact that birth weight predicts later lean mass rather than fat mass, with the same association demonstrated using other body composition methodologies [41].

In addition to its conventional role as a predictor of body water, BIA can also be used to assess fluid distribution. At low frequencies, the current is passed only through extra-cellular water, whereas at high frequencies, the electrical current is passed through intra-cellular water as well. By making measurements across a range of frequencies, it is possible to estimate the relationship between extra- and intra-cellular water, and hence, evaluate fluid distribution [61]. Therefore, multifrequency BIA has the potential to be a valuable clinical tool in monitoring fluid distribution. Research is increasingly focusing on this technique in adults and children; however, it is not yet available for routine clinical application. Other applications of BIA include use of the phase angle to determine physiological quality of the cell mass [62]. Thus, the technique merits further development and is likely to make significant contributions to clinical practice in the future, but more in relation to the quality than the quantity of lean mass.

Two-Component Techniques

A variety of techniques are now available for differentiating the fat and lean components of body weight. These include isotope dilution for measurement of TBW, dual-energy X-ray absorptiometry (DXA), densitometry and total body electrical conductivity (TOBEC). Each technique has its pros and cons, along with a specific theoretical basis which limits the contexts in which the technique will be accurate.

The principle of isotope dilution measurements is that isotopes of water (^{2}H or ^{18}O) can be used to dilute and thus quantify TBW [63]. These isotopes are non-toxic, non-radioactive and naturally occurring, and hence, present no ethical issues. Therefore, making assumptions about the hydration of lean tissue, TBW can be used to estimate lean mass. Of all the body composition techniques, isotope dilution is the most versatile, being practical in virtually all contexts, age groups and disease states. The measurement requires only collection of body fluid samples (saliva, urine or blood) before and after administration of a dose of labelled water. The dose can be given as fruit juice or milk in younger age groups, and through a gastrostomy tube in patients, or if suitably sterilised, through a parenteral nutrition line. The technique is robust for determining body water, though if the subject has oedema, it is necessary to adopt a more sophisticated protocol for sample collection. The main factor limiting its application is the validity of the assumption that lean mass has a known water content. In healthy subjects, hydration is tightly regulated and variability is within ±1.5% [52], though varying in relation to age and sex [7]. However, some disease states exert further effects on hydration. In some diseases, the alteration is of modest magnitude and similar in all individuals. For example, in young female patients with cystic fibrosis, mean hydration is significantly different from that of healthy children, due to delayed puberty, but the variability is similar, allowing a disease-specific correction factor to be applied [Williams, Wells and Fewtrell, unpubl. data]. In these circumstances, isotope dilution remains a relatively accurate approach for assessment of body composition, particularly if an appropriate correction factor can be applied. Where fluid distribution is altered, and the extent of this alteration varies between individuals, isotope dilution needs to be combined with other techniques, as discussed below.

DXA is increasingly available in hospitals, and in some countries, especially the US, is now regarded as a gold standard body composition technique. The method relies on the differential attenuation of X-rays by bone, fat and lean tissue in order to distinguish these three components of body weight [64]. The technique has high precision, but its accuracy is poorer than is often assumed. The method first distinguishes pixels with and without bone. In those pixels lacking bone, the method then distinguishes fat and lean tissue. This information is used to infer soft tissue composition of those pixels containing bone. Thus, the technique only measures soft tissue directly in non-bone pixels, and in the trunk, much of the data is an estimation rather than a measurement. Studies comparing DXA against multicomponent models have generally reported good agreement; however, most of these studies have been conducted in healthy adults within the normal range of weight. Recent evaluations have incorporated a wide range of age, body size and adiposity and have also considered disease states. These studies demonstrated that the bias of DXA varies systematically in relation to adiposity, size, gender and disease state [65]. On this basis, DXA cannot be considered optimal for case-control studies, or for longitudinal evaluations, since the bias will differ between groups or time points. Nevertheless, DXA is capable of contributing to routine patient care, in particular because of its capacity to estimate both total and regional lean mass. Of all the techniques currently available, it remains the most practical for this purpose in routine care. For example, measurements by DXA have recently been used to estimate the TBW for the calculation of dialysis dosages [66]. This approach proved substantially more accurate than the conventional alternative of predicting body water from weight and height.

Densitometry is one of the older approaches to body composition, relying on the theoretical basis that fat and lean tissues have predictable densities [67]. Using Archimedes' principle, measurement of whole-body density can be used to calculate the proportion of fat and lean in body weight. Fat has a constant density in all age groups, but in children, as for lean mass hydration, age- and sex-specific values for lean mass density are required [7]. Body density, requiring measurements of weight and volume, was traditionally measured using underwater weighing. This technique is clearly inappropriate for the majority of the paediatric population, especially patients. However, in the last decade, an alternative technique has been developed, known as whole-body air displacement plethysmography [68]. This technique involves the subject sitting in a small chamber (the Bodpod®) for a couple of minutes while changes in air pressure and temperature are monitored in order to estimate body volume. The technique is well tolerated by children of 4 years upwards and is increasingly widely used in research studies. A smaller plethysmograph suitable for the age range between birth and 6 months has also been recently developed (the Peapod®; fig. 6) [69], and a similar version for the toddler age range is under development. Validation studies suggest that the technique has acceptable accuracy for the measurement of body volume [70, 71]. However, further analyses have identified significant variability, both within populations and between disease states, in the density of lean tissue, due to variability in the water and mineral content [52, 72, 73]. This variability confounds the use of Archimedes' principle for distinguishing fat and lean masses and increases both individual error and group accuracy in any given disease state. Therefore, as a clinical technique, the accuracy of densitometry remains dependent on the accuracy of assumptions about lean mass density. It can be used to evaluate broad trends and may be particularly useful in monitoring changes in obese patients, since changes in their gross body composition are likely to be of considerably greater magnitude than changes in their lean tissue composition. Furthermore, as with isotope probes, disease-specific values for the density of lean mass may be obtained from empirical research and used in subsequent applications to improve accuracy. However, the greatest value of plethysmography is its role in multicomponent techniques (see below).

TOBEC has a theoretical basis similar to BIA, attempting to predict TBW and hence lean mass from bioelectrical properties. The measurement involves the subject being placed inside a solenoid coil. The equipment is not widely available, being restricted to specialist research centres, and although the accuracy of TOBEC is greater than that of BIA, it remains based on empirical studies relating bioelectrical data to body water. The technique loses accuracy when body properties alter, for example, when the subject is suffering from fever.

Total body potassium scanning likewise requires access to specialised instrumentation and is not a widely available technique. Unlike other two-component techniques which quantify lean mass, potassium scanning estimates the body cell mass. The technique is based on the principle that the cell mass contains a predictable level of ^{40}K, which emits a constant gamma signal that can be quantified using sensitive detectors. Due to inconsistencies between individuals in the potassium content of lean mass, the technique is not an accurate method for the quantification of fat or lean masses. However, cell mass is often a more useful outcome than lean mass, being the most functional component of lean mass. For example during malnutrition, the cell mass undergoes considerably greater change than the skeletal or connective tissue. Potassium scanning is used in some hospitals to monitor the composition of weight gain in paediatric patients with eating disorders [74], or to monitor body composition in patients with cystic fibrosis [75]. The technique merits wider application in clinical practice and could make an important contribution in children's hospitals.

Regional body composition can be measured by radiographic techniques such as computerized tomography (CT) scanning or MRI. The former technique is unsuitable for whole-body paediatric use due to the high radiation exposure. However, recently, a peripheral quantitative CT has emerged. CT scans use multiple cross-sectional

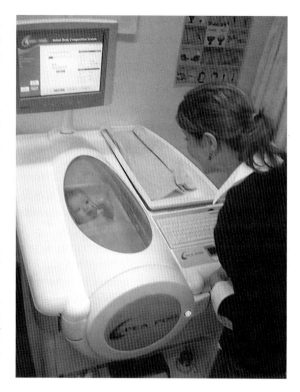

Fig. 6. A whole-body air displacement plethysmograph suitable for infants within the age range from birth to 6 months, known as the Peapod. The instrumentation collects data on body weight and body volume in order to calculate body density for estimation of body fat by the Archimedes principle. The technique can be used on its own as a densitometric method, or combined with isotope dilution and DXA in a multi-component model. Printed with permission from Life Measurements Inc.

X-rays to construct a 3-dimensional volumetric model of bone, muscle and fat tissue. Peripheral quantitative CT is designed to scan only specific limb sites such as the radius or tibia. Measurements are made during a 1- to 2-min period, and the radiation dose is acceptable for children at <2 μSV. Focusing on the limbs, the technique represents a significant contribution to the capacity to measure muscle mass [76], although measurements refer to a cross-sectional area within a given location (similar to arm anthropometry) rather than to total limb lean mass as provided by DXA. Reference data now exist for children [77]; however, care is needed with respect to differences between types of instrumentation [78].

MRI scanning does not involve radiation, and instead, measures the alignment of hydrogen nuclei in a magnetic field. Variability in the density of hydrogen nuclei is proportional to the water content of the tissue, allowing the technique to discriminate tissues of different water content. Raw data are obtained in transverse 'slices', which can be summed in order to provide regional or whole-body volumes. In contrast to the techniques described above, MRI scanning differentiates with high accuracy the location of different tissue types. Of all the techniques, it is the only one that can quantify intra-abdominal adipose tissue, in particular the visceral fat depot [79], which is most strongly associated with adverse health outcomes. It is also the most accurate technique for measurement of regional muscle mass [80] and can be used to quantify the organ masses. However, it should be noted that adipose tissue is not equivalent to fat mass, and hence, the technique measures a different outcome to the other methods discussed above. Again, the technique is only available in specialised centres and is expensive. In the foreseeable future, the main contribution of MRI will be to the evidence base for underpinning clinical practice, providing the most accurate data on regional body composition and tissue composition in research studies.

Multicomponent Models

In healthy individuals, two-component techniques generally offer sufficient accuracy for the measurement of whole-body lean and fat masses. In disease states where the composition of tissues, and hence tissue properties, are altered, it is necessary to combine techniques in order to achieve acceptable accuracy.

Many diseases influence the composition of lean mass, for example altering the mineral or water content. Such changes can be addressed by three- or four-component models, which provide information both on the composition of lean tissue and on properties such as the hydration or density of lean tissue. The three-component model requires measurements of body weight, body volume and body water, by plethysmography and isotope dilution, respectively. These data allow differentiation of fat mass, water mass and the mass of fat-free dry tissue (containing mineral, protein, glycogen and free amino acids) [52]. The four-component model further incorporates measurement of bone mineral mass by DXA, and hence, separates the manual component of fat-free dry tissue [52]. The application of the four-component model in obese children has highlighted many effects of this condition on tissue composition, with obese children having an increased water content and decreased mineral content of lean mass, as well as a lower density of lean tissue [10]. The four-component model represents the most accurate in vivo technique for differentiation of fat and lean tissue and is increasingly used in research studies.

An alternative multi-component approach involves addressing water distribution. In healthy individuals, there is a predictable relationship between intra-cellular and extra-cellular water. Many disease states perturb this relationship, for example, in obesity, the extra-cellular space expands [81]. Water distribution can be evaluated by combining two probes, one for the estimation of TBW and the other for the estimation of extra-cellular water, allowing calculation of intra-cellular water by difference. Extra-cellular water can be quantified by sodium bromide dilution [82], though in the future, multi-frequency BIA may also contribute in this context. Unlike deuterium dilution, bromide dilution requires blood samples before dose administration and after equilibration. The calculation of extra-cellular water is also more difficult than that of TBW, requiring several correction factors and assumptions to be applied [82]. However, this approach is merited in research on critically ill children.

Summary

This review has described a variety of body composition methodologies that can be used in paediatric research and clinical practice. Different techniques are appropriate for different functions and applications [47], but any technique becomes much more valuable for paediatric application if appropriate reference data are available. It is inevitable that routine clinical care will favour simpler, cheaper and more portable techniques; however, it is also clear from rapidly accumulating research studies that body composition is an important indication of health, that it predicts future risk or outcome, and that it merits increased attention. Consequently, there is a need both for continued development of practical and viable techniques, but also for greater incorporation of sophisticated methodologies in research studies to provide the evidence base to underpin practice.

References

1 Reilly JJ, Methven E, McDowell ZC, Hacking B, Alexander D, Stewart L, Kelnar CJ: Health consequences of obesity. Arch Dis Child 2003;88:748–752.
2 Power C, Lake JK, Cole TJ: Measurement and long-term health risks of child and adolescent fatness. Int J Obes Relat Metab Disord 1997;21:507–526.
3 Rauch F, Bailey DA, Baxter-Jones A, Mirwald R, Faulkner R: The 'muscle-bone unit' during the pubertal growth spurt. Bone 2004;34:771–775.
4 Cole TJ: Weight/height^p compared to weight/height^2 for assessing adiposity in childhood: influence of age and bone age on p during puberty. Ann Hum Biol 1986;13:433–451.
5 Gasser T, Ziegler P, Seifert B, Prader A, Molinari L, Largo R: Measures of body mass and of obesity from infancy to adulthood and their appropriate transformation. Ann Hum Biol 1994;21:111–125.
6 Cole TJ, Freeman JV, Preece MA: Body mass index reference curves for the UK, 1990. Arch Dis Child 1995;73:25–29.
7 Fomon SJ, Haschke F, Ziegler EE, Nelson SE: Body composition of reference children from birth to age 10 years. Am J Clin Nutr 1982;35:1169–1175.
8 Ryan AS, Martinez GA, Baumgartner RN, Roche AF, Guo S, Chumlea WC, Kuczmarski RJ: Median skinfold thickness distributions and fat-wave patterns in Mexican-American children from the Hispanic Health and Nutrition Examination Surveys (HHANES 1982–1984). Am J Clin Nutr 1990;51:925S–935S.
9 Rolland-Cachera MF, Deheeger M, Bellisle F, Sempé M, Guilloud-Bataille M, Patois E: Adiposity rebound in children: a simple indicator for predicting obesity. Am J Clin Nutr 1984;39:129–135.
10 Wells JC, Fewtrell MS, Williams JE, Haroun D, Lawson MS, Cole TJ: Body composition in normal weight, overweight and obese children: matched case-control analyses of total and regional tissue masses, and body composition trends in relation to relative weight. Int J Obes (Lond) 2006;30:1506–1513.
11 James WPT, Ferro-Luzzi A, Waterlow JC: Definition of chronic energy deficiency in adults. Eur J Clin Nutr 1994;42:969–981.
12 Garrow JS, Webster J: Quetelet's index (W/H^2) as a measure of fatness. Int J Obes 1985;9:147–153.
13 Wells JCK, Treleaven P, Cole TJ: BMI compared with 3D body shape. The UK National Sizing Survey. Am J Clin Nutr, in press.
14 Savva SC, Tornaritis M, Savva ME, Kourides Y, Panagi A, Silikiotou N, Georgiou C, Kafatos A: Waist circumference and waist-to-height ratio are better predictors of cardiovascular disease risk factors in children than body mass index. Int J Obes Relat Metab Disord 2000;24:1453–1458.
15 Cole TJ, Bellizzi MC, Flegal KM, Dietz WH: Establishing a standard definition for child overweight and obesity worldwide: international survey. BMJ 2000;320:1240–1243.
16 Pietrobelli A, Faith MS, Allison DB, Gallagher D, Chiumello G, Heymsfield SB: Body mass index as a measure of adiposity among children and adolescents: a validation. J Pediatr 1998;132:204–210.
17 Chan YL, Leung SSF, Lam WWM, Peng XM, Metreweli C: Body fat estimation in children by magnetic resonance imaging, bioelectrical impedance, skinfold and body mass index: a pilot study. J Paediatr Child Health 1998;34:22–28.
18 Wells JCK, Cole TJ, ALSPAC study team: Adjustment of fat-free mass and fat mass for height in children aged 8 years. Int J Obes Relat Metab Disord 2002;26:947–952.
19 Wells JCK, Victora CG: Indices of whole-body and central adiposity for evaluating the metabolic load of obesity. Int J Obes (Lond) 2005;29:483–489.

20 Van Itallie TB, Yang MU, Heymsfield SB, Funk RC, Boileau RA: Height-normalised indices of the body's fat-free mass and fat mass: potentially useful indicators of nutritional status. Am J Clin Nutr 1990;52:953–959.
21 Hattori K, Tatsumi N, Tanaka S: Assessment of body composition by using a new chart method. Am J Hum Biol 1997;9:573–578.
22 Wells JCK: A Hattori chart analysis of body mass index in infancy and childhood. Int J Obes Relat Metab Disord 2000;24:325–329.
23 Haschke F: Body composition during adolescence; in Klish WJ, Kretchmer N (eds): Body Composition in Infants and Children: Report of the 98th Ross Conference on Pediatric Research. Columbus, Ross Laboratories, 1989, pp 76–83.
24 Maynard LM, Wisemandle W, Roche AF, Chumlea WC, Guo SS, Siervogel RM: Childhood body composition in relation to body mass index. Pediatrics 2001;107:344–350.
25 Cole TJ: Children grow and horses race: is the adiposity rebound a critical period for later obesity? BMC Pediatr 2004;12:4–6.
26 Deurenberg P, Yap M, van Staveren WA: Body mass index and percent body fat: a meta-analysis among different ethnic groups. Int J Obes Relat Metab Disord 1998;22:1164–1171.
27 Wang J, Thornton JC, Russell M, et al: Asians have lower body mass index (BMI) but higher percent body fat than do whites: comparisons of anthropometric measurements. Am J Clin Nutr 1994;60:23–28.
28 Deurenberg P, Deurenberg-Yap M, Foo LF, Schmidt G, Wang J: Differences in body composition between Singapore Chinese, Beijing Chinese and Dutch children. Eur J Clin Nutr 2003;57:405–409.
29 Eckhardt CL, Adair LS, Caballero B, Avila J, Kon IY, Wang J, Popkin BM: Estimating body fat from anthropometry and isotopic dilution: a four-country comparison. Obes Res 2003;11:1553–1562.
30 Whincup PH, Gilg J, Papacosta O, Seymour C, Miller GJ, Alberti KGM, Cook DG: Early evidence of ethnic differences in cardiovascular risk: cross sectional comparison of British South Asian and white children. BMJ 2002;324:635–638.
31 Wells JCK, Coward WA, Cole TJ, Davies PSW: The contribution of fat and fat-free tissue to body mass index in contemporary children and the reference child. Int J Obes Relat Metab Disord 2002;26:1323–1328.
32 Flegal KM: Defining obesity in children and adolescents: epidemiologic approaches. Crit Rev Food Sci Nutr 1993;33:307–312.
33 Moreno LA, Fleta J, Sarria A, Rodriguez G, Gil C, Bueno M: Secular changes in body fat patterning in children and adolescents of Zaragoza (Spain), 1980–1995. Int J Obes Relat Metab Disord 2001;25:1656–1660.
34 Torun B, Viteri FE: Influence of exercise on linear growth. Eur J Clin Nutr 1994;48(suppl 1):S186–S189.
35 Wells JCK, Mok Q, Johnson AW: Nutritional status in children. Lancet 2001;357:1293.
36 Sullivan PB, Alder N, Bachlet AME, Grant H, Juszczak E, Henry J, Vernon-Roberts A, Warner J, Wells JCK: Gastrostomy feeding in cerebral palsy – too much of a good thing? Dev Med Child Neurol 2006;48:877–882.
37 Parsons TJ, Power C, Logan S, Summerbell CD: Childhood predictors of adult obesity: a systematic review. Int J Obes Relat Metab Disord 1999;23(suppl 8):S1–S107.
38 Baird J, Fisher D, Lucas P, Kleijnen J, Roberts H, Law C: Being big or growing fast: systematic review of size and growth in infancy and later obesity. BMJ 2005;331:929–934.
39 Hediger ML, Overpeck MD, Kuczmarski RJ, McGlynn A, Maurer KR, Davis WW: Muscularity and fatness of infants and young children born small- or large-for-gestational-age. Pediatr 1998;102:E60.
40 Loos RJF, Beunen G, Fagard R, Derom C, Vlietinck R: Birth weight and body composition in young adult men: a prospective twin study. Int J Obes Relat Metab Disord 2001;25:1537–1545.
41 Singhal A, Wells JCK, Cole TJ, Fewtrell MS, Lucas A: Programming of lean body mass: a link between birth weight, obesity and cardiovascular disease? Am J Clin Nutr 2003;77:726–730.
42 Wells JCK, Hallal PC, Wright A, Singhal A, Victora CG: Fetal, infant and childhood growth: relationships with body composition in Brazilian boys aged 9 years. Int J Obes (Lond) 2005;29:1192–1198.
43 Sachdev HS, Fall CH, Osmond C, Lakshmy R, Dey Biswas SK, Leary SD, Reddy KS, Barker DJ, Bhargava SK: Anthropometric indicators of body composition in young adults: relation to size at birth and serial measurements of body mass index in childhood in the New Delhi birth cohort. Am J Clin Nutr 2005;82:456–466.
44 Ekelund U, Ong K, Linne Y, Neovius M, Brage S, Dunger DB, Wareham NJ, Rossner S: Upward weight percentile crossing in infancy and early childhood independently predicts fat mass in young adults: the Stockholm Weight Development Study (SWEDES). Am J Clin Nutr 2006;83:324–330.
45 Wang Y: Cross-national comparison of childhood obesity: the epidemic and the relationship between obesity and socioeconomic status. Int J Epidemiol 2001;30:1129–1136.
46 McCarthy HD, Ashwell M: A study of central fatness using waist-to-height ratios in UK children and adolescents over two decades supports the simple message – 'keep your waist circumference to less than half your height'. Int J Obes (Lond) 2006;30:988–992.
47 Wells JCK, Fewtrell MS: Measuring body composition. Arch Dis Child 2006;91:612–617.
48 Tanner JM, Whitehouse RH: Revised standards for triceps and subscapular skinfolds in British children. Arch Dis Child 1975;50:142–145.
49 Paul AA, Cole TJ, Ahmed EA, Whitehead RG: The need for revised standards for skinfold thickness in infancy. Arch Dis Child 1998;78:354–358.
50 Slaughter MH, Lohman TG, Boileau RA, Horswill CA, Stillman RJ, van Loan MD, Bemben DA: Skinfold equations for estimation of body fatness in children and youth. Hum Biol 1988;60:709–723.
51 Brook CGD: Determination of body composition of children from skinfold measurements. Arch Dis Child 1971;46:182–184.
52 Wells JCK, Fuller NJ, Dewit O, Fewtrell MS, Elia M, Cole TJ: Four-component model of body composition in children: density and hydration of fat-free mass and comparison with simpler models. Am J Clin Nutr 1999;69:904–912.

53 Owens S, Litaker M, Allison J, Riggs S, Ferguson M, Gutin B: Prediction of visceral adipose tissue from simple anthropometric measurements in youths with obesity. Obes Res 1999;7: 16–22.

54 Brambilla P, Bedogni G, Moreno LA, Goran MI, Gutin B, Fox KR, Peters DM, Barbeau P, De Simone M, Pietrobelli A: Crossvalidation of anthropometry against magnetic resonance imaging for the assessment of visceral and subcutaneous adipose tissue in children. Int J Obes (Lond) 2006;30:23–30.

55 McCarthy HD, Jarrett KV, Crawley HF: The development of waist circumference percentiles in British children aged 5.0–16.9 years. Eur J Clin Nutr 2001;55:902–907.

56 Frisancho AR: Triceps skin fold and upper arm muscle size norms for assessment of nutrition status. Am J Clin Nutr 1974;27:1052–1058.

57 Chomtho S, Fewtrell MS, Jaffe A, Williams JE, Wells JCK: Evaluation of arm anthropometry for assessing pediatric body composition: evidence from healthy and sick children. Pediatr Res 2006;59:860–865.

58 Wabitsch M, Braun U, Heinze E, Muche R, Mayer H, Teller W, Fusch C: Body composition in 5–18-y-old obese children and adolescents before and after weight reduction as assessed by deuterium dilution and bioelectrical impedance analysis. Am J Clin Nutr 1996;64: 1–6.

59 Arpadi SM, Wang J, Cuff PA, Thornton J, Horlick M, Kotler DP, Pierson RN: Application of bioimpedance analysis for estimating body composition in prepubertal children infected with human immunodeficiency virus type 1. J Pediatr 1996;129:755–757.

60 Fuller NJ, Fewtrell MS, Dewit O, Elia M, Wells JCK: Segmental bioelectrical impedance analysis in children aged 8–12 years. 1. The assessment of whole-body composition. Int J Obes Relat Metab Disord 2002;26:684–691.

61 Dewit O, Ward L, Middleton SJ, Watson C, Friend PJ, Elia M: Multiple frequency bioimpedance: a bed-side technique for assessment of fluid shift patterns in a patient with severe dehydration. Clin Nutr 1997;16:189–192.

62 Vienna A, Hauser G: A qualitative approach to assessing body compartments using bioelectrical variables. Coll Anthropol 1999;23:461–472.

63 Davies PSW, Wells JCK: Calculation of total body water in infancy. Eur J Clin Nutr 1994;48:490–495.

64 Mazess RB, Barden HS, Bisek JP, Hanson J: Dual-energy X-ray absorptiometry for total-body and regional bone-mineral and soft-tissue composition. Am J Clin Nutr 1990;51:1106–1112.

65 Williams JE, Wells JCK, Wilson CM, Haroun D, Lucas A, Fewtrell MS: Evaluation of lunar prodigy dual-energy X-ray absorptiometry for assessing body composition in healthy individuals and patients by comparison with the criterion four-component model. Am J Clin Nutr 2006;83:1047–1054.

66 Mendley SR, Majkowski NL, Schoeller DA: Validation of estimates of total body water in pediatric dialysis patients by deuterium dilution. Kidney Int 2005;67:2056–2062.

67 Siri WE: Body composition from fluid spaces and density: analysis of methods; in Brozek J, Henschel A (eds): Techniques for Measuring Body Composition. Washington, National Academy of Sciences NRC, 1961, pp 223–244.

68 Dempster P, Aitkens S: A new air displacement method for the determination of human body composition. Med Sci Sports Exerc 1995;27:1692–1697.

69 Urlando A, Dempster P, Aitkens S: A new air displacement plethysmograph for the measurement of body composition in infants. Pediatr Res 2003;53: 486–492.

70 Dewit O, Fuller NJ, Fewtrell MS, Elia M, Wells JCK: Whole-body air-displacement plethysmography compared to hydrodensitometry for body composition analysis. Arch Dis Child 2000;82: 159–164.

71 Wells JCK, Fuller NJ, Wright A, Fewtrell MS, Cole TJ: Evaluation of air-displacement plethysmography in children aged 5–7 years using a three-component model of body composition. Br J Nutr 2003;90:699–707.

72 Haroun D, Wells JCK, Williams JE, Fuller NJ, Fewtrell MS, Lawson MS: Composition of the fat-free mass in obese and non-obese children: matched case-control analyses. Int J Obes (Lond) 2005;29:29–36.

73 Murphy AJ, Wells JC, Williams JE, Fewtrell MS, Davies PS, Webb DK: Body composition in children in remission from acute lymphoblastic leukemia. Am J Clin Nutr 2006;83:70–74.

74 Wells JC, Murphy AJ, Buntain HM, Greer RM, Cleghorn GJ, Davies PS: Adjusting body cell mass for size in women of differing nutritional status. Am J Clin Nutr 2004;80:333–336.

75 Murphy AJ, Buntain HM, Wainwright CE, Davies PS: The nutritional status of children with cystic fibrosis. Br J Nutr 2006;95:321–324.

76 Schoenau E, Neu CM, Mokov E, Wassmer G, Manz F: Influence of puberty on muscle area and cortical bone area of the forearm in boys and girls. J Clin Endocrinol Metab 2000;85:1095–1098.

77 Rauch F, Schoenau E: Peripheral quantitative computed tomography of the distal radius in young subjects – new reference data and interpretation of results. J Musculoskelet Neuronal Interact 2005;5:119–126.

78 Rauch F, Tutlewski B, Schoenau E: Peripheral quantitative computed tomography at the distal radius: cross-calibration between two scanners. J Musculoskelet Neuronal Interact 2001; 2:153–155.

79 Fox K, Peters D, Armstrong N, Sharpe P, Bell M: Abdominal fat deposition in 11-year-old children. Int J Obes Relat Metab Disord 1993;17:11–16.

80 Mitsipoulos N, Baumgartner RN, Heymsfield SB, Lyons W, Gallagher D, Ross R: Cadaver validation of skeletal muscle measurements by magnetic resonance imaging and computerised tomography. J Appl Physiol 1998;85: 115–122.

81 Sartorio A, Malavolti M, Agosti F, Marinone PG, Caiti O, Battistini N, Bedogni G: Body water distribution in severe obesity and its assessment from eight-polar bioelectrical impedance analysis. Eur J Clin Nutr 2005;59:155–160.

82 Planche T, Onanga M, Schwenk A, Dzeing A, Borrmann S, Faucher JF, Wright A, Bluck L, Ward L, Kombila M, Kremsner PG, Krishna S: Assessment of volume depletion in children with malaria. PLoS Med 2004;1:e18.

83 Wells JCK: Lessons from body composition analysis; in Bowman BA, Russell RM (eds): Present Knowledge in Nutrition. Washington, International Life Sciences Institute, 2006, vol 1, pp 23–33.

84 Wells JCK: The evolution of human fatness and susceptibility to obesity: an ethological approach. Biol Rev 2006;81: 183–205.

Metabolic Effects of Growth Hormone

Ulla Feldt-Rasmussen

Initially, growth hormone (GH) was only considered responsible for promoting somatic growth in children, but recent years of investigations have clarified that GH has also very important metabolic actions such as regulation of body composition, muscle and bone metabolism, as well as glucose homeostasis and lipolysis. Some of these GH effects are direct actions, whereas others are mediated via insulin-like growth factor 1 (IGF-1). Recent experiments using gene deletions and transgenic technologies have revealed new information regarding the differential mechanisms of direct actions of GH and indirectly through its growth factors [1–4]. The current hypothesis is that the liver is the principal source of IGF-1 in the circulation but is not required for postnatal body growth, and that autocrine/paracrine IGF-1, but not liver-derived IGF-1 (endocrine IGF-1), is the major determinant of postnatal body growth (fig. 1) [1–6]. In addition, IGF-1 and IGF-2 are important growth factors involved in cellular actions such as proliferation, differentiation and apoptosis.

GH secretion is pulsatile with a circadian rhythm, the maximal release occurring in the second half of the night. GH secretion is regulated by two hypothalamic hormones: GH-releasing hormone, which stimulates gene transcription, and somatostatin, which has an inhibitory effect on the GH secretion from the pituitary gland. Synthetically produced GH-releasing compounds as well as the natural compound, ghrelin, probably affect both systems, thereby resulting in a very powerful stimulation of GH secretion.

The main body of knowledge concerning the metabolic actions of GH in humans comes from studies in adults, but it is important to underline that these metabolic effects are equally important in children. Thus, stress, hypoglycaemia and ingestion of protein stimulate GH secretion, whilst high levels of glucose and free fatty acids (FFAs) inhibit GH secretion, which is restored by acute pharmacological reduction in FFAs [7]; furthermore, GH effects are physiologically modulated by other hormone systems and vice versa [5].

The present chapter will briefly review the effects of GH on intermediary metabolism in adults and present evidence of a relationship between GH deficiency (GHD) and the metabolic syndrome, because this reflects a pathophysiological metabolic consequence of the lack of GH. Other important physiological effects of GH will be dealt with in other chapters of this book.

Department of Medical Endocrinology PE-2132
Rigshospitalet, Copenhagen University Hospital
Blegdamsvej 9, DK–2100 Copenhagen (Denmark)

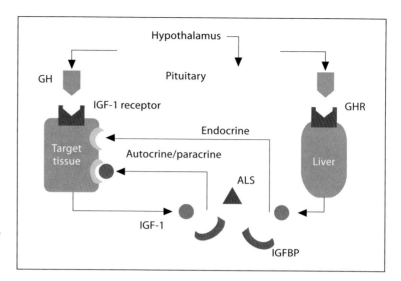

Fig. 1. Schematic presentation of the GH/IGF-1 axis. GHR = GH receptor; ALS = acid-labile subunit.

Metabolic Effectors of the Growth Hormone/Insulin-Like Growth Factor Axis

Effects on Lipids and Lipolysis

The main impact of GH is most probably both in the fasting state, where the pulsatile GH secretion is amplified, and after absorption of meals, which conversely inhibits GH release [6]. GH has further been demonstrated to induce lipolysis in a dose-dependent manner through hormone-sensitive lipase, with elevation of circulatory FFAs and glycerol and increased lipid oxidation rates [8, 9]. These effects occur despite increased insulin levels, indicating that the lipogenic actions of insulin can be overcome by relatively low doses of GH. A recent study presented evidence that the insulin antagonistic effects of GH on fasting glucose metabolism were causally linked to concomitant stimulation of lipolysis [10].

The lipid profile displays show a characteristic pattern in patients with untreated GHD, comprising increased low-density lipoprotein (LDL) cholesterol, in particular the atherogenic small dense particles (VLDL), and triglycerides with normal or reduced high-density lipoprotein (HDL) cholesterol [11–13]. GH replacement in these patients appears to normalize the abnormal lipid profile but may not have an effect on triglyceride levels [11–13]. The mechanisms are not fully understood, but may partly occur through a decreased cholesterol 7α-hydroxylase activity in patients with GHD, leading to increased cholesterol accumulation in the liver and reduced hepatic LDL receptor expression [6]. Another contributing action could be decreased LDL cholesterol clearance in GHD, which might explain why plasma cholesterol goes down following GH treatment [6, 11–13].

Effects on Carbohydrate Metabolism

In the short term, GH is acting in the post-absorptive state by a reduction in plasma glucose and glucose production, and an increase in glucose clearance. On the other hand, sustained GH administration leads to glucose intolerance, secondary to increased hepatic glucose output from gluconeogenesis and glycogenolysis, and to reduced insulin-mediated glucose uptake. The effects of GH on induction of lipolysis, with increased FFA concentrations, may reduce skeletal muscle glucose uptake and account for the reduction in insulin sensitivity [14, 15]. These altera-

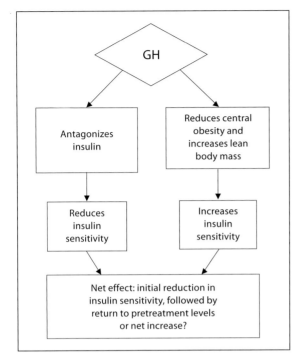

Fig. 2. Possible effect of GH on insulin sensitivity during replacement of patients with GHD.

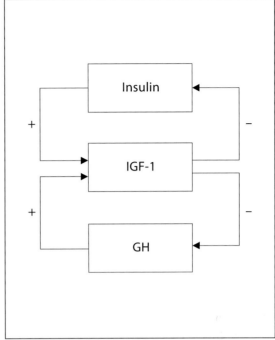

Fig. 3. Relationship between GH, IGF-1 and insulin. + = Stimulation; – = inhibition.

tions in carbohydrate handling are also re-produced in clinical studies of patients with GHD, who have reduced insulin sensitivity compared with controls, though there is no evidence of an increased prevalence of diabetes mellitus [6]. Short-term GH replacement causes further deterioration in insulin sensitivity, which usually returns to baseline with continued treatment for 3–12 months, partly due to the beneficial effects of GH on body composition (fig. 2) [14, 16].

Growth Hormone, Insulin, Insulin-Like Growth Factor 1 and Nutrition

Insulin, GH and IGF-1 are highly interrelated (fig. 3). GH and insulin both stimulate hepatic IGF-1 production, and IGF-1 feeds back to suppress GH and insulin release. The relationships are even more complex, as GH positively regulates IGF-binding protein 3 (IGFBP-3) and the associated acid-labile subunit, whereas IGFBP-1 levels are negatively regulated by insulin [17]. Another important factor in the regulation of IGF-1 may be nutrition [18]. The meal-induced acute increase in glucose and amino acid concentrations in blood causes an acute increase in insulin levels. As a consequence, glucose production by the liver stops, and insulin-mediated uptake of glucose in muscles and the liver is stimulated. Like insulin, dietary amino acids are capable of stimulating GH secretion, while a rise in glucose levels suppresses GH secretion. However, when food intake is too low to meet the needs of the body, insulin secretion decreases and GH secretion increases. This induces insulin resistance and results in increased lipolysis and ketogenesis [18]. Inadequate food intake and/or lack of insulin action both stimulate insulin secretion, but in this situation, GH cannot stimulate insulin and at the same time maintain a sufficient IGF-1 synthesis. Thus, GH actions are only mediated by IGF-1 when they are assisted by insulin and adequate food intake, i.e. anabolic [18]. Thus, in the early postprandial period, GH, IGF-1 and insulin all promote anabolism, with IGF-1 as the main mediator and/or supporter of the effects of both insulin and GH (fig. 2). In the late postprandial period, IGF-1 reduces the GH-induced insulin resistance and stimulates lipolysis by reducing insulin secretion. Essentially, IGF-1 plays a key role in switching the body from using glucose to using FFAs as a source of energy [18].

Role of Decreased Growth Hormone Secretion in the Development of the Metabolic Syndrome

Generally, obese persons have decreased GH secretion, but unlike patients with GHD, they have normal or even high serum IGF-1 levels [19]. As a consequence, prepubertal obese children are generally of normal or tall stature [20]. Thus, diminished GH secretion is not considered the cause of obesity, and patients with GHD respond differently to over-nutrition compared with other obese individuals, without normalization of IGF-1 [21]. GH has several metabolic effects, either directly or indirectly, on adipocytes, which do not seem to be mediated by IGF-1. GH replacement in patients with GHD results in an up-regulation of adipose tissue GH receptor gene expression [22]. GH has opposing effects on glucose and lipid metabolism in adipose tissue, with an insulin-like effect, which is an acute anti-lipolytic action, whereas the GH-mediated insulin-antagonizing action is a long-term effect, inhibiting lipogenesis and glucose transport and increasing lipolysis [23]. The latter may contribute to the development of adiposity in GHD patients.

Abdominal adiposity is a common finding both in patients with GHD and in the metabolic syndrome, and both disorders are associated with high levels of VLDL cholesterol and triglycerides and reduced levels of HDL cholesterol, opposite to what is seen in patients with active acromegaly. As mentioned earlier, GH replacement partly restores these changes with a sustained effect [24]. Another similarity between untreated GHD and the metabolic syndrome is an association with hypertension [6, 11]. A common mechanism may be through increased peripheral arterial resistance and decreased systemic nitric oxide formation, known to be present in both conditions [25]. Treatment with GH decreases peripheral arterial resistance in patients with GHD, probably via IGF-1 stimulation of endothelial nitric oxide formation [25]. Recently, an adipose-derived renin-angiotensin system, which may be responsible for obesity-related hypertension and insulin resistance, has also been described, and it has been suggested that GH treatment may indirectly lower blood pressure by reducing fat mass, thereby down-regulating the activity of the adipose-derived renin-angiotensin system [26]. GH treatment may also lower blood pressure via IGF-1-mediated down-regulation of the angiotensin II type 1 receptor. Finally, decreased serum IGF-1 levels are coupled with increased sympathetic nerve activity, and it has been hypothesized that increased activity of the sympathetic nervous system may be one of the mechanisms responsible for the development of hypertension in the metabolic syndrome [27, 28]. It has been suggested that the insulin resistance in GHD is directly related to the decreased lean body mass, reduced physical activity and increased abdominal obesity that usually characterize this condition [6], although the low serum IGF-1 level may also contribute, as IGF-1 has GH-independent insulin-sensitizing actions.

Thus, GH per se may be responsible for the development of a metabolic syndrome phenotype in patients with GHD, but it is not likely to be involved in the development of the syndrome in the general population.

Interaction between the Metabolic Syndrome and an Imbalance between Cortisol and the Growth Hormone/Insulin-Like Growth Factor 1 Axis

Bjorntorp and Rosmond [29] have previously suggested that the metabolic syndrome is due to elevated cortisol secretion and that the combination of increased cortisol secretion and low GH secretion with decreased IGF-1 levels may even result in the metabolic syndrome. GHD is associated with an increased cortisol production in key target tissues, including liver and adipose tissue, promoting insulin resistance and visceral adiposity [30]. The enzyme type 1 11β-hydroxysteroid dehydrogenase (11β-HSD1) reduces cortisone to cortisol in the liver, adipose tissue and omental adipose tissue, and its overexpression can stimulate glucocorticoid-induced adipocyte differentiation, which may lead to central obesity. The action of cortisol at the tissue level is partially regulated by GH [30], which has an important inhibitory effect on 11β-HSD1 [31, 32]. Thus, patients with GHD have higher levels of cortisol metabolites in the untreated state [31]. Increased concentrations of cortisol in adipose tissue promote lipid accumulation by increasing the expression of lipoprotein lipase. The subsequent increased visceral adipose tissue depots and the FFAs released from these depots induce an increase in insulin resistance [33]. The increased delivery of FFAs to the liver may then add to the generation of other risk factors, such as hyperinsulinaemia, lipoprotein abnormalities and hypertension [33, 34]. GH inhibits lipoprotein lipase expression induced by cortisol and increases lipolysis [30]. GH administration results in a profound reduction in visceral adipose tissue and less marked effects on other adipose tissue depots. The consequences of GH treatment are more evident in visceral than subcutaneous adipose tissues because of a higher cellularity, innervation and blood flow [26]. In summary, elevated cortisol activity and decreased GH secretion are able to induce many of the symptoms and signs of the metabolic syndrome. GH treatment may decrease cortisol activity. This may be partly explained by inhibitory activity on 11β-HSD1.

Is the Metabolic Syndrome due to Adverse Environmental Conditions during Fetal and Postnatal Life?

Increasing experimental evidence suggests that adverse environmental conditions during fetal and/or postnatal life may have long-term consequences for the development of the metabolic syndrome in adult life [35]. It has been found that people who were small or disproportionate (thin or short) at birth have high rates of coronary heart disease, high blood pressure, high cholesterol concentrations and abnormal glucose-insulin metabolism. These effects are independent of the length of gestation, suggesting that the occurrence of the metabolic syndrome is directly linked to fetal growth restriction [35]. Fetal growth is highly dependent on GH, mainly produced by the placenta, in late gestation [36]. Prepubertal children, born small for gestational age (SGA) or with very low body weight (VLBW), prematurely exhibit marked insulin resistance. Both SGA and VLBW children have been exposed to sub-optimal nutritional environments during the last trimester of pregnancy, and both SGA and VLBW groups fail to reach genetic height potential and are recognized causes of short stature in childhood. However, there are differences between the groups with respect to the GH and IGF-1 axis. SGA children have elevated IGF-1 levels, possibly due to either hyperinsulinism or partial IGF-1 resistance, whereas VLBW children have low IGF-1 and IGFBP-3 levels suggestive of GH resistance

[37]. It may be that the nature and timing of the early insult may lead to discordant changes in the metabolic and endocrine axes. These changes could be due to alterations in the environment of the periconceptual embryo resulting in changes in imprinting of genes involved in growth and development.

Studies in rats have suggested that maternal dietary restriction during gestation and lactation may permanently reduce the activity of the GH/IGF-1 axis and up-regulate the hypothalamic-pituitary-adrenal (HPA) axis in the offspring [36]. There is evidence that the GH/IGF-1 axis and the HPA axis may be permanently influenced by events in early life, so-called 'fetal programming', whereby the environmental conditions at a critical, sensitive period of early life have permanent effects on structure, physiology and metabolism in adult life. Fetal programming is likely to involve permanent changes in the 'setpoints' of the endocrine systems. The phenotypic, endocrine and metabolic consequences of alterations in the periconceptual, fetal and early neonatal periods are subject to intense investigation. Future research in this field is likely to focus on the mechanisms through which environmental changes lead to these programmed effects, in order to be able to change their course. Of particular interest in this respect is the finding that treatment with GH (or IGF-1) alleviated obesity, hyperinsulinaemia and hypertension in rats programmed to develop the metabolic syndrome [38].

Summary and Conclusions

The GH/IGF axis has effects on lipids and lipolysis as indicated by GH activation of hormone-sensitive lipase. Furthermore, lipid profiles in patients with untreated GHD have persistently demonstrated increased LDL cholesterol and triglycerides, with normal or reduced HDL cholesterol, and GH replacement usually reduces total and LDL cholesterol, tends to increase HDL cholesterol and in general has no effect on triglyceride levels. However, the detailed mechanisms underpinning these changes are not fully understood. GH signalling pathways have been described in skeletal muscle and adipose tissue in human subjects following exposure to an intravenous bolus injection of GH, providing future means to study mechanisms subserving the in vivo action of GH on substrate metabolism and insulin sensitivity in both muscle and fat [39].

Concerning carbohydrate metabolism, GH has short-lived effects on reducing plasma glucose and glucose production, while sustained GH administration leads to glucose intolerance. Patients with GHD are reported to have reduced insulin sensitivity, and short-term GH replacement causes a further deterioration in insulin sensitivity, which usually returns to baseline after continued treatment.

The metabolic syndrome and GHD share many similarities, and recently, the GH/IGF-1 axis has been focused on in explaining some of the features of this syndrome. It has also been suggested that therapeutic modulation of the GH/IGF-1 system might alleviate the syndrome and its long-term consequences. However, this still has to await further controlled trials.

Prepubertal children, born SGA or with VLBW, prematurely exhibit marked insulin resistance. There is evidence to suggest that the GH/IGF-1 axis and the HPA axis may be permanently influenced by events in early life. This process has been called 'fetal programming', whereby the environmental conditions at a critical, sensitive period of early life have permanent effects on structure, physiology and metabolism in adult life. Fetal programming is likely to involve permanent changes in the setpoints of the endocrine systems.

References

1 Green H, Morikawa M, Nixon T: A dual effector theory of growth hormone action. Differentiation 1985;29:195–198.
2 Liu JL, Grinberg A, Westphal H, Sauer B, Accili D, Karas M, LeRoith D: Insulin-like growth factor-I affects perinatal lethality and postnatal development in a gene dosage-dependent manner: manipulation using the Cre/loxP system in transgenic mice. Mol Endocrinol 1998;12:1452–1462.
3 Sjögren K, Liu JL, Blad K, Skrtic S, Vidal O, Wallenius V, LeRoith D, Tornell J, Isaksson OG, Jansson JO, Ohlsson C: Liver-derived insulin-like growth factor I (IGF-I) is the principal source of IGF-I in blood but it is not required for postnatal growth in mice. Proc Natl Acad Sci USA 1999;96:7088–7092.
4 Yakar S, Liu J, Stannard B, Butler A, Accili D, Sauer B, LeRoith D: Normal growth and development in the absence of hepatic insulin-like growth factor I. Proc Natl Acad Sci USA 1999;96:7324–7329.
5 Behringer RR, Lewin TM, Quaife CJ, Palmiter RD, Brinster RL, Ercole AJ: Expression of insulin-like growth factor I stimulates normal somatic growth in growth hormone-deficient transgenic mice. Endocrinology 1990;127:1033–1040.
6 Feldt-Rasmussen U, Abs R (eds): Growth Hormone Deficiency in Adults: 10 Years of Experience: 1994–2004. Oxford, Oxford PharmaGenesis™ Ltd., 2004, pp 1–361.
7 Pontiroli AE, Manzoni MF, Malighetti ME, Lanzi R: Restoration of growth hormone (GH) response to GH-releasing hormone in elderly and obese subjects by acute pharmacological reduction of plasma free fatty acids. J Clin Endocrinol Metab 1996;81:3998–4001.
8 Copeland KC, Nair KS: Acute growth hormone effects on amino acid and lipid metabolism. J Clin Endocrinol Metab 1994;78:1040–1047.
9 Dietz J, Schwartz J: Growth hormone alters lipolysis and hormone-sensitive lipase activity in 3T3-F442A adipocytes. Metabolism 1991;40:800–806.
10 Norrelund H, Nielsen S, Christiansen JS, Jorgensen JO, Moller N: Modulation of basal glucose metabolism and insulin sensitivity by growth hormone and free fatty acids during short-term fasting. Eur J Endocrinol 2004;150:779–787.
11 Abs R, Feldt-Rasmussen U, Mattsson AF, Monson JP, Bengtsson BA, Goth MI, Wilton P, Koltowska-Haggstrom M: Determinants of cardiovascular risk in 2589 hypopituitary GH-deficient adults – a KIMS database analysis. Eur J Endocrinol 2006;155:79–90.
12 Abdul Shakoor SK, Shalet SM: Effects of GH replacement on metabolism and physical performance in GH-deficient adults. J Endocrinol Invest 2003;26:911–918.
13 McCallum RW, Petrie JR, Dominiczak AF, Connell JM: Growth hormone deficiency and vascular risk. Clin Endocrinol (Oxf) 2002;57:11–24.
14 Svensson J, Bengtsson BÅ: Growth hormone replacement therapy and insulin sensitivity. J Clin Endocrinol Metab 2003;88:1453–1454.
15 Rosenfalck AM, Maghsoudi S, Fisker S, Jorgensen JOL, Christiansen JS, Hilsted J, Vølund AA, Madsbad S: The effect of 30 months of low-dose replacement therapy with recombinant human growth hormone (rhGH) on insulin and C-peptide kinetics, insulin secretion, insulin sensitivity, glucose effectiveness, and body composition in GH-deficient adults. J Clin Endocrinol Metab 2000;85:4173–4181.
16 Jorgensen JO, Vestergaard E, Gormsen L, Jessen N, Norrelund H, Christiansen JS, Moller N: Metabolic consequences of GH deficiency. J Endocrinol Invest 2005;28:47–51.
17 Bondy CA, Underwood LE, Clemmons DR, Guler HP, Bach MA, Skarulis M: Clinical uses of insulin-like growth factor I. Ann Intern Med 1994;120:593–601.
18 Froesch ER: Insulin-like growth factor: endocrine and autocrine/paracrine implications and relations to diabetes mellitus; in Zahnd GR, Wollheim CB (eds): Contributions of Physiology to the Understanding of Diabetes. Berlin, Springer, 1997, pp 127–147.
19 Nam SY, Marcus C: Growth hormone and adipocyte function in obesity. Horm Res 2000;53:87–97.
20 Dietz WH Jr, Hartung R: Changes in height velocity of obese preadolescents during weight reduction. Am J Dis Child 1985;139:705–707.
21 Thissen JP, Ketelslegers JM, Underwood LE: Nutritional regulation of the insulin-like growth factors. Endocr Rev 1994;15:80–101.
22 Kamel A, Margery V, Norstedt G, Thorén M, Lindgren AC, Bronnegard M, Marcus C: Growth hormone (GH) treatment up-regulates GH receptor mRNA levels in adipocytes from patients with GH deficiency and Prader-Willi syndrome. Pediatr Res 1995;38:418–421.
23 Davidson MB: Effect of growth hormone on carbohydrate and lipid metabolism. Endocr Rev 1987;8:115–131.
24 Götherström G, Svensson J, Koranyi J, Alpsten M, Bosæus I, Bengtsson B, Johannsson G: A prospective study of 5 years of GH replacement therapy in GH-deficient adults: sustained effects on body composition, bone mass, and metabolic indices. J Clin Endocrinol Metab 2001;86:4657–4665.
25 Boger RH, Skamira C, Bode-Boger SM, Brabant G, von zur Muhlen A, Frolich JC: Nitric oxide may mediate the hemodynamic effects of recombinant growth hormone in patients with acquired growth hormone deficiency. A double-blind, placebo-controlled study. J Clin Invest 1996;98:2706–2713.
26 Vickers MH, Ikenasio BA, Breier BH: Adult growth hormone treatment reduces hypertension and obesity induced by an adverse prenatal environment. J Endocrinol 2002;175:615–623.
27 Sverrisdottir YB, Johannsson G, Jungersten L, Wallin BG, Elam M: Is the somatotropic axis related to sympathetic nerve activity in healthy ageing men? J Hypertens 2001;19:2019–2024.
28 Reaven GM, Lithell H, Landsberg L: Hypertension and associated metabolic abnormalities – the role of insulin resistance and the sympathoadrenal system. N Engl J Med 1996;334:374–381.
29 Bjorntorp P, Rosmond R: Hypothalamic origin of the metabolic syndrome X. Ann N Y Acad Sci 1999;892:297–307.
30 Bjorntorp P: The regulation of adipose tissue distribution in humans. Int J Obes Relat Metab Disord 1996;20:291–302.

31 Gelding SV, Taylor NF, Wood PJ, Noonan K, Weaver JU, Wood DF, Monson JP: The effect of growth hormone replacement therapy on cortisol-cortisone interconversion in hypopituitary adults: evidence for growth hormone modulation of extrarenal 11β-hydroxysteroid dehydrogenase activity. Clin Endocrinol (Oxf) 1998;48:153–162.

32 Paulsen SK, Pedersen SB, Jorgensen JO, Fisker S, Christiansen JS, Flyvbjerg A, Richelsen B: Growth hormone (GH) substitution in GH-deficient patients inhibits 11β-hydroxysteroid dehydrogenase type 1 messenger ribonucleic acid expression in adipose tissue. J Clin Endocrinol Metab 2006;91:1093–1098.

33 Bjorntorp P: 'Portal' adipose tissue as a generator of risk factors for cardiovascular disease and diabetes. Arteriosclerosis 1990;10:493–496.

34 Johannsson G, Bjorntorp P, Bengtsson BÅ: Is GH therapy indicated in the metabolic syndrome?; in Monson J (ed): Growth Hormone Therapy. Oxford, Blackwell Science, 1999, pp 264–281.

35 Godfrey KM, Barker DJ: Fetal nutrition and adult disease. Am J Clin Nutr 2000; 71:1344–1352.

36 Barker DJP: Programming the baby; in Barker DJP (ed): Mothers, Babies, and Disease in Later Life. London, BMJ Publishing Group, 1994, pp 14–36.

37 Miles HL, Hofman PL, Cutfield WS: Fetal origin of adult disease: a paediatric perspective. Rev Endocr Metab Disord 2005;6:261–268.

38 Vickers MH, Ikenasio BA, Breier BH: IGF-I treatment reduces hyperphagia, obesity, and hypertension in metabolic disorders induced by fetal programming. Endocrinology 2001;142:3964–3973.

39 Jorgensen JO, Jessen N, Pedersen SB, Vestergaard E, Gormsen L, Lund SA, Billestrup N: Growth hormone receptor signalling in skeletal muscle and adipose tissue in human subjects following exposure to an intravenous GH bolus. Am J Physiol Endocrinol Metab 2006;291:E899–E905.

The Growth Plate

Ola Nilsson

Longitudinal bone growth occurs at the growth plate. The growth plate contains one cell type, the chondrocyte, at different stages of differentiation. Resting zone chondrocytes replicate at a slow rate [1] and act as the stem-like cells that replenish the pool of proliferative chondrocytes [2]. Proliferative zone chondrocytes replicate at a high rate [1], and the resulting daughter cells line up along the long axis of the bone. As a result, clones of chondrocytes are arranged in columns parallel to this axis, a process critical to the formation of bones with an elongated shape [2].

At a certain point, the cells stop dividing and terminally differentiate into hypertrophic chondrocytes [1]. During the hypertrophic process, chondrocytes increase their height about 6- to 10-fold, and thus, hypertrophic differentiation makes an important contribution to longitudinal growth [3]. The hypertrophic chondrocytes calcify the surrounding extracellular matrix and produce factors, including vascular endothelial growth factor, that attract the invading bone cells and blood vessels [4]. Hypertrophic chondrocytes undergo apoptosis shortly before the blood vessels invade the chondrocyte lacuna [5] (fig. 1).

The Developmental Program of Growth Plate Cartilage: Growth Plate Senescence

The rate of longitudinal bone growth decreases dramatically with age [1]. This age-dependent decline in growth rate is due to a decline in chondrocyte proliferation, matrix production and hypertrophic cell size [6]. In rats, the growth rate of the proximal tibial growth plate decreases approximately 20-fold from 3 to 26 weeks of age. Simultaneously, proliferation in the proliferative zone decreases approximately 9-fold, and hypertrophic cell size decreases 2-fold (fig. 2). Thus, the decline in growth rate is, in large part, caused by a decline in chondrocyte proliferation [6]. In addition to these functional senescent changes, the growth plate also undergoes structural senescent changes (fig. 3). As the animal ages, there is a decrease in the overall height of the growth plate, associated with a decline in the number of proliferative and hypertrophic chondrocytes per column. In addition, the columns become more widely spaced with more intervening cartilage matrix [7, 8].

Pediatric Endocrinology Unit, Q2:08
Department of Woman and Child Health
Karolinska Institutet
Karolinska University Hospital
SE–171 76 Stockholm (Sweden)

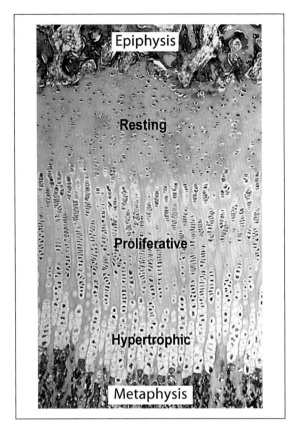

Fig. 1. Histology of the growth plate. The growth plate is a thin layer of cartilage located between the epiphysis and metaphysis of long bones. The growth plate contains three histologically distinct layers: the resting, proliferative and hypertrophic zones.

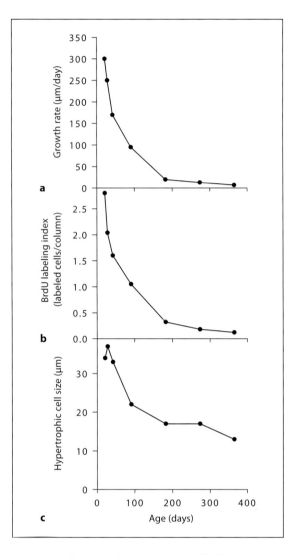

Fig. 2. Developmental decline in growth plate function. In rats, the growth rate of the proximal tibial growth plate decreases approximately 20-fold from 3 to 26 weeks of age (**a**). Simultaneously, proliferation in the proliferative zone decreases approximately 9-fold (**b**), and hypertrophic cell size decreases 2-fold (**c**). BrdU = Bromodeoxyuridine. Curves were created from data published by Walker and Kember [6].

This gradual decline in growth plate function appears to be due to a mechanism intrinsic to the growth plate rather than to a hormonal or other systemic mechanism. Consequently, when growth plates are transplanted among rabbits of different ages, the growth rate of the transplanted growth plate depends on the age of the donor animal, not the age of the recipient [9]. The term 'growth plate senescence' [10] has been used to describe this intrinsic process that involves both a decline in the function (e.g., cell proliferation and hypertrophic cell size) (fig. 2) and cellularity (fig. 3) of the growth plate. Clinical observations and experimental evidence suggest that growth plate senescence is associated with chondrocyte proliferation. In other words, stem-like cells in the resting zone may have a finite proliferative

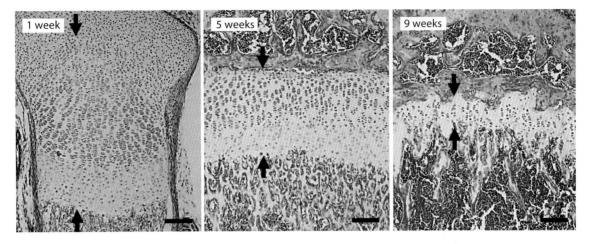

Fig. 3. Developmental changes in growth plate histology. Proximal tibial growth plates from 1-, 5-, and 9-week-old mice. With age, there is a gradual decline in the overall height of the growth plate due to a decline in the number of cells in the resting, proliferative and hypertrophic zones, and a decrease in the size of the individual hypertrophic cells. Arrows indicate growth plate height. Scale bar = 150 μm.

capacity that is gradually exhausted, causing chondrocyte proliferation to decline and eventually come to a complete stop [8, 11].

Adults Do Not Grow Taller

In humans, longitudinal bone growth ceases permanently in late adolescence; adults do not grow taller over time. Why does longitudinal bone growth cease? Careful observation indicates that growth ceases before fusion occurs [8, 12], suggesting that fusion is the result and not the cause of growth cessation [8, 13]. Instead, growth cessation appears to be the culmination of a progressive decline in the growth rate that begins early in life, years prior to fusion. For example, in humans, the linear growth rate exceeds 100 cm/year in the fetus, but then declines to about 5 cm/year by midchildhood. In humans, the decline is briefly interrupted by a pubertal growth spurt, after which the deceleration resumes. In other mammals, a similar dramatic decline in growth rate occurs. The shape of the curve is similar to that in humans in that the initial decline is rapid, but then, the decline slows as the growth rate approaches zero. However, the time scale involved varies greatly. In small mammals, the decline occurs over weeks to months, whereas in large mammals, the decline occurs over months to years (fig. 4).

The Final Act: Epiphyseal Fusion

In some mammals, including humans, the growth plate is resorbed at the time of sexual maturation; the growth plate cartilage is replaced by bone. Estrogen is pivotal for epiphyseal fusion in both young men and women [14]. This key role for estrogen was confirmed with the recognition of two genetic disorders, i.e. estrogen deficiency due to mutations in the aromatase gene [15] and estrogen resistance due to mutations in the estrogen receptor-α gene [16]. In both of these conditions, the growth plate fails to fuse and growth persists, albeit slowly, into adulthood. Conversely, premature estrogen exposure, e.g., precocious puberty, leads to premature epiphyseal fusion.

The mechanism by which estrogen promotes epiphyseal fusion is not well understood. Early studies suggested that estrogen induces growth plate ossification by stimulating vascular and bone cell invasion of the growth plate cartilage causing ossification to advance beyond the hypertrophic zone into the proliferative and resting zones [17, 18]. However, a more recent study suggests that estrogen does not stimulate ossification of cartilage directly but instead accelerates the normal process of growth plate senescence, secondarily causing earlier fusion [5]. In young ovariectomized rabbits, estrogen treatment accelerates the normal senescent decline in the longitudinal growth rate, the chondrocyte proliferation rate, the growth plate height, the number of proliferative and hypertrophic chondrocytes per column, the size of the hypertrophic chondrocytes, and the column density. In addition, estrogen treatment induces earlier growth plate fusion. These findings suggest that estrogen may not stimulate fusion directly. Instead, it may accelerate the senescence program, thus secondarily triggering fusion earlier. In particular, in this animal model, fusion occurs when the chondrocyte proliferation rate approaches zero. This temporal association suggests that fusion is triggered when the proliferative potential of the growth plate chondrocytes is finally exhausted. Estrogen, by accelerating senescence, may hasten replicative exhaustion and thus cause earlier fusion [8].

This model may also apply to humans, providing an explanation for certain clinical observations. It may, for example, explain why the magnitude of estrogen exposure needed to cause epiphyseal fusion depends on the age of the individual. In a 1-year-old child with precocious puberty, 8–10 years of estrogen exposure are required to cause fusion [19]. In contrast, if the estrogen exposure occurs later in life, then fusion occurs after a shorter exposure time. An extreme example is adult men with estrogen deficiency due to aroma-

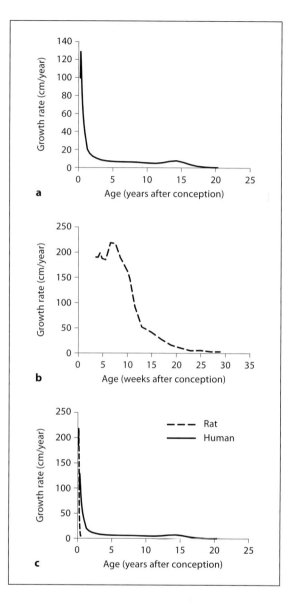

Fig. 4. Linear growth rates of rats and humans. The growth rates of rats (**a**, **c**) and humans (**b**, **c**) decrease dramatically with age. The shapes of the curves are similar in that the initial decline is rapid, but then the decline slows as the growth rate approaches zero. However, the time scale involved varies greatly. In rats, the decline occurs over weeks to months, whereas in humans, the decline occurs over months to years. Reproduced with kind permission of Springer Science and Business Media [114].

tase mutations in whom fusion occurs after less than 1 year of estrogen exposure [20, 21]. This difference in time scale may be explained by the hypothesis that estrogen accelerates growth plate senescence leading to earlier exhaustion of replicative capacity of the growth plate, and thus, secondarily, to earlier fusion. In a young child, there would be a very large proliferative capacity which would need to be exhausted before fusion can occur. Thus, it might require years of estrogen exposure to exhaust this large capacity. In an older individual, there would remain less proliferative capacity, and therefore, it might require a shorter exposure to estrogen before proliferative exhaustion and fusion would occur.

The model also provides an explanation for the observation that girls with precocious puberty who are treated with gonadotropin-releasing hormone (GnRH) analog often have a poor growth velocity. Prior to treatment, these children grow at an abnormally high rate. Treatment with a GnRH analog suppresses the gonadal axis. However, growth does not just return to normal but actually declines to subnormal rates. Previous studies have sought ongoing hormonal abnormalities in these children to explain the slow growth. However, on GnRH analog, the levels of growth hormone (GH), insulin-like growth factor 1 (IGF-1) and estrogen appear not to be deficient [22–24]. Instead, the explanation appears to involve accelerated growth plate senescence [25]. Prior to treatment, the elevated estrogen levels apparently accelerate the senescent decline in proliferative potential, and thus, even when the hormones are normalized by GnRH analog treatment, the growth plates are excessively senescent for age and do not grow at a normal rate [26].

Paracrine Regulation of the Growth Plate

The unique cellular architecture and kinetics of the growth plate requires both patterning and differentiating factors that act in concert to regulate the process of growth plate chondrogenesis. The understanding of these regulatory signals has increased substantially over the past few years. The role of parathyroid hormone-related protein (PTHrP), Indian hedgehog (Ihh), bone morphogenetic proteins (BMPs) and fibroblast growth factors (FGFs) in growth plate chondrogenesis will be discussed below. The role of Ihh and PTHrP has been outlined by careful studies using genetically modified animals and fetal organ culture systems. The importance of BMP and FGF signaling in endochondral bone formation is clear, but the large number of ligands and receptors in these systems has not permitted a straightforward approach to elucidate the exact role of individual proteins.

Parathyroid Hormone-Related Protein
In the growth plate, PTHrP, signaling through its receptor PTH1R, inhibits differentiation of proliferative chondrocytes, thus maintaining them in a proliferative mode. Mice in which either the PTHrP or the PTH1R gene was ablated exhibit similar abnormalities in the growth plate. Both have short limbs and thin proliferative zones with hypertrophic chondrocytes close to the ends of the bones, suggesting accelerated chondrocyte maturation [27, 28]. Conversely, overexpression of PTHrP results in short limbs due to a delay in chondrocyte maturation [29]. In chimeric mice containing both wild-type and PTH1R–/– chondrocytes, the PTH1R–/– proliferative chondrocytes underwent hypertrophic differentiation, while still located in the proliferative zone, confirming the important role of PTH1R signaling in chondrocyte differentiation in vivo [30].

The PTH1R appears to play a similar role in human skeletal development since mutations in the PTHrP receptor cause at least three different conditions with altered chondrocyte maturation. Null mutations of the PTH1R, as in Blomstrand lethal osteochondrodysplasia, are associated with accelerated maturation and ossification of the developing skeleton [31, 32] and thereby resemble the skeletal phenotype of PTH1R–/– mice. Jansen metaphyseal dysplasia, an autosomal dominant disorder that is characterized by short-limb dwarfism, hypercalcemia and hypophosphatemia, is caused by activating mutations of PTH1R [33]. A recent report also associates a substitution in the extracellular domain of the PTH1R with enchondromatosis. The mutant receptor elevated the basal levels of cAMP and caused an enchondromatosis-like chondrodysplasia when introduced into mice [34].

Indian Hedgehog
Genetic targeting of Ihh, PTHrP and PTH1R have revealed a mechanism by which the balance between proliferation and differentiation is controlled, at least during fetal development [35]. Ihh is predominantly secreted by early hypertrophic chondrocytes, PTHrP by periarticular chondrocytes, whereas the PTH1R is expressed on proliferative chondrocytes [36, 37]. Ihh produced by newly formed hypertrophic chondrocytes signals to epiphyseal chondrocytes, which are induced to produce PTHrP. PTHrP then act on the PTHR1 on proliferative chondrocytes to inhibit their differentiation into hypertrophic chondrocytes, thus forming a feedback loop that acts to stabilize the rate of chondrocyte differentiation and consequently the height of the proliferative columns [35, 36, 38, 39]. During fetal development, the PTHrP expression moves into the resting zones, and the feedback loop may thus be maintained when the secondary ossification center is formed [40] (fig. 5).

Independent of PTHrP signaling, Ihh stimulates chondrocyte proliferation and promote differentiation of resting chondrocytes [36, 40]. In addition, Ihh signaling is required for the formation of bone collars and directly stimulates osteoblast maturation [30, 36].

Fibroblast Growth Factors
The discovery that achondroplasia, the most common form of human dwarfism, is caused by point mutations in the transmembrane domain of an FGF receptor, FGFR3 [41, 42], was the start of a number of discoveries attributing several skeletal dysplasias to mutation in the genes encoding FGFR1, FGFR2 and FGFR3 [43–46].

Similar to humans, mice that express activating mutations of the FGFR3 gene exhibit syndromes including short-limb dwarfism due to decreased chondrocyte proliferation and disor-

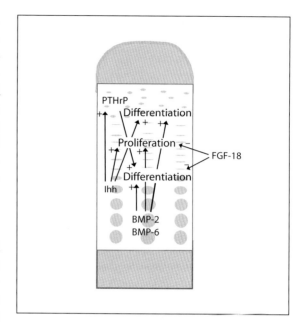

Fig. 5. Paracrine regulation of growth plate. PTHrP secreted in the resting zone inhibits differentiation of proliferative chondrocytes. PTHrP production is in turn stimulated by Ihh secreted by early hypertrophic chondrocytes. Thus, Ihh and PTHrP form a feedback loop that acts to delay hypertrophic differentiation and consequently increases the height of the proliferative columns. Ihh also stimulates chondrocyte differentiation of resting zone chondrocytes and proliferation of proliferative chondrocytes directly. FGFs, exemplified by FGF-18 that is expressed in the perichondrium, inhibit both proliferation and differentiation of growth plate chondrocytes. BMPs, here exemplified by BMP-2 and BMP-6 that are expressed in hypertrophic chondrocytes, stimulate differentiation and proliferation. + = Stimulatory effect; – = inhibitory effect.

ganization of the proliferative columns [47]. Conversely, FGFR3 null mice show increased longitudinal bone growth, increased chondrocyte proliferation and taller proliferative columns in the growth plate [48]. FGFR3 is thus regarded as a negative regulator of longitudinal bone growth at the level of the growth plate. Mice with targeted disruption of FGF-18 exhibit, like FGFR3–/– mice, expanded proliferative and hypertrophic zones. Based on these findings, FGF-18 is suggested to be a natural ligand of FGFR3 in growth plate cartilage [49].

Bone Morphogenetic Protein
BMPs, a subfamily of the transforming growth factor-β protein family, were first discovered as the component of demineralized bone matrix that is able to induce new bone formation in intramuscular sites [50]. These proteins were later found to exhibit diverse roles during early embryogenesis and organogenesis by their ability to regulate cell proliferation, differentiation, apoptosis and cell fate [51, 52]. BMP signaling governs numerous aspects of limb formation and outgrowth, including mesenchymal condensation, chondrocyte differentiation and apoptosis [53, 54]. To be able to play these diverse roles during development, BMP signaling has to be locally restricted by distinct expression of BMP antagonists. Genetic targeting in mice has revealed that loss of BMP antagonism by Gremlin results in defective patterning and outgrowth of limbs and that the BMP antagonist Noggin is required for proper allocation of limb mesenchyme to the cartilage compartment and for specification of joints. In humans, heterozygous mutations of Noggin result in a variety of skeletal abnormalities, including synostosis, symphalangism and joint formation. In the postnatal growth plate, BMP signaling promotes chondrocyte differentiation at multiple steps, as well as proliferation [55, 56]. The mechanisms for these effects are not elucidated, but are, at least in part, independent of the Ihh-PTHrP system [56].

Hormonal Regulation of the Growth Plate

Longitudinal bone growth at the growth plate is governed by a complex network of endocrine signals (fig. 6). Most of these signals regulate growth plate function by acting locally on growth plate chondrocytes and indirectly by modulating other endocrine signals in the network (fig. 3). Some of the local effects of hormones are mediated by changes in paracrine factors that control chondrocyte proliferation and differentiation.

Our improved understanding in this field has provided insight into the molecular genetic causes of human growth failure. For example, human mutations affecting the GH-IGF-1 system at many different levels have recently been shown to cause short stature, including mutations in genes encoding the GH-releasing hormone receptor [57], GH [58], STAT5b [59], IGF-1 [60], acid-labile subunit [61] and IGF-1 receptor [62]. Molecular genetic defects affecting other endocrine regulators of growth can also cause growth plate dysfunction and short stature but often in conjunction with dysfunction of other tissues and organs, for example, mutations involving thyroid hormone receptor-β [63].

GH and IGFs
GH and IGFs are potent stimulators of longitudinal bone growth. GH excess, due to pituitary adenomas in childhood, results in gigantism. Conversely, GH deficiency or insensitivity due to GH receptor mutations or defects in GH signaling pathways markedly impairs postnatal growth [59, 64, 65]. Final height data on patients with untreated isolated GH deficiency suggest that it leads to an average final height standard deviation score of –4.7 (–6.1 to –3.9) [65]. GH deficiency and insensitivity do not significantly impair prenatal growth. In contrast, both pre- and postnatal growth deficits occurred in the only reported cases of IGF-1 deficiency due to a mutation in the *igf-1* gene [60] and of IGF-1 resistance due to mutations in the type 1 IGF receptor gene [62].

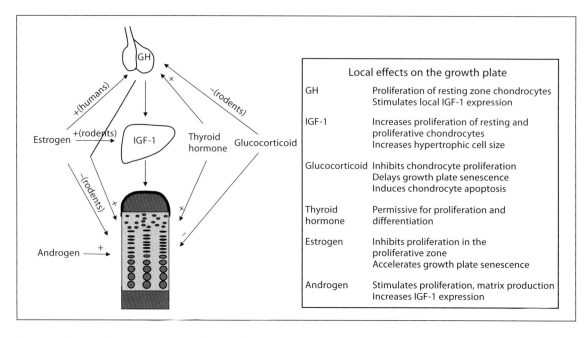

Fig. 6. Endocrine signals that regulate longitudinal bone growth. Arrows indicate direct action on the growth plate and indirect action by modulating other endocrine signals. + = Stimulatory effect; – = inhibitory effect.

The role of the GH-IGF axis in longitudinal bone growth has been evaluated by genetic targeting of its components in mice. Mice lacking the GH gene exhibit normal birth weight but a reduction in postnatal growth [66]. Mice lacking either the *igf-1* or *igf-2* genes show intrauterine growth retardation with birth weights of approximately 60% compared with wild-type littermates [67]. Mice deficient in the type 1 IGF receptor have even more severe reduction in birth weight (45% of wild-type) and die soon after birth due to respiratory failure [67].

The original somatomedin hypothesis stipulates that the effect of GH on linear growth is mediated by liver-derived IGF-1 [68]. The role of circulating IGF-1 has recently been evaluated using tissue-specific gene targeting. Liver-specific ablation of *igf-1* in mice using the cre/lox system reduces circulating IGF-1 levels by approximately 80%, but has no appreciable effect on postnatal growth. However, in these mice, changes in IGF binding proteins may have preserved bioactive IGF-1 levels [69]. Combined deficiency in liver-derived IGF-1 and knockout of acid-labile substance (a component of the circulating IGF-1 complex) further reduces circulating IGF-1 levels and inhibits linear growth and growth plate height. In addition, in both mice and humans with inactivating mutations in the GH receptor, increased circulating IGF-1 can markedly improve linear bone growth, supporting a role for circulating IGF-1 [70, 71].

GH can also stimulate longitudinal bone growth by a local action on the growth plate. Injection of GH into the tibial growth plate accelerates longitudinal growth in the injected growth plate compared with the vehicle-injected contralateral growth plate [72]. Part of the local action of GH on the growth plate may be mediated by increased local production of IGF-1 which then acts in a paracrine/autocrine fashion to increase chondrogenesis [73, 74]. In addition, GH may also have an effect on the growth plate that is independent of both endocrine and paracrine IGF-1. The dual effector hypothesis states that GH acts locally at the growth plate to recruit resting chondrocytes into a proliferative state [75], as well as stimulating local IGF-1 production which then stimulates proliferation of proliferative zone chondrocytes [74–76]. However, detailed in vivo labeling experiments suggest that IGF-1, like GH, can stimulate proliferation of resting zone chondrocytes and chondrocyte hypertrophy [77]. In contrast, studies in IGF-1-deficient mice suggest that IGF-1 acts primarily to increase hypertrophic cell height with little effect on proliferation [78].

Glucocorticoid
Glucocorticoids are widely used as anti-inflammatory and immunosuppressive drugs in children. Long-term, high-dose glucocorticoid treatment often leads to growth failure. Similarly, systemic administration of glucocorticoid in mice, rats and rabbits decreases the rate of longitudinal bone growth by inhibiting growth plate chondrocyte proliferation [11, 79]. In addition, glucocorticoid may stimulate apoptosis of growth plate chondrocytes [79, 80].

Glucocorticoid inhibits longitudinal bone growth, in part, through a direct effect on growth plate chondrocytes. Glucocorticoid receptor is expressed by growth plate chondrocytes [79]. Furthermore, glucocorticoid inhibits proliferation of growth plate chondrocytes in vitro [81]. In addition, local infusion of dexamethasone into the growth plate causes a local inhibition of longitudinal bone growth [82].

The local effects of glucocorticoid on growth plate chondrocyte proliferation may be mediated, in part, by changes in the local IGF-1 system. Short-term systemic administration of glucocorticoid in rodents decreases IGF-1 expression in the growth plate [83]. In contrast, long-term treatment of rodents increases IGF-1 expression in the growth plate [84], and growth-suppressive doses of dexamethasone given to rabbits actually increase GH receptor mRNA expression in the growth plate [85]. In vitro, glucocorticoid suppresses GH receptor expression in cultured rat growth plate chondrocytes, while type 1 IGF receptor expression is not affected [81].

In addition to its direct action on the growth plate, glucocorticoid may also suppress longitudinal bone growth through an indirect action, involving other endocrine signals. In humans, glucocorticoid excess has been associated with reduced GH secretion in some studies [86], but not in all [87]. The interpretation of these findings is complicated by the presence of the underlying disease requiring glucocorticoid treatment and by the suppressive effect of obesity per se on GH secretion. In humans, plasma IGF-1 and IGF binding protein 3 levels have been found to be either normal [86] or increased [88].

Thyroid Hormone
Thyroid hormone is necessary for normal skeletal growth and maturation. Hypothyroidism slows longitudinal bone growth and endochondral ossification, while hyperthyroidism accelerates both processes [89, 90]. In hypothyroid animals, there is a decrease in the heights of the proliferative and hypertrophic zones and a decrease in chondrocyte proliferation, chondrocyte hypertrophy and vascular/bone cell invasion [91]. In addition, the normal columnar organization of the growth plate is disrupted [91].

Some of the skeletal effects of thyroid hormone appear to be due to a direct action on the growth plate. In fetal mouse tibia organ culture, thyroid hormone promotes longitudinal growth with the largest effect seen in the hypertrophic zone [92]. In cell culture, thyroid hormone stimulates hypertrophic differentiation but often diminishes proliferation [93]. Local conversion of T_4 to T_3 by thyroid hormone deiodinase 2 in the growth plate may contribute to local effects [92].

Growth plate chondrocytes express thyroid hormone receptor isoforms TR-α_1, TR-α_2 and

TR-β_1 [94]. Knocking out TR-β isoforms in mice has little effect on the skeleton. In contrast, ablation of TR-α impairs longitudinal bone growth and endochondral ossification, effects that resemble hypothyroidism [95]. In humans, one family with homozygous deletion of TR-β showed epiphyseal stippling and some delayed skeletal maturation, suggesting that TR-β may mediate some of the effects of thyroid hormone on human skeletal development [63]. Most cases of thyroid hormone resistance in humans are caused by dominant-negative mutations of the TR-β gene that may also affect TR-α function and show variable skeletal effects [63].

In addition to its local action on the growth plate, thyroid hormone may have indirect effects on the growth plate, mediated by GH and IGF-1. In hypothyroid humans and mice, GH and IGF-1 levels are reduced [96]. Replacing GH in hypothyroid rats or in mice lacking TR-α improves longitudinal bone growth. However, GH does not normalize growth plate endochondral ossification or morphology [96].

Estrogen
During puberty, sex steroids induce a pubertal growth spurt in humans. This growth acceleration may be primarily induced by estrogen since a near-normal growth spurt occurs in patients with androgen insensitivity [97], whereas little or no growth spurt appears to occur in patients with aromatase deficiency [98]. In addition, low-dose estrogen treatment can accelerate growth in both prepubertal boys and girls [99], and the accelerated growth in patients with familial male-limited precocious puberty is curtailed by the administration of an aromatase inhibitor [100]. The pubertal growth spurt has a better temporal correlation with the increase in estrogen levels than with the increase in androgen levels [101]. Much of the growth acceleration is mediated by estrogen-induced stimulation of the GH-IGF-1 axis [98].

Estrogen may act directly on the growth plate. Three lines of evidence support this hypothesis.

First, estrogen receptor-α and -β are expressed in growth plate cartilage [102]. Second, estrogen inhibits longitudinal bone growth of gonadohypophysectomized female rats [103]. Third, human growth plate chondrocytes placed in primary culture reportedly respond to estrogen stimulation [104]. In addition, Gunther et al. [105] were able to inhibit estrogen-induced bone maturation using ICI 182,780, a pure anti-estrogen, thus suggesting that estrogen acts to advance bone maturation, at least in part, through a classical estrogen receptor.

Androgen
Androgen also contributes to the pubertal growth spurt. Some of this effect is probably due to aromatization of androgens to estrogens in peripheral tissues. Aromatase, the enzyme that converts androgens to estrogens, is expressed in growth plate cartilage [106], suggesting that some of the effects of androgen may be due to local conversion into estrogen. However, androgen per se, without conversion into estrogen, also appears to stimulate longitudinal bone growth. In boys, dihydrotestosterone, a nonaromatizable androgen, can accelerate linear growth [107]. This effect does not appear to be associated with increased circulating GH or IGF-1 [107]. Similarly, in gonadohypophysectomized rats, testosterone stimulates growth in the absence of GH [103, 108]. These GH-independent effects of androgen may be due to a direct action of androgen on growth plate chondrocytes. Androgen receptor expression has been detected in rat [109] and human growth plate cartilage [102, 110]. Local administration of testosterone reportedly increases unilateral rat tibial epiphyseal growth plate width [111]. Furthermore, in vitro, dihydrotestosterone can stimulate proliferation and proteoglycan synthesis in growth plate chondrocytes [112]. Similarly, testosterone and, to a lesser extent, dihydrotestosterone stimulate chondrocyte proliferation in the mouse mandibular condyle, an organ culture model of endochondral ossification

[113]. These local effects may be mediated, in part, by increased local IGF-1 expression [112, 113].

Conclusions

Longitudinal bone growth is governed by a large system of endocrine signals that interact with a complex system of paracrine signals within the growth plate. Whereas knowledge of the endocrine systems involved in the regulation of longitudinal bone growth is fairly good, the complexity of the local regulation is just starting to unfold. New experimental approaches including inducible and tissue-specific gene targeting, traditional and laser-assisted microdissection, microarray analysis and linkage studies exploiting the full sequence of the human and mouse genomes promise to accelerate progress in the understanding of the paracrine regulatory system as well as the interaction of endocrine and paracrine signals. These advances will lead to improved understanding of human skeletal growth disorders and are, combined with stem cell biology and tissue engineering, likely to yield new therapeutic approaches.

References

1 Kember NF: Cell population kinetics of bone growth: the first ten years of autoradiographic studies with tritiated thymidine. Clin Orthop Relat Res 1971;76: 213–230.
2 Abad V, Meyers JL, Weise M, Gafni RI, Barnes KM, Nilsson O, Bacher JD, Baron J: The role of the resting zone in growth plate chondrogenesis. Endocrinology 2002;143:1851–1857.
3 Hunziker EB: Mechanism of longitudinal bone growth and its regulation by growth plate chondrocytes. Microsc Res Tech 1994;28:505–519
4 Gerber HP, Vu TH, Ryan AM, Kowalski J, Werb Z, Ferrara N: VEGF couples hypertrophic cartilage remodeling, ossification and angiogenesis during endochondral bone formation. Nat Med 1999;5:623–628.
5 Farnum CE, Wilsman NJ: Cellular turnover at the chondro-osseous junction of growth plate cartilage: analysis by serial sections at the light microscopical level. J Orthop Res 1989;7: 654–666.
6 Walker KV, Kember NF: Cell kinetics of growth cartilage in the rat tibia. 2. Measurements during ageing. Cell Tissue Kinet 1972;5:409–419.
7 Kember NF: Aspects of the maturation process in growth cartilage in the rat tibia. Clin Orthop Relat Res 1973;95: 288–294.
8 Weise M, De-Levi S, Barnes KM, Gafni RI, Abad V, Baron J: Effects of estrogen on growth plate senescence and epiphyseal fusion. Proc Natl Acad Sci USA 2001;98:6871–6876.
9 Stevens DG, Boyer MI, Bowen CV: Transplantation of epiphyseal plate allografts between animals of different ages. J Pediatr Orthop 1999;19:398–403.
10 Baron J, Klein KO, Colli MJ, Yanovski JA, Novosad JA, Bacher JD, Cutler GB Jr: Catch-up growth after glucocorticoid excess: a mechanism intrinsic to the growth plate. Endocrinology 1994; 135:1367–1371.
11 Gafni RI, Weise M, Robrecht DT, Meyers JL, Barnes KM, De-Levi S, Baron J: Catch-up growth is associated with delayed senescence of the growth plate in rabbits. Pediatr Res 2001;50:618–623.
12 Moss ML, Noback CR: A longitudinal study of digital epiphyseal fusion in adolescence. Anat Rec 1958;131:19–32.
13 Parfitt AM: Misconceptions. 1. Epiphyseal fusion causes cessation of growth. Bone 2002;30:337–339.
14 Grumbach MM, Auchus RJ: Estrogen: consequences and implications of human mutations in synthesis and action. J Clin Endocrinol Metab 1999;84:4677–4694.
15 Morishima A, Grumbach MM, Simpson ER, Fisher C, Qin K: Aromatase deficiency in male and female siblings caused by a novel mutation and the physiological role of estrogens. J Clin Endocrinol Metab 1995;80:3689–3698.
16 Smith EP, Boyd J, Frank GR, Takahashi H, Cohen RM, Specker B, Williams TC, Lubahn DB, Korach KS: Estrogen resistance caused by a mutation in the estrogen-receptor gene in a man. N Engl J Med 1994;331:1056–1061.
17 Silberberg M, Silberberg R: Further investigations concerning the influence of estrogen on skeletal tissues. Am J Anat 1941;69:295–325.
18 Sutro CJ: Effects of subcutaneous injection of estrogen upon skeleton in immature mice. Proc Soc Exp Biol Med 1940;44:151–154.
19 Sigurjonsdottir TJ, Hayles AB: Precocious puberty. A report of 96 cases. Am J Dis Child 1968;115:309–321.
20 Bilezikian JP, Morishima A, Bell J, Grumbach MM: Increased bone mass as a result of estrogen therapy in a man with aromatase deficiency. N Engl J Med 1998;339:599–603.
21 Carani C, Qin K, Simoni M, Faustini-Fustini M, Serpente S, Boyd J, Korach KS, Simpson ER: Effect of testosterone and estradiol in a man with aromatase deficiency. N Engl J Med 1997;337:91–95.

22 Kamp GA, Manasco PK, Barnes KM, Jones J, Rose SR, Hill SC, Cutler GB Jr: Low growth hormone levels are related to increased body mass index and do not reflect impaired growth in luteinizing hormone-releasing hormone agonist-treated children with precocious puberty. J Clin Endocrinol Metab 1991; 72:301–307.

23 Klein KO, Baron J, Barnes KM, Pescovitz OH, Cutler GB Jr: Use of an ultrasensitive recombinant cell bioassay to determine estrogen levels in girls with precocious puberty treated with a luteinizing hormone-releasing hormone agonist. J Clin Endocrinol Metab 1998; 83:2387–2389.

24 Pescovitz OH, Rosenfeld RG, Hintz RL, Barnes K, Hench K, Comite F, Loriaux DL, Cutler GB Jr: Somatomedin-C in accelerated growth of children with precocious puberty. J Pediatr 1985;107: 20–25.

25 Weise M, Flor A, Barnes KM, Cutler GB Jr, Baron J: Determinants of growth during gonadotropin-releasing hormone analog therapy for precocious puberty. J Clin Endocrinol Metab 2004; 89:103–107.

26 Weise M, Flor A, Barnes KM, Cutler GB Jr, Baron J: Determinants of growth during gonadotropin-releasing hormone analog therapy for precocious puberty. J Clin Endocrinol Metab 2004; 89:103–107.

27 Karaplis AC, Luz A, Glowacki J, Bronson RT, Tybulewicz VL, Kronenberg HM, Mulligan RC: Lethal skeletal dysplasia from targeted disruption of the parathyroid hormone-related peptide gene. Genes Dev 1994;8:277–289.

28 Lanske B, Karaplis AC, Lee K, Luz A, Vortkamp A, Pirro A, Karperien M, Defize LH, Ho C, Mulligan RC, Abou-Samra AB, Juppner H, Segre GV, Kronenberg HM: PTH/PTHrP receptor in early development and Indian hedgehog-regulated bone growth. Science 1996;273:663–666.

29 Weir EC, Philbrick WM, Amling M, Neff LA, Baron R, Broadus AE: Targeted overexpression of parathyroid hormone-related peptide in chondrocytes causes chondrodysplasia and delayed endochondral bone formation. Proc Natl Acad Sci USA 1996;93:10240–10245.

30 Chung UI, Lanske B, Lee K, Li E, Kronenberg H: The parathyroid hormone/parathyroid hormone-related peptide receptor coordinates endochondral bone development by directly controlling chondrocyte differentiation. Proc Natl Acad Sci USA 1998;95:13030–13035.

31 Jobert AS, Zhang P, Couvineau A, Bonaventure J, Roume J, Le Merrer M, Silve C: Absence of functional receptors for parathyroid hormone and parathyroid hormone-related peptide in Blomstrand chondrodysplasia. J Clin Invest 1998;102:34–40.

32 Karaplis AC, He B, Nguyen MT, Young ID, Semeraro D, Ozawa H, Amizuka N: Inactivating mutation in the human parathyroid hormone receptor type 1 gene in Blomstrand chondrodysplasia. Endocrinology 1998;139:5255–5258.

33 Schipani E, Langman CB, Parfitt AM, Jensen GS, Kikuchi S, Kooh SW, Cole WG, Juppner H: Constitutively activated receptors for parathyroid hormone and parathyroid hormone-related peptide in Jansen's metaphyseal chondrodysplasia. N Engl J Med 1996;335:708–714.

34 Hopyan S, Gokgoz N, Poon R, Gensure RC, Yu C, Cole WG, Bell RS, Juppner H, Andrulis IL, Wunder JS, Alman BA: A mutant PTH/PTHrP type I receptor in enchondromatosis. Nat Genet 2002;30: 306–310.

35 Chung UI, Schipani E, McMahon AP, Kronenberg HM: Indian hedgehog couples chondrogenesis to osteogenesis in endochondral bone development. J Clin Invest 2001;107:295–304.

36 St Jacques B, Hammerschmidt M, McMahon AP: Indian hedgehog signaling regulates proliferation and differentiation of chondrocytes and is essential for bone formation. Genes Dev 1999;13: 2072–2086.

37 Vortkamp A, Pathi S, Peretti GM, Caruso EM, Zaleske DJ, Tabin CJ: Recapitulation of signals regulating embryonic bone formation during postnatal growth and in fracture repair. Mech Dev 1998;71:65–76.

38 Kobayashi T, Soegiarto DW, Yang Y, Lanske B, Schipani E, McMahon AP, Kronenberg HM: Indian hedgehog stimulates periarticular chondrocyte differentiation to regulate growth plate length independently of PTHrP. J Clin Invest 2005;115:1734–1742.

39 Vortkamp A, Lee K, Lanske B, Segre GV, Kronenberg HM, Tabin CJ: Regulation of rate of cartilage differentiation by Indian hedgehog and PTH-related protein. Science 1996;273:613–622.

40 Koziel L, Wuelling M, Schneider S, Vortkamp A: Gli3 acts as a repressor downstream of Ihh in regulating two distinct steps of chondrocyte differentiation. Development 2005;132:5249–5260.

41 Rousseau F, Bonaventure J, Legeai-Mallet L, Pelet A, Rozet JM, Maroteaux P, Le Merrer M, Munnich A: Mutations in the gene encoding fibroblast growth factor receptor-3 in achondroplasia. Nature 1994;371:252–254.

42 Shiang R, Thompson LM, Zhu YZ, Church DM, Fielder TJ, Bocian M, Winokur ST, Wasmuth JJ: Mutations in the transmembrane domain of FGFR3 cause the most common genetic form of dwarfism, achondroplasia. Cell 1994; 78:335–342.

43 Britto JA, Chan JC, Evans RD, Hayward RD, Thorogood P, Jones BM: Fibroblast growth factor receptors are expressed in craniosynostotic sutures. Plast Reconstr Surg 1998;101:540–543.

44 Cohen MM Jr: Achondroplasia, hypochondroplasia and thanatophoric dysplasia: clinically related skeletal dysplasias that are also related at the molecular level. Int J Oral Maxillofac Surg 1998;27:451–455.

45 Muenke M: Finding genes involved in human developmental disorders. Curr Opin Genet Dev 1995;5:354–361.

46 Naski MC, Ornitz DM: FGF signaling in skeletal development. Front Biosci 1998;3:D781–D794.

47 Chen L, Adar R, Yang X, Monsonego EO, Li C, Hauschka PV, Yayon A, Deng CX: Gly369Cys mutation in mouse FGFR3 causes achondroplasia by affecting both chondrogenesis and osteogenesis. J Clin Invest 1999;104:1517–1525.

48 Colvin JS, Bohne BA, Harding GW, McEwen DG, Ornitz DM: Skeletal overgrowth and deafness in mice lacking fibroblast growth factor receptor 3. Nat Genet 1996;12:390–397.

49 Liu JP, Baker J, Perkins AS, Robertson EJ, Efstratiadis A: Mice carrying null mutations of the genes encoding insulin-like growth factor I (Igf-1) and type 1 IGF receptor (Igf1r). Cell 1993;75:59–72.

50 Urist MR: Bone: formation by autoinduction. Science 1965;150:893–899.
51 Hogan BL: Bone morphogenetic proteins: multifunctional regulators of vertebrate development. Genes Dev 1996;10:1580–1594.
52 Zhao GQ: Consequences of knocking out BMP signaling in the mouse. Genesis 2003;35:43–56.
53 Zou H, Wieser R, Massague J, Niswander L: Distinct roles of type I bone morphogenetic protein receptors in the formation and differentiation of cartilage. Genes Dev 1997;11:2191–2203.
54 Zou H, Niswander L: Requirement for BMP signaling in interdigital apoptosis and scale formation. Science 1996;272:738–741.
55 De Luca F, Barnes KM, Uyeda JA, De Levi S, Abad V, Palese T, Mericq V, Baron J: Regulation of growth plate chondrogenesis by bone morphogenetic protein-2. Endocrinology 2001;142:430–436.
56 Kobayashi T, Lyons KM, McMahon AP, Kronenberg HM: BMP signaling stimulates cellular differentiation at multiple steps during cartilage development. Proc Natl Acad Sci USA 2005;102:18023–18027.
57 Wajnrajch MP, Gertner JM, Harbison MD, Chua SC Jr, Leibel RL: Nonsense mutation in the human growth hormone-releasing hormone receptor causes growth failure analogous to the little (lit) mouse. Nat Genet 1996;12:88–90.
58 Wagner JK, Eble A, Hindmarsh PC, Mullis PE: Prevalence of human GH-1 gene alterations in patients with isolated growth hormone deficiency. Pediatr Res 1998;43:105–110.
59 Kofoed EM, Hwa V, Little B, Woods KA, Buckway CK, Tsubaki J, Pratt KL, Bezrodnik L, Jasper H, Tepper A, Heinrich JJ, Rosenfeld RG: Growth hormone insensitivity associated with a STAT5b mutation. N Engl J Med 2003;349:1139–1147.
60 Woods KA, Camacho-Hubner C, Savage MO, Clark AJ: Intrauterine growth retardation and postnatal growth failure associated with deletion of the insulin-like growth factor I gene. N Engl J Med 1996;335:1363–1367.
61 Domene HM, Bengolea SV, Martinez AS, Ropelato MG, Pennisi P, Scaglia P, Heinrich JJ, Jasper HG: Deficiency of the circulating insulin-like growth factor system associated with inactivation of the acid-labile subunit gene. N Engl J Med 2004;350:570–577.
62 Abuzzahab MJ, Schneider A, Goddard A, Grigorescu F, Lautier C, Keller E, Kiess W, Klammt J, Kratzsch J, Osgood D, Pfaffle R, Raile K, Seidel B, Smith RJ, Chernausek SD: IGF-I receptor mutations resulting in intrauterine and postnatal growth retardation. N Engl J Med 2003;349:2211–2222.
63 Takeda K, Sakurai A, Degroot LJ, Refetoff S: Recessive inheritance of thyroid hormone resistance caused by complete deletion of the protein-coding region of the thyroid hormone receptor-β gene. J Clin Endocrinol Metab 1992;74:49–55.
64 Rosenfeld RG, Rosenbloom AL, Guevara-Aguirre J: Growth hormone (GH) insensitivity due to primary GH receptor deficiency. Endocr Rev 1994;15:369–390.
65 Wit JM, Kamp GA, Rikken B: Spontaneous growth and response to growth hormone treatment in children with growth hormone deficiency and idiopathic short stature. Pediatr Res 1996;39:295–302.
66 Zhou Y, Xu BC, Maheshwari HG, He L, Reed M, Lozykowski M, Okada S, Cataldo L, Coschigamo K, Wagner TE, Baumann G, Kopchick JJ: A mammalian model for Laron syndrome produced by targeted disruption of the mouse growth hormone receptor/binding protein gene (the Laron mouse). Proc Natl Acad Sci USA 1997;94:13215–13220.
67 Baker J, Liu JP, Robertson EJ, Efstratiadis A: Role of insulin-like growth factors in embryonic and postnatal growth. Cell 1993;75:73–82.
68 Daughaday WH, Hall K, Raben MS, Salmon WD Jr, van den Brande JL, van Wyk JJ: Somatomedin: proposed designation for sulphation factor. Nature 1972;235:107.
69 Butler AA, LeRoith D: Minireview: tissue-specific versus generalized gene targeting of the igf1 and igf1r genes and their roles in insulin-like growth factor physiology. Endocrinology 2001;142:1685–1688.
70 Guevara-Aguirre J, Rosenbloom AL, Vasconez O, Martinez V, Gargosky SE, Allen L, Rosenfeld RG: Two-year treatment of growth hormone (GH) receptor deficiency with recombinant insulin-like growth factor I in 22 children: comparison of two dosage levels and to GH-treated GH deficiency. J Clin Endocrinol Metab 1997;82:629–633.
71 Sims NA, Clement-Lacroix P, Da Ponte F, Bouali Y, Binart N, Moriggl R, Goffin V, Coschigano K, Gaillard-Kelly M, Kopchick J, Baron R, Kelly PA: Bone homeostasis in growth hormone receptor-null mice is restored by IGF-I but independent of Stat5. J Clin Invest 2000;106:1095–1103.
72 Isaksson OG, Jansson JO, Gause IA: Growth hormone stimulates longitudinal bone growth directly. Science 1982;216:1237–1239.
73 Isgaard J, Moller C, Isaksson OG, Nilsson A, Mathews LS, Norstedt G: Regulation of insulin-like growth factor messenger ribonucleic acid in rat growth plate by growth hormone. Endocrinology 1988;122:1515–1520.
74 Schlechter NL, Russell SM, Spencer EM, Nicoll CS: Evidence suggesting that the direct growth-promoting effect of growth hormone on cartilage in vivo is mediated by local production of somatomedin. Proc Natl Acad Sci USA 1986;83:7932–7934.
75 Ohlsson C, Nilsson A, Isaksson O, Lindahl A: Growth hormone induces multiplication of the slowly cycling germinal cells of the rat tibial growth plate. Proc Natl Acad Sci USA 1992;89:9826–9830.
76 Isaksson OG, Lindahl A, Nilsson A, Isgaard J: Mechanism of the stimulatory effect of growth hormone on longitudinal bone growth. Endocr Rev 1987;8:426–438.
77 Hunziker EB, Wagner J, Zapf J: Differential effects of insulin-like growth factor I and growth hormone on developmental stages of rat growth plate chondrocytes in vivo. J Clin Invest 1994;93:1078–1086.
78 Wang J, Zhou J, Bondy CA: Igf1 promotes longitudinal bone growth by insulin-like actions augmenting chondrocyte hypertrophy. FASEB J 1999;13:1985–1990.

79 Silvestrini G, Ballanti P, Patacchioli FR, Mocetti P, Di Grezia R, Wedard BM, Angelucci L, Bonucci E: Evaluation of apoptosis and the glucocorticoid receptor in the cartilage growth plate and metaphyseal bone cells of rats after high-dose treatment with corticosterone. Bone 2000;26:33–42.

80 Chrysis D, Ritzen EM, Savendahl L: Growth retardation induced by dexamethasone is associated with increased apoptosis of the growth plate chondrocytes. J Endocrinol 2003;176:331–337.

81 Jux C, Leiber K, Hugel U, Blum W, Ohlsson C, Klaus G, Mehls O: Dexamethasone impairs growth hormone (GH)-stimulated growth by suppression of local insulin-like growth factor (IGF)-I production and expression of GH- and IGF-I-receptor in cultured rat chondrocytes. Endocrinology 1998; 139:3296–3305.

82 Baron J, Huang Z, Oerter KE, Bacher JD, Cutler GB Jr: Dexamethasone acts locally to inhibit longitudinal bone growth in rabbits. Am J Physiol 1992; 263:489–492.

83 Smink JJ, Gresnigt MG, Hamers N, Koedam JA, Berger R, van Buul-Offers SC: Short-term glucocorticoid treatment of prepubertal mice decreases growth and IGF-I expression in the growth plate. J Endocrinol 2003;177: 381–388.

84 Smink JJ, Koster JG, Gresnigt MG, Rooman R, Koedam JA, van Buul-Offers SC: IGF and IGF-binding protein expression in the growth plate of normal, dexamethasone-treated and human IGF-II transgenic mice. J Endocrinol 2002;175:143–153.

85 Heinrichs C, Yanovski JA, Roth AH, Yu YM, Domene HM, Yano K, Cutler GB Jr, Baron J: Dexamethasone increases growth hormone receptor messenger ribonucleic acid levels in liver and growth plate. Endocrinology 1994;135: 1113–1118.

86 Magiakou MA, Mastorakos G, Gomez MT, Rose SR, Chrousos GP: Suppressed spontaneous and stimulated growth hormone secretion in patients with Cushing's disease before and after surgical cure. J Clin Endocrinol Metab 1994;78:131–137.

87 Crowley S, Hindmarsh PC, Matthews DR, Brook CG: Growth and the growth hormone axis in prepubertal children with asthma. J Pediatr 1995;126:297–303.

88 Borges MH, Pinto AC, DiNinno FB, Camacho-Hubner C, Grossman A, Kater CE, Lengyel AM: IGF-I levels rise and GH responses to GHRH decrease during long-term prednisone treatment in man. J Endocrinol Invest 1999;22: 12–17.

89 Buckler JM, Willgerodt H, Keller E: Growth in thyrotoxicosis. Arch Dis Child 1986;61:464–471.

90 Leger J, Czernichow P: Congenital hypothyroidism: decreased growth velocity in the first weeks of life. Biol Neonate 1989;55:218–223.

91 Stevens DA, Hasserjian RP, Robson H, Siebler T, Shalet SM, Williams GR: Thyroid hormones regulate hypertrophic chondrocyte differentiation and expression of parathyroid hormone-related peptide and its receptor during endochondral bone formation. J Bone Miner Res 2000;15:2431–2442.

92 Miura M, Tanaka K, Komatsu Y, Suda M, Yasoda A, Sakuma Y, Ozasa A, Nakao K: Thyroid hormones promote chondrocyte differentiation in mouse ATDC5 cells and stimulate endochondral ossification in fetal mouse tibias through iodothyronine deiodinases in the growth plate. J Bone Miner Res 2002;17:443–454.

93 Robson H, Siebler T, Stevens DA, Shalet SM, Williams GR: Thyroid hormone acts directly on growth plate chondrocytes to promote hypertrophic differentiation and inhibit clonal expansion and cell proliferation. Endocrinology 2000;141:3887–3897.

94 Ballock R, Mita BC, Zhou X, Chen DH, Mink LM: Expression of thyroid hormone receptor isoforms in rat growth plate cartilage in vivo. J Bone Miner Res 1999;14:1550–1556.

95 Gauthier K, Chassande O, Plateroti M, Roux JP, Legrand C, Pain B, Rousset B, Weiss R, Trouillas J, Samarut J: Different functions for the thyroid hormone receptors TRα and TRβ in the control of thyroid hormone production and post-natal development. EMBO J 1999; 18:623–631.

96 Kindblom JM, Gothe S, Forrest D, Tornell J, Tornell J, Vennstrom B, Ohlsson C: GH substitution reverses the growth phenotype but not the defective ossification in thyroid hormone receptor α_1-/-β-/- mice. J Endocrinol 2001; 171:15–22.

97 Zachmann M, Prader A, Sobel EH, Crigler JF Jr, Ritzen EM, Atares M, Ferrandez A: Pubertal growth in patients with androgen insensitivity: indirect evidence for the importance of estrogens in pubertal growth of girls. J Pediatr 1986;108:694–697.

98 Grumbach MM: Estrogen, bone, growth and sex: a sea change in conventional wisdom. J Pediatr Endocrinol Metab 2000;13(suppl 6):1439–1455.

99 Cutler GB Jr: The role of estrogen in bone growth and maturation during childhood and adolescence. J Steroid Biochem Mol Biol 1997;61:141–144.

100 Laue L, Kenigsberg D, Pescovitz OH, Hench KD, Barnes KM, Loriaux DL, Cutler GB Jr: Treatment of familial male precocious puberty with spironolactone and testolactone. N Engl J Med 1989;320:496–502.

101 Klein KO, Martha PM Jr, Blizzard RM, Herbst T, Rogol AD: A longitudinal assessment of hormonal and physical alterations during normal puberty in boys. 2. Estrogen levels as determined by an ultrasensitive bioassay. J Clin Endocrinol Metab 1996;81:3203–3207.

102 Nilsson O, Chrysis D, Pajulo O, Boman A, Holst M, Rubinstein J, Martin RE, Savendahl L: Localization of estrogen receptors-α and -β and androgen receptor in the human growth plate at different pubertal stages. J Endocrinol 2003;177:319–326.

103 Jansson JO, Eden S, Isaksson O: Sites of action of testosterone and estradiol on longitudinal bone growth. Am J Physiol 1983;244:135–140.

104 Blanchard O, Tsagris L, Rappaport R, Duval-Beaupere G, Corvol M: Age-dependent responsiveness of rabbit and human cartilage cells to sex steroids in vitro. J Steroid Biochem Mol Biol 1991;40:711–716.

105 Gunther DF, Calikoglu AS, Underwood LE: The effects of the estrogen receptor blocker, Faslodex (ICI 182,780), on estrogen-accelerated bone maturation in mice. Pediatr Res 1999;46:269–273.

106 Oz OK, Millsaps R, Welch R, Birch J, Zerwekh JE: Expression of aromatase in the human growth plate. J Mol Endocrinol 2001;27:249–253.

107 Keenan BS, Richards GE, Ponder SW, Dallas JS, Nagamani M, Smith ER: Androgen-stimulated pubertal growth: the effects of testosterone and dihydrotestosterone on growth hormone and insulin-like growth factor-I in the treatment of short stature and delayed puberty. J Clin Endocrinol Metab 1993;76:996–1001.

108 Phillip M, Maor G, Assa S, Silbergeld A, Segev Y: Testosterone stimulates growth of tibial epiphyseal growth plate and insulin-like growth factor-1 receptor abundance in hypophysectomized and castrated rats. Endocrine 2001;16:1–6.

109 van der Eerden BC, van Til NP, Brinkmann AO, Lowik CW, Wit JM, Karperien M: Gender differences in expression of androgen receptor in tibial growth plate and metaphyseal bone of the rat. Bone 2002;30:891–896.

110 Abu EO, Horner A, Kusec V, Triffitt JT, Compston JE: The localization of androgen receptors in human bone. J Clin Endocrinol Metab 1997;82:3493–3497.

111 Ren SG, Malozowski S, Sanchez P, Sweet DE, Loriaux DL, Cassorla F: Direct administration of testosterone increases rat tibial epiphyseal growth plate width. Acta Endocrinol (Copenh) 1989;121:401–405.

112 Krohn K, Haffner D, Hugel U, Himmele R, Klaus G, Mehls O, Schaefer F: 1,25(OH)2D3 and dihydrotestosterone interact to regulate proliferation and differentiation of epiphyseal chondrocytes. Calcif Tissue Int 2003;73:400–410.

113 Maor G, Segev Y, Phillip M: Testosterone stimulates insulin-like growth factor-I and insulin-like growth factor-I-receptor gene expression in the mandibular condyle – a model of endochondral ossification. Endocrinology 1999;140:1901–1910.

114 Nilsson O, Baron J: Impact of growth plate senescence on catch-up growth and epiphyseal fusion. Pediatr Nephrol 2005;20:319–322.

Pharmacogenetics of Growth Hormone Therapy

Linda B. Johnston   Adrian J.L. Clark

The availability of recombinant human growth hormone (GH) therapy since the 1980s has meant that the supply of GH is not limited. This has allowed treatment of children with various growth disorders, and studies of efficacy have led to the recommendation of specific standard doses based on the patient's diagnosis and weight or body surface area. However, there remains wide variability in patients' responses to GH treatment. It is logical that individualisation of the GH dose could be used to optimise patient therapy. This may have additional benefits in terms of improving cost-effectiveness and reducing adverse events.

The large number of GH-treated patients entered into the KIGS database has allowed the identification of some of the factors which influence the variability in response to GH therapy in different disorders [1–3]. These prediction models, generated by multiple regression analysis, have provided the first opportunity to rationally individualise patient therapy, but do not explain all of the observed variability. It has been proposed that part of the variability, not explained by the prediction models, could relate to the influence of genetic factors. The study of GH pharmacogenomics is a new emerging field.

Definition – What Is Pharmacogenomics?

Pharmacogenomics is a broad term. In relation to GH therapy, it involves the elucidation of genetic factors influencing the variable clinical response seen. However, the term pharmacogenomics can also refer to the identification of potential new drug targets through understanding the genomic basis of the disease. A relevant endocrine example is the development of Pegvisomant® for the treatment of acromegaly [4].

Genetic Factors Influencing Growth Hormone Response

The GH/insulin-like growth factor 1 (IGF-1) axis is the predominant regulator of the childhood growth phase. The GH ligand binds to the GH

Department of Endocrinology, William Harvey Research Unit
John Vane Science Centre, Charterhouse Square
Barts and the London Queen Mary School of Medicine
London EC1M 6BQ (UK)

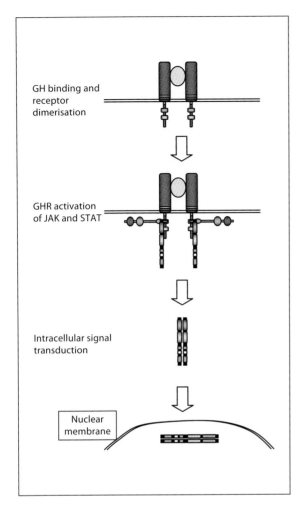 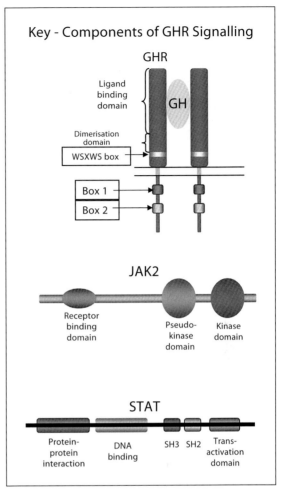

Fig. 1. GH signalling cascade demonstrating the dimerised GHR and its interaction with JAK2 and signal transducers and activators of transcription (STAT).

receptor (GHR) to mediate both its direct effects and its stimulatory effect on IGF-1 production and secretion. The GHR has extracellular, transmembrane and intracellular domains and is a member of the cytokine receptor superfamily. Normal signal transduction involves GH binding to a receptor molecule at one site and to another GHR molecule at a second GH site, thus inducing receptor homodimerisation and the conformational changes essential for GHR activation [5, 6]. Janus tyrosine kinase 2 (JAK2) association with the proline-rich box 1 region of the intracellular domain induces phosphorylation of JAK2 and the receptor, which in turn activates divergent signalling pathways including the cytoplasmic signal transducers and activators of transcription proteins 1, 3 and 5, and the mitogen-activating peptide kinase pathway (fig. 1). It is possible that genetic variation of any of the factors involved in this signalling pathway may influence GH therapy responsiveness.

Recombinant human GH is now licensed to treat growth failure in several disorders, including GH deficiency (GHD), small for gestational age (SGA) with short stature, Turner syndrome, chronic renal failure, Prader-Willi syndrome, achondroplasia (Japan only) and idiopathic short stature (USA only). Given the different genetic bases of these disorders, it is likely that the specific genes influencing the response to GH therapy and their magnitude of effect will vary between the disorders.

Growth Hormone Receptor

Studies of patients with severe GH insensitivity syndrome (GHIS, Laron syndrome), where subjects either have deletions or deleterious mutations of the GHR and severe short stature, have shown that they do not respond to endogenous or exogenous GH [7, 8]. Thus, clinical observations in GHIS demonstrate that the GHR is essential for growth.

The human GHR exists in several isoforms, among which are two classes that differ by the retention (GHRfl) or exclusion of exon 3 (GHRd3). While originally thought to be the result of alternative splicing, this variation has been recently shown to arise from a homologous recombination event occurring between retroviral repetitive sequence elements flanking exon 3 [9, 10]. The recombination event results in the loss of exon 3 and some flanking intronic sequence generating the so-called GHRd3 allele from the GHRfl allele. Once this event has occurred, the GHRd3 allele follows the normal mendelian pattern of inheritance in subsequent generations. This event appears to be specific to humans, as the retroviral elements originate from an endogenous human retrovirus.

The 22 amino acid region of the GHR encoded by exon 3 is in the extracellular domain and not in close proximity to the GH binding domain [11]. The GHRd3 allele shows similar binding properties and similar receptor internalisation to GHRfl [12, 13]. In addition, the study of a GHIS family demonstrated that one normal allele of GHRd3 or GHRfl in the heterozygous parents was sufficient for normal growth [14].

The first publication on the influence of GHRd3 on GH responsiveness came from Dos Santos et al. [15] in a study of two mixed cohorts of short SGA and idiopathic short stature phenotypes. This study showed that GHRd3 in heterozygous or homozygous form correlated with greater growth acceleration after 1 and 2 years of therapy (table 1). Fibroblast transfection experiments by this group found greater luciferase activation when cells expressing either GHRd3 alone or GHRd3 and GHRfl were stimulated at various GH concentrations. These functional data, showing higher GH signal transduction in the presence of GHRd3 homo- or heterodimer receptors, support the clinical finding of a dominant effect of GHRd3 on GH responsiveness.

While this report was highly exciting, it was criticised for not being prospective, showing no effect on adult height and not reporting IGF-1 levels [16]. Furthermore, the results from cohort 1 are not in Hardy-Weinberg equilibrium, and this is not explained. However, it has stimulated many other publications, which are on the whole supportive of similar findings in different phenotypes (table 1). Still, this does not take into account the publication biases in negative studies, several of which have been presented but not published [17, 18].

GHRd3 and Growth Hormone Deficiency

The first-year response prediction model for GHD patients shows that a combination of peak GH to provocation, age, current height to target height deficit, body weight, GH dose and birth weight explains 61% of responsiveness, with peak GH being the most important single predictor

Table 1. Summary of published associations of GHRd3/GHRfl with first-year growth response

Phenotype	Patients	Age at treatment start, years	Height SDS at treatment start	HV SDS at treatment start	GH dose µg/kg/day	Allele distribution, %		First-year Δ height SDS		First-year HV cm/year		First-year Δ HV cm/year		Reference
Mixed	76	5.8 ± 0.4	−2.5 ± 0.1		1.11 ± 0.06	fl/fl	47						3.6 ± 0.3	15
ISS	51	7.9 ± 0.4	−2.6 ± 0.1		1.04 ± 0.06	fl/d3	32						6.3 ± 0.6	
SGA	25	6.4 ± 0.6	−2.6 ± 0.2		1.03 ± 0.08	d3/d3	21						6.5 ± 0.8	
Mixed	96	7.6 ± 0.3	−2.7 ± 0.1		0.71 ± 0.05	fl/fl	52						2.6 ± 0.2	15
ISS	61	7.7 ± 0.4	−2.8 ± 0.1		0.70 ± 0.06	fl/d3	40						4.3 ± 0.3	
SGA	35	7.9 ± 0.7	−2.8 ± 0.1		0.72 ± 0.2	d3/d3	8						4.9 ± 0.3	
SGA	60	7.1 ± 2.3	−3.4 ± 0.9	−1.0 ± 1.3	56 ± 11	fl/fl	48	fl/fl	0.8 ± 0.3			fl/fl	3.4 ± 1.6	22
						fl/d3	38	fl/d3	0.9 ± 0.4			fl/d3	4.3 ± 1.9	
						d3/d3	13	d3/d3	1.0 ± 0.3			d3/d3	3.9 ± 1.6	
Turner syndrome	53	8.9 ± 3.1	−3.2 ± 1.0	−1.9 ± 1.9	38 ± 8	fl/fl	51	fl/fl	0.5 ± 0.4			fl/fl	2.8 ± 1.5	22
						fl/d3	28	fl/d3	0.5 ± 0.4			fl/d3	3.4 ± 1.5	
						d3/d3	21	d3/d3	0.6 ± 0.4			d3/d3	4.6 ± 1.5	
GHD	54	7.8 ± 4.0	−1.9 ± 0.7	−1.5 ± 1.3	28.5	fl/fl	52	0.6 ± 0.4				5.3 ± 3.0		20
						fl/d3 or d3/d3	48	no difference				no difference		
GHD	58	8.9 ± 3.8	−4.2 ± 1.5		31 ± 5	fl/fl	47	fl/fl	0.9 ± 0.5	fl/fl	10.6 ± 2.3			19
						fl/d3	41	fl/d3 or d3/d3	1.4 ± 0.6	fl/d3 and d3/d3	12.3 ± 2.6			
						d3/d3	12							
GHD	44	11 ± 3.5	−4.4 ± 1.5		fl/fl 34 ± 8 fl/d3 and d3/d3 36 ± 6	fl/fl	50	fl/fl	0.8 ± 0.5	fl/fl	9.3 ± 2.3			19
						fl/d3	41	fl/d3 or d3/d3	1.2 ± 0.6	fl/d3 and d3/d3	10.8 ± 2.5			
						d3/d3	9							

SDS = Standard deviation score; HV = height velocity; ISS = idiopathic short stature.

[1]. This leaves 39% of variation in response unaccounted for. The inter-individual differences in GH responsiveness can be great and in part explained by different underlying diagnoses. Thus, severe GHD offers a more homogenous group to study, as in severe cases, timely replacement of GH should result in complete recovery of a patient's growth failure.

Jorge et al. [19] have reported on two cohorts with severe GHD (peak GH <3.3 μg/l), i.e. one prepubertal group during the first year of GH therapy and another slightly older group with final height data (table 1). While similar at baseline, they found that the patients with GHRd3 in both groups had a greater first-year growth response, and in addition, the second group achieved a significantly greater mean adult height (final height standard deviation score –0.8 ± 1.1 with GHRd3 and –1.7 ± 1.2 with GHRfl only). This suggests that GHRd3 influences both the short-term response to GH therapy and the final height gains.

However, Pilotta et al. [20] reported no significant effect of GHRd3 or other common polymorphisms, alone or in combination, on GH responsiveness in a similar sized cohort to that of Jorge et al. [19] (table 1). There is no obvious explanation for these differences but they may relate to the difference in definition of GHD or population genetic differences.

GHRd3 and Small for Gestational Age

In the first year of GH therapy in SGA subjects, the GH dose, age and weight at treatment start, as well as the midparental height standard deviation score account for 52% of the variability of clinical response, with the GH dose alone accounting for 35% [3]. The remaining 48% are unaccounted for and may relate to the heterogenous factors underlying the original diagnosis of SGA and poor postnatal growth in this group. The heterogeneity within this group may make it harder to identify significant single genetic effects. However, short SGA patients formed a significant part of the Dos Santos cohorts [21], and more recently, Binder et al. [22] have reported on a group of 60 short SGA patients. They found that carriers of GHRd3 grow faster than predicted by the KIGS-based prediction model and GHRfl homozygotes have a slower than predicted growth. This suggests that addition of the GHR genotype could further augment the prediction model. Further studies are required to confirm this finding in other SGA populations and to investigate GHRd3 associations with birth size or spontaneous postnatal growth.

Turner Syndrome

The prepubertal Turner syndrome prediction model shows that GH dose, age, current height to target height deficit, birth weight, number of injections per week and inclusion of oxandrolone therapy explain 46% of the variation in GH response seen in these subjects [2]. Binder et al. [22] reported that Turner patients who are GHRd3 carriers are more responsive to GH therapy, growing a mean of 1.5 cm more in the first year compared with GHRfl homozygotes. In addition, GHRd3 carriers grew faster than predicted using the prediction model, and GHRfl homozygotes grew slower than predicted. However, there were no differences in IGF-1 levels, which leaves the mechanism of improved growth open to question. GHRd3 had a greater effect in Turner syndrome patients compared with short SGA patients, potentially explained by the differences in the underlying pathology of growth failure, but the exact factors involved remain to be discovered.

Although these reports demonstrate that GHRd3 is the first pharmacogenomic factor involved in GH therapy responsiveness, many questions remain. Is there an effect on the response to endogenous GH, does the presence of a less responsive allele result in alteration of endogenous GH secretion in those who are not GH deficient, and what is the mechanism by which GHRd3 influences GHR signal transduction? The small sample sizes reflect the availability of patients within clinical settings but hamper the study power. Larger studies are required to confirm these findings and explore other potential genetic influences.

Other Genetic Influences

Turner Syndrome
Analysis of the KIGS data by karyotype did not show any significant differences in GH response [2]. However, the Canadian randomised controlled trial of GH therapy response to adult height in Turner syndrome has recently reported that the parent of origin of the intact X chromosome in Turner syndrome patients has a significant effect on GH responsiveness [23]. In 35 patients who had received GH therapy, those with an intact X chromosome of maternal origin grew a mean of 3.4 cm more than those with paternal origin of the intact X chromosome. Overall, the parental origin accounted for 36% of the response to GH therapy, and in the 45X karyotype patients (69% of the treated group), it accounted for 53% of the variation in response. Age and height at the start of treatment were also strongly correlated with response, as previously published [2, 23]. A further report failed to show any effect of parental origin of the X chromosome, perhaps due to the lower proportion of subjects with a single X chromosome (55%) [24]. This region clearly needs further study in other populations, in addition to further investigation of imprinted candidate genes on the X chromosome that influence GH responsiveness.

Noonan Syndrome
Protein tyrosine phosphatase, nonreceptor type 11 (PTPN11) was identified as one of the genes involved in Noonan syndrome, with mutations in this gene found in 33–60% of patients [25–27]. PTPN11 encodes Src homology protein tyrosine phosphatase 2, which is ubiquitously expressed and acts predominantly as a tyrosine phosphatase. The mutations seen in Noonan syndrome are predicted to result in gain of function, increasing the capacity of dephosphorylation [25]. Both GH and IGF-1 signalling involves phosphorylation of receptors and postreceptor signalling molecules. Thus, an increase in phosphatase activity is expected to reduce GH and IGF-1 signalling efficiency [28, 29]. However, genotype-phenotype studies do not consistently report a higher frequency of short stature in Noonan syndrome cases with PTPN11 mutations [26, 30, 31].

There are three reports of reduced GH therapy effectiveness in mutation-positive cases (table 2) [30–32]. It would appear that mutation-positive cases have features suggestive of GH resistance, namely higher GH levels with lower basal IGF-1 and IGF binding protein 3 levels and a smaller increment of IGF-1 levels on GH therapy [30, 32]. This GH insensitivity could be explained by the interference of increased phosphatase activity (as a result of the PTPN11 mutation) on postreceptor signalling efficiency. Thus, PTPN11 mutations are another pharmacogenetic factor influencing the clinical response to GH therapy.

Future Directions

GH pharmacogenomics is still in its infancy. It is likely that new genetic factors will be identified that influence GH therapeutic action under different circumstances. While to date candidate gene approaches have been used, new factors could also be identified through genome screening or in vitro mRNA expression profiling. These latter approaches are unlimited by current knowledge and hypotheses.

Table 2. Noonan syndrome: response to GH therapy according to PTPN11 genotype

Reference:	Ferreira et al. [32], 2005		Binder et al. [30], 2005		Limal et al. [31], 2006	
PTPN11 mutation:	positive	negative	positive	negative	positive	negative
Patients	7	7	8	3	15	10
Age at treatment start, years	12.9 ± 4	11.7 ± 3	5.1 ± 2.7**	10.3 ± 5.2**	10.4 ± 3.1	10.3 ± 3.3
Patients in puberty	2	2				
GH dose, μg/kg/day	48 ± 5	46 ± 7	42	50	43–67	43–67
Genetic target height SDS	−0.7 ± 0.6	−0.8 ± 0.8			−0.6 ± 0.8	−1.2 ± 1.0
Height SDS at treatment start	−3.6 ± 1	−3.4 ± 1	−3.2 ± 0.5	−3.0 ± 1.4	−3.5 ± 0.9	−3.0 ± 0.8
Height SDS at the end of the first year					−3.1 ± 1.2	−2.4 ± 0.7
First-year Δ height SDS	0.3 ± 0.4	0.4 ± 0.4	0.7 ± 0.2**	1.3 ± 0.4**		
HV at treatment start, cm/year	4.3 ± 1.0	3.9 ± 1.4			4.3 ± 0.9	5.2 ± 1.4
HV at the end of the first year, cm/year	6.8 ± 1.5	7.6 ± 1.9			7.4 ± 1.6	8.5 ± 1.7
Basal IGF-1 SDS	−2.2 ± 1.0	−1.9 ± 1.8	−2.0 ± 0.7**	−1.1 ± 0.9**	−1.9 ± 0.9	−1.3 ± 1.1
IGF-1 SDS after the first year	−1.2 ± 0.8*	0.1 ± 1.5*			0.0 ± 1.1	0.7 ± 1.1

SDS = Standard deviation score; HV = height velocity. *p = 0.03, statistically significantly different from baseline; ** p < 0.05, statistically significantly different between the two groups.

Conclusions

Pharmacogenomics is a tool to individualise therapy with the aim of increasing efficacy, minimising risk of adverse events, and thus, improving disease management and therapeutic outcome. It is likely to increase cost-effectiveness and has the potential to reduce health care costs. While there is still a lot of research to be done, it seems likely that pharmacogenetics will play a role in the future in drug selection, combination and dosing, in addition to the identification of new drug targets for further study, in many fields of medicine.

GHR isoforms were the first reported pharmacogenomic markers with some predictive value for GH responsiveness. Clinical studies are ultimately required to evaluate the utility of any genetic information on personalising GH doses to optimise growth response.

References

1 Ranke MB, Lindberg A, Chatelain P, et al: Derivation and validation of a mathematical model for predicting the response to exogenous recombinant human growth hormone (GH) in prepubertal children with idiopathic GH deficiency. KIGS International Board. Kabi Pharmacia International Growth Study. J Clin Endocrinol Metab 1999;84:1174–1183.

2 Ranke MB, Lindberg A, Chatelain P, et al: Prediction of long-term response to recombinant human growth hormone in Turner syndrome: development and validation of mathematical models. KIGS International Board. Kabi International Growth Study. J Clin Endocrinol Metab 2000;85:4212–4218.

3 Ranke MB, Lindberg A, Cowell CT, et al: Prediction of response to growth hormone treatment in short children born small for gestational age: analysis of data from KIGS (Pharmacia International Growth Database). J Clin Endocrinol Metab 2003;88:125–131.

4 Kopchick JJ: Discovery and mechanism of action of pegvisomant. Eur J Endocrinol 2003;148(suppl 2):S21–S25.

5 Gent J, Van Den EM, Van Kerkhof P, Strous GJ: Dimerization and signal transduction of the growth hormone receptor. Mol Endocrinol 2003;17:967–975.

6 Brown RJ, Adams JJ, Pelekanos RA, et al: Model for growth hormone receptor activation based on subunit rotation within a receptor dimer. Nat Struct Mol Biol 2005;12:814–821.

7 Rosenfeld RG, Rosenbloom AL, Guevara-Aguirre J: Growth hormone (GH) insensitivity due to primary GH receptor deficiency. Endocr Rev 1994;15:369–390.

8 Woods KA, Dastot F, Preece MA, et al: Phenotype: genotype relationships in growth hormone insensitivity syndrome. J Clin Endocrinol Metab 1997;82:3529–3535.

9 Stallings-Mann ML, Ludwiczak RL, Klinger KW, Rottman F: Alternative splicing of exon 3 of the human growth hormone receptor is the result of an unusual genetic polymorphism. Proc Natl Acad Sci USA 1996;93:12394–12399.

10 Pantel J, Machinis K, Sobrier ML, Duquesnoy P, Goossens M, Amselem S: Species-specific alternative splice mimicry at the growth hormone receptor locus revealed by the lineage of retroelements during primate evolution. J Biol Chem 2000;275:18664–18669.

11 Bass SH, Mulkerrin MG, Wells JA: A systematic mutational analysis of hormone-binding determinants in the human growth hormone receptor. Proc Natl Acad Sci USA 1991;88:4498–4502.

12 Sobrier ML, Duquesnoy P, Duriez B, Amselem S, Goossens M: Expression and binding properties of two isoforms of the human growth hormone receptor. FEBS Lett 1993;319:16–20.

13 Urbanek M, Russell JE, Cooke NE, Liebhaber SA: Functional characterization of the alternatively spliced, placental human growth hormone receptor. J Biol Chem 1993;268:19025–19032.

14 Pantel J, Grulich-Henn J, Bettendorf M, Strasburger CJ, Heinrich U, Amselem S: Heterozygous nonsense mutation in exon 3 of the growth hormone receptor (GHR) in severe GH insensitivity (Laron syndrome) and the issue of the origin and function of the GHRd3 isoform. J Clin Endocrinol Metab 2003;88:1705–1710.

15 Dos Santos C, Essioux L, Teinturier C, Tauber M, Goffin V, Bougneres P: A common polymorphism of the growth hormone receptor is associated with increased responsiveness to growth hormone. Nat Genet 2004;36:720–724.

16 Rosenfeld RG: Editorial: the pharmacogenomics of human growth. J Clin Endocrinol Metab 2006;91:795–796.

17 Blum WF, Machinis K, Shavrikova EP, Stobbe H, Pfaeffle RW, Amselem S: The growth response to growth hormone (GH) treatment in children with isolated GH deficiency is independent of the presence of the exon 3-minus isoform of the GH receptor (GHR) (abstract). Horm Res 2005;64(suppl 1):OR3-71.

18 Ito Y, Makita Y, Matsuo K, et al: Influence of the exon 3 deleted isoform of GH receptor gene on growth response to GH in Japanese children (abstract). Horm Res 2005;64(suppl 1):P1-150.

19 Jorge AA, Marchisotti FG, Montenegro LR, Carvalho LR, Mendonca BB, Arnhold IJ: Growth hormone (GH) pharmacogenetics: influence of GH receptor exon 3 retention or deletion on first-year growth response and final height in patients with severe GH deficiency. J Clin Endocrinol Metab 2006;91:1076–1080.

20 Pilotta A, Mella P, Filisetti M, et al: Common polymorphisms of the growth hormone (GH) receptor do not correlate with the growth response to exogenous recombinant human GH in GH-deficient children. J Clin Endocrinol Metab 2006;91:1178–1180.

21 Dos SC, Essioux L, Teinturier C, Tauber M, Goffin V, Bougneres P: A common polymorphism of the growth hormone receptor is associated with increased responsiveness to growth hormone. Nat Genet 2004;36:720–724.

22 Binder G, Baur F, Schweizer R, Ranke MB: The d3-growth hormone receptor polymorphism is associated with increased responsiveness to GH in Turner syndrome and short SGA children. J Clin Endocrinol Metab 2006;91:659–664.

23 Hamelin CE, Anglin G, Quigley CA, Deal CL: Genomic imprinting in Turner syndrome: effects on response to growth hormone and on risk of sensorineural hearing loss. J Clin Endocrinol Metab 2006;91:3002–3010.

24 Tsezou A, Hadjiathanasiou C, Gourgiotis D, et al: Molecular genetics of Turner syndrome: correlation with clinical phenotype and response to growth hormone therapy. Clin Genet 1999;56:441–446.

25 Tartaglia M, Mehler EL, Goldberg R, et al: Mutations in PTPN11, encoding the protein tyrosine phosphatase SHP-2, cause Noonan syndrome. Nat Genet 2001;29:465–468.

26 Tartaglia M, Kalidas K, Shaw A, et al: PTPN11 mutations in Noonan syndrome: molecular spectrum, genotype-phenotype correlation, and phenotypic heterogeneity. Am J Hum Genet 2002;70:1555–1563.

27 Yoshida R, Hasegawa T, Hasegawa Y, et al: Protein-tyrosine phosphatase, nonreceptor type 11 mutation analysis and clinical assessment in 45 patients with Noonan syndrome. J Clin Endocrinol Metab 2004;89:3359–3364.

28 Stofega MR, Herrington J, Billestrup N, Carter-Su C: Mutation of the SHP-2 binding site in growth hormone (GH) receptor prolongs GH-promoted tyrosyl phosphorylation of GH receptor, JAK2, and STAT5B. Mol Endocrinol 2000;14:1338–1350.

29 Maile LA, Clemmons DR: Regulation of insulin-like growth factor I receptor dephosphorylation by SHPS-1 and the tyrosine phosphatase SHP-2. J Biol Chem 2002;277:8955–8960.

30 Binder G, Neuer K, Ranke MB, Wittekindt NE: PTPN11 mutations are associated with mild growth hormone resistance in individuals with Noonan syndrome. J Clin Endocrinol Metab 2005;90:5377–5381.

31 Limal JM, Parfait B, Cabrol S, et al: Noonan syndrome: relationships between genotype, growth, and growth factors. J Clin Endocrinol Metab 2006;91:300–306.

32 Ferreira LV, Souza SA, Arnhold IJ, Mendonca BB, Jorge AA: PTPN11 (protein tyrosine phosphatase, nonreceptor type 11) mutations and response to growth hormone therapy in children with Noonan syndrome. J Clin Endocrinol Metab 2005;90:5156–5160.

Author Index

Abs, R. 176
Albertsson-Wikland, K. 319
Butler, G.E. 6
Clark, A.J.L. 500
Clayton, P. E. 163
Cutfield, W.S. 136, 145, 277, 389
Czernichow, P. 286
Darendeliler, F. 213, 319
Dunger, D.B. 400
Feldt-Rasmussen, U. 477
Ferrández-Longás, A. 56
Frisch, H. 108
Fujieda, K. 16
Gastaldi, R. 93
Geffner, M.E. 176
Gleeson, H. 163
Haffner, D. 407
Hána, V. 176
Hertel, T. 356
Höybye, C. 176
Iorgi di, N. 93
Jönsson, P. 176
Johnston, L.B. 500
Jostel, A. 240
Juul, A. 70
Karagiannis, G. 145
Karlsson, H. 202, 261
Kelnar, C.J.H. 340
Koltowska-Häggström, M. 176
Labarta, J.I. 56
Lindberg, A. 23, 319, 332, 407, 422
Lindgren, A.C. 369
Lorini, R. 93

Maghnie, M. 93
Mayayo, E. 56
Mehls, O. 407
Monson, J.P. 176
Mullis, P.E. 189
Nilsson, O. 485
Nissel, R. 407
Noordam, K. 347
Nyberg, F. 450
Otten, B.J. 347
Polak, M. 269
Price, D.A. 116, 207, 261, 319
Ranke, M.B. 23, 29, 60, 83, 116, 183, 202, 250, 277, 319, 332, 422
Reiter, E.O. 116, 136, 145, 292, 304, 319, 389
Romo, A. 56
Rose, S.R. 38
Rosenfeld, R.G. 326
Rossi, A. 93
Schaefer, F. 407
Schnabel, D. 296
Shalet, S.M. 240
Stabler, B. 442
Tanaka, T. 16
Tauber, M. 47, 377
Tönshoff, B. 407
Tortori-Donati, P. 93
Underwood, L.E. 442
Wells, J.C.K. 461
Wilton, P. 1, 319, 432
Wit, J.M. 309
Wühl, E. 407

Subject Index

Aarskog syndrome
   clinical features and diagnosis 214, 215
   gene defects 215
   growth characteristics 215, 218
   growth hormone therapy 218
Achondroplasia, growth hormone therapy 356, 357, 359, 365
Acquired growth hormone deficiency
   causes 250
   growth hormone therapy
      adult height outcomes 255, 260
      first-year response 253, 255
      patient characteristics at start of treatment 250, 253
   KIGS classification 18
Adiponectin, small-for-gestational-age levels 393
Adult height
   growth hormone therapy outcomes
      acquired growth hormone deficiency 255, 260
      ethnic factors 138
      leukemia/lymphoma 262, 265–267
      overview 137, 138
      Prader-Willi syndrome 382, 385, 386
      sex differences 138
   idiopathic growth hormone deficiency response to growth hormone therapy 148–150, 152–157, 159, 160
   prediction
      bone age 12, 13
      disability effects 13
      overview 12, 24
   target height calculation 12
Adverse events, growth hormone therapy
   brain tumor 435, 436, 438
   chronic kidney disease 416–418, 437
   congenital growth hormone deficiency 433, 434
   craniopharyngioma 434, 435, 438
   diabetes 438, 439
   idiopathic growth hormone therapy 433
   idiopathic intracranial hypertension 439
   idiopathic short stature 437
   Langerhans cell histiocytosis 435
   leukemia 436–438
   Noonan syndrome 353
   Prader-Willi syndrome 437
   secondary neoplasms 436
   seizures 439
   slipped capital femoral epiphysis 439
   small for gestational age 404, 436
   Turner syndrome 436
   types reported in KIGS 433, 434
Androgens, growth plate regulation 494, 495
Anthropometry
   adult height 24
   birth size 24
   body composition analysis 467–469
   body mass index 24
   body surface area 26
   data analysis
      group comparisons 27
      growth hormone dose calculation 28
      means and standard deviation 27
      medians and ranges 27
      missing data 27
      standard deviation scores 27
   disease-specific references 26, 27
   height velocity 24
   standards 23, 24
   target height calculation 26
Appetite, growth hormone therapy response 455
Arachnoid cyst, growth hormone therapy 230
Aromatase inhibitors, growth hormone combination therapy 140, 141
Arthritis, *see* Juvenile idiopathic arthritis; Juvenile rheumatoid arthritis

Bayley-Pinneau method, adult height prediction 13
Bioelectric impedance analysis (BIA), body composition assessment 469, 470
Bioinactive growth hormone syndrome
    features 198
    KIGS classification 32
Birth complications, growth hormone deficiency 56–58, 61, 63
Birth size
    anthropometry 24
    KIGS data 60–68
Body composition
    assessment
        anthropometric markers 467–469
        bioelectric impedance analysis 469, 470
        computed tomography 472
        densitometry 471
        dual-energy X-ray absorptiometry 470, 471
        isotope dilution 470
        magnetic resonance imaging 472, 473
        multicomponent models 473, 474
        total-body electrical conductivity 472
    clinical requirements 467
    equations 463
    growth hormone therapy effects 170, 171, 290, 291
    Hattori charts 464–466
    Prader-Willi syndrome 370–372
Body mass index (BMI)
    age dependence in children 462
    anthropometry 24
    calculation 461, 463
    classification in adults 463
    growth hormone therapy effects 381, 382, 386
    limitations in body composition assessment 466, 467
    population variability 466
Body surface area, calculation 26
Bone
    growth hormone therapy effects 168–170, 301, 302
    growth plate, see Growth plate
Bone age
    adult height prediction 12, 13
    estimation 24, 187
    idiopathic growth hormone deficiency 111, 112
Bone morphogenetic proteins (BMPs), growth plate regulation 491
Brain tumors, see also specific tumors
    classification 240, 241
    clinical presentation 240
    epidemiology 241, 242
    growth hormone deficiency and therapy in childhood survivors 244–247, 435, 436, 438
    imaging 242
    magnetic resonance spectroscopy 244
    molecular diagnostics 243, 244
    secondary malignant neoplasms from treatment 247, 248
    treatment 242–244
Breech delivery, growth hormone deficiency risks 56–58, 61

Caesarean section, trends 56, 57
Carotid artery, growth hormone therapy effects 171
Cartilage-hair hypoplasia
    clinical features and diagnosis 227
    genetic defects 227
    growth characteristics 227, 228
    growth hormone therapy 228
Central malformation, KIGS classification 18, 34
Childhood brain tumors, see Brain tumors
Chronic kidney disease (CKD)
    growth disturbances 407, 408
    growth hormone resistance 408–410
    growth hormone therapy
        adverse events 416–418, 437
        efficacy 410–412
        final height 415, 416
        predictive factors 412–415
Computed tomography (CT)
    body composition assessment 472
    growth hormone deficiency evaluation 94
Congenital growth hormone deficiency
    adverse events of growth hormone therapy 433, 434
    KIGS classification 17
Cornelia de Lange syndrome
    clinical features and diagnosis 218, 219
    gene defects 219
    growth characteristics 219
    growth hormone therapy 219
Cortisol
    effects on growth in idiopathic growth hormone deficiency 129, 133–135
    metabolic syndrome and cortisol/growth hormone axis imbalance 481
Craniopharyngioma
    epidemiology 207
    growth hormone therapy
        adverse events 434, 435, 438
        comparison with idiopathic growth hormone deficiency outcomes 210
        first-year response 208, 283
        prepubertal growth 208, 210, 211
        tumor treatment mode and outcomes 210
Cystic fibrosis (CF)
    epidemiology 296
    growth hormone therapy
        body composition effects 299, 300

bone metabolism 301, 302
exercise capacity 301
growth velocity 297, 305, 307
insulin-like growth factor-1 response 297
protein metabolism effects 297, 299
pulmonary function effects 300, 302
quality of life 300
rationale 297, 304, 305
side effects 302
growth retardation 296, 297, 304
malnutrition 296
treatment 296

Densitometry, body composition assessment 471
Diabetes
    growth hormone therapy risks 438, 439
    small-for-gestational-age association 393, 394
Diamond-Blackfan anemia
    clinical features and diagnosis 228, 229
    genetic defects 229
    growth characteristics 229
    growth hormone therapy 229
Down syndrome
    clinical features and diagnosis 220
    genetic defects 220
    growth characteristics 220, 221
    growth hormone therapy 221
Dual-energy X-ray absorptiometry (DXA), body composition assessment 470, 471
Dyschondrosteosis, growth hormone therapy 360, 366

Empty sella syndrome (ESS)
    growth hormone therapy 203–206, 230–232
    magnetic resonance imaging 229
Estrogen, growth plate regulation 494

Familial isolated growth hormone deficiency
    classification
        overview 193, 194
        type IA 193, 194
        type IB 194–196
        type II 196, 197
        type III 197
    epidemiology 192, 193
    growth hormone insensitivity 198
    post-genomic defects 198, 199
    syndrome of bioinactive growth hormone 198
Fanconi anemia
    clinical features and diagnosis 225
    genetic defects 225
    growth characteristics 225, 226

growth hormone therapy 226
Fat mass index, calculation 463
Fibroblast growth factors (FGFs), growth plate regulation 490, 491
Final height, see Adult height
Floating-harbor syndrome
    clinical features and diagnosis 221, 222
    genetic defects 222
    growth characteristics 222
    growth hormone therapy 222

GATA-2, pituitary development role 190, 192
Gender bias, KIGS 20, 21
Glucocorticoids
    growth plate regulation 493
    growth retardation 288
Gonadotropin-releasing hormone agonists, growth hormone combination therapy 139, 140, 314
Growth charts
    disease-specific charts 8, 9
    height velocity assessment and calculation 9, 10
    problems 8
    standards 6, 7
    users 7, 8
Growth hormone (GH)
    biology 164, 340, 341
    brain function
        aging changes 455
        appetite response 455
        blood-brain barrier permeability 451–453
        cognition and memory 455, 456
        extrapituitary sources 452
        history of study 450, 451
        mechanism of action 453, 454
        neuroprotection 456, 457
        receptors 450–453
    gene defects 193–197
    growth plate regulation 491–493
    insensitivity 198
    levels in transition period between childhood and adulthood 165–167
    metabolic actions
        carbohydrate metabolism 478, 479
        insulin-like growth factor-1 479, 480
        lipid metabolism 478
        metabolic syndrome and deficiency 480, 481
        overview 477
    receptor
        GHRd3 isoform and growth hormone therapy response
            growth hormone deficiency 502, 504
            small for gestational age 504
            Turner syndrome 504, 505

Growth hormone (GH) (continued)
    isoforms 502
    signaling 501
    testing
        assay standardization 41
        limitations 42–44
        KIGS data
            characteristics of children 50, 52
            idiopathic growth hormone deficiency 48, 49
            stimuli 48, 52
            tests by etiology 49, 54
            trends 47, 48
        spontaneous secretion 41, 42, 55
        stimulation tests 40, 41
Growth hormone deficiency (GHD), *see also* Familial isolated growth hormone deficiency; Idiopathic growth hormone deficiency
    birth complications and risks 56–58, 61, 63
    childhood-onset versus adult-onset 164, 165
    diagnosis, *see also* Growth hormone; Insulin-like growth factor
        clinical manifestations 38, 39
        imaging 39
        laboratory studies 39–42
        testing limitations 42–44
    history of study 38
    pharmacogenomics of growth hormone therapy 502, 504
    transition period between childhood and adulthood 165–167
Growth hormone-releasing hormone (GHRH)
    familial isolated growth hormone deficiency and receptor gene mutations 195, 196
    tests 42
Growth hormone therapy, *see also* specific diseases
    adult height outcomes
        ethnic factors 138
        overview 137, 138
        sex differences 138
    adverse events, *see* Adverse events, growth hormone therapy
    childhood dosing 178, 181
    dosing
        calculation 28
        regimens 136, 137
    effects
        body composition 170, 171
        bone 168–170
        cardiac changes 171
        carotid artery 171
        lipid profile 171, 178, 179, 181
        quality of life 172, 178, 179, 181
    estrogen action decrease
        aromatase inhibitor therapy 140, 141
        gonadotropin-releasing hormone agonist therapy 139, 140
    idiopathic growth hormone deficiency and KIGS analysis
        extreme-weight-categorized patients
            first-year growth response 118, 120
            near-adult height 121, 122
        final height 148–150, 152–157, 159, 160
        first year on growth hormone therapy
            head circumference 122, 123
            overview 147, 148
            sitting height 122
        patient features at start of growth hormone therapy 116–118, 147
        prepuberty
            growth hormone dosing 125
            height velocity before and during growth hormone therapy 127, 138, 139
        puberty
            dosing 125, 127, 139
            response 150–152, 157–159
    idiopathic growth hormone deficiency response 113
    insulin-like growth factor-1 monitoring
        adults 76, 77
        children 75, 76
        KIGS database 84, 87, 89–91
    patient expectations for outcome 446–448
    pharmacogenomics, *see* Pharmacogenomics
    pituitary-derived hormone 136
    prediction of growth
        KIGS cohorts 426
        long-term growth prediction 429, 430
        model validation 426
        overview 422, 423
        predictors 427, 428
        prospects 430
        response and responsiveness 424–426
        short-term response variables 428, 429
        variables in response 426, 427
    safety 172
    termination by patient
        patient demographics 187
        reasons 184–186
        study design 83
    transition period between childhood and adulthood 167, 168, 172, 173
Growth plate
    epiphyseal fusion 487–489
    growth cessation in adults 487
    histology 485
    hormone regulation
        androgen 494, 495
        estrogen 494

glucocorticoids 493
growth hormone 491–493
insulin-like growth factor-1 491–493
thyroid hormone 493, 494
paracrine regulation
bone morphogenetic proteins 491
fibroblast growth factors 490, 491
Indian hedgehog 490
parathyroid-hormone-related peptide 489, 490
senescence 485–487

Head circumference, growth hormone therapy effects in first year 122, 123
Heart, growth hormone therapy effects 171
Height velocity
assessment and calculation 9, 10, 24
idiopathic growth hormone deficiency and growth hormone therapy effects 127
HESX1, mutation and magnetic resonance imaging 101
Hydrocephalus
growth hormone deficiency in congenital disease 230
growth hormone therapy 233
Hypochondroplasia, growth hormone therapy 359, 360, 365, 366

Idiopathic growth hormone deficiency (IGHD)
bone age 111, 112
clinical presentation 111, 146
endocrinological features 108, 109
KIGS
adverse events 433
etiological classification 16, 17, 22, 31, 32, 34, 146
extreme-weight-categorized patients
first-year growth response 118, 120
near-adult height 121, 122
final height 148–150, 152–157
first year on growth hormone therapy
head circumference 122, 123
overview 113, 147, 148
sitting height 122
patient features at start of growth hormone therapy 116–118, 147
prepuberty
blood laboratory findings 135
growth hormone dosing 125
height velocity before and during growth hormone therapy 127
patient characteristics 118
thyroxin and cortisol effects on growth 129, 133–135

puberty
growth hormone dosing 125, 127, 139
growth hormone response 150–152, 157–159
testing 48, 49
magnetic resonance imaging findings 96–99
neonatal characteristics and complications 109, 110
Idiopathic intracranial hypertension, growth hormone therapy risks 439
Idiopathic short stature (ISS)
definition 309
growth hormone therapy
adverse events 437
gonadotropin-releasing hormone agonist combination therapy 314
growth outcomes 312–314
outcome prediction
adult height determinants 321, 324, 325
first-year response 321
study design 319, 321
prospects 314, 315
KIGS classification 32, 33, 35, 319
pathophysiology 310–312
spontaneous growth and height prognosis 312
Indian hedgehog, growth plate regulation 490
Insulin-like growth factor (IGF)
binding proteins
IGFBP-3 and diagnostic utility 73, 74
overview 71
biology 40, 70, 71
growth hormone therapy monitoring
adults 76, 77
children 75, 76
growth plate regulation 491–493
IGF-1
adult growth hormone deficiency diagnosis 74, 75
KIGS database features
basal levels 84
diagnostic use 89, 90
growth hormone treatment monitoring 84, 87, 89–91
measurement 83
neuroprotection 456, 457
normal levels 71, 72
testing 40, 72, 73
metabolism effects 479, 480
structure 70
Interleukin-6, inflammation and growth retardation 292
Intrauterine growth retardation (IUGR), *see also* Small for gestational age
definition 389
KIGS classification 33, 35

515

Isl-1, pituitary development role 190
Isotope dilution, body composition assessment 470

Janus kinase, growth hormone signaling in brain 454, 456
Juvenile idiopathic arthritis (JIA)
　growth hormone therapy
　　efficacy 289, 290
　　prospects 290, 291
　　rationale 288, 289
　　safety 290
　growth retardation 286–288
Juvenile rheumatoid arthritis (JRA)
　growth hormone therapy 292, 294, 295
　inflammation and growth retardation 292

Kabuki syndrome
　clinical features and diagnosis 222, 223
　genetic defects 223
　growth characteristics 223
　growth hormone therapy 223
KIGS
　Aetiology Classification List
　　bioinactive growth hormone syndrome 32
　　central malformation 18, 34
　　hierarchy of diagnoses 30
　　idiopathic growth hormone deficiency 16, 17, 22, 31, 32, 34
　　idiopathic short stature 32, 33, 35
　　intrauterine growth retardation 33, 35
　　neurosecretory dysfunction 32
　　organic growth hormone deficiency 17–19, 34
　　other causes of short stature 19, 20, 34
　　overview 16, 30, 31
　　psychogenic short stature 34, 37
　　requirements 29, 30
　　skeletal dysplasia 20, 33, 34, 36
　data management
　　collection 3
　　processing 4
　　quality control 3, 4
　gender bias 20, 21
　growth 2, 20
　prospects 4, 5
　rationale 1, 3
　reporting of data 2, 3
　scientific organization 2
KIMS database, pediatric growth hormone effects on serum lipids and quality of life 176–181
Klippel-Feil syndrome
　clinical features and diagnosis 228
　genetic defects 228
　growth characteristics 228
　growth hormone therapy 228

Langerhans cell histiocytosis (LCH)
　clinical manifestations 269, 278
　growth hormone deficiency 269, 270
　growth hormone therapy
　　dosing 270, 271
　　first-year response 283
　　growth response 271
　　patient characteristics at initiation 281
　　safety 271, 272, 435
Lean mass index, calculation 463
Learning and memory, growth hormone therapy effects 455, 456
Leukemia
　epidemiology 261
　growth hormone therapy
　　adult height 262, 265–267
　　adverse events 436–438
　　age at diagnosis and treatment initiation 266
　　first-year response 262
　　patient characteristics at initiation 262
　　radiation schedule influences 265, 266
LHX3 mutation and magnetic resonance imaging 101, 102
LHX4 mutation and magnetic resonance imaging 102
Lipid profile, growth hormone therapy effects 171, 178, 179, 181, 478
Lipoprotein(a), small-for-gestational-age levels 393
Lymphoma
　epidemiology 261
　growth hormone therapy
　　adult height 262, 265–267
　　age at diagnosis and treatment initiation 266
　　first-year response 262
　　patient characteristics at initiation 262
　　radiation schedule influences 265, 266

Magnetic resonance imaging (MRI)
　body composition assessment 472, 473
　brain tumors 242
　empty sella syndrome 229
　pituitary
　　familial growth hormone deficiency 99, 100
　　growth hormone deficiency findings 39
　　HESX1 mutation 101
　　idiopathic growth hormone deficiency 96–99
　　LHX3 mutation 101, 102
　　LHX4 mutation 102
　　morphology after adult height achievement 103

normal anatomy 94
normal appearance 94–96
normal size 96
POU1F1 mutation 100
PROP1 mutation 100, 101
prospects 105
SOX2 mutation 102, 103
SOX3 mutation 102
principles 93, 94
Magnetic resonance spectroscopy, brain tumors 244
Metabolic syndrome
cortisol/growth hormone axis imbalance 481
fetal stress 481, 482
growth hormone deficiency 480, 481
Metaphyseal chondrodysplasia 364
N-methyl-D-aspartate (NMDA) receptor, growth hormone effects in brain 453, 454
Midline palatal cleft
growth hormone deficiency 229
growth hormone therapy 232, 233

Near-adult height, *see* Adult height
Neurofibromatosis type 1
central nervous system tumors 277
clinical manifestations 272, 273, 277
growth hormone deficiency 273, 274
growth hormone therapy
first-year response 283
growth response 274
patient characteristics at initiation 278, 279
safety 275
progression 274
Neurosecretory dysfunction, KIGS classification 32
Noonan syndrome
anthropometric parameters 26, 27
clinical features 340, 347
epidemiology 340
genetic defects 340, 347, 505
growth hormone therapy
benefits 344
KIGS analysis
cardiac adverse effects 353
dosing 352, 354
efficacy 348, 349, 354
gender effects 349, 352
patient characteristics at initiation 348
termination 353, 354
literature review 341, 342
pharmacogenomics 505
rationale 341
safety 343, 344
study limitations 343

Organic growth hormone deficiency, KIGS classification 17–19, 34
Other causes of short stature, KIGS classification 19, 20, 34

Parathyroid-hormone-related peptide (PTHrP), growth plate regulation 489, 490
Pharmacogenomics
definition 500
growth hormone receptor
GHRd3 isoform and growth hormone therapy response
growth hormone deficiency 502, 504
small for gestational age 504
Turner syndrome 504, 505
isoforms 502
signaling 501
Noonan syndrome growth hormone therapy response 505
prospects 505, 506
Turner syndrome genotype and growth hormone therapy response 505
Pit1, pituitary development role 190, 192
Pituitary
development 189, 190, 192
hormones and cell function 192
imaging, *see* Magnetic resonance imaging
POU1F1 mutation and magnetic resonance imaging 100
Prader-Willi syndrome (PWS)
anthropometric parameters 26, 27
body composition and growth 370–372
clinical features 369
diagnosis 369
genetic defects 370
growth hormone axis 372
growth hormone therapy
adverse events 437
efficacy 372, 373
indications 377
KIGS analysis
adult height 382, 385, 386
age effects 381
body mass index changes 381, 382, 386
first-year response 379–382
obese versus nonobese children 381
study design 377, 379
side effects 373
treatment 373, 374
Prediction, growth in growth hormone therapy
adult height prediction
bone age in prediction 12, 13
disability effects 13

Prediction, growth in growth hormone therapy (continued)
    overview 12, 24
    chronic kidney disease factors 412–415
    idiopathic short stature
        adult height determinants 321, 324, 325
        first-year response 321
        study design 319, 321
    KIGS cohorts 426
    long-term growth prediction 429, 430
    model validation 426
    overview 422, 423
    predictors 427, 428
    prospects 430
    response and responsiveness 424–426
    short-term response variables 428, 429
    small-for-gestational-age response 402, 403
    Turner syndrome outcome 327, 328, 332, 333, 335, 337, 338
    variables in response 426, 427
PROP1
    defects 189, 192
    mutation and magnetic resonance imaging 100, 101
Pseudoachondroplasia, growth hormone therapy 363, 364, 366, 367
Psychogenic short stature, KIGS classification 34, 37
Psychology, growth delay
    expectations for growth hormone therapy outcome 446–448
    pediatric endocrinologists
        interventions 446
        opinions 443, 444
    prospective studies 444–446
    societal perception of short stature 442, 443
Puberty
    age of onset 10, 11
    growth hormone therapy in idiopathic growth hormone deficiency
        dosing 125, 127, 139
        response 150–152, 157–159
    growth in late maturers and short individuals 11, 12
    small-for-gestational-age effects 392, 393
Pulmonary function, growth hormone therapy effects in cystic fibrosis 300, 302

Quality of life
    growth hormone therapy effects 172, 178, 179, 181
    prospective studies of short individuals 444–446

Renal disease, *see* Chronic kidney disease
Rubinstein-Taybi syndrome
    clinical features and diagnosis 226
    genetic defects 226
    growth characteristics 227
    growth hormone therapy 227

Seizures, growth hormone therapy risks 439
Septo-optic dysplasia (SOD), growth hormone therapy 203–206
Silver-Russell syndrome, *see also* Small for gestational age
    anthropometric parameters 26, 27
    auxology 390, 391
    clinical features 390
    etiology 390
    growth hormone axis defects 392
    growth hormone therapy 403, 404
Skeletal dysplasia
    causes 356
    growth hormone therapy
        achondroplasia 356, 357, 359, 365
        dyschondrosteosis 360, 366
        hypochondroplasia 359, 360, 365, 366
        metaphyseal chondrodysplasia 364
        pseudoachondroplasia 363, 364, 366, 367
        spondyloepiphyseal dysplasia 362, 363, 366
    KIGS classification 20, 33, 34, 36, 364, 365
Slipped capital femoral epiphysis (SCFE), growth hormone therapy risks 439
Small for gestational age (SGA)
    auxology 390, 391
    definition 389, 390
    etiology 390
    growth hormone axis defects 391, 392
    growth hormone therapy
        adverse effects 404, 436
        KIGS outcomes 404, 405
        literature review 394, 395
        pharmacogenomics 504
        prediction models 402, 403
        prospects for study 395
        Silver-Russell syndrome 403, 404
    KIGS classification 400, 401
    metabolic syndrome risks 481, 482
    metabolism defects 393, 394
    pubertal and gonadal function 392, 393
Social acceptability, short stature and gender bias 21
Societal perception, short stature 442, 443
SOCS, growth hormone signaling in brain 454
Solitary median maxillary central incisor
    growth hormone deficiency 229, 230
    growth hormone therapy 233
SOX2 mutation and magnetic resonance imaging 102, 103
SOX3 mutation and magnetic resonance imaging 102

Spondyloepiphyseal dysplasia, growth hormone therapy 362, 363, 366
Standard deviation (SD), anthropometric data analysis 27
STATs, growth hormone signaling in brain 454

Tanner-Whitehouse methods, adult height prediction 13
Target height, calculation 12, 26
Thyroid hormone, growth plate regulation 493, 494
Thyroxin, effects on growth in idiopathic growth hormone deficiency 129, 133–135
Total-body electrical conductivity, body composition assessment 472
Turner syndrome
    anthropometric parameters 26, 27
    genetic defects 326
    growth hormone therapy
        adverse events 436
        first-year response 333
        guidelines 329, 330
        literature review 328, 329
        patient characteristics at initiation 333
        pharmacogenomics 504, 505
        prediction factors in outcome 327, 328, 332, 333, 335, 337, 338
        prospects 330
    height prognosis 327
    karyotypes in KIGS patients 333
    spontaneous growth 327

Williams-Beuren syndrome
    clinical features and diagnosis 223, 224
    genetic defects 224
    growth characteristics 224
    growth hormone therapy 224